W9-AOD-769

PERSONAL HEALTH: A MULTICULTURAL APPROACH

Patricia A. Floyd

Sandra E. Mimms

Caroline Yelding-Howard

Alabama State University

Morton Publishing Company

925 W. Kenyon Ave., Unit 12
Englewood, CO 80110

In honor of my father, James Aubrey Alford, and to the memory of my mother, Cleone Rhodes Alford, with love, respect, appreciation, and admiration.

Patricia Alford Floyd

To my mother and first health educator, Rosa Malone Mimms, and to the memory of my father, Cornelius Mimms, and my grandmother, Robbie Malone.

Sandra E. Mimms

To my family, Leon, Ravi, and Jai Howard, my mother, Clara Lucious Yelding, and in memory of my father, Bailey Yelding, and nephew, Coley Bolton, and to my friends Lorain Harmon and Willie O. Lewis.

Caroline Yelding-Howard

Book Team

Publisher:	Douglas Morton
Senior Editor:	Ruth Horton
Production Manager/Designer:	Joanne Saliger
Consulting Editor:	Carolyn Acheson
Contributing Editor:	Kathryn Frandsen
Cover:	Bob Schram
Cover Photo:	John Crawley
Back Cover Photos:	Robinson's Photography
Illustrators:	Jennifer Johnson, Randy Nelson
Reviewers:	Sharon Dittman, Dr. John Gormley, Brent Hafen, Dr. Werner Hoeger, Dr. Virginia Utermohlen, Janice Talbot
Photo Models:	Natalie Alley-Christensen, Shireen Brown, Jamie M. Cook, Traci Fong, Hema Heimuli, James P. Hyde, Stanley Y. Kamimoto, Ellen Martin, Neil Martin, Lawanda McGhee, Alicia Ormsby, Douglas Rollins, Vielane Parker, Leslie Peabody, Mindy Shoemaker, Chris Siebert, Ya-Hui Shih, Kauri Thompson, Natalie Wilson, Kingsley Au You

Special Photo Credits:

Chapter 2: p. 13, John Crawley; p. 27, Ann Little
Chapter 3: pp. 41 and 42, John Crawley
Chapter 4: p. 67, 68, 69, John Crawley
Chapter 6: pp. 131, 134, Robinson's Photography; p. 139, John Crawley
Chapter 8: p. 211, Robinson's Photography
Chapter 9: pp. 233, 257, 258, Robinson's Photography
Chapter 10: p. 207, Ann Little
Chapter 11: p. 313, Ann Little; p. 314, 319, John Crawley; p. 320-323, 325, Robinson's Photography; p. 326, Universal Equipment, Inc., Nautilus Sports/Medical Industries
Chapter 12: pp. 345, 360, John Crawley
Chapter 13: p. 397, John Crawley
Chapter 15: p. 461, John Crawley

Copyright © 1995 by Morton Publishing Company

All rights reserved. No part of this publication may be reproduced, stored in a retrieval system, or transmitted, in any form or by any means, electronic, mechanical, photocopying, recording, or otherwise, without the prior written permission of the publisher.

Printed in the United States of America

10 9 8 7 6 5 4 3 2 1

ISBN: 0-89582-285-7

RA
776
.F569
1995

Preface

Attention to one's health is no longer an option. It is a necessity. The state of health in today's world depends more on lifestyle and behaviors than on treatment of disease as it did in the past. The current focus is on preventing illness before it occurs, taking control of one's own life. Before people can adopt an optimum lifestyle, they must have the information necessary to know what to do and how to do it.

Personal Health: A Multicultural Approach provides relevant information that will allow readers to make wise decisions regarding their health throughout life. The book actually goes a step further than mere health by promoting wellness as a physical and psychological quality of living life to its fullest.

The objectives at the beginning of each chapter provide a guide to the contents. Summaries at the end of each chapter present a succinct synopsis. Key terms appear in boldface type and, together with their definitions, appear in boxes within the text. The terms also are combined in a glossary at the end of the book.

In addition to being factual and current, the book represents an attempt to be "reader-friendly" in writing style. The emphasis is on practicality, highlighted by the Tips for Action feature throughout. The sidebars capture the reader's attention with information of special interest. In keeping with the theme of *personal* health, the self-assessments at the end of the chapters allow the readers to evaluate themselves regarding the chapter content. "Call for Information" phone numbers enable anyone to access more information and gain assistance for specific concerns. Photographs, figures, and tables are sprinkled throughout the book to clarify, extend, and summarize important concepts.

This book is flexible enough to accommodate courses that carry from one to three hours of credit. It highlights the major health issues: personal relationships, sexuality and contraception, stress and emotional health, communicable and noncommunicable diseases, physical fitness and exercise, nutrition and weight management, substance use and abuse, aging and death, and consumer and environmental issues.

We take the subtitle seriously and have attempted to make this book truly multicultural. Literally hundreds of agencies, associations, organizations, and libraries are sources of the information herein. In accumulating research, we requested the most up-to-date data on every cultural grouping. In many cases the data were available on only selected subpopulations. If the book seems lacking in regard to any ethnic minority, it reflects the absence of data underlying those omissions.

In figures and tables we adhered to the usage in the original source. In text the terminology generally used is African American, Anglo American, Hispanic, and American Indian. While researching this book, we came to truly appreciate the concept of diversity. Hispanics are heterogenous, with distinct differences between Cubans, Puerto Ricans, and Mexicans, for example. The Bureau of Indian Affairs indicated that American Indian is the preferred term for the some

500 tribes that comprise the larger population. In their unique cultures these tribes have health issues that are as disparate as any ethnic group, and, like any minority group, they resist stereotyping and generalization.

With all these considerations as a foundation, we hope that you, the readers, utilize this information to embrace a healthy lifestyle. We trust that this book will be a helpful tool on your path to personal health and wellness.

Supplements

✻ The Morton Test III Personal Health **Computerized Testbank** with the following options: (a) over 600 multiple choice questions, (b) additional multiple choice, true-false or essay test questions can be added by the course instructors, (c) previously generated tests can be recalled — creating new exam versions — because all multiple choice answers rotate with each new test generated, (d) capability to generate tests using a LaserJet printer, and (e) answer sheets can be formatted to be read by a scanner.

✻ Sixty color **overhead transparency acetates** of the book's most important illustrations and figures to facilitate class instruction and help explain key fitness and wellness concepts.

✻ An **instructor's manual** to aid with the implementation of your personal health and includes additional transparency masters.

✻ A comprehensive **video program**. Ask our representatives for details. Call 1-800-348-3777.

ACKNOWLEDGMENTS

We are grateful to those who participated in the preparation of this book. We wish to thank Jean A. Thompson, Courtney Floyd, Mrs. George Haggerty, Jai Howard, William Duey, Evelyn Nettles, Linda Hockett McClellan, Comprehensive Sickle Cell Center—Meharry Medical College; and Mary Smith, Alabama Department of Public Health.

Further, we wish to thank the members of the Department of Health, Physical Education, and Recreation, especially Barbara Williams, James Oliver, Johnny Mitchell, Ronald Mitchell, Roger Pritchard, Andrea Pent, and Roger Totten, instructors of Personal Health and Wellness at Alabama State University, for their comments and assistance. We also thank Ann Little and Robinson's Photography for their contributions to the book.

We are grateful to the following for their technical assistance:

Nekesha Bowden	Jerry Floyd	Lawanda McGhee
Diane Brisbon	Betty Freeman	Jesse McKinnon
Marzell Brown	Jacqueline Hill	Kenny Smith
James Cowan	William Jones	Amanda Thompson
Zack Duey	Peggy Keebler	Taylor Thompson
Mona East	Kelvin Mack	Sam Whatley

We especially want to thank Doug Morton for his ability to recognize the need for a textbook emphasizing the multicultural approach to personal health. We appreciate his staff, primarily Ruth Horton, who shepherded the project to completion, and to the editorial and technical expertise of Carolyn Acheson and Joanne Saliger. Thank you all.

Contents

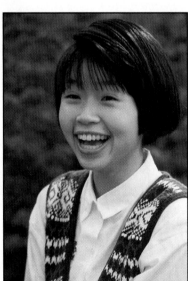

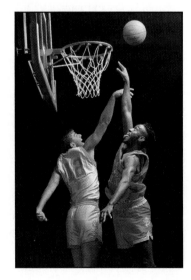

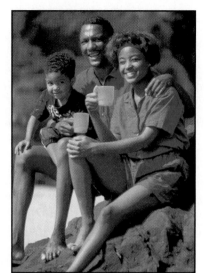

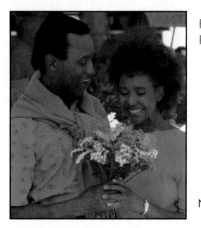

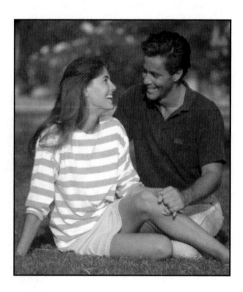

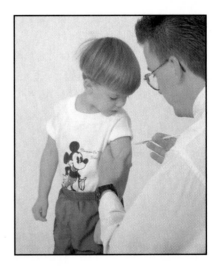

✳ 6   **Communicable Diseases**   **131**

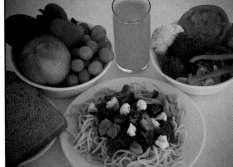

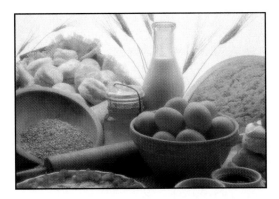

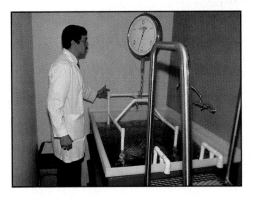

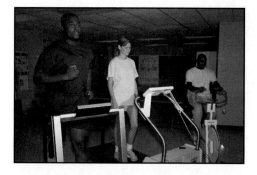
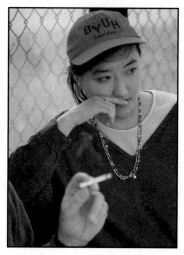

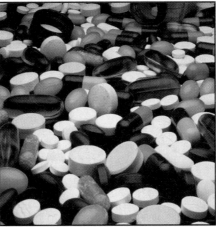

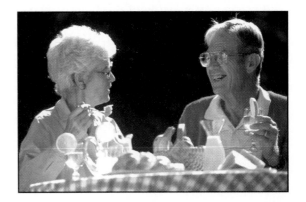

✳ 14 **Aging, Death, and Dying   407**

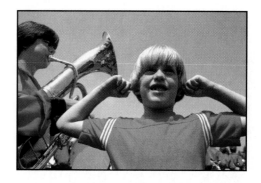

Introduction to Personal Health

1

* Give several definitions or descriptions of health.
* Define wellness and list its dimensions.
* Differentiate the three phases of prevention.
* Name the ten leading causes of death for adults in the United States.
* List the top ten underlying causes of death.
* Suggest some measures to combat violence.

*P*ersonal health is just that—personal. Health is a quality that is unique to each person. At the same time, health is a universal quality that applies to everyone. Health is defined in Webster's Dictionary as "the condition of being sound in body, mind, and spirit...freedom from physical disease or pain." The most widely quoted definition, by the World Health Organization, is similar. WHO defines health as "a state of complete physical, mental, and social well-being, not merely the absence of disease or infirmity."

The definition of health has evolved over the years. The earliest definitions were

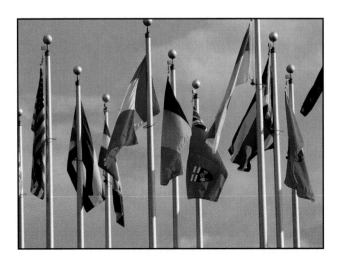

※ 1

synonymous with hygiene and sanitation, in keeping with the major concerns at the time — the devastating toll taken by highly infectious diseases carried throughout community water supplies and in sewage. With most of the deadliest infectious diseases under control, the emphasis on the meaning of health has changed. **Health** no longer means simply the absence of illness. It has shifted to the positive. Contemporary Americans are more likely to define health as "the energy to do the things I care about."

A definition of wellness that has been widely used is: the adoption of healthy lifestyle habits that will enhance your well-being while decreasing the risk of disease. Wellness obviously encompasses more than physical health. It is a state of being with several interrelated dimensions.

DIMENSIONS OF WELLNESS

The dimensions of wellness are physical, mental, emotional, social, intellectual, and spiritual, as depicted in Figure 1.1. Balancing these dimensions is necessary to achieve a high level of wellness.

1. *Physical*. Physical health is the dimension most often associated with health. It has the attributes of good cardiovascular endurance, muscular flexibility, muscular strength and endurance, and body composition (discussed in Chapters 10 and 11).

2. *Mental/intellectual*. Philosophers such as Homer, Plato, and Aristotle speculated more than 5,000 years ago that the mind exerts a powerful influence over the body, and therefore on wellness. Among the components of high mental wellness are alertness, creativity, logic, curiosity, open-mindedness, and keen memory.

3. *Emotional*. Emotions, the topic of Chapter 2, bridge the gap between the mind and the body. Emotions cause complex physical changes that affect the immune system. Negative emotions such as chronic stress (the topic of Chapter 3) can lead to serious illness and death. In brief, emotional wellness entails the ability to adjust to

change, face challenges and problems, and enjoy life.

In writing the Declaration of Independence, Thomas Jefferson specified three rights: life, liberty, and the pursuit of happiness. He did not promise happiness itself, because he knew that the government could not provide it. The individual alone can make choices that will lead to a deep underlying sense of contentment, or happiness.

4. *Social*. Social wellness is characterized by a concern and affinity for others and the world in general. Social wellness requires the ability to relate to other people, communicate effectively with them, show respect, and give of oneself. Socially healthy people have friends and are members of groups — families, neighborhoods, churches. The old axiom applies here: Before you can love others, you must be able to love yourself.

5. *Spiritual*. Spiritual wellness combines one's personal ethics, values, and morals. This dimension of wellness is what gives life meaning and purpose. It is based on faith, hope, love, optimism, and forgiveness.

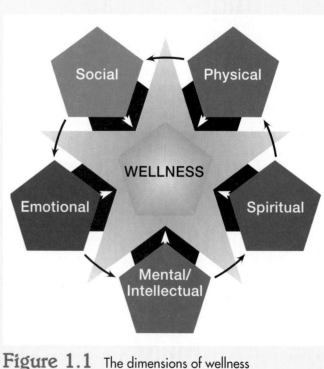

Figure 1.1 The dimensions of wellness

Wellness, then, encompasses the entire lifestyle: sound nutrition, fitness, stress management, avoidance of tobacco and other psychoactive drugs, moderate use of alcohol, weight management, sexuality, safety and spirituality. How well people manage these lifestyle factors determines in large part how well they will be.

Health and wellness range along a continuum, illustrated in Figure 1.2. At one end is the condition of total illness or disease, ending in death. At the opposite extreme is the condition of total well-being or wellness. Each person moves back and forth along this continuum from day to day as his or her health status fluctuates. Fortunately, people can do much to prevent illness and promote health and wellness by taking responsibility for their health through wise lifestyle choices, behavior patterns, and behavior modification.

PREVENTION

The emphasis on prevention in promoting wellness is clear. This emphasis is reflected in the *Healthy People 2000: National Health Promotion and Disease Prevention Objectives*, scattered throughout the chapters of this book. Crucial to prevention is a change in attitude by health-care providers and patients alike. Patients have to stop demanding medication and hospitalization and surgery for every ache and pain. Health-care providers have to be less eager to dispense medication and advise hospitalization and surgery for conditions that can be treated in less extreme ways.

Joseph Califano, former Secretary of Health and Human Services, stated that American doctors should be "more skeptical in resorting to surgery and less promiscuous in dispensing pills." Of the people who die each year in the United States, only 10% die because of inadequate health care. Only 20% die because of biological and environmental factors combined. The remaining 70% die from a combination of lifestyle behaviors.

Preventive measures include getting recommended immunizations, never starting to smoke, getting the right kind and amount of exercise, eating nutritionally, using contraceptives wisely to prevent sexually transmitted diseases, and following recommended safety procedures. These measures fall into the category of **primary prevention**, taking measures to stop a health problem before it begins.

In **secondary prevention** a health problem is detected early so intervention may deter or lessen the negative consequences of an undesirable condition. For example, a long-term smoker who develops a chronic cough, attends a clinic, and subsequently quits smoking has reduced his or her risks for acquiring cancer, heart disease, and other diseases attributable to smoking.

Tertiary prevention, taking care of people after they get ill, unfortunately is the established pattern

KEY TERMS

Health the condition of being sound in body, mind, and spirit, free from pain or disease

Wellness adoption of healthy lifestyle habits that enhance well-being and reduce the risk of disease

Primary prevention taking steps to prevent health problems from developing

Secondary prevention early detection and intervention to reduce the consequences of a health problem

Tertiary prevention taking care of a sick person

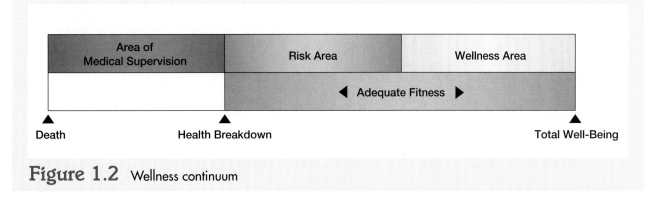

Figure 1.2 Wellness continuum

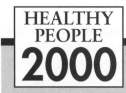

SELECTED HEALTH OBJECTIVES

I. Physical Activity and Fitness

1. Increase the proportion of people who engage regularly, preferably daily, in *light* to *moderate* physical activity for at least 30 minutes per day.
2. Increase the proportion of people who engage in *vigorous* physical activity that promotes the development and maintenance of cardiorespiratory fitness 3 or more days per week for 20 or more minutes per occasion.
3. Increase the proportion of people who regularly perform physical activities that enhance and maintain muscular strength, muscular endurance, and flexibility.
4. Reduce the proportion of people who engage in no leisure-time physical activity.
5. Reduce overweight to a prevalence of no more than 20% among people aged 20 and older and no more than 15% among adolescents aged 12 through 19.
6. Increase to at least 50% the proportion of overweight people aged 12 and older who have adopted sound dietary practices combined with regular physical activity to attain an appropriate body weight.

II. Nutrition

1. Reduce dietary fat intake to an average of 30% of calories or less and average saturated fat intake to less than 10% of calories among people aged 2 and older.
2. Increase complex carbohydrate and fiber-containing foods in the diets of adults to 5 or more daily servings for vegetables and fruits, and to 6 or more daily servings for grain products.
3. Increase calcium consumption in the diet.
4. Reduce iron deficiency among children 1 through 4 and women of childbearing age.
5. Decrease salt and sodium intake in the diet.
6. Increase to at least 85% the proportion of people aged 18 and older who use food labels to make nutritious selections.

III. Chronic Diseases

1. Increase years of healthy life to at least 65 years.
2. Reduce coronary heart disease deaths.
3. Reduce the mean serum cholesterol level among adults to no more than 200 mg/dL.
4. Increase the proportion of adults with high blood cholesterol who are aware of their condition and are taking action to reduce their blood cholesterol to recommended levels.
5. Increase the proportion of people with high blood pressure whose blood pressure is under control.
6. Increase the proportion of people with high blood pressure who are taking action to help control their blood pressure.
7. Reverse the rise in cancer deaths.
8. Slow the rise in lung cancer deaths.
9. Reduce the rate of breast cancer deaths.
10. Reduce colorectal cancer deaths.
11. Reduce diabetes-related deaths.
12. Reduce the proportion of people with asthma who experience activity limitation.
13. Reduce deaths from cirrhosis of the liver.
14. Reduce hip fractures among older adults.
15. Reduce activity limitation due to chronic back conditions.
16. Reduce the proportion of people who experience a limitation in major activity due to chronic conditions.

IV. Mental Health and Disorders

1. Reduce the prevalence of mental disorders.
2. Reduce the suicide rate.

3. Reduce the proportion of people who experience adverse health effects from stress.
4. Decrease the proportion of people who experience stress who do not take steps to reduce or control their stress.

V. Tobacco

1. Reduce the incidence of cigarette smoking.
2. Reduce the initiation of cigarette smoking by children and youth.
3. Reduce the proportion of children who are regularly exposed to tobacco smoke at home.
4. Reduce smokeless tobacco use.
5. Increase the proportion of worksites with a formal smoking policy that prohibits or severely restricts smoking at the workplace.

VI. Alcohol and Other Drugs

1. Reduce the proportion of young people who have used alcohol, marijuana, and cocaine.
2. Reduce the proportion of high school seniors and college students engaging in recent occasions of heavy drinking of alcoholic beverages.
3. Reduce alcohol consumption by people aged 14 and older to an annual average of no more than 2 gallons of ethanol per person.
4. Increase the proportion of high school seniors who associate risk of physical or psychological harm with the heavy use of alcohol, occasional use of marijuana, and experimentation with cocaine.
5. Reduce the proportion of male high school seniors who use anabolic steroids.
6. Reduce deaths caused by alcohol-related motor vehicle crashes.
7. Reduce drug-related deaths.
8. Increase the proportion of all intravenous drug abusers who are in drug abuse treatment programs.
9. Increase the proportion of intravenous drug abusers not in treatment who use only uncontaminated drug paraphernalia ("works").

VII. AIDS, HIV Infection, and Sexually Transmitted Diseases

1. Confine annual incidence of diagnosed AIDS cases to no more than 98,000 cases.
2. Confine the prevalence of HIV infection to no more than 800 per 100,000 people.
3. Increase the proportion of sexually active, unmarried people who used a condom at last sexual intercourse.
4. Reduce the incidence of gonorrhea.
5. Reduce the incidence of chlamydia.
6. Reduce the incidence of primary and secondary syphilis.
7. Reduce the incidence of genital herpes and genital warts.
8. Reduce the incidence of pelvic inflammatory disease.
9. Reduce the incidence of sexually transmitted hepatitis B infection.

VIII. Family Planning

1. Reduce the number of pregnancies that are unintended.
2. Reduce the proportion of adolescents who have engaged in sexual intercourse.
3. Increase the proportion of sexually active, unmarried people aged 19 and younger who use contraception, especially combined method contraception that both effectively prevents pregnancy and provides barrier protection against disease.

IX. Unintentional Injuries

1. Reduce deaths caused by unintentional injuries.
2. Increase use of occupant protection systems, such as safety belts, inflatable safety restraints, and child safety seats among motor vehicle occupants.
3. Increase use of helmets among motorcyclists and bicyclists.

---

* Adapted from the U.S. Department of Health and Human Services, Public Health Service. *Healthy People 2000: National Health Promotion and Disease Prevention Objectives*. Boston, Jones and Bartlett Publishers, 1992. Refer to this publication for further information on these objectives.

of medical delivery. The cost of health care could be reduced dramatically if the focus were to change to primary and secondary prevention.

LEADING CAUSES OF DEATH

The significance of the three degrees of prevention is illustrated clearly in the leading causes of death in the United States as percentages of overall deaths, depicted in Figure 1.3. Factors over which a person has absolutely no control account for only a fraction of the total deaths, whereas more than half of all disease can be entirely self-controlled.

"It is much cheaper and more effective to maintain good health than it is to regain it once it is lost."
— Kenneth H. Cooper, M.D.

At the beginning of the century, almost a third of all deaths in the United States resulted from tuberculosis, influenza, and pneumonia. Fewer than 5% of deaths were the result of cancer, and only about 10% were from cardiovascular diseases. In the 1990s, according to the U. S. Department of Health and Human Services, approximately 70% of all deaths in the United States are attributable to cardiovascular disease and cancer. Up to 80% of those deaths might have been prevented by lifestyle changes as basic as eating a diet lower in fat, getting regular exercise, not abusing alcohol, and not smoking.

From another perspective, the *Journal of the American Medical Association* has translated the actual numbers of deaths into underlying causes of death. These are shown in Figure 1.4. Ahead of microbial infections are the three lifestyle-related factors of tobacco, poor diet coupled with inactivity, and alcohol.

Of the leading causes of death, the fastest rising is AIDS. Many of the current deaths represent individuals who contracted HIV a decade ago. In early 1995, AIDS surpassed accidents and injury as the leading cause of death in the 25-44 age group.

HOMICIDE

Homicide appears on charts as the tenth leading cause of death. A report of the Secretary's Task Force on Black and Minority Health has linked homicide rates with the health factors listed in Table 1.1. Homicide is the leading cause of death

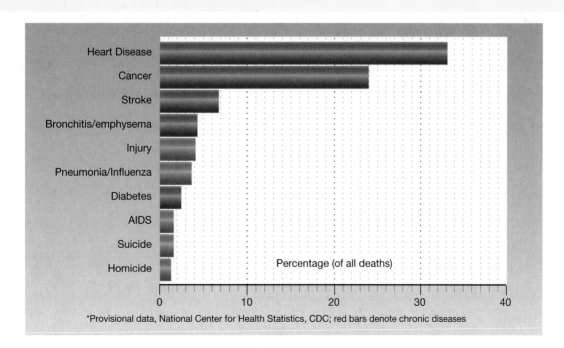

Figure 1.3 Top ten causes of death in United States

Table 1.1
Health Factors Related to Homicide

Health Factor	Characteristics
Physiology	male, youth, biological dysfunction
Psychology	commitment to violent lifestyle, impaired inhibitions against violence, repressed aggression, goal-oriented violence, and reaction to provocative conditions
Environment	depressed urban surrounding, cultural acceptance of violence in United States, and violence in the media
Lifestyle	alcohol abuse, illegal drug use, antisocial behavior, and value system emphasizing violence

in African American males ages 15-44. The rate is over seven times that of Anglo Americans. African American males have a lifetime chance of 1 in 21 of dying by homicide compared to 1 in 131 for Anglo American males. The rate of homicide for Hispanics is about two and a half times that for Anglo Americans. The high rate of homicide in the Hispanic population may reflect socioeconomic factors. Most Hispanics live in large cities, where homicide rates are high for all groups.

Although poverty is a strong correlate of homicide in African Americans and Anglo Americans, it may not be the most important factor. The high African American homicide rate might be attributed in part to anger, frustration, and low self-esteem resulting from racism, as well as society's historical disregard for violent crime against African Americans. These issues may make African Americans more aggressive in defending their integrity.

PREVENTING VIOLENCE

Violence often is the end product of exposure to violence in the home, in schools, and in

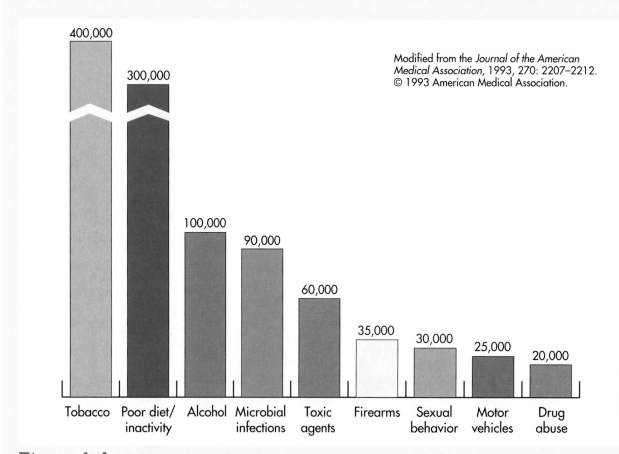

Modified from the *Journal of the American Medical Association*, 1993, 270: 2207–2212. © 1993 American Medical Association.

Figure 1.4 Underlying causes of death

communities. Violent ways of living are not inevitable or immutable. Some suggestions for preventing violence, set forth by the Task Force, are:

* *Informing and educating.* Media campaigns make the public aware of the enormity of the problem and convey the message that violence is not an acceptable way to deal with problems.

* *Building coalitions.* Consortia of civic, religious, political, youth, and community leaders could meet regularly to exchange ideas and develop programs.

* *Reducing television violence.* Various consumer, professional, and political groups are advocating reduction of violence as entertainment on television.

* *Reducing family violence.* Programs to assist in parenting and providing effective discipline that avoids excessive punishment should be developed.

* *Teaching nonviolence.* Health education curricula extending from elementary through high school should include teaching children how to manage hostility and aggression by nonviolent means. Good role models are needed in this effort.

* *Improving mental health programs.* Because aggressive and antisocial behaviors in children often are associated with later violence, improved and targeted mental health interventions are needed where appropriate.

* *Fighting chemical dependence.* Programs to reduce violence should include segments on the proper use of alcohol and drugs.

> "Good health is a duty to yourself, to your contemporaries, to your inheritors, to the progress of the world."
> —Gwendolyn Brooks

SAFETY ISSUES

A final health issue is safety at home and in the workplace. Violence in the workplace is receiving much attention lately, and security is being tightened to try to prevent sprees of violence of this nature. In addition, the **Occupational Safety and Health Administration (OSHA)** strives to provide American workers with a job environment as free as possible from health and safety hazards. Specific regulations have been put in place to protect workers from the occupational risks of blood-borne pathogens such as AIDS and hepatitis B. Most workplaces are smoke-free by now.

On their own initiative, many companies are installing fitness programs. Others have health clubs for their employees' use. Private enterprises are increasingly realizing that healthy employees are productive employees. A healthy workforce has less absenteeism, takes fewer sick days, has fewer accidents on the job, and places fewer demands on insurance policies.

THE FUTURE

As the 21st century nears, health issues are at the forefront. Advances in medicine and research are continuing. We know what the problems are. We also know the solutions to many of the problems. In large measure they entail imposing self-discipline and taking charge of one's life. People can do their part to reverse the rising costs of health care by taking charge of their personal health rather than depending on the health care community to deal with health problems after they have developed. With these kinds of changes, the 21st century might well be proclaimed "the era of health."

KEY TERMS

Occupational Safety and Health Administration (OSHA) government agency that regulates health and safety in the workplace

Summary

1 The most widely accepted definition of health, by the World Health Organization, is: "the state of complete physical, mental, and social well-being, not merely the absence of disease or infirmity."

2 Wellness has been defined as the adoption of healthy lifestyle habits that will enhance your well-being while decreasing the risk of disease.

3 The dimensions of wellness are physical, mental/intellectual, emotional, social, and spiritual.

4 The three phases of prevention are primary (prevention), secondary (early detection and treatment), and tertiary (treatment after becoming ill).

5 Whereas the leading causes of death at the turn of the century were largely infectious diseases, the leading causes of death today—heart disease, cancer, stroke, and chronic lung disease—are primarily the result of poor lifestyle habits.

6 The "hidden killers" are tobacco, poor diet coupled with inactivity, alcohol, and unsafe sexual practices.

7 Violence can be counteracted by informing and educating, building coalitions, reducing television violence, reducing family violence, teaching nonviolence, improving mental health programs, and reducing and preventing psychoactive drug use.

8 OSHA regulations protect workers from health and safety hazards, and most workplaces are now smoke-free.

Select Bibliography

Cooper, K. H. *The Aerobics Program for Total Well-Being*. New York: Mount Evans and Co., 1982.

Corbin, C. B., and R. Lindsey, *Concepts of Physical Fitness with Laboratories*, 8th edition. Dubuque, IA: Wm. C. Brown, 1994.

Floyd, P. A., et al. *Wellness: A Lifetime Commitment*. Winston-Salem, NC: Hunter Publishing, 1993.

Floyd, P. A., and J. E. Parke. *Walk, Jog, Run for Wellness Everyone*, 2d edition. Winston-Salem, NC: Hunter Publishing, 1993.

Hafen, Brent Q., and Werner W. K. Hoeger. *Wellness: Guidelines for a Healthy Lifestyle*. Englewood, CO: Morton Publishing, 1994.

Hoeger, W. W. K. *Principles and Labs*, 3d edition. Englewood, CO: Morton Publishing, 1994.

Robbins, G., D. Powers, and S. Burges. *A Wellness Way of Life*. Dubuque, IA: Wm. C. Brown, 1991.

World Health Organization. "Constitution of the World Health Organization." *Chronicle of the World Health Organization*. Geneva, Switzerland; WHO, 1947.

Wellness Lifestyle Questionnaire

NAME _____ DATE _____

COURSE _____ SECTION _____

Please circle the appropriate answer to each question and total your points as indicated at the end of the questionnaire. Circle 5 if the statement is ALWAYS true, 4 if the statement is FREQUENTLY true, 3 if the statement is OCCASIONALLY true, 2 if the statement is SELDOM true, 1 if the statement is NEVER true.

1. I am able to identify the situations and factors that overstress me.   5   4   3   2   1

2. I eat only when I am hungry.   5   4   3   2   1

3. I don't take tranquilizers or other drugs to relax.   5   4   3   2   1

4. I support efforts in my community to reduce environmental pollution.   5   4   3   2   1

5. I avoid buying foods with artificial colorings.   5   4   3   2   1

6. I rarely have problems concentrating on what I'm doing because
    of worrying about other things.   5   4   3   2   1

7. My employer (school) takes measures to ensure that my work
    (study) place is safe.   5   4   3   2   1

8. I try not to use medications when I feel unwell.   5   4   3   2   1

9. I am able to identify certain bodily responses and illnesses
    as my reactions to stress.   5   4   3   2   1

10. I question the use of diagnostic x-rays.   5   4   3   2   1

11. I try to alter personal living habits that are risk factors
    for heart disease, cancer, and other life-style diseases.   5   4   3   2   1

12. I avoid taking sleeping pills to help me sleep.   5   4   3   2   1

13. I try not to eat foods with refined sugar or corn sugar ingredients.   5   4   3   2   1

14. I accomplish goals I set for myself.   5   4   3   2   1

15. I stretch or bend for several minutes each day to keep my
    body flexible.   5   4   3   2   1

Source: Edlin and Golanty: Health & Wellness, fourth edition, © 1992, Boston: Jones and Bartlett Publishers. Reprinted by permission.

16. I support immunization of all children for common childhood diseases. 5 4 3 2 1

17. I try to prevent friends from driving after they drink alcohol. 5 4 3 2 1

18. I minimize extra salt intake. 5 4 3 2 1

19. I don't mind when other people and situations make me wait or lose time. 5 4 3 2 1

20. I walk four or fewer flights of stairs rather than take the elevator. 5 4 3 2 1

21. I eat fresh fruits and vegetables. 5 4 3 2 1

22. I use dental floss at least once a day. 5 4 3 2 1

23. I read product labels on foods to determine their ingredients. 5 4 3 2 1

24. I try to maintain a normal body weight. 5 4 3 2 1

25. I record my feelings and thoughts in a journal or diary. 5 4 3 2 1

26. I have no difficulty falling asleep. 5 4 3 2 1

27. I engage in some form of vigorous physical activity at least three times a week. 5 4 3 2 1

28. I take time each day to quiet my mind and relax. 5 4 3 2 1

29. I am willing to make and sustain close friendships and intimate relationships. 5 4 3 2 1

30. I obtain an adequate daily supply of vitamins from my food or vitamin supplements. 5 4 3 2 1

31. I rarely have tension or migraine headaches, or pain in the neck or shoulders. 5 4 3 2 1

32. I wear a safety belt when driving. 5 4 3 2 1

33. I am aware of the emotional and situational factors that lead me to overeat. 5 4 3 2 1

34. I avoid driving my car after drinking any alcohol. 5 4 3 2 1

35. I am aware of the side effects of the medicines I take. 5 4 3 2 1

36. I am able to accept feelings of sadness, depression, and anxiety, knowing that they are almost always transient. 5 4 3 2 1

37. I would seek several additional professional opinions if my doctor recommended surgery for me. 5 4 3 2 1

38. I agree that nonsmokers should not have to breathe the smoke from cigarettes in public places. 5 4 3 2 1

39. I agree that pregnant women who smoke harm their babies.   5   4   3   2   1

40. I feel I get enough sleep.   5   4   3   2   1

41. I ask my doctor why a certain medication is being prescribed
    and inquire about alternatives.   5   4   3   2   1

42. I am aware of the calories expended in my activities.   5   4   3   2   1

43. I am willing to give priority to my own needs for time and
    psychological space by saying "no" to others' requests of me.   5   4   3   2   1

44. I walk instead of drive whenever feasible.   5   4   3   2   1

45. I eat a breakfast that contains about one-third of my daily need
    for calories, proteins, and vitamins.   5   4   3   2   1

46. I prohibit smoking in my home.   5   4   3   2   1

47. I remember and think about my dreams.   5   4   3   2   1

48. I seek medical attention only when I have symptoms or feel
    that some (potential) condition needs checking, rather than
    have routine yearly check-ups.   5   4   3   2   1

49. I endeavor to make my home accident-free.   5   4   3   2   1

50. I ask my doctor to explain the diagnosis of my problem until
    I understand all that I care to.   5   4   3   2   1

51. I try to include fiber or roughage (whole grains, fresh fruits
    and vegetables, or bran) in my daily diet.   5   4   3   2   1

52. I can deal with my emotional problems without alcohol
    or other mood-altering drugs.   5   4   3   2   1

53. I am satisfied with my school/work.   5   4   3   2   1

54. I require children riding in my car to be in infant seats
    or in shoulder harnesses.   5   4   3   2   1

55. I try to associate with people who have a positive attitude about life.   5   4   3   2   1

56. I try not to eat snacks of candy, pastries, and other "junk" foods.   5   4   3   2   1

57. I avoid people who are "down" all the time and bring down
    those around them.   5   4   3   2   1

58. I am aware of the calorie content of the foods I eat.   5   4   3   2   1

59. I brush my teeth after meals.   5   4   3   2   1

60. (for women only) I routinely examine my breasts.   5   4   3   2   1

    (for men only) I am aware of the signs of testicular cancer.   5   4   3   2   1

How to Score

Enter the numbers you've circled next to the question number and total your score for each category. Then determine your degree of wellness for each category using the wellness status key.

Emotional health	Fitness and body care	Environmental health	Stress	Nutrition	Medical self-responsibility
6 _____	15 _____	4 _____	1 _____	2 _____	8 _____
12 _____	20 _____	7 _____	3 _____	5 _____	10 _____
25 _____	22 _____	17 _____	9 _____	13 _____	11 _____
26 _____	24 _____	32 _____	14 _____	18 _____	16 _____
36 _____	27 _____	34 _____	19 _____	21 _____	35 _____
40 _____	33 _____	38 _____	28 _____	23 _____	37 _____
47 _____	42 _____	39 _____	29 _____	30 _____	41 _____
52 _____	44 _____	46 _____	31 _____	45 _____	48 _____
55 _____	58 _____	49 _____	43 _____	51 _____	59 _____
57 _____	59 _____	54 _____	53 _____	56 _____	60 _____
Total _____	Total _____	Total _____	Total _____	Total _____	Total _____

Wellness Status

To assess your status in each of the six categories, compare your total score in each to the following key:

0–34 Need improvement;   **35–44** Good;   **45–50** Excellent.

Personality and Emotional Health

2

OBJECTIVES

* Define *personality*.
* Describe psychoanalytic theory.
* Explain the main premise of developmental psychology.
* Describe the cultural differences in interpersonal needs.
* Identify the levels in Maslow's hierarchy of needs.
* Explain the "toxic core."
* Identify personality types and their relation to emotional health.
* Cite the attributes of emotional health.
* Identify various emotional disorders.
* Identify demographics of suicide.
* Identify methods, agencies, and personnel designed to alleviate emotional disturbances.

*A*ll humans are similar in many ways, yet each person is totally and uniquely different, with a distinct personality. Each individual is the author of his or her life's performance, or "production." People develop not just biologically but also through their interaction with physical, social, and spiritual environments. Each day is different from the day before, and each interaction is a learning experience. Interactions allow individuals to meet their physical and emotional needs.

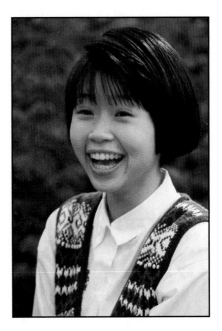

Personality is the total of individual characteristics that make each person unique. It includes all the traits, including mental processes, feelings, and behaviors, that influence how a person deals with the realities of the world. More than 100 personality variables — predispositions to behave and respond in certain ways to certain situations — have been identified. Personality is not static, though. It is influenced by many factors, both internal and external, including environment, culture, heredity, and socialization by institutions such as family, church, school, and peer groups.

THEORIES OF PERSONALITY

Various theories have attempted to explain why people are the way they are. Among these theories are psychoanalytic, behavioral, developmental, and humanistic.

Psychoanalytic Theory

In the late 1800s Sigmund Freud sought to explain the human **psyche**, the sum of all mental activity, including conscious and unconscious functions. **Psychology** is the study of the psyche, and Freud is the father of **psychoanalysis** — literally "analyzing the psyche." He defined three aspects of the psyche: the **id**, which constantly seeks pleasure and satisfaction of instinctual drives; the **ego**, which controls and regulates these drives and determines appropriate behavior; and the **superego**, an internal "voice" or conscience that tells the person what is and is not acceptable behavior. Freud emphasized early childhood events and the sex drive, or **libido**, as major forces propelling the person throughout life.

Behavioral Psychology

The field of psychology branched off in a different direction with the advent of **behavioral psychology**. In the view of its originator, B. F. Skinner, all behavior is learned. Human actions can be explained in terms of stimuli (external factors) that prompt responses. Through conditioning, desired behaviors can be learned through rewards, and undesirable behaviors can be extinguished through punishment.

Thus, behavioral psychology explains behavior as being a product of external forces rather than a consequence of processes in the mind. It relies on quantifiable, tangible measures rather than subjective interpretations. For example, in attempting to reduce a child's tantrum behavior, a behaviorist would count the number of tantrums in a given time and note the increase or decrease in tantrums as measured against aversive (negative) reinforcement.

Developmental Psychology

A third branch of psychology focuses on the stages in life and the necessity of completing certain **developmental tasks** to achieve a complete personality and emotional health. Among adherents of this theory was Erik Erikson. He took the psychoanalytic theory of his mentor, Freud, into a broader social and cultural perspective. He also emphasized successful psychological development versus Freud's emphasis on the abnormal personality.

Erikson postulated that human development throughout the lifespan proceeds through eight stages, each characterized by a crisis to be resolved. Successful resolution of the conflict enables the person to advance to the next stage. Erikson's stages are shown in Figure 2.1.

From birth to age 1 the conflict to be resolved is trust versus mistrust. An infant who is fed and comforted will more likely develop trust than one who is not. In the toddler stage the dilemma centers on the need to explore and gain independence, offset by frequent self-doubt. This conflict is well illustrated by the "terrible twos." During the

What Is Maturity?

According to Father John Powell, the three-step process toward maturity is:

✳ Accept yourself.

✳ Be yourself.

✳ Forget yourself.

These steps represent a gradually widening circle beginning with self-acceptance and expanding to the point at which we are able to put others ahead of ourselves, forgetting ourselves in the process.

Source: Professional Counselor, December 1993, p. 37.

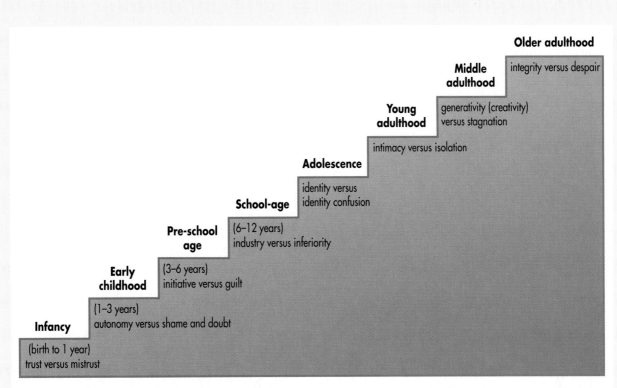

Adapted from Erik Erikson, *Childhood and Society* (New York: W. W. Norton, 1963), p. 52.

Figure 2.1 Erikson's developmental conflict stages

preschool stage the child develops a conscience, alternating between taking initiative and harboring guilt. During the elementary school ages the child develops a newfound appreciation for accomplishment, often negated by feelings of insecurity when he or she does not succeed.

Adolescence is marked by identity confusion: Who am I? Ideally resolved by adulthood, this crisis is replaced by one involving the balance of needs for intimacy and for "my own space." By middle age the person is conflicted by altruistic motivations in being a parent and doing community work versus maintaining one's own creativity, which essentially requires self-centeredness. Toward the end of the lifespan, if the person has advanced developmentally through each of the previous phases, the task to be resolved centers on integrity versus despair, a time when the person has to affirm the value of life and its ideals. People at this stage reflect on their life and assess what they have done. Successful resolution of this stage brings a sense of contentment and fulfillment.

Sometimes a person becomes stuck at a stage. For example, a certain amount of self-love, or narcissism, is healthy, but if the person does not develop empathy or the ability to give of self, this person may not be able to develop satisfying intimate relationships. According to Erikson, then, to be psychologically healthy requires a person to resolve issues successfully at each of the eight stages before that stage is negotiated successfully.

KEY TERMS

Personality the total of all individual characteristics that make each person unique

Psyche all conscious and unconscious mental functions

Psychology the study of the human psyche

Psychoanalysis literally, "analyzing the psyche"

Id the part of the psyche that seeks pleasure and satisfaction of basic drives

Ego the part of the psyche that controls and regulates basic drives

Superego internal voice or conscience; determines acceptable and unacceptable behavior

Libido sex drive

Behavioral psychology theory that all behavior is learned

Developmental tasks work to be done at various stages in a person's life

Humanistic Psychology

Humanistic psychology is based on the premise that behavior is motivated by a desire for personal growth and achievement. One well-known contributor to humanistic psychology was Carl Rogers. His **client-centered therapy** gave the client's beliefs and needs more weight than the therapist's. The person most often associated with this branch of psychology, however, is Abraham Maslow.

Maslow's Hierarchy of Needs

Maslow developed the hierarchy of needs depicted in Figure 2.2. Like Erikson, he believed that each stage builds upon the previous one. In his pyramid the most basic needs must be met first, enabling the person to advance to the next level. Unlike Erikson, however, Maslow saw the person's climb toward the top as less age-related and as fluctuating between stages depending on the circumstances in the person's life.

The first level of needs, according to Maslow, is physiological. These needs include the necessity for air, water, food, shelter, sleep, sex, and survival. Once these needs are fulfilled, the person develops a need for safety and security, to be protected from harm. After those needs have been met, the person looks for social acceptance and belonging, love and affection. Positive self-esteem (or ego fulfillment in the Freudian schema) hinges on these needs being met. The ultimate level is **self-actualization**, or the fulfillment of one's potential. People at this stage accept reality, themselves, and others, are both independent and creative, appreciate people and the world around them, and have vitality.

Schutz's Interpersonal Needs

Psychologist William Schutz theorized that every person has three categories of needs that can be met only through interaction with other people. Whereas Maslow's categories included physical needs, Schutz addressed only psychological needs. These are: inclusion, control, and affection.

The inclusion need emphasizes the drive to establish and maintain satisfactory relationships. The control need is met by attaining influence, power,

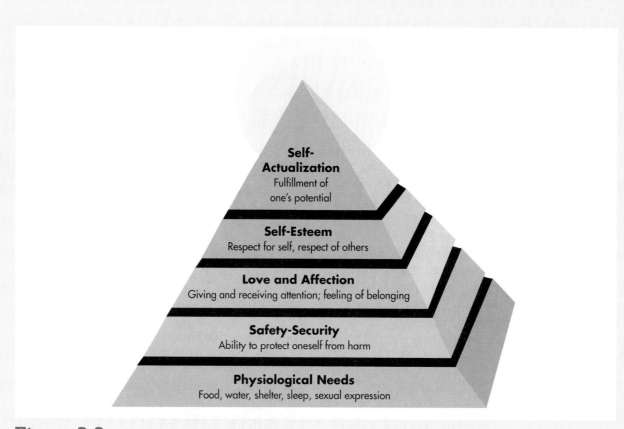

Figure 2.2 Maslow's hierarchy of needs

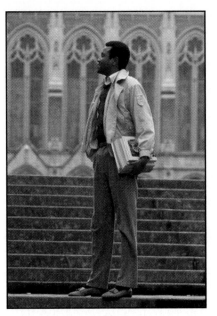

The drive for success is a strong interpersonal need.

leadership, authority, intellectual superiority, high achievement, and independence. The need for affection goes beyond inclusion and refers to intimacy, a topic explored further in Chapter 4. Schutz developed the FIRO-B (Fundamental Interpersonal Relations Orientation-Behavior) scale to measure the extent to which these three needs are being met in a person.

Cultural differences appear in these three needs. According to intercultural experts Donald Klopf and Donald Cambra, Americans have much stronger inclusion needs than the Japanese, Koreans, Chinese, Micronesians, and Australians. One reason may relate to family life. The Asians, Micronesians, and Australians maintain stronger family bonds, and family relationships are close, satisfying their needs for inclusion, control, and affection. Americans, on the other hand, are acculturated to be more independent. Children are encouraged to leave home sooner and are trained to assume larger roles in society. Therefore, Americans are more likely to have unmet interpersonal needs and look for non-family individuals and groups to fulfill these needs.

PERSONALITY TYPES

Personality can be classified in other ways, too. In recent years the connection between personality and health has become a topic of high interest, and most researchers now seem to accept the likelihood of an **immune-prone personality** that enables a

person to resist pressures without becoming ill. Likewise, researchers continue to investigate the **disease-prone personality**, which tends toward illness.

Type A and Type B Personalities

During the 1950s Dr. Meyer Friedman and Dr. Ray Rosenman studied risk factors that could lead to coronary heart disease. These doctors coined the term **Type A personality** to describe people who were impatient, quick-tempered, hard-driven, aggressive, ambitious. Type A's developed heart attacks in greater numbers than people without that constellation of traits.

By now researchers have identified, in addition to the Type A, a **Type B personality**. Type B's are calm, casual, relaxed, easy-going. The informal term "laid back" is often applied to them. They take one thing at a time, are not bothered by pressures, and do not get hurried. The Type A and Type B personality types are compared in Table 2.1.

More recent research by Duke University researcher Redford Williams and others identified one facet of the type A personality — antagonistic hostility — as the factor most associated with risk for heart disease. The other characteristics, such as competitiveness and impatience, seem to be less dangerous.

Stemming from this finding is the concept of the **toxic core**, a group of traits that are most "poisonous" to physical health. The most toxic traits are believed to be:

1. Cynical beliefs that others are bad, selfish, mean, and untrustworthy.

KEY TERMS

Humanistic psychology theory that behavior is motivated by a desire for personal growth and achievement

Client-centered therapy a focus on clients and their beliefs and needs as more important than the counselor's

Self-actualization fulfillment of one's potential

Immune-prone personality personality that enables a person to handle pressure without becoming ill

Disease-prone personality personality that tends toward illness

Type A personality characterized by being impatient, aggressive, ambitious, hot-tempered, and hard-driving

Type B personality characterized by being calm, casual, and relaxed

Toxic core group of personality traits most detrimental to physical health: cynicism, frequent anger, aggression

Table 2.1
Comparison of Type A and Type B Personality Traits

Type A	Type B
Hard-driving	Easy-going
Must finish tasks	Can leave tasks
Never late for appointments	Late for appointments
Highly competitive	Cooperative
Tends to interrupt others	Listens well
Always in a hurry	Not hurried
Uneasy when waiting	Content to wait
Eats, walks fast	Does things slowly
Sets own deadlines; self-motivated	Tends to not set deadlines
Goal-oriented	Methodical

2. Frequent angry feelings when these negative feelings arise.

3. Aggressive acts toward others when these angry feelings arise.

Type A's may be at greater risk for heart disease because their bodies make unusually small amounts of HDL ("good") cholesterol, according to Dr. Michael Miller, director of preventive cardiology at the University of Maryland. He cautions, however, that the association between these variables does not prove a cause-and-effect relationship.

To Blow Off Anger the Healthy Way

❋ Recognize anger for what it is. Don't be afraid of it or try to suppress it.

❋ Figure out what made you so angry — then figure out whether it's really worth being so upset about.

❋ Stop before you act. Calm down first. Take a deep breath. Mentally rehearse something distracting. *Then* get ready to deal with the anger.

❋ If you're angry at another person, use calm contact to explain why. Try to negotiate.

❋ Be generous with other people. Try to understand where they're coming from.

❋ When all else fails, forgive the other person. Everyone makes mistakes — and carrying a grudge will hurt *you* more than anyone else.

Anger and hostility are not the same. **Anger** is a temporary emotion that combines physiological arousal with physical arousal. Everyone experiences anger. It can range from exasperation to intense rage.

Cultural differences become apparent in the ways people feel and express anger. Latin and Arab cultures, for example, encourage free expression of anger. Utku Eskimos, on the other hand, ostracize people who lose their temper, regardless of the reason. The Japanese people assume a neutral expression and polite demeanor when they are angry. The Mbuti gatherer-hunters of northeast Zaire laugh when they are angry. Some American Indians brood silently.

In contrast to anger, **hostility** is an ongoing accumulation of irritation, a chronic form of anger. The Latin term *hostis* means enemy. For hostile people enemies seem to abound. They are everywhere: at the office, in the classroom, on the elevator, in the supermarket checkout line, on the freeway, in the next apartment. Hostility is marked by lack of trust in others in general and the belief that others are "out to get me."

Because of the health-damaging effects of hostility, people literally become their own worst enemy. The mechanism that translates emotions into physical problems is explained in Chapter 3, along with the physical consequences of stress-related hostility.

Explanatory Style

Another way of looking at personality is **explanatory style**, the way people perceive the events in their lives. It is a habitual way of thinking. The two major styles are pessimistic and optimistic. The pessimistic explanatory style has three thought patterns:

1. Assuming that a problem is never-ending; it will never go away.

2. Believing the problem affects everything, not just an isolated incident.

3. Internalizing everything ("It's my fault"), often placing the wrong blame at the wrong time.

Tips for action

To reduce hostility:

1 **Monitor your destructive thoughts**. Keep a log of incidents that trigger your anger so you learn to recognize and arrest them.

2 **Share your hostility problem with someone**. Let your spouse, or a close friend, know that you recognize you have a problem with hostility, and that you hope he or she will support your efforts to change.

3 **Stop those hostile thoughts**. As soon as you realize you are having cynical thoughts, say loudly to yourself, "STOP!" Those thoughts will stop, and the anger may cease also.

4 **Reason with yourself**. Because you are a rational being, try to reason with yourself.

5 **Put yourself in the other person's shoes**. Empathy and anger are incompatible.

6 **Learn to laugh at yourself**. Humor is an excellent strategy to deflect cynical mistrust and defuse your anger.

7 **Learn to relax**.

8 **Practice trust**. Trusting others makes them feel good about you and in turn allows you to feel good about them.

9 **Learn to listen**. By not interrupting others, you will learn to value their opinion, and they, in turn, will value you and your ideas.

10 **Learn to be assertive**. A measured response to injustice is more effective than a hostile one.

11 **Pretend today is your last**. Which would you rather be remembered for — angry feelings and aggressive acts, or joyful feelings and acts of kindness?

12 **Practice forgiving**. By letting go of resentment, you may find the weight of anger lifting, helping you to forget the wrong.

Source: *Executive Health Report*, 26:5 (February 1990), p. 5. Developed by Dr. Redford Williams. Used by permission.

Explanatory style has an extremely powerful influence on health and wellness. A negative explanatory style affects both emotional and physical well-being and it can lead to anxiety, depression, guilt, anger, and hostility.

In contrast, an optimistic explanatory style promotes emotional and physical health. Optimistic people tend to have a sense of personal control. They also have outgoing personalities. In study after study **extroverts** report greater happiness and satisfaction with life than **introverts**. Extroverted people are obviously more involved with people. They have a larger circle of friends.

KEY TERMS

Anger temporary, negative emotion that combines physiological and emotional arousal

Hostility exasperation; characterized by lack of trust in others

Explanatory style the way people perceive the events in their lives — optimistic or pessimistic

Extrovert outgoing personality

Introvert reflective, inner-centered personality

A Key to Success

In his senior year at a tiny high school in Texarkana, Arkansas, Willie Davis was voted "least likely to succeed." Four years later he was the only male from his class to graduate from college. In the winter of 1968 he was an All-Pro standout with the Green Bay Packers football team, arguably the best defensive player in the game at the time.

What was the factor that propelled a high school student with a poor self-image and lack of direction into a world-class athlete? As he tells it, he was walking home from school and passed a city work crew digging ditches. He noticed their disdain for their job, reflected in how weary and worn their faces looked. He shuddered at the thought of switching places with them. He didn't want to dig ditches, but if he had to, he would be the best ditch digger in town. Then and there he decided that *attitude means everything*. And beyond that is a *positive mental attitude*, a deep belief that whatever the difficulty, no matter what the obstacles, whatever goals are set are attainable.

After his football career Willie Davis got a master's degree in marketing, went on to become the owner and operator of Schlitz's largest beer distributorship on the West Coast, and in 1970 served on the board of directors of the parent company. He also acquired five highly profitable radio stations and was invited to sit on the board of directors of some of the nation's most successful companies.

The words of Willie Davis sum it up: "I knew that my attitude, more than any other factor, would determine my success or failure."

Source: *Think and Grow Rich*, by Dennis Kimbro and Napoleon Hill (New York: Fawcett Columbine, 1991).

Locus of Control

The concept of **locus of control** originated several years ago with the work of Julian Roberts. It involves the belief that a person's actions are effective enough to master or control the environment. Control does not mean a need to control everything around us — other people, the environment, our circumstances, good or bad. Control *does* entail a deep-seated belief that we can impact a situation by how we look at the problem. We can choose how we react and respond. If we view it as a chance for growth and opportunity, we minimize its ability to hurt us.

As far as a sense of control is concerned, a person is somewhere along a continuum. At one end of the continuum is the *external locus of control*. At the opposite end is the *internal locus of control* (see Figure 2.3).

People with external locus of control believe that the things that happen to them are unrelated to their own behavior and, therefore, are beyond their control. At the opposite end of the spectrum are the people with an internal locus of control, who believe that negative events are a consequence of personal actions and, thus *potentially* can be controlled.

The results of a host of studies show the importance of control. As a whole, people with greater sense of control are at less risk for illness. As new research is completed, scientists are realizing that an internal locus of control has an even more profound role in protecting health than we once thought.

Former *Saturday Review* editor Norman Cousins, renowned for his work linking attitudes and health, maintained that, in general, "Anything that restores a sense of control to a patient can be a

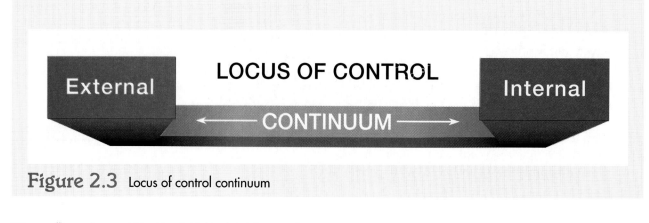

Figure 2.3 Locus of control continuum

To boost your optimism:

✳ Surround yourself with optimistic people so you will begin to "catch" their attitude.

✳ Try to genuinely like all sorts of people, regardless of ethnic and cultural differences.

✳ Be patient with yourself.

✳ Get past disappointments and look at these as challenges.

✳ Set small, attainable goals. Reward yourself when you meet those goals.

✳ Look beyond yourself. Become "other-centered."

✳ Gather all the facts before you form a conclusion. Be open-minded. Stretch your thinking.

✳ Face your problems and develop strategies for solving them instead of trying to escape them.

✳ Have fun, and relax. Learn to laugh at yourself, enjoy yourself, and respect yourself.

profound aid to a physician treating serious illness." That sense of control is more than a mere mood or attitude. It may well be a vital pathway between the brain, the endocrine system, and the immune system (see Chapter 3).

Shyness

Shyness is a personality trait. It may have its roots in low self-worth, lack of social skills, or even heredity. Shy people usually avoid speaking up in public and in social gatherings. They avoid attention. Although we should not mistakenly assume that all shy people are unhappy or maladjusted, shyness in some cases can lead to loneliness or depression.

ASSESSING PERSONALITY

Sometimes an assessment of personality is helpful when personality variables are being related to other areas, such as education, counseling, and career satisfaction. One such scale was developed by Andrew L. Comrey. The Comrey Personality Scale is a self-administering instrument consisting of

180 items, 20 per scale, for each of eight personality dimensions. These are: trust versus defensiveness, orderliness versus lack of compulsion, social conformity versus rebelliousness, activity versus lack of energy, emotional stability versus neuroticism, extroversion versus introversion, masculinity versus femininity, and empathy versus egocentrism.

Another widely used personality scale is the Myers-Briggs Type Indicator. Katherine Briggs and, later, Isabel Briggs Myers and her husband Clarence Meyers expanded Carl Jung's theories of people's inclinations and preferences for dealing with life. Their sixteen-box matrix consists of the personality variables of extroversion versus introversion, sensing versus intuition, thinking versus feeling, and judging versus perception. Combining the four preferred modes, the result is a person who is, for example, introverted, intuitive, feeling, and perceptive in style. Each of these styles can be related to work environments, optimal relationships, and learning style, among other practical applications.

KEY TERMS

Locus of control the extent to which a person believes he or she can control the external environment

Tips for action

For Shy People:

To overcome shyness:

✻ Improve your social skills by introducing yourself at a party. Then ask questions of the other person and let him or her do most of the talking. Listening is a valued skill.

✻ Take part in discussions with small groups of people with whom you are comfortable. This should enable you to gain confidence so you eventually can branch out to other discussion groups.

✻ Take an assertiveness-training class or a public-speaking course.

✻ Join a club in which you are interested, and volunteer to be on a committee.

✻ Always try to think positively about yourself.

EMOTIONAL HEALTH

Feelings may run the gamut of extreme happiness to extreme sadness. At times a person feels accepted, loved, safe, joyful, pleased, warm, and excited. At other times a person may feel unloved, sad, angry, frustrated, rejected, jealous, and unsafe. Everyone encounters conflict, criticism, and loneliness during the lifespan.

Life is highly complicated, with many challenging situations, each of which evokes a different feeling or emotion. Within the total spectrum, emotions can reflect disruptive interpersonal relationships, the frustrations and disappointments of school and work, the need for supportive financial and social resources, or peer pressure.

Emotional health has been described as the capacity to live life to its fullest in ways that enable us to realize our own potential. Emotional health begins with a person's true understanding of how he or she feels about himself or herself. Emotionally healthy individuals place positive value or worth on the self. They develop a sense of loving others and being loved by others. They feel confident about their ability to communicate effectively and to achieve success. They respect and demonstrate strength, usefulness, and competency. They exhibit reasonable and healthy attitudes about life and living.

Emotionally healthy people have high self-esteem. **Self-esteem** is a way of looking at oneself. A person with high self-esteem has confidence, a sense of positive self-regard, belief in self. Self-esteem has been called the blueprint for behavior, as it guides what a person thinks he or she can do, and thus a person's goals.

Much research attests to the value of healthy self-esteem to overall health, both mental and physical. It can boost the immune system, protect against disease, and aid in healing. It often has a bearing on whether people do or do not get sick, and how long they stay sick. Some evidence, for example, shows that recovery from mononucleosis is related to ego strength; the higher the self-esteem, the more rapid the recovery.

Continuing emotional health depends upon many factors. Among them are:

✻ a true perception of reality

✻ adaptation to change

✻ social relationships

✻ job satisfaction

✻ recreational satisfaction

✻ spirituality

A True Perception of Reality

Emotionally healthy people are able to face reality whether it is pleasant or unpleasant. They cope realistically with the problems they encounter rather than escape and retreat to unrealistic means such as drug misuse and abuse or overindulgence in foods or sex, or suicide.

Tips for action

The Need To Belong

To instill a sense of belonging in children and families:

✳ Spend quality time with each other.

✳ Express love both verbally and nonverbally.

✳ Be open and honest.

✳ Set reasonable limits for children and take *reasonable* disciplinary measures when needed.

✳ Relate your own experiences and feelings with which family members can identify.

✳ Don't allow one child to verbally tear down a sibling.

✳ Make sure all members have specific responsibilities within the family.

✳ Don't show favoritism.

✳ Validate each family member's feelings.

✳ Don't be overly protective of any member.

✳ Value all family members' opinions and values as worthy even though you may not agree with them.

✳ Maintain eye contact during communication whenever possible.

✳ Praise positive behaviors and attitudes.

Adaption to Change

Emotionally healthy people realize that nothing is absolute or unchangeable. Adaptable people deal with life as they find it and do not expect it to change at a whim. Though individuals often become secure in familiar situations and environments, emotionally healthy people adapt to changing circumstances when necessary. They have a continuous and positive interest in what goes on around them. They realize that the world is a special place to inhabit — even though it can stand some improvement.

Emotionally healthy people take responsibility for their behaviors, their feelings, and their actions. They work at solving problems with a positive attitude. They do not dwell on negative aspects of the past, other than to learn from them. These individuals solve problems as they arise and also make long-range plans, accept new experiences, make individual and independent decisions, and set realistic goals for themselves.

Social Relationships

People learn early that much satisfaction is derived from communicating and associating with other people. Most people want the approval of other people. They have a strong need for love and acceptance. Social relationships range along a continuum from familial relationships to romantic and sexual unions to platonic to co-worker relationships to acquaintances. In keeping with Maslow's theory, people have a strong need and desire for love and belonging. We want others' approval. The ability to form satisfying relationships develops early in life. Ideally, children receive love and acceptance from their parents, relatives, and other caring, giving adults. From this they learn to accept and express love in a positive, constructive manner.

KEY TERMS

Self-esteem a way of looking at oneself; may be high or low

Are Emotions Tangible?

Researchers have come to realize that emotional brain circuits are just as tangible as circuits for seeing, hearing, and touching, and neuroscientists are beginning to describe the biological processes involved in emotions and feelings. Emotions are largely the brain's interpretation of our visceral reaction to the world. Among the recently uncovered concepts:

✳ Emotions are integral to the ability to reason. Although too much emotion can impair reasoning, lack of emotion can be just as harmful.

✳ Gut feelings and intuition are indispensable for rational decision making.

✳ Many psychiatric disorders — including anxiety, phobias, posttraumatic stress syndrome, and panic attacks — involve malfunctions in the brain's ability to control fear.

Source: "Brainy Love?" by Sandra Blakeslee, *New York Times*, reprinted in the *Denver Post*, December 6, 1994.

They learn early that they derive much satisfaction from communicating and associating with other people.

Further, *intimate relationships* are to be desired. Intimate relationships are based on shared interests, friendship, and concern for the other person. This sort of relationship might incorporate a mutually satisfying sexual relationship with another person. In addition, lasting love relationships include ingredients such as commitment, open communication, realistic expectations, appreciation for one another, and the ability to work through conflicts. Intimate relationships involve recognition that the love the individuals feel for each other means accepting the other as a uniquely different person. This knowledge, plus commitment to the relationship, can be a source of understanding of differences, growth, and maturity for both. These concepts are explored further in Chapter 4.

Vocational Satisfaction

Another indicator of emotional health is to be productive and efficient in one's chosen vocation. When setting vocational goals, young people often have difficulty recognizing attainable career goals. Each person should take into consideration his or her abilities and limitations. Further, each person should realize that he or she must expend unremitting effort to reach goals. Nothing remains static. Constant changes in chosen vocations demand continuous professional growth and flexibility.

Recreational Satisfaction

A prime indicator of emotional health is the enjoyment of constructive activities other than work. Recreational activities can play a vital role in a person's life. Recreation may reduce mental stressors and sometimes overcome physical disabilities. If done with others, it allows people to meet, know, understand, and appreciate other people. Recreation is a valuable educational tool, and people learn more when the subject is enjoyable. Involvement in recreational activities, especially outdoor recreation, tends to make a person aware and appreciative of the environment. Recreational activities may consist of sports, traveling, hunting, fishing, dancing, cooking, reading, gardening, and enjoying music and other art forms.

Spirituality

Spirituality is a belief in a power higher than oneself. It occupies multiple facets in one's life. Spirituality is not just a covenant, doctrine, ritual, or ceremonial activity in a church, synagogue, mosque, or place of worship. It is a thought, a feeling, a personal experience that is extremely individual.

Spirituality grows out of individual needs, especially during times of crisis. It can be vital and

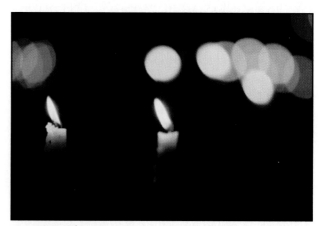

Spirituality recognizes a power higher than oneself.

active during sickness and sorrow, in despair, during failures, in the face of baffling complexities, injustices, and numerous inconsistencies. Spirituality teaches respect for existence, respect for the conscience of others, and aligns what is best in you against what is worst in you. It is tied to forgiveness, altruism, and volunteerism, hope, faith, and love.

Spiritual belief can nurture a person throughout life — from the humblest beginning to the complex end. Spirituality can kindle zeal, bestow wisdom, strengthen virtue. It can illuminate knowledge, preserve immortality, and surround one with various forms of protection.

Although belief in a higher power indeed can be a positive and helpful attribute, spirituality can leave many questions unanswered and many needs unmet. The purpose of spirituality is not to make people certain and sure about everything. It does not relieve people from the duty of thought. It enables an individual to begin thinking.

Spiritual health brings tremendous freedom, says Bernie Segal, Yale surgeon and cancer specialist. You always have a choice about how you feel, he says. Jesse Jackson says that you may not have chosen to be down, but you have a choice as to whether you try to get up. Therefore, you have a choice about how you behave whether you are in prison, whether you are sick, or whether you are on a college campus. You have a choice.

A Secret of Longevity

"Daddy Bruce" was the only name he needed. By the time he died in 1994, he was a household name in Denver. The owner of Daddy Bruce's Bar-B-Q, he organized giant Thanksgiving dinners for 30 years for thousands of needy people who had nowhere else to go for the holiday. His philanthropy didn't end there. He often served free meals on Christmas and on his birthday. He collected and distributed clothing for the poor, and he organized Easter egg hunts in the park for children. A street was named in his honor.

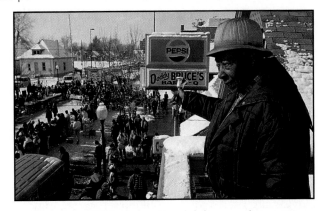

In the early 1960s Bruce Randolph was almost 60 years old and nearly broke when he headed to Denver to be near his son. He began his little barbecue restaurant out of a house, using his mother's "secret" sauce recipe. Four years later he started the holiday meal tradition, feeding a few hundred people out of the back of a truck.

Now, after his death at age 93, a handpainted sign on the closed restaurant reads, "It is more blessed to give than to receive." No one would argue that one of Daddy Bruce's secrets to a long life was altruism, a giving spirit.

MENTAL/EMOTIONAL DISORDERS

A National Center for Health Statistics survey in 1992 showed that approximately 3.3 million adult Americans have mental disorders that interfere seriously with one or more aspects of daily life. Approximately 50,000 to 60,000 people reside in mental hospitals, and other people with emotional disabilities are found among the nursing home and homeless populations. Although precise numbers are not obtainable, the recorded statistics provide some indication of the prevalence of emotional disturbances at any given time. These numbers are not static. They ebb and flow, as emotional disturbance is not a static condition.

If psychological problems could be identified, classified, and compartmentalized like infectious diseases or other health problems, the solutions would be vastly simplified. In the past, psychiatrists, psychologists, and other mental health professionals relied on the classifications of neurosis and psychosis to differentiate psychological disorders.

By definition, a **neurosis** is an emotional disorder caused by unresolved conflicts, which produces

KEY TERMS

Neurosis emotional disorder caused by unresolved conflicts and characterized by irrational behavior anxiety. Neurotic people do not distort reality grossly (they recognize what is real), but they have irrational thoughts and may act irrationally. Because neurotic people have not lost touch with reality, they recognize their thoughts and actions as irrational. They may have difficulty, however, making changes in their behavior that are considered rational and correct.

Psychosis refers to the severe emotional condition at the other end of the continuum. This general term actually refers to a number of mental disorders caused by organic (physical) or emotional disturbances, or both. The psychotic person has lost contact with reality and has *delusions*, *hallucinations*, or *illusions*.

Even as you read these descriptions, you are forming mental images. Your image of neurosis may be of individuals and behaviors that are unusual to the point of being eccentric. You may have labeled a behavior as "strange" or a person as "weird." Your impressions of psychosis probably are more intense, and "insane" or "crazy" may come to mind. Expressions such as "His elevator doesn't go to the top floor" or "She's not playing with a full deck" are part of the lexicon surrounding psychosis.

The classifications of neurosis and psychosis are much too limiting, and are certainly stereotypical. Even people who are considered "normal" display atypical behaviors at times. The American Psychiatric Association (APA) now uses a classification of mental disorders that is more useful. The APA has updated and classified emotional disorders in the *Diagnostic and Statistical Manual of Mental Disorders* (DSM–IV). The representative categories discussed here are:

✳ schizophrenic disorders

✳ anxiety disorders

✳ mood disorders

Schizophrenic Disorders

Schizophrenic disorders are mental conditions characterized by severe disturbances in perception, thought, mood, or behavior, in some combination. Theories as to the cause of schizophrenia include (a) a congenital or stress-induced biochemical imbalance, (b) family environment, and (c) a family history of mental illness.

Deterioration in functioning is a mark of schizophrenic disorders. The person's thought processes are disorganized, and conversations may seem illogical and hard to follow. Social relationships, performance at school and work, and personal appearance may decline noticeably. The schizophrenic person may exhibit inappropriate facial expressions or emotions and display psychomotor disturbances such as rapid pacing or rocking movements. *Thought disturbances* include delusions of being grand, important, or able to "save the world." *Perceptual disturbances* encompass auditory, visual, and tactile hallucinations.

Mental health is the capacity to live life to the fullest.

Schizophrenic disorders range from mild to severe and may affect up to 2 million Americans. These disorders should be diagnosed and treated promptly and professionally by a psychiatrist. Treatment may be on an outpatient basis or may require hospitalization. Overall, treatment may consist of antipsychotic medications and support therapy for the affected person as well as family members.

Anxiety Disorders

Anxiety disorders are characterized by alarm, fear, or even terror that certain circumstances evoke in a person. Obviously, if the circumstance poses a serious threat or a real danger, being afraid is a natural response. Our lifespan surely would be shorter if we did not learn what situations or circumstances were dangerous and take action to avoid them. Individuals with anxiety disorders, however, experience feelings of fear or anxiety in the presence of things or situations that do not cause anxiety for most people. To reduce the anxiety the perceived threat causes, these people tend to avoid the situation that precipitates it. Examples of anxiety disorder are specific phobias (formerly simple phobia), panic disorder, obsessive compulsive disorder, and post-traumatic stress disorder.

Panic Disorder

A **panic disorder** is a condition in which a person is overwhelmed suddenly by feelings of anxiety and loss of control. Physical symptoms include rapid heartbeat, breathing difficulties (as if one is suffocating), and mental confusion. People who have had panic attacks sometimes describe the experience as claustrophobic.

These episodes can occur while shopping at the mall, while driving a car, or even when the person is alone. Some people can anticipate the onset of the panic attack and avoid the situations that most likely will trigger it; others cannot.

Obsessive Compulsive Disorder

In the *obsession* component of **obsessive compulsive disorder**, the person has recurring thoughts that become all-consuming and affect the person's productivity. At this point obsession becomes a problem. Extreme obsessive thoughts might be to repeatedly think of killing or hurting a dearly loved or highly respected person.

Compulsion may be thought of as a complement to obsession. People who are compulsive are emotionally driven to constantly perform acts that other people view as unnecessary and a waste of time. Classic examples of compulsive behavior are repeated hand washing and an intense need for order and cleanliness. Returning many times to the dormitory to ensure that the door to the room is secured and locked is another example of compulsive behavior.

Post-Traumatic Stress Disorder

Post-traumatic stress disorder is characterized by mentally reexperiencing a traumatic event again and again after the occurrence. The person may have been a victim, for example, of rape, incest, or some other type of sexual assault. People involved in natural disasters, combat, automobile accidents, and victims of social violence such as physical assault, car-jackings, gay bashing, or cross burning may develop this condition. These individuals keep reliving the traumatic event and dream about the trauma. When encountering a situation or being in an environment similar to the one involving the trauma, they may become mentally and physically distressed and have nightmares. To cope, they avoid conversations that remind them of the traumatic event.

Mood Disorders

A **mood disorder** is a condition characterized by emotional highs or lows. In combination, this might be diagnosed as manic depression, or bipolar

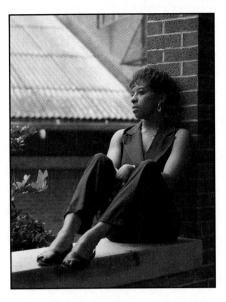

Depression can range from a mild form of the blues to severe clinical depression.

illness. This disorder involves sudden, dramatic shifts in the extremes of emotion, seemingly without relation to external variables. The manic, or "high," phase is characterized by ecstasy, bursts of energy, and hyperactivity. This phase usually is followed by severe depression, the "low" phase. Between cycles — which last days, weeks, or months — the person can have normal moods.

More common is depression by itself. In its mildest form, the "blues," the person often looks sad or unhappy and presents an aura of gloom. Sometimes, however, people hide the problem so well that even those who are close to them are not aware of it. Symptoms of the blues include:

❋ pessimism

❋ trouble concentrating

KEY TERMS

Psychosis mental disorder characterized by loss of contact with reality

Schizophrenic disorders psychological conditions characterized by severe disturbances in perceptions, thoughts, moods, and behaviors

Anxiety disorders psychological conditions characterized by exaggerated fear

Panic disorder a condition in which a person is overwhelmed by feelings of anxiety and loss of control

Obsessive compulsive disorder an anxiety disorder in which a person has constant unpleasant and unacceptable thoughts and performs repetitive acts that are unnecessary

Post-traumatic stress disorder condition in which a person mentally reexperiences a violent event

Mood disorder psychological condition characterized by emotional highs or lows

Risk Factors for Depression

The causes of depression vary from one person to another. Any of the following could contribute.

* Stressful life changes
* Susceptibility to biochemical imbalance
* Family history of depression
* Pessimistic outlook on life
* Excessive alcohol or drug use
* Painful childhood experiences

---

* temporary withdrawal from family and friends
* apathy (an "I don't care" attitude)
* episodes of sadness and crying
* temper flare-ups
* low-energy

Everyone feels "down" from time to time. The best course of action is to try to isolate the cause and find viable solutions. Isolation from others may not be constructive. True friends with a positive outlook can help.

Some people suffer from more than the blues. They have **clinical depression**. At times the cause of depression is identifiable, resulting from death of a loved one, for example. Dr. Alan Romenoski of Johns Hopkins University found that nearly nine in ten cases of major depression were associated with life events. In other cases the cause is unknown.

Symptoms of severe depression may include:

* feelings of confusion, hopelessness, and loneliness
* lack of interest in physical appearance and well-being
* loss of interest in activities that formerly were considered important
* fatigue and insomnia
* menstrual changes and lack of interest in sex
* self-doubting
* gloomy, negative, or suicidal thinking
* compulsive spending
* escaping through alcohol or drugs

Symptoms of severe depression should not be ignored. If they persist, a competent medical professional should be consulted. Depression can be treated with medication, psychotherapy, or both. If the depression stems from a physical health problem such as an underactive thyroid or a chemical intolerance in the brain, specific medication might resolve the problem. If this is not the case, a referral can be made to a competent psychiatrist.

According to the National Depressive and Manic-Depressive Association (DMDA), African Americans seek treatment for depression less than any other statistical category. If they do seek help, they most commonly turn to clergy, who are not trained in medical aspects of depression or its treatment. The reasons African Americans are less likely to seek help from mental health professionals are influenced by historical, cultural, and economic factors. In the past, as a matter of protection, it was more prudent for African Americans to guard emotions rather than discuss them. For many African Americans, cultural differences (even body language), social distance, and stereotyping may continue to be barriers and may hinder proper diagnosis in "cross-racial interactions" of client and therapist.

One form of depression that became recognized by the American Psychiatric Association in 1987 is **seasonal affective disorder (SAD)**. It is associated with less exposure to sunlight during the winter months. Up to 10% of people living in the northern United States may have this disorder, contrasted with less than 2% in the southern states, reflecting the differences in sunlit hours.

People with SAD are irritable and apathetic, sleep more, and are less active than normal. Women are about four times more susceptible to SAD than men are, and it seems to be most prevalent in the 20- to 40-year age range. This disorder also tends to run in families.

Some scientists believe SAD is related to a malfunctioning hypothalamus gland. The most beneficial treatment (for about 80% of patients) is light

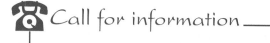

Call for information

National Depressive and Manic-Depressive Association
800-826-3632

Tips for action

How to Beat the Blues

✳ **Sit back and enjoy (or at least tolerate) the tumble.** "Realize that feeling a little bad is no big deal," says William Knaus, a psychologist in Long Meadow, Massachusetts. The "blues" is a temporary condition in life.

✳ **Do something active.** Hanging around the house and moping is sure to make you more depressed, says Jonathan Stewart, a research psychiatrist at the New York State Psychiatric Institute in New York City. Go for a walk. Take a bike ride. Turning the knob on the TV set is not being active.

✳ **Search your memory for fun things to do.** A suggestion from Eugene Walker, professor of psychology at the University of Oklahoma Health Sciences Center, is to jot down a list of things you enjoyed before you got depressed. Then pick one and do it!

✳ **Talk it out.** It's always helpful to share your feelings with someone, says Bonnie Strickland, professor of psychology at the University of Massachusetts at Amherst. "Find friends who care about you and tell them what's on your mind."

✳ **Have a good cry.** According to Robert Jaffe, a marriage and family therapist in Sherman Oaks, California, "Crying is a wonderful release — especially if you know what you're crying about."

✳ **Analyze the situation.** If you can pinpoint the source of your depression, you'll feel a lot better, says Fred Strassburger, associate clinical professor of psychiatry and behavioral sciences, George Washington University School of Medicine. Once you understand the problem, you can begin to figure out what you need to do about it.

Source: *Doctors Book of Home Remedies* (Emmaus, PA: Rodale Press, 1990).

---

therapy, in which a person is exposed for a period of time each day to a light source that mimics the sun. Treatments also considered might be dietary changes, stress management techniques, exercise, and prescribed antidepressants.

SUICIDE

The tragic end to severe depression may be suicide. According to the Mental Health Association, up to 35,000 Americans commit suicide every year. The American Association of Suicidology puts the figure at 30,000. A more precise statistic is not possible because in many cases (single-car automobile fatalities, for example), the true cause may never be known.

The figures for teens and young adults are particularly grim. Some 5,000 teens commit suicide annually. Suicide is reported as the third leading cause of death among 15–19 year olds, behind teen accidents and homicides. Suicide transcends socioeconomic boundaries, and its causes are multiple. Some conditions that may place young people at particular risk are:

✳ family breakdown and domestic violence

✳ feelings of being isolated and unappreciated by family members

✳ depression

✳ pressure to compete and succeed

KEY TERMS

Clinical depression extreme emotional low characterized by feelings of hopelessness, thoughts of suicide, and other symptoms

Seasonal affective disorder (SAD) form of depression caused by lack of exposure to sunlight during the winter

✳ alcohol or other drug dependencies

✳ previous attempted suicide

In terms of other demographics, males commit suicide three to four times as often as females. Suicide rates for Anglo Americans are approximately twice those of non-Anglos (see Figure 2.4). American Indians have the highest suicide rates overall, but wide tribal differences are apparent. The lowest rates are in African American females. The most often utilized method of suicide by all demographic groups is by firearms. Nationwide, rates of suicide are highest in the West and specifically the Mountain States. The highest suicide rates of all are in the over-65 group (see Table 2.2). The elderly comprised 12.6% of the 1991 population but committed about 20% of the suicides.

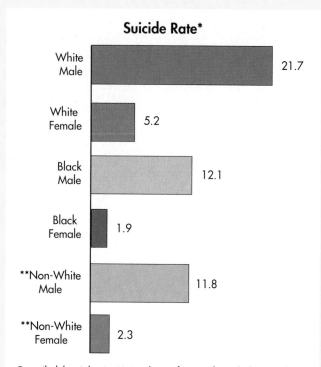

Suicide Rate*

White Male	21.7
White Female	5.2
Black Male	12.1
Black Female	1.9
**Non-White Male	11.8
**Non-White Female	2.3

Compiled by John L. McIntosh, Professor of Psychology, Indiana University, South Bend, from data provided by the National Center for Health Statistics, "Advance Report of Final Mortality Statistics, 1991," *NCHS Monthly Vital Statistics Report, 42* (2, Supplement), 1993; and U. S. Bureau of the Census, "U. S. Population Estimates by Age, Sex, Race, and Hispanic Origin: 1980–1991," *Current Population Reports, Series p–25, No. 1095, 1993.*

*Rate = $\dfrac{\text{number of suicides by group}}{\text{population of group}} \times 100{,}000$

** All non-White groups including Blacks

Figure 2.4 Comparison of white and non-white suicide rates in United States by gender, 1991

Table 2.2
U.S. Suicide Rates by Age, 1991

Age Group	Rates per 100,000 population
5–14	0.7
15–24	13.1
25–34	15.2
35–44	14.7
45–54	15.5
55–64	15.4
65–74	16.9
75–84	23.5
65+	24.0
85+	19.7
Total	12.2

Source: National Center for Health Statistics, 1993.

Suicide is usually a planned or premeditated act. Most suicidal individuals give some warning or signal of their intention, such as an unexplained and very high mood after a period of depression or giving away personal possessions that the suicidal person cherishes. Contrary to popular belief, discussing the person's feelings and possible suicide plan may deter the act. In addition, the person might be assisted in seeking help from the family physician or a mental health professional. Emergency sources include paramedics, police, and community mental health centers.

MENTAL HEALTH PROFESSIONALS, FACILITIES, AND ORGANIZATIONS

At times daily activities and other events may overwhelm us and affect our state of mind. During these times we usually take "mental health breaks" to restore equilibrium to our psyche. These activities could include meditating, taking a long walk, getting engrossed in a hobby, exercising, or talking with a close friend or family member.

Mental health problems sometimes become too serious to be left to self-diagnosis

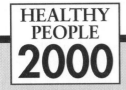

HEALTHY PEOPLE 2000 — OBJECTIVES FOR MENTAL HEALTH

❋ Reduce the prevalence of mental disorders among children and adolescents.

❋ Reduce suicides among the following groups:

Youth ages 15-19
Men aged 20-34
Anglo-American men aged 65 and older
American Indian/Alaska Native men on reservations

❋ Reduce incidence of injurious suicide attempts among adolescents ages 14 through 17

and treatment. In these cases professional intervention should be sought before the problem becomes unmanageable. If anxiety or depression begins to interfere markedly, causing problems on the job, at school, and with interpersonal relationships, the person should see a mental health professional. Obviously, any person who has attempted or dwells on the notion of suicide should be seen immediately.

A **psychiatrist** is a physician (M.D.) who specializes in the diagnosis and treatment of mental disorders, using psychotherapy as well as medication. Because psychiatrists are physicians, they have the expertise to make a medical diagnosis.

A **clinical psychologist** holds the Ph.D degree in psychology and treats psychological problems through various psychotherapies. Clinical psychologists are not physicians and may not prescribe medications for treatment.

The **psychiatric registered nurse** is responsible for the nursing care of patients in the hospital or other clinical settings. The psychiatric registered nurse (R.N. or B.S.N.) has additional clinical training in nursing and mental health problems.

The **psychiatric social worker** is responsible for coordinating available resources for the patient/client and family. This professional assists in making the transition from treatment to community as smooth as possible. The psychiatric social worker usually holds the degree of Master of Social Work (MSW).

A variety of facilities and organizations specialize in diagnosing and treating mental health problems or provide mental health services. They are categorized as:

❋ Psychiatric hospitals (public or private)

❋ Community mental health centers, which may be supported in some part by taxes and grants.

❋ Voluntary agencies such as the Mental Health Association, with local chapters in major cities throughout the United States.

Anyone is subject to stresses that can cause temporary emotional instability. Emotionally healthy people usually are able to adjust, solve the problem, and get on with life. If emotional problems become more complex or disabling, however, professional assistance may be needed.

KEY TERMS

Psychiatrist physician who specializes in the diagnosis and treatment of mental disorders

Clinical psychologist mental health professional with a Ph.D. in psychology who treats psychological problems through psychotherapy

Psychiatric registered nurse a registered nurse (R.N. or B.S.N.) who has additional training in mental health and cares for patients in a clinical setting

Psychiatric social worker mental health professional with a Master of Social Work degree who coordinates patient resources

Summary

1 Among the various psychological theories that have been proposed to explain the personality are psychoanalytic, behavioral, developmental, and humanistic.

2 Erik Erikson postulated that human development proceeds through eight crises stages, each of which must be resolved successfully for emotional health.

3 Abraham Maslow's hierarchy has five levels of needs that humans must have met on their way to self-actualization.

4 Personality types and physical health are related, as exemplified by the toxic core of the type A personality, which carries greater risk for heart disease and other illnesses.

5 Whether a person has a pessimistic or an optimistic overall way of thinking has an effect on physical health.

6 Locus of control ranges along a continuum from external (factors outside of myself determine my lot in life) to internal (many things in life are within my control).

7 Emotional health is based on having a true perception of reality, being adaptable to change, having social relationships, having job satisfaction, enjoying recreational activities, and being spiritual.

8 Mental/emotional disorders range from mild, such as occasional "blues," to severe disorders in which the person loses touch with reality, such as schizophrenia.

9 Anxiety disorders include panic disorder, obsessive compulsive disorder, and post-traumatic stress disorder.

10 Suicide is a serious problem in young people and requires professional intervention.

Select Bibliography

Adessa, Mia. "Sad Hearts." *Psychology Today*, August 1988, p. 23.

Adler, Valerie. "Accentuate the Positive." *American Health*, May, 1989.

American Psychiatric Association. *Diagnostic and Statistical Manual of Mental Disorders* (DSM–IV). Washington, DC: APA.

Angell, Marcia. "Disease as a Reflection of the Psyche." *New England Journal of Medicine*, 312 (1985), 1570-1572.

Benson, Herbert, and Eileen M. Stuart. *The Wellness Book*. New York: Birch Lane Press, 1992.

Berger, Amy H. "Are You a Chronic Worrier?" *Complete Woman*, October 1987, p. 58.

Black, D. W., G. Winokur, and A. Nasrallah. "Mortality in Patients with Primary Unipolar Depression, Secondary Unipolar Depression, and Bipolar Affective Disorder: A Comparison with General Population Mortality." *International Journal of Psychiatric Medicine*, 17 (1987), 351-360.

Carney, R. M., M. W. Rich, K. E. Freedland, J. Saini, A. TeVelde, C. Simeone, and K. Clark, "Major Depressive Disorder Predicts Cardiac Events in Patients with Coronary Artery Disease." *Psychosomatic Medicine*, 50 (1988), 627-633.

Comrey, Andrew L. *Comrey Personality Scales*. San Diego: Educational and Industrial Testing Service.

Fackelmann, Kathy A. "Hostility Boosts Risk of Heart Trouble." *Science News*, 135 (January 28, 1989), 60.

Flannery, Raymond B. "The Stress-Resistant Person." *Harvard Medical School Health Letter*, February 1989, pp. 1-3.

Freidman, Howard S. *The Self-Healing Personality*. New York: Henry Holt & Co., 1991.

Gallagher, Winifred. "The Dark Affliction of Mind and Body." *Discover*, May 1986, pp. 66-76.

Goode, Erica E. "Accounting for Emotion. *U.S. News and World Report*, June 27, 1988, p. 53.

Groër, Maureen. "Psychoneuroimmunology." *American Journal of Nursing*, August 1991, p. 33.

"Hearts and Minds." *Longevity*, April 1989, p. 14.

"How Your Personality Affects Your Health." *Good Housekeeping*, June 1983.

"Is Yours a Hostile Heart?" *Men's Health*, 5:7/8 (August/September 1989).

Jacobs, M. A., A. Spilken, and M. Norman. "Relationship of Life Change, Maladaptive Aggression, and Upper Respiratory Infection in Male College Students." *Psychosomatic Medicine*, 31:1 (1969), pp. 31-44.

Jung, Carl. *Psychological Types*. New York: Harcourt Brace, 1923.

Justice, Blair. *Who Gets Sick: Thinking and Health*. Houston: Peak Press, 1987.

Kimbro, Dennis, and Napoleon Hill. *Think and Grow Rich*. New York: Fawcett Columbine, 1991.

Klopf, Donald W., and Donald E. Cambra. *Personal and Public Speaking*. Englewood, CO: Morton Publishing, 1993.

Lehmann, C. "Racism Often at Root of Misdiagnosing Minority Patients." *Psychiatric News*, 29 (Dec. 16, 1994), p. 9.

Locke, Steven, and Douglas Colligan. *The Healer Within: The New Medicine of Mind and Body*. New York: E. P. Dutton, 1986, p. 140.

Maranto, Gina. "Emotions: How They Affect Your Body." *Discover*, November 1984, p. 35.

Maslow, Abraham. *Motivation and Personality*, 2d edition. New York: Harper & Row, 1970.

McKinnon, D. "The Development of Personality." In *Personality of the Behavior Disorders*, edited by M. V. Hunt. New York: Ronald Press, 1994.

McMillen, S. I. *None of These Diseases*, rev. edition. Old Tappan, NJ: Fleming H. Revell Co., 1984.

Mossey, Jana M., Elizabeth Mutran, Kathryn Knott, and Rebecca Craik. "Recovery After Hip Fractures: The Importance of Psychosocial Factors." *Advances*, 6:4 (1989), 23-25.

Myers, David. *The Pursuit of Happiness: Who is Happy — and Why*. New York: William Morrow & Co., 1992.

Myers, I.B. *The Myers-Briggs Type Indicator*. Palo Alto, CA: Consulting Psychologists Press, 1962.

Ornstein, Robert, and David Sobel. *The Healing Brain*. New York: Simon and Schuster, 1987.

Padus, Emrika. *The Complete Guide to Your Health and Your Emotions*. Emmaus, PA: Rodale Press, 1986.

Powell, Barbara. *Good Relationships Are Good Medicine*. Emmaus, PA: Rodale Press, 1987.

Remen, Rachel Naomi. "Feeling Well: A Clinician's Casebook." *Advances*, 6:2, 43-49.

Rodgers, Joann. "Longevity Predictors: The Personality Link." *Omni*, February 1989, p. 25.

Rosenman, Ray. "Do You Have Type 'A' Behavior?" *Health and Fitness* (supplement), 1987.

Schutz, William. *FIRO-B*. Palo Alto, CA: Consulting Psychologists Press, 1967.

Stanwyck, Douglas J., and Carol A. Anson. "Is Personality Related to Illness? Cluster Profiles of Aggregated Data." *Advances*, 3:2 (Spring 1986), pp. 4-15.

Siegel, Bernie. "Mind Over Cancer." *Prevention*, March 1988, pp. 61-62.

Suinn, R. M. "The Cardiac Stress Management Program for Type A Patients." *Cardiac Rehabilitation*, 5 (1975), pp. 13-15.

Tavris, Carol. *Anger: The Misunderstood Emotion*. New York: Touchstone, 1982.

Tavris, Carol. "On the Wisdom of Counting to Ten." *Review of Personality and Social Psychology*, 5 (1984), 170–191.

Thoresen, Carl E. "The Hostility Habit: A Serious Health Problem?" *Healthline*, April 1984, p. 5.

Wallis, Claudia. "Stress: Can We Cope?" *Time*, June 6, 1983, pp. 48-54.

Weisinger, Hendrie. "Mad? How to Work Out Your Anger." *Shape*, January 1988, pp. 86-93.

Williams, Redford. "Hostility, Anger, and Heart Disease." *Drug Therapy*, August 1986, p. 43.

Williams, Redford. *The Trusting Heart: Great News About Type A Behavior*. New York: Times Books, Division of Random House, 1989, p. 120.

Wood, Clive. "The Cold Character." *Psychology Today*, April 1988, p. 13.

Vaughan, Christopher. "The Depression-Stress Link." *Science News*, 134 (September 3, 1988), p. 155.

Symptoms of Depression

NAME _____ DATE _____

COURSE _____ SECTION _____

Check any symptoms you have had for 2 weeks or more:

❑ Loss of interest in things you used to enjoy.

❑ Feeling sad, blue, or down in the dumps.

❑ Feeling slowed down or restless and unable to sit still.

❑ Feeling worthless or guilty.

❑ Changes in appetite or weight loss or gain.

❑ Thoughts of death or suicide; suicide attempts.

❑ Trouble concentrating, thinking, remembering, or making decisions.

❑ Trouble sleeping or sleeping too much.

❑ Loss of energy or feeling tired all of the time.

❑ Feeling pessimistic or hopeless.

❑ Being anxious or worried.

If you have had five or more of these symptoms for at least 2 weeks, you may have major depression. See your health care provider. Even if you have only a few depressive symptoms, your health care provider can be of help.

Adapted from U.S. Department of Health and Human Services booklet, *Depression Is a Treatable Illness, A Patient's Guide.*

Self-Esteem Checklist

NAME _____ DATE _____

COURSE _____ SECTION _____

AA = Almost Always   O = Occasionally   R = Rarely   N = Never

1. Do you find yourself bragging or exaggerating the importance of your role?	AA	O	R	N
2. Are you jealous of the possessions, opportunities, or positions of others?	AA	O	R	N
3. Do you find yourself judging your behavior by other people's standards or expectations rather than your own?	AA	O	R	N
4. Are you possessive in your relationships with friends or family members?	AA	O	R	N
5. Is it difficult for you to acknowledge your own mistakes?	AA	O	R	N
6. Do you resort to bullying and intimidation in your dealings with others?	AA	O	R	N
7. Do you "put people down" so that you can feel "one up?"	AA	O	R	N
8. Are you a perfectionist?	AA	O	R	N
9. Must you be a "winner" in recreational activities to have fun?	AA	O	R	N
10. When faced with new opportunities, do you feel inadequate or insecure?	AA	O	R	N
11. Do you have difficulty accepting compliments?	AA	O	R	N
12. Do you refrain from expressing your feelings and opinions?	AA	O	R	N
13. Do you shy away from trying new things for fear of failure or looking dumb?	AA	O	R	N
14. Do you neglect your own needs to respond to others needs?	AA	O	R	N

"ALMOST ALWAYS" or "OFTEN" answers to any of these questions may indicate that your self-esteem needs attention.

Reprinted by permission from Structured Exercises in Stress Management, Volume 2, © 1984, 1994 by Donald A. Tubesing. Published by Whole Person Associates, 210 West Michigan, Duluth, MN 55842-1908, 218-727-0500.

Assessing Hostility

NAME_____ DATE_____

COURSE _____ SECTION _____

Each question describes a specific or general situation that you probably have encountered. If you haven't, imagine as vividly as you can how you would react in the situation.

Following each description are two responses, A or B, describing how that situation might affect you, or how you might behave under those circumstances. In some instances neither response may seem to fit, or both may appear equally desirable. Go ahead and answer anyway, choosing the single response that is *more likely* for you in that situation. Choose only *one* response for each situation described.

Take as much time as you need to make your choice for each item, but remember, what seems right at first glance — your "gut reaction" — usually represents your true position.

1. A teenager drives by my yard with the car stereo blaring acid rock.
   A. I begin to understand why teenagers can't hear.
   B. I can feel my blood pressure starting to rise.

2. The person who cuts my hair trims off more than I wanted.
   A. I tell him or her what a lousy job he or she did.
   B. I figure it'll grow back, and I resolve to give my instructions more forcefully next time.

3. I'm in the express checkout line at the supermarket, where a sign reads: "No more than ten items please!"
   A. I pick up a magazine to pass the time.
   B. I glance ahead to see if anyone has more than ten items.

4. Many large cities have a visible number of homeless people.
   A. I believe that the homeless are down and out because they lack ambition.
   B. The homeless are victims of illness or some other misfortune.

5. There have been times when I was very angry with people.
   A. I was always able to stop short of hitting them.
   B. I have, on occasion, hit or shoved them.

6. The newspaper contains a prominent news story about drug-related crime.
   A. I wish the government had better educational/drug programs, even for pushers.
   B. I wish we could put every drug pusher away for good.

7. The prevalence of AIDS has reached epidemic proportions.
   A. This is largely the result of irresponsible behavior on the part of a small proportion of the population.
   B. AIDS is a major tragedy.

8. I sometimes argue with a friend or relative.
   A. I find profanity an effective tool.
   B. I hardly ever use profanity.

9. I'm stuck in a traffic jam.
   A. I usually am not particularly upset.
   B. I quickly start to feel irritated and annoyed.

10. There is a really important job to be done.
    A. I prefer to do it myself.
    B. I'm apt to call on my friends or co-workers to help.

11. Sometimes I keep my angry feelings to myself.
    A. Doing so can often prevent me from making a mountain out of a molehill.
    B. Doing so is usually a bad idea.

12. Another driver butts ahead of me in traffic.
    A. I usually flash my lights or honk my horn.
    B. I stay farther back behind such a driver.

13. Someone treats me unfairly.
    A. I usually forget it rather quickly.
    B. I'm apt to keep thinking about it for hours.

14. The cars ahead of me on an unfamiliar road start to slow and stop as they approach a curve.
    A. I assume that there's a construction site ahead.
    B. I assume someone ahead had a fender bender.

15. Someone expresses an ignorant belief.
    A. I try to correct him or her.
    B. I'm likely to let it pass.

16. I'm caught in a slow-moving bank or supermarket line.
    A. I usually start to fume at people who dawdle ahead of me.
    B. I seldom notice the wait.

17. Someone is being rude or annoying.
    A. I'm apt to avoid that person in the future.
    B. I might have to get rough with the person.

18. An election year rolls around.
    A. I learn anew that politicians are not to be trusted.
    B. I'm caught up in the excitement of pulling for my candidate.

19. An elevator stops too long on a floor above where I'm waiting.
    A. I soon start to feel irritated and annoyed.
    B. I start planning the rest of my day.

20. I'm around someone I don't like.
    A. I try to end the encounter as soon as possible.
    B. I find it hard not to be rude to the person.

21. I see a very overweight person walking down the street.
    A. I wonder why this person has such little self-control.
    B. I think the person might have a metabolic defect or a psychological problem.

22. I'm riding as a passenger in the front seat of a car.
    A. I take the opportunity to enjoy the scenery.
    B. I try to stay alert for obstacles ahead.

23. Someone criticizes something I've done.
    A. I feel annoyed.
    B. I try to decide whether the criticism is justified.

24. I'm involved in an argument.
    A. I concentrate hard so I can get my point across.
    B. I can feel my heart pounding, and I breathe harder.

25. A friend or co-worker disagrees with me.
    A. I try to explain my position more clearly.
    B. I'm apt to get into an argument with him or her.

26. Someone is speaking very slowly during a conversation.
    A. I'm apt to finish his or her sentences.
    B. I'm apt to listen until he or she finishes.

27. If they were put on the honor system, most people wouldn't sneak into a movie theater without paying.
    A. That's because they're afraid of being caught.
    B. It's because it would be wrong.

28. I have strong beliefs about rearing children.
    A. I try to reward mine when they behave well.
    B. I make sure they know what the rules are.

29. I hear news of another terrorist attack.
    A. I feel like lashing out.
    B. I wonder how people can be so cruel.

30. I'm talking with my mate, boyfriend, or girlfriend.
    A. I often find my thoughts racing ahead to what I plan to say next.
    B. I find it easy to pay close attention to what he or she is saying.

31. There have been times in the past when I was really angry.
    A. I have never thrown things or slammed a door.
    B. At times I have thrown something or slammed a door.

32. Life is full of little annoyances.
    A. They often seem to get under my skin.
    B. They seem to roll off my back unnoticed.

33. I disapprove of something a friend has done.
    A. I usually keep the disapproval to myself.
    B. I usually let my friend know about it.

34. I'm requesting a seat assignment for an airline flight.
    A. I usually request a seat in a specific area of the plane.
    B. I generally leave the choice to the agent.

35. I feel a certain way nearly every day of the week.
    A. I feel grouchy some of the time.
    B. I usually stay on an even keel.

36. Someone bumps into me in a store.
    A. I pass it off as an accident.
    B. I feel irritated at the person's clumsiness.

37. My mate, boyfriend, or girlfriend is preparing a meal.
    A. I keep an eye out to make sure nothing burns or cools too long.
    B. I either talk about my day or read the paper.

38. A boyfriend or girlfriend calls at the last minute to say that he or she is "too tired to go out tonight," and I'm stuck with a pair of $15 tickets.
    A. I try to find someone else to go with.
    B. I tell my friend how inconsiderate he or she is.

39. I recall something that angered me previously.
    A. I feel angry all over again.
    B. The memory doesn't bother me nearly as much as the actual event did.

40. I see people walking around in shopping malls.
    A. Many of them are shopping or exercising.
    B. Many of them are just wasting time.

41. Someone is hogging the conversation at a party.
    A. I look for an opportunity to put him or her down.
    B. I soon move to another group.

42. At times I have to work with incompetent people.
    A. I concentrate on my part of the job.
    B. Having to put up with them ticks me off.

43. My mate, boyfriend, or girlfriend is going to get me a birthday present.
    A. I prefer to pick it out myself.
    B. I prefer to be surprised.

44. I hold a poor opinion of someone.
    A. I keep it to myself.
    B. I let him or her know it.

45. In most arguments I have, the roles are consistent.
    A. I'm the angrier one.
    B. The other person is angrier than I am.

46. Slow-moving lines often can be found in banks and supermarkets.
    A. They are an unavoidable part of modern life.
    B. They often are because of someone's incompetence.

SCORING KEY

CYNICISM	_____
ANGER	_____
AGGRESSION	_____
- - - - - - - - - - - - - - - - -	
TOTAL **HOSTILITY**	_____

To score your Cynicism level, turn back to the test and look at the following items and responses: 3(B), 4(A), 7(A), 10(A), 14(B), 18(A), 21(A), 22(B), 27(A), 30(A), 34(A), 37(A), 40(B), 43(A), and 46(B). Give yourself one point every time your answer agrees with the letter in parentheses after each item number. Thus, if your answers matched the letters in the parentheses for 8 of the 15 Cynicism questions, your Cynicism score would be 8.

Enter your Cynicism score on the appropriate line at the end of the test.

❋ If your score is 0 to 3, your Cynicism level is very low.

❋ If your score is 4 to 6, your Cynicism level is probably high enough to be of some concern.

❋ If your score is 7 or more, your Cynicism level is very high.

To score your Anger level, give yourself one point for each answer that agrees with the letter in parentheses after these items: 1(B), 6(B), 9(B), 13(B), 16(A), 19(A), 23(A), 24(B), 29(A), 32(A), 35(A), 36(B), 39(A), 42(B), and 45(A). Enter the total on the line marked "Anger" in the scoring key.

❋ If your score is 0 to 3, your Anger level is very low.

❋ If your score is 4 to 6, your Anger level is probably high enough to deserve your attention.

❋ If your score is 7 or higher, your Anger level is very high.

To score your Aggression level, give yourself one point for each answer that agrees with the letter in parentheses after these items: 2(A), 5(B), 8(A), 11(B), 12(A), 15(A), 17(B), 20(B), 25(B), 26(A), 28(B), 31(B), 33(B), 38(B), 41(A), and 44(B). Write the total on the "Aggression" line of the scoring key.

❋ If your score is 0 to 3, your Aggression level is very low.

❋ If your score is 4 to 6, your Aggression level is borderline and you may want to consider way to reduce it.

❋ If your score is 7 or more, you probably need to take serious steps to reduce your Aggression level.

Your Total Hostility score is the sum of the three aspects you have just scored. Add your Cynicism, Anger, and Aggression scores and enter the total on the "Total Hostility" line of the scoring key. Any score above 10 is high enough to increase your risk of health problems.

Source: *Anger Kills*, © by Redford Williams and Virginia Williams, 1993. Reprinted by permission of Times Books, a division of Random House.

Stress and Health

3

The 1949 Conference on Life and Stress and Heart Disease provided the first formal recognition that stress could precipitate chronic disease. Practitioners who gathered at that conference also were among the first to formally define stress by stating that it is a force that induces distress or strain upon both the emotional and physical make-up.

Our understanding of stress has come a long way in the last four or five decades. Despite the volumes that have been written about it and the years of research dedicated to it, however, we are in some ways still hovering on the edge of understanding all of

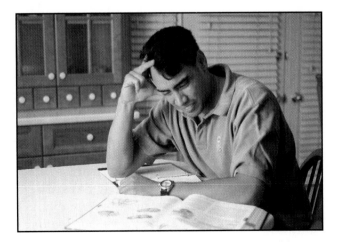

its complexity. Austrian-born Hans Selye, considered the father of **stress** research, pointed out that stress "is a scientific concept which has suffered from the mixed blessing of being too well known and too little understood."

Selye himself defined stress as "the nonspecific response of the human organism to any demand placed upon it." Stress results from any physical, emotional, social, or spiritual event or condition that causes us to adapt — to adjust to a certain situation. Simply stated, *stress occurs whenever something changes and we are forced to adapt to the change.* Our adaptation is sometimes successful, sometimes unsuccessful. Stress is not the same as frustration, anxiety, or conflict — though it can lead to all of those emotions. In popular jargon, "stress" is used in a negative way — but situations that cause stress can be either happy (such as the birth of a baby) or sad (such as the death of a loved one). What Selye says in his definition of stress is critical to understand: The body reacts to stress the same way, regardless of the event that precipitates the response. Your heart may pound and your stomach may churn with excess acid whether you just landed a new job or got in trouble with your boss.

Stress is no respecter of persons or situations. No one can escape it, wish it away, or even live without it. The only way to be completely free of stress is to be dead. The American Institute of Stress claims that 90% of all American adults experience high levels of stress one or two times a week and a fourth of all American adults are subject to crushing levels of stress nearly every day. It can happen at home, in the classroom, on the job, in families, between friends or associates, and even between us and our surroundings in the form of extreme heat or cold, noise, pollution, or overcrowding. **Stressors**, the factors that cause stress, can be:

❋ Physical (fatigue or a bacterial infection)

❋ Emotional (pent-up anger or hostility)

❋ Social (rejection or embarrassment)

❋ Intellectual (confusion)

❋ Spiritual (guilt)

The very process of living entails change. Therefore, people of all ages, both sexes, all races, every culture, and every socioeconomic group are susceptible to stress. The problem occurs with *unremitting*

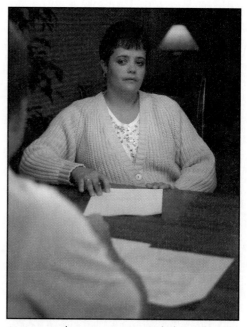
Many people encounter stress daily on the job.

stress — the kind that requires constant adaptation to chronic change. Unremitting stress can become a threat to health, because maintaining lifelong wellness is difficult when much of the body's energy is channeled into coping with stress.

Researchers at the American Institute of Stress estimate that 75% to 90% of all visits to health care providers result from stress-related disorders. The National Council on Compensation Insurance reports that stress-related claims account for almost one-fifth of all occupational disease. Fully one-fourth of all Worker Compensation claims are for stress-related injuries, and researchers estimate that 60% to 80% of all industrial accidents in the United States are related to stress.

Stress is not limited to what goes on in our thoughts. Stress is a nonspecific automatic biological response to demands made upon an individual. Scientifically speaking, stress is any challenge to **homeostasis**, the body's internal sense of balance. Stress is a biological and biochemical process that begins in the brain and spreads through the autonomic nervous system, causing the release of hormones and exerting eventual influence over the immune system.

DISTRESS AND EUSTRESS

All stress is not negative. Hans Selye coined the term **eustress** to denote positive, desirable stress.

This is in contrast to **distress**, or negative stress — too much stress in a short time, chronic stress over a long time, or a combination of stressors that throw the body out of balance.

Eustress is the stress that keeps life interesting and provides opportunity for growth. Positive stress is associated with happy occasions, such as family get-togethers, class reunions, graduations, victorious athletic competitions, weddings, births, and baptisms. Other good stressors may be finally getting a driver's license, buying the first car, landing the first job, or moving into the first apartment. Eustress is a challenging force that helps a person feel successful, loved, secure, accepted, and protected.

Some stress promises curiosity and exploration. Some stressful situations are challenging, stimulating, and rewarding. Competitive sport is an excellent example. To gear up for a football game, worry about winning, and then pound across the field for 3 hours is extremely stressful, both physically and emotionally. The athletes who do it believe the rewards and thrill are well worth the stress — and millions of fans couldn't agree more.

Distress, on the other hand, is associated with the kinds of changes that disrupt homeostasis. For example, leaving home for the first time brings with it many sources of distress — interacting with

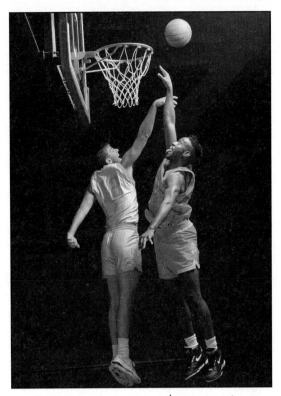

Positive stress can occur on happy occasions such as an athletic competition.

unfamiliar people, missing the established social support system, having too little money, and experiencing conflicts in social relationships. People of color in the United States — especially African American, American Indian, and Hispanic — are more likely than the general population to be subjected to stressors such as discrimination, unemployment, access to career opportunities, access to educational advancement, limited resources, poor nutritional status, and undesirable living conditions.

SOURCES OF STRESS

Psychological stress can come from almost anywhere — missing a bus, not having enough money to make ends meet, having an argument with a

Eustress Versus Distress

How can you tell if you're being affected more by "good stress" or "bad stress?" One way is to compare the results of each:

Eustress inspires	Distress inspires
Good health	Poor health
Regular exercise	Sedentary lifestyle
Good relationships	Poor relationships
High self-esteem	Low self-esteem
Intellectual vibrancy	Stagnation
Emotional stability	Emotional instability
Ability to give love	Inability to love
Ability to receive love	Rejection
Enjoyment of life	Diminished purpose
and results in	**and results in**
Contentment	Discontentment
Happiness	Sadness
Longer life	Disease
Wellness	Premature death

KEY TERMS

Stress demand that places physical and emotional strain on an individual

Stressors factors that cause stress

Homeostasis the body's internal sense of balance

Eustress positive stress

Distress negative stress

friend. *Environmental stressors* range from the relatively common — air pollution, temperature extremes, overcrowding, unsanitary conditions, lack of security, water pollution — to the catastrophic — an earthquake, a flood. Although stressors such as hurricanes and forest fires are certainly dramatic, they are not necessarily the most damaging in the long-term. Chronic exposure to noise or the threat of living in a high-crime neighborhood, for example, could have much greater long-term effects than one-time exposure to a disaster such as a chemical spill.

Some of the most pervasive stressors are called **hassles** — the seemingly minor, irritating annoyances that happen every day, such as losing the car keys, getting stuck behind a disorganized shopper in a supermarket line, forgetting about an important exam, waking up to a miserable snowstorm, being kept waiting for an appointment, or getting stuck in a traffic jam.

In his now-famous book *Future Shock*, Alvin Toffler listed, among the top ten hassles, rising consumer prices, yard work, losing things, and having too many things to do. These seemingly trivial problems may be more damaging to health and wellness than major stressors, partly because they disturb us constantly, piling up until no end is in sight ("at wits end").

Stressors also may be *physiological*, arising from injury, illness, surgery, genetic weaknesses, prolonged exercise, physical disabilities, or inadequate nutrition, as examples.

Psychosocial stressors are those that stem from interpersonal relationships, from living, working, and playing with other people. Some examples are stress from the expectations others impose on us, discriminatory behavior from others, intense social interactions, and social isolation. Possibly the most common is conflict, the stress that results from two opposing and incompatible goals, demands, or needs.

Although researchers had recognized the presence of stress decades earlier and even linked it specifically to disease, not until early in the 1950s was anyone able to categorize specific contributors to stress. During the early 1950s, University of Washington psychiatrist Thomas Holmes noted that the most common denominator for stress was significant change in the life pattern. He began to search for specific links between disease and what he called social "life events," the things in life that

The Holmes-Rahe Scale

Holmes and Rahe listed approximately four dozen social changes that are considered "major" contributors to stress and illness. The top ten are:

1. Death of a spouse
2. Divorce
3. Marital separation
4. Jail term
5. Death of a close family member
6. Personal injury or illness
7. Marriage
8. Fired at work
9. Marital reconciliation
10. Retirement

call for the greatest adjustment. He discovered that the more major life events a person was subjected to within a brief period, the more likely the person was to become ill — in essence, to be depleted from the exhaustion of stress.

Holmes teamed up with his colleague, Richard Rahe, to develop what they called the "social-readjustment rating scale." More commonly known as the **Holmes-Rahe Scale**, it assigns a numerical score to the four dozen or so life changes that most increase the risk for disease. By adding the scores assigned to each life event that happens within a year, the likelihood of someone developing a stress-related illness may be predicted.

Not all the items on the Holmes-Rahe Scale are "bad." Marriage, an outstanding personal achievement, a vacation, and Christmas are positives. Some of the items on the scale can be *either* negative or positive. For example, a "change" in the number of arguments with a mate might mean fewer arguments and less stress or a record number of arguments and teetering on the brink of divorce. The key word is *change*. Each item on the Holmes-Rahe Scale describes a change in social routine — a need to adapt.

A significant source of stress for students is pressure — to get the best grades, to be the type of child that parents had always dreamed of, to keep pace with peers in achievement. That kind of pressure often comes from the people around us: parents, mates, friends. More commonly, however, it comes from within, from the fear of what others may think, from a desire to achieve important goals, or from a host of expectations that we all place on ourselves.

Every period of life presents different challenges. If we meet the challenges successfully, they are eustress. If we fail to meet the challenges, we become distressed. Some of the challenges that can occur during various life stages include:

✳ For children: separation from a parent, death of a parent, divorce of parents, lack of adult supervision, inferior daycare, struggles to become independent, child abuse, socialization, birth of a sibling, anxieties about school, bullies, changing schools, conflicts with teachers, forced competitiveness, difficulty with classmates, fads, dares by classmates, failing to make an athletic team, parental pressure to achieve, lack of parental interest in achievements, discrimination (relating to race, weight, hair color, disability), witnessing violence

✳ For adolescents: physical changes during puberty, heightened sexual awareness, peer pressure, the desire to be independent, the need to establish identity, lack of supportive relationships, changing relationships with parents and siblings, physical or sexual abuse, divorce of parents, loss of a parent, confusion about sexual identity, low self-esteem

✳ For college students: academic pressure, course overload, career decisions, self-doubt, feelings of anonymity, financial struggles, measuring up to expectations (from self and others), loneliness, isolation, intimidation, separation from parents and established social networks, dramatic changes in environment, developing sexual intimacy with a partner

✳ For adults: marriage, parenthood, step-parenting, family planning, responsibility for others (including aging parents), changing roles within the family, career challenge, dual-career marriage, loss of a job, financial struggles, marital stress, mate abuse, divorce, death of a spouse, death of a child, death of a parent, complex interpersonal relationships

✳ For the elderly: retirement, memory loss, physical deterioration, loss of independence, financial struggles, death of a spouse, death of a child, death of established friends, loneliness, boredom, aging, dying, and death

THE GENERAL ADAPTATION SYNDROME

When the body becomes stressed, regardless of the source of the stress, it undergoes the stress response, or **general adaptation syndrome**, the body's attempt to react and adapt to stressors that disrupt its normal balance. It is the same response that primitive people used when facing the various threats in their environment, called **fight or flight**. It is the collection of physiological changes that occurred in rapid-fire succession when a cave-dweller was confronted with a saber-toothed tiger. The body systems sped up, and hormones started surging through the bloodstream. The senses sharpened, and energy levels were high. Everything combined to enable cave-dwellers to conquer their enemies or run for their life. While society has become more civilized, the human body has not. A student giving an oral presentation to a classroom full of sleepy students and a mild-mannered professor have the same physiological response as the cave-dweller who faced the saber-toothed tiger.

The general adaptation syndrome (GAS) occurs in three general stages: alarm, resistance, and exhaustion. These are discussed next and are graphed in Figure 3.1.

Alarm

The stress response begins the second the brain perceives any kind of stress or threat. An alarm sounds inside the body. Immediately the sympathetic branch of the autonomic nervous system — the same complex set of nerves that operate independently of conscious thought to control heart rate, digestion, breathing, and other automatic body functions — takes over. Control centers in the brain act with spilt-second speed and accuracy in a chain reaction.

KEY TERMS

Hassles various minor annoyances that occur daily

Holmes-Rahe Scale assessment used to determine who is at risk for developing a stress-related illness

General adaptation syndrome body's attempt to react to and adapt to stressors

Fight-or-flight collection of physiological changes evoked by stress

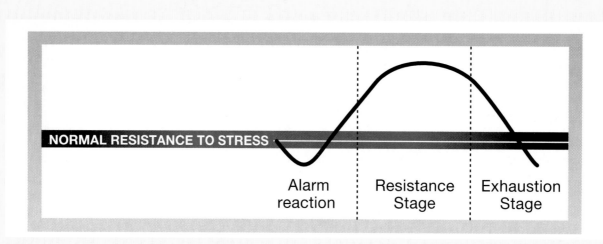

Figure 3.1 Stages of general adaptation syndrome

* The hypothalamus directs the pituitary gland to release **adrenocorticotropic hormone** (ACTH).

* ACTH stimulates the adrenal glands to release **cortisol** and other key hormones.

* Sympathetic nerves stimulate the adrenal glands to release **epinephrine** and **norepinephrine**.

* The brain releases **endorphins** (natural pain-killers) in case of injury.

The custom mixture of hormones surging through the bloodstream triggers a rapid and immediate series of changes throughout the body, also illustrated in Figure 3.2.

* The mucous membranes in the nose and throat shrink to widen the air passages; the air sacs in the lungs dilate so more air can enter the lungs.

* The heart pumps harder and faster to circulate more oxygen throughout the body; blood pressure increases dramatically, and the spleen releases red blood cells to increase the blood's oxygen-carrying capacity.

* Digestion stops so much-needed blood will not be diverted to the stomach; as part of that process, the mouth gets dry, digestive juices from the pancreas diminish, and muscles in the intestines relax.

* Blood vessels in the skin constrict, and goosebumps arise on the skin.

* The liver releases sugar into the bloodstream to provide instant energy.

* Perspiration increases; the palms get sweaty.

* The muscles get tense, prepared for a workout.

* The senses — sight, hearing, smell, and taste — become acute, ready to identify any "danger."

Defense Mechanisms for Coping with Stress

People learn to cope with stress in various ways — some of them healthy, some not. The more common defense mechanisms include:

* Daydreaming about pleasurable situations.

* Repression — the process of purposely or selectively forgetting unpleasant experiences.

* Denial — flat refusal to believe or recognize that a stressful situation is true.

* Rationalization — coming up with socially acceptable justifications for behavior or situations.

* Reaction formation — adopting behaviors and attitudes that are exactly the opposite of how the person really feels.

* Projection — placing the blame for one's weaknesses or problems on someone else.

* Displacement — redirecting socially unacceptable behavior from the true source to a less threatening substitute.

* Regression — reverting or retreating to childish or child-like behaviors.

* Altruism — giving of oneself to others.

* Isolation — detaching oneself from the underlying cause of a stressor.

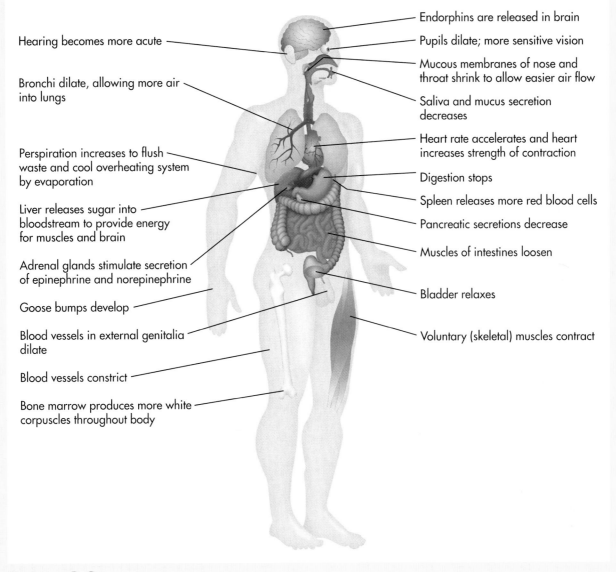

Figure 3.2 The alarm reaction

Hearing becomes more acute

Endorphins are released in brain

Pupils dilate; more sensitive vision

Mucous membranes of nose and throat shrink to allow easier air flow

Bronchi dilate, allowing more air into lungs

Saliva and mucus secretion decreases

Heart rate accelerates and heart increases strength of contraction

Perspiration increases to flush waste and cool overheating system by evaporation

Digestion stops

Spleen releases more red blood cells

Liver releases sugar into bloodstream to provide energy for muscles and brain

Pancreatic secretions decrease

Muscles of intestines loosen

Adrenal glands stimulate secretion of epinephrine and norepinephrine

Goose bumps develop

Bladder relaxes

Blood vessels in external genitalia dilate

Voluntary (skeletal) muscles contract

Blood vessels constrict

Bone marrow produces more white corpuscles throughout body

During the alarm stage a person can have "super-human" strength. The physiological reactions of the alarm stage are what enable a small woman to lift a car weighing several tons off the chest of a toddler.

Resistance

The alarm and resistance stages of the stress response evoke more than 1,400 known physio-chemical reactions. During the second stage of the stress response, resistance, the person actually meets

KEY TERMS

Adrenocorticotropic hormone (ACTH) hormone released by the pituitary gland that stimulates the adrenal glands to release other hormones in the initial stage of stress

Cortisol hormone released by the adrenal glands in the first stage of stress

Epinephrine hormone released by the adrenal glands during the first stage of stress that affects metabolism, the muscles, and circulation

Norepinephrine hormone released by the adrenal glands during the first stage of stress that affects circulation.

Endorphins natural painkillers released by the brain

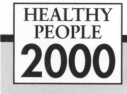

OBJECTIVES FOR STRESS REDUCTION

❋ Reduce the proportion of people age 18 and older who experience adverse health effects from stress.

❋ Decrease the proportion of people aged 18 and older who report experiencing significant levels of stress who do not take steps to reduce or control their stress.

the perceived challenge. The adrenal glands continue to release adrenaline, the thyroid gland pumps out thyroid hormones, the hypothalamus releases endorphins, and the adrenal gland inhibits the release of sex hormones (to prevent the possibility of any diversion). Glucose and cholesterol enter the bloodstream, providing instant energy and endurance. Heart and breathing rates become more rapid to boost the oxygen supply to the body. The blood thickens and the skin "crawls" and sweats.

Once the perceived challenge passes, the parasympathetic branch of the autonomic nervous system signals the alarm reaction to stop. The body tries to adapt — to once again achieve the balance (homeostasis) that existed before the stress occurred. That is a substantial challenge. The body maintains its vital functions (such as heartbeat) within a *very* narrow range considered normal. The dynamic physical reactions to stress push the body to the limit. During resistance, then, the body is on guard, trying to resist the ill effects of the stress and return the body to normal. The body quickly repairs any damage that occurred during the alarm phase.

The resistance stage of the stress response is ideally suited to meeting the challenges of short-term stress. If the stress is short-term, the body usually is able to adapt and return to a state of balance. If the stress becomes chronic, however, the body eventually loses its ability to adapt.

Exhaustion

Although most people experience the alarm and resistance stages of the stress response frequently, only those under chronic stress experience exhaustion, a stage in which the body's resources are

If stress becomes chronic, the body eventually loses its ability adapt.

depleted and its adaptive abilities are lost. Exhaustion occurs when the body is traumatized by one stress after another for a prolonged time.

During the exhaustion stage, many of the events of the alarm stage occur again as the body attempts to adjust to higher levels of stress, but the resulting wear and tear knock out the immune system, injure body systems and organs, and lead to illness and disease. The exhaustion stage is when long-term effects of stress emerge.

The result is literal exhaustion, a depletion of the body's energy stores. The incredible series of physiological reactions involved in the alarm and resistance stages demand vast stores of energy. Probably most significant is that the body's ability to adapt is exhausted, resulting in a life-threatening inability to maintain normal balance. The obvious conclusion is disease and premature death.

RESPONSES TO CHRONIC STRESS

With more than a thousand physical reactions taking place within a few minutes, stress and the general adaptation syndrome obviously impact most body systems. The brain is the first to recognize a stressor. It immediately instructs the rest of the body how to adjust to the stressor. The brain continues to stimulate the stress reaction as long as 72 hours following a stressful incident.

The brain is not a discriminator of stressors. It reacts the same whether the stress is physical (almost being hit by a car) or emotional (finding out while walking into class that you studied the wrong material for the test). The resulting deluge of hormones and brain chemicals takes its toll. Elevated levels of stress hormones destroy vitally important brain cells.

The brain is not the only thing that suffers from chronic stress. The endocrine system works overtime, pumping out excess hormones that increase blood pressure, damage the lining of the heart and blood vessels, inhibit vitamin D activity, deplete calcium, increase the risk of diabetes, and suppress the immune system.

Stress impacts every part of the digestive system. The mouth stops producing saliva. The regular rhythmic contractions of the esophagus are disrupted, so swallowing becomes difficult. The stomach slows down and gets bathed in gastric acid; its lining becomes fragile and engorged with blood. The liver overproduces glucose, and the pancreas becomes chronically inflamed. Production of hydrochloric acid increases and normal peristaltic (wavelike) action is disrupted throughout the intestinal tract.

In the cardiovascular system the heart speeds up, blood pressure rises, serum cholesterol levels increase, and the blood thickens. Over time these effects seriously impair body functioning and can lead to premature death.

Because of the physical responses to stress, certain behavioral signs characteristically accompany stress. Changes in appetite are manifested in overeating or undereating. Sleep disturbances may be demonstrated in either insomnia or excessive sleep. Other common behavioral responses include inability to concentrate, lack of creativity, loss of memory, sexual problems, and impulsive behavior. Many people turn to tobacco, alcohol, and other drugs for relief.

Common emotional signs and symptoms include:

    nervousness
    forgetfulness
    unexplained fearfulness
    severe mood swings
    anxiety
    tearfulness
    emotional instability
    urge to hide
    depression
    difficulty completing tasks
    irritability

Table 3.1 summarizes the physical and emotional signs of stress.

✳ Table 3.1
Signs and Symptoms of Stress

Body System	Symptoms
Cardiovascular	Pounding and racing of the heart High blood pressure Irregular heartbeat Chest pain Cold, sweaty hands
Respiratory	Shortness of breath Rapid breathing Asthma attacks
Musculoskeletal	Twitching or shakiness Neck or back pain Headache (tension, migraine) Stiffness of muscles
Digestive	Dryness of mouth and throat Difficulty swallowing Grinding of teeth Indigestion Nausea or queasiness Vomiting Loss of appetite or excessive appetite Diarrhea or constipation Abdominal pain Cravings for food Frequent urination
Sleep Disorders	Insomnia Fatigue Nightmares
Skin	Acne Dry skin Rashes Excessive perspiration
Emotional/Mental	Nervousness Unexplained fearfulness Anxiety Emotional instability Impulsive behavior Depression Irritability Forgetfulness Severe mood swings Tearfulness Difficulty in completing tasks Changes in eating habits Increased dependence on drugs Inability to concentrate Lack of creativity Loss of memory Low self-esteem

Source: *Wellness: Guidelines for a Healthy Lifestyle*, by Brent Q. Hafen and Werner W. K. Hoeger (Englewood, CO: Morton Publishing, 1994).

THE SCIENCE OF PSYCHONEUROIMMUNOLOGY

A growing body of evidence indicates that virtually every illness known in contemporary times — from arthritis to migraine headaches, from the common cold to cancer — is influenced for good or bad by our emotions. Illnesses do not just happen. Many are caused by bacteria, viruses, fungi, or other pathogens. What factors, however, ascertain whether we will or will not fall ill when these microscopic trouble-makers enter our lives? What determines our immunity?

Emotions, particularly stress, impact our susceptibility to disease. The American Medical Association has estimated that half of all disease is preventable because it is related to behavioral lifestyle factors. The way we react to what comes along in life can determine in great measure how we will react to the disease-causing organisms. One of the reasons strong emotions can lead to illness — even infectious disease — is that they may weaken the immune system over time. The fight-or-flight response to stress is especially damaging to immunity. Emotions such as stress send chemical messages to the brain that alter involuntary physiologic responses, which may affect the way the brain responds to messages from the immune system in the presence of disease.

The scientific investigation of how the brain affects the body's immune system is called **psychoneuroimmunology**, a term coined in 1964 by Dr. Robert Ader, director of the division of behavioral and psychosocial medicine at New York's University of Rochester. The science of psychoneuroimmunology (PNI) focuses on the links between the mind, the brain, and the immune system. As a science, it has received the endorsement of the National Institutes of Health.

Although some controversy still surrounds the science itself and some skepticism about the concepts behind it, proponents can cite solid examples that support PNI theories. One example is the late Norman Cousins, former editor of the *Saturday Review* and member of the UCLA medical faculty, who twice intrigued the medical community and the public alike by overcoming usually fatal conditions — a massive heart attack and a degenerative spinal disease. Cousins followed his physicians' regimen each time but also surrounded himself with positive people, positive emotions, and laughter. According to Cousins, he was healed not only by the miracle of modern medicine but also by the healing emotions of love, hope, faith, confidence, and a tremendous will to live.

The theories behind PNI are not new. Chinese physicians noted more than 4,000 years ago that physical illness often followed episodes of frustration. Some of the world's greatest physicians and philosophers — including Hippocrates, Galen, and Descartes — believed that a fundamental link exists between the body and the mind. Only in the 1980s, however, did immunologists finally begin to seriously consider the possibility of anatomical links between the brain, the nervous system, and the immune system. Based on overwhelming evidence, they found that the brain literally "talks" to the cells of the immune system.

Today, much more evidence exists of a neurological connection to the immune system. For example:

✳ After conducting a long-term analysis of thousands of hospital patients, University of Rochester researcher George L. Engel and his colleagues found that the majority of people hospitalized for a physical illness had a psychological upset shortly before they got sick.

✳ A research team from several London hospitals gave questionnaires to more than 200 middle-aged men who had newly registered as patients at a general-practice clinic. The questionnaires helped the research team identify emotions such as worry, sadness, anxiety, and depression. Based on those questionnaires alone, and not on the men's medical condition or history, the researchers predicted which men were most likely to have a heart attack within a year. They were 81% accurate in their predictions.

✳ The Health Insurance Plan (HIP) of Greater New York did a follow-up study of 2,000 men who had suffered a heart attack. They found that those men who were under a great deal of emotional stress were four times more likely to have a second, fatal heart attack. The telling factor was stress. The researchers determined that the hormones released during stress had crippled or damaged the heart.

Even though PNI is still considered to be in its infancy, a number of medical schools already have

Stress and Disease: A Pandora's Box

As research continues into the link between stress and the immune system, scientists have come up with a veritable shopping list of conditions caused or aggravated by stress:

coronary heart disease	arteriosclerosis
hypertension	angina
coronary thrombosis	stroke
respiratory ailments	ulcers
irritable bowel syndrome	pancreatitis
ulcerative colitis	gastritis
diabetes	migraine headache
myasthenia gravis	kidney disease
epileptic attacks	chronic backache
chronic tuberculosis	allergies
rheumatoid arthritis	eczema
systemic lupus erythematosus	psoriasis
cold sores	shingles
hives	multiple sclerosis
asthma	Raynaud's disease
cancer	

integrated it into their curricula and many federal grants are underwriting PNI research. Almost every important conference on immunology now includes at least one seminar on the relationship between the brain and the immune system. More and more physicians are acknowledging that the way a patient thinks and feels can be a powerful determinant of physical health. Herpes viruses such as Epstein-Barr offer a helpful model for studying the effects of stress on immunity. These viruses are common and, unlike some other viruses, herpes viruses are simply held in check by the immune response and never eliminated completely. Diseases caused by herpes viruses often come and go as the virus advances and retreats. Specific herpes viruses are responsible for recurring oral cold sores and genital lesions, as well as chicken pox and its recurring form, **shingles**. A discussion of herpes virus infections is found in Chapter 6. Having more herpes antibodies, or lower immunity, has been associated with many kinds of stress. For example, studies have indicated that students have more herpes antibodies while undergoing exams than they do after summer vacation.

Research provides strong evidence that microorganisms alone do not cause infectious disease. The condition of the person exposed to the microorganism also matters. Scientists are studying, more exactly, how stress might affect the immune systems of people at different stages of life and, in turn, how these immune changes might affect health and disease.

Where stress seems to have the greatest impact on health is on individuals who already have poor immune function because of age or diseases that impair the immune system, and individuals who already have been chronically stressed for reasons other than health."

The link applies to noncommunicable as well as communicable diseases. Yale oncologist and surgeon Bernie Siegel pointed out in *Love, Medicine, and Miracles* that stresses we *choose* evoke a response totally different from those we would like to avoid but cannot. That is probably why the rate of cancer is higher for African Americans than for Anglo Americans, and why cancer is associated with grief and depression.

HARDINESS

Some people seem incapacitated by the smallest degree of stress, and others seem to endure enormous strains and pressures. Suzanne Ouellette Kobasa, a psychologist at the City University of New York's graduate school, conducted a number of pioneering studies that identified what she called **hardiness**, a set of beliefs about how we interact with the world. Hardiness is what spells the difference between getting sick from stress and being resilient to stress. Kobasa defined the personality traits of hardiness according to the "three Cs": commitment, control, and challenge.

Commitment

Commitment — an attitude of curiosity and improvement — means commitment to self, work, family, and other important values in life. This is

---

KEY TERMS

Psychoneuroimmunology science of how the brain affects the immune system

Shingles Herpes blisters appearing on the trunk of the body caused by herpes zoster virus

Hardiness personality traits characteristic of people who are resistant to stress

---

not a fleeting involvement but, rather, a deep and abiding interest. The important commitment may be to an ideal greater than self. For some it may be a commitment to religion. For others it may be a commitment to a certain philosophy, to political reform, or even to something as simple as a hobby.

Control

Control is the belief that individuals can influence the extent to which life events will hurt them. It is the belief that a person can cushion the hurtful impact of a situation by the way he or she looks at it and reacts to it. Control is the opposite of helplessness. Control is the firm belief that one can influence one's reactions, and the willingness to act on that basis. It is the refusal to be victimized. Control is not the belief that you can control your environment. Instead, it is the knowledge that you can control *how you react to your environment*.

Challenge

Challenge is the capacity to see change as an opportunity for growth and excitement. People who are not hardy look at change with helplessness and alienation. Healthy, hardy people face change with confidence, self-determination, eagerness, and excitement. To them, change becomes an eagerly sought-after challenge, not a threat.

MANAGING STRESS

One's ability to cope with stress depends not only on inherent qualities but also on specific coping strategies — such as eating right, getting plenty of exercise, and managing time effectively. Coping with stress successfully does not just happen. It requires planning and work. Sometimes it involves changing attitudes, ideologies, values, or goals. It may even require making gradual but significant lifestyle changes to eliminate sources of stress. Managing stress entails strategies developed ahead of time, strategies that will improve one's physical and emotional condition and give one an edge in meeting stressful situations when they do arise.

A Balanced Diet

Overeating, undereating, or eating the wrong foods can upset the body's balance, making all body systems more likely to suffer the ill effects of stress. A poor diet not only makes a person more susceptible to disease in general but also makes a person more vulnerable to the negative effects of stress. Certain foods can even exaggerate stress by making a person more uptight.

The battering the body takes from stress can change its nutritional requirements. Chronic stress may:

— deplete the body's stores of important vitamins and minerals.

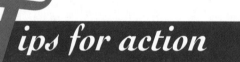

Tips for action

Utilizing Stress Strategies

To use stress reduction strategies wisely:

❋ Don't try to incorporate too many strategies at once. Changing old habits and developing new ways of dealing with things takes time. If you take on too much at once, you'll end up feeling frustrated and stressed. Too much change — even positive change — becomes stressful itself.

❋ Before you decide on the strategies you want to use, consider your strengths and skills. Think about what you'd *enjoy*. Assess what kind of social support you'll have.

❋ Be flexible, be willing to change your coping strategies, and never stop assessing.

❋ Don't expect a single coping strategy to provide you with enough coping power. You'll need several strategies.

❋ Recognize that even negative stress can have a positive outcome if you meet it head-on and use it as an opportunity for learning and growth.

Tips for action

Move to Beat Stress

To get the most benefits from exercise:

❋ Choose a form of exercise you *like*.

❋ Find an activity suited to your personality. Do you want something that will let you daydream? Something that involves a partner?

❋ Consider how much equipment the exercise requires. Walking requires nothing more than a good pair of shoes. Golf requires a set of clubs, a handful of tees, and plenty of fresh balls.

❋ Consider *where* you can exercise. You can walk or bicycle almost anywhere, unlike golfing, skiing, racquetball, and tennis.

❋ Don't feel limited to what you can do already. If you think fencing sounds fun, take a class!

❋ Consider team sports. They provide social support, a proven stress buster!

— increase the need for protein.

— increase the amount of fats in the blood-stream.

— boost calorie needs.

Stressed people should eat foods that are low in fat, high in fiber, and rich in vitamins and minerals. Most of the calories should come from complex carbohydrates, such as whole-grain breads, rice, pasta, fruits, and vegetables. People under chronic stress should boost their protein intake with the leanest sources of protein possible: fish, poultry, lean cuts of beef, and low-fat or skim dairy products. Nutrition is discussed in depth in Chapter 9.

Experts advise against the use of nutritional supplements touted as stress remedies or "anti-stress" formulas. The vitamins in these products are generally seventy or eighty times the U.S. Daily Values, which can produce side effects ranging from mild to severe. Research has even linked deaths to amino acid supplements advertised as remedies for anxiety, stress, depression, and premenstrual syndrome.

Regular Exercise

Exercise, discussed further in Chapter 11, is a natural antidote to stress. Regular aerobic exercise:

— eases muscle tension caused by stress.

— reduces the amount of adrenaline circulating in the bloodstream.

— decreases the intensity of stress.

— lessens the effects of stress.

— reduces the amount of time necessary to recover from stress.

— minimizes the physiological reactions of the stress response.

— reduces the risk of getting sick, even for those under severe or chronic stress.

Sleep

In coping with stress, sleep is essential. Sleep offers the relaxation so important to minimizing the effects of the stress response.

When the body is deprived of sleep, physical, mental, and emotional processes gradually deteriorate. The person who lacks sleep has difficulty concentrating, making decisions, recalling things to memory, and utilizing full intellectual abilities. Lack of sleep itself is a significant source of stress. Severe sleep deprivation can even cause psychosis.

Most people need 6 to 8 hours of sleep a night to function well and feel refreshed. This requirement varies from one person to another. Some need more, and some need less.

Tips for action

A Good Night's Sleep

To find out how much sleep you *really* need, go to sleep at the same time every night, then sleep until you awaken. (It will take a couple of weeks to determine what you need.)

※ Establish a sleep pattern: go to bed at the same time every night, and wake up at the same time every morning — even on the weekends when you can.

※ If you take a nap, limit it to 20 minutes; longer will interfere with sleep at night.

※ Don't exercise, use caffeine, or smoke late in the day. These stimulate the body.

※ Have a light snack before bedtime. You'll sleep more soundly if you're not hungry.

※ Use your bed and bedroom only for sleeping. Don't watch television, study, eat, read, or do work in bed.

※ Deal with worries and pressures before you go to bed. Take notes on possible solutions then forget about the problem until morning.

※ Take a warm bath an hour before bedtime. It will slow down your metabolism.

※ If you don't fall asleep within 20 minutes get up, leave the bedroom, and do something quiet and relaxing until you feel sleepy. Don't toss and turn in bed, getting stressed because you can't fall asleep.

Insomnia involves problems falling asleep or staying asleep. Almost everyone has insomnia at some time in life. Insomnia can be caused by stress. Other common causes are medical problems (respiratory conditions) or various lifestyle factors (overloading on caffeine within a few hours of bedtime). Short-term, temporary insomnia usually is not a serious problem. Long-term insomnia, on the other hand, can cause serious medical problems and can contribute to chronic stress.

Managing Your Time

One of the most common stressors is simply too much to do in too little time. We are living in the fastest-paced society of this century, and the mere speed at which we move can be a significant stressor. In a Gallup Poll conducted at the beginning of this decade, eight of ten Americans felt that time moves too fast — and more than half felt intense pressure to get things done. Learning to manage available time can alleviate stress and reduce anxiety.

A key to effective time management is determining how time is spent. The following steps might be taken to begin the process.

1. Keep a diary for 2 weeks. You might be stunned to find out how much time you are spending on the phone or in front of the television. You cannot outline realistic goals until you know what you are really doing.

2. Try to figure out your peak time. Are you a "morning person," or do you get your second wind when most people are quitting for the day? Plan your most demanding tasks — studying, working — for the time you are at your

Time Killers

In every schedule you'll find things that eat up your time. Necessary activities such as eating and sleeping can become time-killers if you overdo them. Other time-killers are *not* necessary. Try to eliminate:

indecision	watching television
procrastination	lengthy talking on the phone
worry	interruptions
confusion	too much socializing
perfectionism	

Time Management

To get the most out of time-management efforts:

✳ Tackle one thing at a time. If you have a long list of things to do, move through it calmly, one item at a time. Don't move on to the next item until you've finished the first one.

✳ Set realistic goals; break long-term goals into short-term ones.

✳ Delegate the tasks that other people can do for you instead of trying to do everything yourself.

✳ If you're faced with a difficult task, mentally "rehearse" it first. You'll approach it with less stress and apprehension if you have some concrete solution in mind.

✳ Take advantage of little chunks of time that crop up in your schedule; have a handful of short tasks you can plug in.

✳ Stay flexible, and plan for disruptions. Never schedule anything so tightly that an unexpected wrench will throw everything off.

✳ Reward yourself often.

✳ Protect yourself against boredom; set a satisfying, realistic goal, then do something toward it every day.

peak. If you have to take a particularly challenging class and are generally sluggish in the morning, try to schedule it for the afternoon, or find out if it is offered at night.

3. Learn to prioritize, and be mature in distinguishing priorities. Not every demand is a top

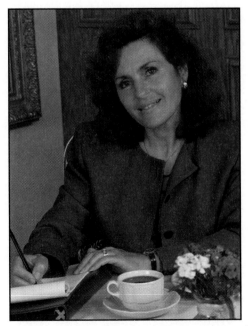

A daily planner is a helpful time-management tool.

priority. You usually can split tasks into those that are essential, important, and unimportant or trivial. Spend your time and attention on the things that are essential and important. If you have time left over, you can go for the trivial things.

4. Judge *realistically* how long a task will take. Most people underestimate by about 50%, so get into the habit of adding 50% to the time you think it will take. Once you learn how to estimate realistically the time different tasks take, you can stop overcrowding your day with too much to handle.

5. Use a daily planner to help organize commitments. Various kinds are available on the market. Look for one that includes everything needed under one cover — a place to write addresses, phone numbers, references, appointments, tasks, and goals.

6. Before you go to bed at night, assess what went on that day. Did you meet all your goals? Were you able to accomplish all your top priorities? If

KEY TERMS

Insomnia inability to fall asleep or stay asleep

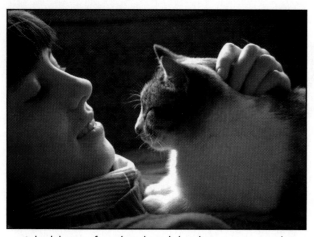
Schedule time for a break and do what you want to do.

not, pinpoint what went wrong, then develop a strategy for change.

7. Write down your schedule for the next day. Before anything else, schedule time for breaks. Include several periods to do what you *want* to do — soak in a hot tub, read a good book, watch a football game on television, or talk to a friend. Knowing you can look forward to a few breaks can help you face the more stressful periods of the day.

8. Think through what *has* to be done — classes you have to attend, the hours you need to spend at your job, a commitment at the community crisis center. Determine which are most important, and make the time for those.

You can do only so much in a single day or week. If you start to get overwhelmed, back off. Do not feel guilty if you have to say "no." Going to the movie with friends might be fun, but not if you have to stay up half the night to study for an exam in exchange for a good time.

Reframing Thought

Reframing entails changing the way of looking at things, learning to be an optimist instead of a pessimist. The way a person thinks often determines what really happens. Under stress, it can help change the way stress impacts the body.

In Suzanne Kobasa's study of AT&T executives, during the period of reorganization of the telecommunications company, the employees who did not get sick were the ones who had a positive perspective on the situation. They saw it as a unique opportunity for meeting a challenge instead of a

Tips for action

Stress-Fighters

Along with long-term strategies, try these quick fixes:

✳ Confide in someone.

✳ Get a massage.

✳ Listen to some soft, relaxing, mellow music.

✳ Take a 20-minute nap.

✳ Lie down and put a warm compress on your eyes.

✳ Stand up and stretch.

✳ Luxuriate in a nice, long soak in a tub filled with hot water.

✳ Have a good cry — followed by a good laugh!

✳ Read a few pages in a good book.

✳ Listen to a tape of birds chirping, the wind whistling, or the waves lapping on the shore.

✳ Close your eyes and gently massage your temples.

Make Your Thoughts Your Allies

To get the most from your thoughts:

❋ Get rid of unimportant details. Keep your mind uncluttered so you can concentrate on what's really important.

❋ While you're at it, let go of the past. Everyone makes mistakes; if you're going to spend time remembering, concentrate on your victories and pleasures, not your defeats and miseries.

❋ Choose your worries. Stop worrying about things you can't change. Concentrate instead on worrying about the things that matter.

❋ Galvanize your worries into action. Figure out how to solve the problem, then tackle the steps one at a time.

❋ Learn to laugh. A good laugh is great for your mental outlook, and it gives your whole body a workout.

❋ Stop "beating up" yourself. Think of yourself as a winner, a person who can cope with stress.

❋ Stop worrying about what everyone else thinks of you or wants out of you. The most important person you need to please is yourself. Be your own best friend.

---

life-altering change that would destroy them and their careers.

To reframe one's own thoughts, the following suggestions may be helpful:

1. Listen carefully to the words you use to describe yourself and your situation. Are they positive or negative? Listen for a few weeks. If you need to, use different phrases and descriptions.

2. Role play, either by yourself or with a friend. Start by relating a stressful situation you have experienced lately. Tell how you reacted. Then come up with different ways in which you could have reacted to the situation. If you are role playing with a friend, ask for feedback or suggestions. Next, imagine some plausible stressful situations and outline how you would handle them. Concentrate on positive responses.

3. For one week look for the good in every person and every situation you encounter. You always can find something. This kind of exercise is like conditioning your attitudes. Before long it can become a habit.

4. Avoid words that signal defeat: *always, never, should have, ought to.* Replace them with more benign choices. Instead of saying, "I *always* fail

quizzes in classes," change your statement to, "I'm *sometimes* not prepared when the teacher springs a quiz on us."

Relaxation Techniques

One of the most *immediate* ways of breaking the stress response is to use a relaxation technique to instigate what Harvard Medical School researcher Herbert Benson calls the **relaxation response**. This promotes an inborn bodily reaction that counteracts the harmful effects of stress.

Invoking the relaxation response not only alleviates stress, but it also bestows a more positive mental outlook, eases anxiety, and instills a sense of control — essential to overcoming the negative aspects of stress. Regular relaxation exercises can:

— reduce stress.

— increase resistance to stress-induced illness.

— minimize the symptoms of illness (such as headache).

KEY TERMS

Reframing changing the way a person looks at things
Relaxation response an inborn bodily reaction that counteracts the harmful effects of stress

— lower blood pressure.

— alleviate pain.

Of the number of relaxation exercises, some are based on deep relaxation. Others, such as deep breathing or a quick massage, reduce stress and are good ways to lead into more extensive relaxation exercises. As with physical exercise, learning about various relaxation exercises takes some time. Decisions should be based on one's likes and dislikes, personality, and situation. Some techniques can be learned independently. Others require some training.

Meditation

Meditation is an exercise that enables a person to gain control over his or her thoughts. During meditation the meditator focuses on some thought or object and banishes all other thoughts. As a consequence, heartbeat and breathing slow, blood pressure drops (often for as long as 12 hours after the meditation), and metabolism slows, decreasing the body's need for oxygen and other nutrients.

As the body relaxes, blood flow to the arms and legs increases, which helps ease muscle tension. Laboratory studies have shown that people who meditate have fewer blood enzymes associated with stress and anxiety. More than 700 studies have proven that meditation induces the relaxation response and alleviates the harmful effects of stress.

The most essential element of meditation is something on which to focus: a word or phrase silently repeated (a **mantra**) or an unchanging object on which to focus. To be effective, meditation has to be done in a comfortable position in a quiet place, free of distractions. No specific posture is required for meditation.

For the best effects from meditation, the person should avoid any stimulants — cigarettes, coffee, tea, cola drinks — for the hour or two before meditating. The best times to meditate are early in the morning (before breakfast) and before dinner. Eating a meal just before meditating diverts blood to the stomach and inhibits the relaxation response.

Progressive Relaxation

Progressive relaxation was pioneered by Edmund Jacobson, a physician who wanted to help patients who had tense muscles associated with stress. His three-step technique was simple:

1. Contract (tense) a small muscle group.
2. Relax the muscle group.
3. Concentrate on determining how different the two sensations felt.

Tips for action

Steps in Meditation

Find a quiet room as free from distraction as possible; turn off the phone. Regulate lights and temperature so you're comfortable.

1. Loosen your clothing if it is tight, especially at the wrists, neck, and waist. Sit in the most comfortable position for you. Place your feet flat on the floor. Rest your hands in your lap.

2. Inhale slowly and deeply, through your nose, hold your breath briefly, then exhale slowly. As you begin to breathe deeply, let the tension flow out of your body.

3. If you are concentrating on an object, partially close your eyes so the object appears blurred. If you are focusing on a mantra, begin repeating it silently and rhythmically as you breathe in and out.

4. Gradually focus all your attention on that one thing.

5. Continue mediating for approximately 20 minutes.

6. When you are finished, give yourself time to readjust. Open your eyes, focus on various objects around the room, and gradually return to your normal pace of breathing. While still seated, stretch your arms, legs, back, shoulders, and neck. Finally, stand up slowly.

Progressive Relaxation

Regardless of the routine used for progressive relaxation, follow these guidelines:

❋ Lie on your back in the most comfortable position possible.

❋ Take off your shoes, and loosen any restrictive clothing.

❋ Close your eyes, rotate your ankles outward, and place your arms at your sides.

❋ Make sure you move all major muscle groups in the body. Don't forget your face, including your forehead, eyes, nose, mouth, cheeks, and tongue.

❋ As you move each muscle group, contract the muscles as tightly as you can, and hold the contraction for 30 seconds.

❋ If you experience pain or cramping during a contraction release the contraction immediately.

❋ Concentrate on the dramatic difference in feeling between a tensed muscle and a relaxed one.

Progressive relaxation is simple. It involves contracting, then relaxing the muscles of the body. The progression can be from head to toes or from feet to head. It does not matter as long as all major muscle groups in the body are involved and eventually relax.

When doing progressive relaxation, the person should first tense the muscles as hard as possible, then relax them. With a little practice, this becomes effortless and the muscles can be relaxed without having to contract them first.

Unlike meditation, in which the person should *not* think about what is happening to the body, progressive relaxation requires the person to *concentrate on what is happening to the muscles.* Acute awareness of the relaxed condition of the body yields the best results.

Biofeedback training

Essentially, **biofeedback training** is a method of measuring physiological functions a person normally is not aware of — such as skin temperature, heart rate, and blood pressure — that are controlled by the involuntary (autonomic) nervous system. This information then is converted into something meaningful so the responses can be controlled.

Unlike some other forms of relaxation exercises, people cannot learn biofeedback training on their own. It requires monitoring by extremely sensitive equipment, then teaching people to regulate their own physiological responses. Biofeedback training is extremely valuable as a stress management technique because it allows the person to control the body's response to stress. Most people can learn effective biofeedback techniques in a few sessions from a trained therapist using monitoring devices.

Yoga

An ancient exercise known to induce calm and invigorate the mind, **yoga** reduces the biological effects of stress. In addition, it is an excellent exercise for improving strength, flexibility, and endurance.

Unlike other relaxation exercises, people cannot design their own technique or routine in yoga. It is composed of precise postures done in a specific sequence combined with an exact breathing rhythm designed to reduce tension and inflexibility.

KEY TERMS

Meditation relaxation exercise that enables a person to control all thought

Mantra word or phrase repeated silently during meditation

Progressive relaxation exercise to relieve stress; involves tensing and relaxing muscle groups

Biofeedback training method of measuring physiological functions that usually are not noticeable

Yoga exercise performed to calm and stimulate the mind

The yoga postures are difficult and complex and require training and practice. Few people can assume the postures at first, and many are not able to complete the sequence properly for as long as 3 months. A number of good yoga instruction books are available in the marketplace, and yoga classes might be taught at the college, university, or recreation center.

AVOIDING BURNOUT

Stress, especially chronic stress, can lead quickly to **burnout**, a state of physical and mental exhaustion in which the person has few remaining resources. The physical signs and symptoms of burnout can include:

— headache
— indigestion
— fatigue
— muscle soreness

Emotional symptoms can include depression, apathy, or loss of enjoyment in life.

To prevent burnout:

1. Surround yourself with a strong social support network. Have at least one friend in whom you can confide.

2. Distract yourself from your routine by developing a new interest, trying a new hobby, or volunteering for something new. Two hours a week telling animated stories to a group of captivated preschoolers at the local library might be just what you need to get a fresh perspective.

3. Take the time to have fun. With all the demands of everyday life, you can get bogged down in things that are not always enjoyable. Go fly a kite, blow bubbles, or have a picnic in the middle of a downtown park. Aim for fun, silly things you can laugh over at least once a day.

KEY TERMS

Burnout physical and mental exhaustion caused by chronic stress

Summary

1 Stressors can be physical, emotional, social, intellectual, or spiritual.

2 Stress can range from mild to severe and can be positive and desirable (eustress) or negative and undesirable (distress).

3 Seemingly minor stresses, or hassles, can have negative effects in the long-term if they are unremitting over time.

4 Social changes that cause stress have been rated, in the Holmes-Rahe Scale, according to their potential for causing illness.

5 Stresses are different throughout the lifespan.

6 The three stages of the general adaptation syndrome are: alarm, resistance, and exhaustion.

7 The science of psychoneuroimmunology studies the link between activity in the brain and the immune system.

8 Hardiness has three components: commitment, control, and challenge.

9 Stress management components include a balanced diet, regular exercise, sufficient sleep, and wise use of time.

10 Techniques for stress reduction include reframing thoughts and relaxation techniques such as meditation, progressive relaxation, biofeedback training, and yoga.

11 Burnout may be manifested by headache, indigestion, fatigue, and muscle soreness.

Select Bibliography

Kiev, Arie. "Managing Stress to Achieve Success." *Executive Health*, 24:1 (October 1987), pp. 1-4.

Knapp, Peter. In "Stress Success and Samoa" by John Tierney. *Hippocrates*, May/June 1987, p. 84.

Lewen, Marc K., and Harold L. Kennedy. "The Role of Stress in Heart Disease." *Hospital Medicine*, August 1986, pp. 125-138.

Maranto, Gina. "Emotions: How They Affect Your Body." *Discover*, November 1984, p. 35.

O'Regan, Brendan, Caryle Hirshberg, Nola Lewis, Barbara McNeill, and Winston Franklin. *The Heart of Healing*. Atlanta: Turner Publishing, 1993.

Pearsall, Paul. *Super Immunity*. New York: McGraw-Hill, 1987.

Rosch, Paul. "Good Stress: Why You Need It to Stay Young." *Prevention*, April 1986, p. 29.

Sagan, Leonard A. *The Health of Nations*. New York: Basic Books, 1987.

Selye, Hans. *Stress Without Distress*. New York: Lippincott, 1974.

Siegel, Bernie S. *Love, Medicine, and Miracles*. New York: Harper and Row, 1986.

Silver, Nan. "Long Term Stress: Does Your Body Fight Back?" *American Health*, May 1986, p. 20.

Toffler, Alvin. *Future Shock*. New York: Random House, 1970.

Weider, Betty. "The Stress-Free Personality." *Shape*, July 1990, p. 18.

Wickramasekera, Ian. "Risk Factors Leading to Chronic Stress-Related Symptoms." *Advances*, 4:1 (1987), p. 21.

"Workplace Warning: Stress May Speed Brain Aging." *New Sense Bulletin*, 16:11, August 1991, p. 1.

Scoring Your Stress:
A Test to Pinpoint What's Eating You

NAME _____ DATE _____

COURSE _____ SECTION _____

How stressed are you?

The answer depends in part on what's going on in your life. But it also depends on some other factors — like what your *attitudes* are about those events and how much control you feel over what happens.

The first step in managing stress, of course, is to *identify* it — and the test below will help you do just that. It's simple: read each question, then circle the number that most closely describes your situation or attitude. If you're completely neutral, circle **5**; if a question doesn't apply to you at all, skip it.

Ready?

Sharpen your pencil, and go to work:

1 How often do you suffer stress-related physical symptoms, such as headaches, jaw pain, neck pain, back pain, indigestion, abdominal pain, diarrhea, loss of appetite, excessive perspiration, fatigue, or a pounding in your chest?

Rarely or never   Every day

1   2   3   4   5   6   7   8   9   10

2 Do you wash your hands before you eat?

Always   Rarely or never

1   2   3   4   5   6   7   8   9   10

3 Do you take measures to keep your food safe, such as cooking it adequately, storing it properly, and avoiding obvious contaminants?

Almost always   Rarely or never

1   2   3   4   5   6   7   8   9   10

4 How often do you eat fresh fruits, fresh vegetables, whole grains, and foods high in fiber?

Every day   Rarely or never

1   2   3   4   5   6   7   8   9   10

5 How often do you eat high fat or high-sugar foods — including candy, pastry, soft drinks, and food from fast-food restaurants?

Occasionally   Every day

1   2   3   4   5   6   7   8   9   10

6 How often do you exercise?

Every day   Rarely or never

1   2   3   4   5   6   7   8   9   10

7 How many hours of sleep do you get each day?

Eight or more   Less than four

1   2   3   4   5   6   7   8   9   10

(continued)

8 How many cups of coffee or caffeinated soft drinks do you drink each day?

None

Five or more

| 1 | 2 | 3 | 4 | 5 | 6 | 7 | 8 | 9 | 10 |

9 How often do you use alcohol, tobacco, over-the-counter drugs, or prescription drugs to relieve stress?

Never

Every day

| 1 | 2 | 3 | 4 | 5 | 6 | 7 | 8 | 9 | 10 |

10 If you have a relationship with a significant other, how would you describe that relationship?

Mutually satisfying in many ways

Marked by jealousy or insecurity

| 1 | 2 | 3 | 4 | 5 | 6 | 7 | 8 | 9 | 10 |

11 How do you feel when you have to say "no" to a request for your time, energy, talents, or money?

Confident and at ease

Anxious and guilt-ridden

| 1 | 2 | 3 | 4 | 5 | 6 | 7 | 8 | 9 | 10 |

12 How would you characterize your support system?

Broad-based, many sources

Limited or no sources

| 1 | 2 | 3 | 4 | 5 | 6 | 7 | 8 | 9 | 10 |

13 What kinds of friendships do you have?

At least several close friends/confidants

No close friends

| 1 | 2 | 3 | 4 | 5 | 6 | 7 | 8 | 9 | 10 |

14 What do you do if you have a problem you can't solve on your own?

Seek help immediately

Suffer on my own

| 1 | 2 | 3 | 4 | 5 | 6 | 7 | 8 | 9 | 10 |

15 How many major changes (such as entering or ending an intimate relationship, the death of a family member, a change in your financial status, moving, starting a new job, a change in sleeping habits, a change in living conditions, or a change in the number of arguments you have with roommates) have occurred in your life during the last year.

None

Many

| 1 | 2 | 3 | 4 | 5 | 6 | 7 | 8 | 9 | 10 |

16 How do you react when confronted with a problem or stressful situation?

Put it aside to gain perspective, then focus on solutions

Feel overwhelmed or panic-stricken

| 1 | 2 | 3 | 4 | 5 | 6 | 7 | 8 | 9 | 10 |

17 How often do you "retreat" temporarily when you start to feel overwhelmed by stress?

Most of the time

Never

| 1 | 2 | 3 | 4 | 5 | 6 | 7 | 8 | 9 | 10 |

18 How do you normally feel at the end of the day?

I got the important things done

I didn't accomplish anything

| 1 | 2 | 3 | 4 | 5 | 6 | 7 | 8 | 9 | 10 |

19 How many "hassles" do you have in a typical day?

A few

A lot

| 1 | 2 | 3 | 4 | 5 | 6 | 7 | 8 | 9 | 10 |

(continued)

20 How much noise are you exposed to every day?

Not very much   Most of the day is noisy

 1   2   3   4   5   6   7   8   9   10

21 How comfortable is your environment? (Consider temperature extremes, humidity, crowding, and environmental pollutants.)

Very comfortable   Very uncomfortable

 1   2   3   4   5   6   7   8   9   10

22 Overall, how satisfying is your life?

Very satisfying   Very disappointing

 1   2   3   4   5   6   7   8   9   10

Scoring

Time to take a look at your stress level. This exercise will tell you *two* things: first, it will indicate your general stress level. Then it will help pinpoint the specific things that are causing you stress.

First, total up your score by adding every number you circled. Now divide it by the number of questions you answered. This is one test on which you don't want a high score: The closer your average creeps toward 10, the higher your stress level is likely to be. (By the way, it's important to "average" your stress score this way; a high level of stress in a few areas won't cause your *general* stress level to skyrocket.

Next, go back and isolate what's causing you problems. Look back through your responses. Find those in which you circled a number higher than 5. Simple — you've found your problem areas.

Finally, determine some stress-busting strategies. Check out your problematic question number, then find the corresponding number among the tips below. The rest is up to you!

Stress-Savvy Tips

1 Obviously, stress-related physical symptoms are just that: related to stress. The best way to get rid of them is to get rid of the stress that causes them. In the meantime, there are a few things you *can* do to manage your most troublesome symptoms. For headaches: keep a "headache diary"; it will help you identify what triggers your headaches, a first step in prevention. Until you can do that, try deep breathing, relaxation, stretching muscles to relieve tension in your neck and jaw, or a warm bath. For back pain: try deep breathing combined with gentle stretching exercises, soaking in a warm bath, or meditation. For irritable bowel syndrome: stay away from high-fat foods, avoid caffeine (including chocolate), add fiber to your diet (eat plenty of whole grains), and try relaxation exercises. For indigestion: eat smaller meals more often during the day; stick to foods that are mild and easy to digest. Watching what you eat can also ease fatigue — eat foods rich in vitamins, potassium, calcium, iron, and zinc.

2 Washing your hands before you eat dramatically reduces your chance of picking up an infection — an obvious stressor. Other simple things you can do: Keep your hands out of your mouth, don't share eating utensils or drinking glasses, avoid contact with people you know are ill, limit sexual contact and use safe sexual practices, and make sure your immunizations are up to date.

3 You can avoid the physical stress of food-borne illness by scrubbing fruits and vegetables thoroughly; preparing raw meat on surfaces that can be easily cleaned; preparing raw meats separate from other foods; avoiding raw or rare meats or fish; cooking hamburger until it's no longer pink; boiling canned foods before you eat them; refrigerating leftovers immediately; avoiding foods that contain raw eggs; avoiding foods that are obviously spoiled; and avoiding wild nuts, berries, mushrooms, and plants unless you are certain they are edible.

4 Stress robs your body of certain nutrients — if you're under stress from *any* source you need an extra shot of certain vitamins and minerals. Especially important are the B vitamins (found in nuts, seeds, beans, peas, meat, and whole grains), vitamin C (found in citrus fruits, green peppers, dark-green vegetables, strawberries, and tomatoes), calcium (found in milk and dairy products, citrus fruits, dark-green leafy vegetables, and dried beans), and protein (found in meat, fish, poultry, dairy products, and eggs). Don't forget that you can get a "complete" protein by combining certain plant foods — rice with legumes, wheat with soybeans, or legumes with corn, rice, wheat, or oats, for example.

(continued)

5 Stress robs your body of some vital nutrients, and sugars and fats speed up the process! Sugars, in fact, tend to strip out certain B vitamins and actually make you more *susceptible* to stress. Concentrate on eating a balanced diet of foods low in fats and sugars; check labels, and steer clear of foods that list sugar in any form as the first or second ingredient. Avoid skipping meals; eat a hearty breakfast and light supper; drink plenty of water; and check with your physician about nutritional supplements if you're under a lot of stress.

6 Research proves that regular exercise diminishes the effects of stress — even stress you can't avoid. The best kind of stress-busting exercise is continuous, rhythmic, aerobic exercise — walking, running, bicycling, swimming, or cross-country skiing are good choices. To avoid injury, make sure you allow for warm-up and cool-down time. And if your joints are a little creaky from inactivity, start slowly and build up gradually. Wear light-colored clothing in the summer, and several light layers of dark-colored clothing in the winter. Drink plenty of fluid before and after you exercise. You should feel energized, not tired, when you finish exercising; you're pushing too hard if you feel a heaviness in your arms or legs, soreness in your muscles or joints, or extreme fatigue.

7 Sleep relieves stress. How? While you're asleep, you breathe more deeply, your heart slows down, your blood pressure drops, and your muscles relax. To get better sleep, review the suggestions earlier in this section; in a nutshell, try to relax for an hour or so before you go to bed, do your best to stick to a regular sleep schedule, avoid eating a big meal right before you go to sleep, and do what you can to make your sleep environment comfortable.

8 Caffeine actually *increases* your sensitivity to stress by stimulating the central nervous system, charging up the autonomic nervous system, and lowering your ability to tolerate stress. Avoid caffeine or use it only in moderation. Remember, too, that caffeine is found in more than just coffee and cola drinks — cut back on chocolate, cocoa, and over-the-counter medications that contain caffeine, too. Try drinking decaffeinated coffee, or switching to a soothing herbal tea.

9 Alcohol might relax you at first — but research shows that, over the long term, alcohol actually *increases* stress by causing your body to churn out stress-related hormones. Keep a diary of your alcohol intake for a few weeks; if you're drinking too much (more than an occasional drink, or more than 12 ounces of beer or 4 ounces of wine at a time), take measures to stop. Find some other ways to relieve stress, and try substituting another kind of drink for alcohol — exotic fruit juices or sparkling mineral water can be fun.

And don't forget tobacco: we know that smoking causes a long list of health problems. What you may not know is that smoking *combined with stress* escalates the situation. Take measures to stop; ask your doctor or the college health center about local programs that can help you quit.

10. The least stressful relationship is one in which your companion is also your *friend* — someone with whom you share your feelings, triumphs, disappointments, goals, and dreams. If appropriate, healthy sexual expression should be part of that relationship; aside from being a way to communicate within a committed relationship, the physiological processes involved in sex work to relieve stress and tension. Finally, remember that no matter how well matched you are, no two people can fill *every* need for each other; maintain separate friends and interests to avoid becoming too dependent on each other.

11. The ability to assert yourself means you usually meet your own needs without destroying interpersonal relationships. Assertive behavior allows you to protect your own rights — essential to avoiding stress. If you're not very assertive now, start by respecting yourself. You're responsible for yourself, and others need to live with your decisions. If you need to say "no," just say it; don't feel obligated to offer excuses. And remember the nonverbals that go along with it: speak in a firm, steady voice without hesitation, stand straight, and look at the other person directly in the eye.

12 The larger your network of support the better you will be able to manage stress. Ideally, your network of support should be broad, stemming from your family, church, neighborhood, school, social and political organizations, and friends. Try organizing or joining a study group (students in a class or within a major area of study), service group, sports team, hobby group, campaign team, social group, or simply a group of friends who share a favorite activity — bicycling, kite-flying, or watercolors, for example. Remember — the most valuable type of social support from groups like these often happens from the informal contacts, such as riding to a meeting with someone or getting together for dinner after the meeting.

13 Research shows that one of the best ways to prevent stress-related illness is to have good friends — people you can really talk to, people with whom you can share your joys, concerns, apprehensions, and love. If you need to expand your circle of friends, start by expanding your contacts: in other words, go where the people are. Draw people into conversation, invite people to informal get-togethers, show people you care, and get involved with others.

14 An important part of social support — and stress reduction — is your willingness to seek help when you need it *and* the assurance that there are people who can help you. Close friends can act as confidants, but you should also know that there are others in your support network to whom you can turn — a clergyman, school counselor, or therapist.

(continued)

15 Research has shown that your chance of developing a stress-induced illness increases with the number of "life crises" you have during any given time. (Check the list of specific crises earlier in this section for an idea of what we're talking about.) Whenever you can, avoid too many changes at once: If you've just ended an important relationship, for example, don't move to a new apartment and start a part-time job, too. For the best coping strategy, try to anticipate likely changes — then slow down your pace, be gentle on yourself, avoid as many new commitments as you can, and stay flexible. Still another strategy is called *stress-inoculation*: in essence, you imagine —vividly — the worst thing that could happen, then map out how you'd handle it. Then, no matter what happens, you know you can do *something* to cope.

16 Your ability to *adapt* to situations and problems directly affects your ability to manage stress. Boost your odds by trying the following: Put the problem aside long enough to get perspective — what long-range effects will it have? Who does it involve? Then focus in on what you can do to solve the problem, and try to come up with several different alternatives. (Having several different plans for confronting the situation gives you flexibility and removes the anxious possibility of your *only* plan failing.) Above all, relax and keep a sense of humor; and, when you've successfully met the challenge, reward yourself for succeeding!

17 There's nothing wrong with retreat — it's a coping skill that can help you buffer the effects of stress. Don't run away from problems or avoid responsibility — that's not what we're talking about. But when you're feeling overwhelmed, buy yourself some breathing space by going for a long walk, taking in a new movie, putting together a challenging puzzle, going to lunch with a friend, reading a favorite book, or taking a nap. The key is to get a mini-escape or time-out: something that will divert your thoughts and recharge your batteries. You'll go back to the problem renewed and strong enough to handle the challenge!

18 If you want to manage stress, learn to manage your time. There are some excellent pointers earlier in this section. One of the most important tactics is prioritizing: figure out which tasks are most important, then *do those things first*. It helps to make a list of everything you need to do — then assign each a "priority" (for example, **1** for things you *must* get done today if you want to avoid problems, **2** for things that *must* be done but that could wait, and **3** for things you'd like to do but that are not essential). Start out with the things that are the highest priority; get them done first. Then move to the second category;. If you have time left over, start on the last category — but, if not, no big deal. For maximum effectiveness, schedule your time, delegate things that someone else could do for you, limit the number of interruptions you have, and plan for some breaks.

19 *Hassles* are defined as the irritants and annoyances — most of them fairly minor — that all of us encounter on a daily basis. Simply stated, they're part of living. Hassles can include things like having to wait for someone, getting caught in traffic, not being able to find a parking space, having to stand in lines, being bothered by a fly, not being able to find the book you need at the library, conflicts with a roommate, having to endure a boring professor, sleeping in and missing breakfast, or not having enough change to do laundry. One or two aren't bad. But when your day gets filled with hassles, your stress skyrockets.

There's not a lot you can do to prevent hassles — but you *can* work smart to defuse them. Think ahead; anticipate what you can. If you think you might get stuck in traffic, leave fifteen minutes early. If you know the parking on campus is a nightmare, ride the bus, ride your bike, walk, or join a carpool. If it's laundry day, stop at the bank on the way home and buy a couple of rolls of quarters. If you've had trouble finding resource materials for a paper, start early. For the rest — those things you can't circumvent — try to change your expectations. Don't expect to avoid traffic problems; don't expect to get your groceries without standing in line. If you learn to look at things differently, you'll be able to wait patiently, sit calmly, and think of something pleasant instead of getting uptight.

20 Everyone knows that noise is irritating. But did you know that *noise actually increases stress?* How? It boosts the heart rate, increases blood pressure, tenses the muscles, and causes the body to secrete stress-related hormones. At certain decibels (a jet plane engine, a pneumatic riveter, a guitar amplifier), noise can permanently damage hearing; if you're trying to concentrate on a difficult task, even a little noise can be stressful. The most stressful is noise that constantly changes in intensity, frequency, or pitch.

There's a lot you can do to reduce your stress from noise. If you can, choose an apartment away from a busy street, a convenience store, a fast-food restaurant, or an industrial area. Look for a carpeted apartment — you at least want carpet in the rooms that are directly adjacent to other units. Choose upholstered instead of hard-surfaced furniture, heavy drapes instead of aluminum blinds. Put a small foam pad under noisy appliances, such as blenders. Turn down the TV and the stereo. And, if you're exposed to chronic noise, use cotton or ear plugs to protect your ears and filter out some of the sound.

21 The environment you live in can either soothe you or add to your stress. You can't control some things — like air pollution — but you *can* clean up clutter, keep your room at the most comfortable temperature, and use adequate lighting, for example. Do whatever you can to limit your exposure to pollutants, insecticides, pesticides, food additives, gasoline exhaust, industrial wastes, and glazes or paints that contain lead.

22 You'll do best at coping with stress if you are generally satisfied: you feel some control over your life, you are able to set and meet goals, you have aspirations you believe you'll fulfill, the people closest to you are affectionate and caring, you feel valued, and you are able to make a meaningful contribution. Generally, satisfaction leads to optimism — and optimists suffer fewer symptoms of stress. If you're not optimistic and satisfied, try to figure out why. Change the things you can. Work to accept the things you can't change. Most importantly, learn to concentrate on your successes and use what you learned from them to meet your challenges head-on.

Personal Relationships

4

*P*ersonal relationships start the moment we are born. They begin by bonding with our parents, then branch out to friends in the neighborhood and at school, and finally in the world at large. Relationships include social groups, work associates, and mates. The commonality is that healthy relationships are essential to physical and emotional health. They increase our well-being and longevity.

Relationships within the family are the foundation for future relationships. Some people believe the American family is in trouble because of the diminishing quality of parent-child relationships, manifested in

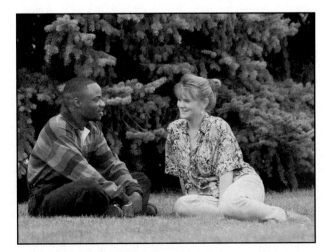

divorce and the two-parent working family. The problem is not that simple, but a child does need a loving, secure, constant environment in which to learn to trust and develop the self-esteem needed to thrive and eventually become autonomous.

FRIENDSHIPS

The first relationships we form outside the family are friendships. Friendship is a vehicle by which we move out of ourselves. We learn to share ourselves with others and, in turn, discover others. Friendships are characterized by respect, trust, affection, and loyalty. Friends like to be together. In some cases, particularly when the family is absent or dysfunctional, friendships can assume a more important role than family.

Sometimes the absence of friends portends loneliness. **Loneliness** has been defined as a condition in which a person's social network is significantly

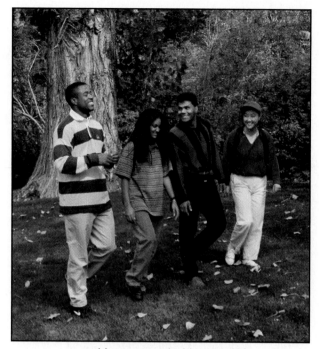

Friendships are a valuable part of life, particularly when family is absent.

A Secret to Longevity

Japanese people who moved to the United States but retained their former family values have among the highest life expectancies in the world. In contrast, Japanese immigrants who adopted American lifestyles started becoming sick and dying in the same patterns that American-born natives do. This happened within a single generation.

Various researchers concluded that Japan's emphasis on the group was a key to health and longevity. The Japanese culture places high priority on the family, and Japanese people develop lifelong friendships as well. Friends contribute to health by providing the same functions as families.

※　　　※　　　※

Another study focused on the close-knit Italian-American community of Roseto, Pennsylvania. Men and women alike had much lower mortality rates from heart disease than random population groups in the United States. Researchers concluded that the protective factor was the strong social support provided in this community. Family ties were exceptionally strong.

When the younger generations started changing — moving away, marrying outside the community, severing the close emotional ties to the original town — their physical health began to deteriorate and their mortality rates soon compared to that of surrounding Pennsylvania communities.

Source: *Wellness: Guidelines for a Healthy Lifestyle*, by Brent Q. Hafen and Werner W. K. Hoeger (Englewood, CO: Morton Publishing, 1994).

lacking in quality or quantity. Loneliness has been associated with higher rates of cancers and heart attack, among other diseases. Loneliness may compromise the immune system and leave lonely people vulnerable to various physical and mental illnesses.

We should point out that loneliness and being alone are not the same thing. Being alone can be generative. After the loss of her husband Charles, Anne Morrow Lindbergh wrote, in *Gift from the Sea*:

> I find there is a quality to being alone that is incredibly precious. Life rushes back into the void, richer, more vivid, fuller than before. It is as if in parting one did actually lose an arm. And then, like starfish, one grows it anew; one is whole again, complete and round — more whole, even, than before, when the other people had pieces of one.

Loneliness is associated with the quality, not the quantity, of relationships. It can stem from lack of attachments to others.

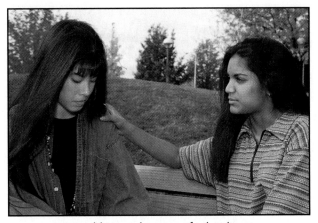
Friendship can be a cure for loneliness.

INTIMACY AND SEXUALITY

Attachments to others require that the person have a capacity for **intimacy**, marked by a very close association, contact, or familiarity. Intimacy may or may not have a sexual component, and many friendships exist without sexual intimacy. In other cases, friendships exist with a sexual component or evolve into a sexual relationship.

In the broadest meaning of the term, **sexuality** encompasses the biological, psychological, emotional, social, environmental, and cultural components of sexual behavior. Our identity, sense of self, roles — all involve sexuality. This chapter is concerned with the facets of sexuality manifested in relationships. The physical activities of sex and reproduction are discussed in Chapter 5.

Sexuality is present in a person from — and even before — birth. For example, male babies have been observed to have erections while in the uterus. From birth both sexes have the capacity for orgasm, although many do not experience it. As they grow, some children discover orgasm through self-exploration. Sexual stimulation by manipulating one's genitals is **masturbation**.

The first milestone in one's evolving sexuality is puberty. This is a time of major physiological changes dominated by the increased production of sex hormones. Thus, adolescents begin to show much more interest in the physical aspects of sex. Teenage boys begin to experience nocturnal emissions ("wet dreams"), and some girls have orgasmic dreams. At this stage teenagers are adults biologically. In psychological and social terms, however, they are still children and need at least 5 more years to reach a level of maturity commensurate with their physical status.

According to the Center for Population Options, the average age of first sexual intercourse was 16.2 years for girls and 15.7 for boys as of 1990. Among inner-city African American males in 1994, the average age of first intercourse was 11.8. The percentages of boys and girls having sex are shown in Table 4.1.

Table 4.1
Adolescents Having Sex

Age	Females	Males
15	27%	33%
16	34%	50%
17	52%	66%
18	70%	72%
19	78%	86%

Note: From National Survey of Family Growth (males) and Urban Institute (females). Figures reflect teens in metropolitan areas.

Source: *Kids Still Having Kids: People Talk About Teen Pregnancy* (New York: Franklin Watts, 1992), p. 17.

The current high rate of teen pregnancy and birth to adolescent mothers has reached crisis proportions. Each year approximately 1 million adolescent girls became pregnant (1 in every 10 girls under age 20), and approximately 500,000 give birth. The United States has the highest adolescent childbearing rate in the industrialized world.

Further facts provided by the Child Welfare League of America include the following:

❋ Adolescents age 17 and younger are twice as likely to deliver low birthweight babies (less than 5½ pounds at birth), who are 40 times more likely to die in the first 4 weeks of life than are newborns of normal weight.

KEY TERMS

Loneliness feeling of emptiness when a person's social network is significantly lacking in quality or quantity

Intimacy a close association, contact, or familiarity with someone

Sexuality the total biological, psychological, emotional, social, environmental, and cultural aspects of sexual behavior

Masturbation self-stimulation of genitals or other erogenous areas

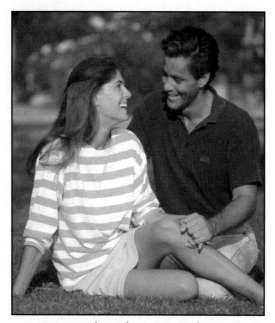

Intimate relationships create a closeness in which two people share their thoughts and feelings.

❋ Teenage girls who give birth are less likely to complete a high school education than their nonparent peers.

❋ Only half of the females who have their first child at age 17 or younger will have graduated from high school by age 30.

❋ Teenagers who become mothers are disproportionately poor and dependent on public assistance.

Many parents, and teens themselves, believe teens are under too much pressure to have sex. The pressure comes from TV, music videos, and movies that promote sex without considering the consequences. Once teens know their friends are having sex, many follow their lead to avoid feeling left out. Girls often say they have sex to feel "loved."

Love is a difficult concept because it means different things to different people at different stages in life. During adolescence love tends to be romantic and synonymous with passion and intense feelings. Teens typically develop infatuations and "fall in love." Although sex and love are obviously different, they tend to become confused because they are new concepts at this developmental age, and they also may have different meanings for boys and girls. Sorting out these differences while developing intimate relationships is one of the tasks of adolescence.

☎ Call for information

Planned Parenthood Federation of America
800-829-7732

National Life Center/Pregnancy Hotline
800-848-5683

Sexual Orientation

Sexual orientation often becomes apparent during puberty, when hormonal changes are taking place in the body. **Heterosexuality**, or being "straight," is the most common orientation. A heterosexual's physical attraction and sexual relationships are to and with members of the opposite sex. **Homosexuality** is characterized by sexual attraction to members of the same sex. A homosexual male usually is referred to as gay. A homosexual female is referred to as a lesbian or gay. Homosexuality encompasses individuals of every socioeconomic level, educational background, ethnicity, and religious preference. A third orientation is called **bisexuality** or **ambisexuality**. Bisexuals are sexually attracted to and may have sexual relationships with members of either sex.

A term often heard in regard to homosexuality is **homophobe**. It denotes a person with exaggerated fear, dislike, and hatred for homosexuals. Homophobia has led to discriminatory practices toward gays in employment, housing, and military services. As of 1974 the American Psychiatric Association stopped listing homosexuality as a psychosexual disorder in its *Diagnostic and Statistical Manual (DSM)*. This was the first "official" step in continuing efforts by gay people to be accepted as equal members of society.

Sexual Deviations

Paraphilia is a sexual disorder in which a person's sexual arousal and sexual gratification are dependent upon objects, acts, or imagery that is unusual or atypical. Table 4.2 contains a listing of selected atypical sexual behaviors and their definitions.

☎ Call for information

SIECUS (Sexuality Information and Education Council of the U.S.):
212-819-9770

Table 4.2
Atypical Sexual Behaviors

Behavior	Description
Exhibitionism	Showing one's genitals to unwilling observers and achieving sexual gratification by observing their responses.
Fetishism	Becoming sexually aroused by inanimate objects (e. g., brassieres, panties) or body parts (e. g., lips, feet, hair).
Frotteurism	Obtaining sexual gratification by rubbing or pressing against an unwilling person's body.
Incest	Sexual intercourse and other forms of sexual activities between close relatives such as father-daughter, mother-son, sister-brother (incest is illegal and prohibited in the United States).
Klismaphilia	Obtaining sexual pleasure from receiving enemas.
Masochism	Experiencing sexual gratification while receiving physical or emotional pain and attendant suffering and humiliation at the hands of another.
Necrophilia	Obtaining sexual gratification by having sexual intercourse with a corpse.
Pedophilia	An adult's sexual attraction to children, which can include victimization of children for sexual gratification.
Sadism	Being sexually gratified by inflicting physical pain or cruelty upon another.
Sadomasochism (S & M)	Mutually participating in masochistic and sadistic acts.
Transsexualism	Feeling, thinking, and acting as a person of the opposite sex (this is not homosexuality); feeling trapped in the wrong body.
Transvestism	Becoming sexually aroused by dressing in clothing worn normally by individuals of the opposite gender.
Voyeurism	Obtaining gratification by secretly gazing at others as they dress, undress, or engage in sexual activities; variation is obscene phone calls, in which men (extremely few women) are aroused sexually by anonymous communication and may masturbate during the phone call or immediately afterward.

DATING

Dating usually begins during the teen years. Many times the partners explore several forms of intimacy such as kissing, hugging, and intimate touching, which can easily lead to sexual intercourse. Too often teens emulate adult sexual behavior without being aware of its responsibilities and consequences. In this day and age, sexual intimacy is a risky proposition because of the heightened chances of contracting sexually transmitted diseases, including AIDS — not to mention the potential for young girls' becoming pregnant.

KEY TERMS

Sexual orientation determined by whether a person is physically attracted to members of the same sex or the opposite sex

Heterosexuality physical attraction to the opposite sex

Homosexuality physical attraction to the same sex

Bisexuality/ambisexuality physical attraction to both the same sex and the opposite sex

Homophobe exaggerated fear and hatred for homosexuals

Paraphilia atypical sexual behaviors using unusual objects, acts, or imagery to achieve gratification

Dating Violence

Dating does not always go smoothly, and sometimes it is even physically dangerous. Further, violence in dating relationships tends to carry over into more permanent arrangements. Battered spouses often were battered dates. In the early teen years the perpetrators are more often girls than boys. As the boys become physically larger and stronger than girls, that statistic reverses itself, and males continue to be the perpetrators of violence more often than females in subsequent years.

Studies by the Child Welfare League involving dating violence, based largely on FBI statistics, reveal the following:

- 12% of high school daters reported experiencing some form of dating violence.
- The incidence of physical violence in college dating relationships is reported as 20% to 50%, varying from slapping and hitting to more life-threatening violence.
- The rate of severe violence among dating couples ranges from about 1% to 27% each year.

Table 4.3 shows the types of violence and threatened violence that occurred among teens in one study.

Table 4.3
Types of Teen Violence

	Victims (66)		Perpetrators (62)	
Violence Tactic	**#**	**%**	**#**	**%**
Thrown an object	13	19.7	15	24.2
Pushed or shoved	23	34.8	20	32.3
Slapped	30	45.5	30	48.4
Kicked	7	10.6	11	17.7
Punched	10	15.2	17	27.4
Struck with an object	2	3.0	4	6.5
Beaten up	1	1.5	4	6.5
Threatened with or used a knife or gun	3	4.5	1	1.6
Threatened to hit but did not	30	45.5	28	45.2

Source: "Teen Dating Violence," by Nona O'Keefe, Karen Brockopp, and Esther Chew, *Social Work*, November/December 1986.

Date Rape

A related phenomenon in modern dating is the frequency of what has been termed **date rape** or acquaintance rape. Essentially defined as sex without the consent of both participants, it is particularly widespread in college settings. Minnesota Representative Jim Ramstad introduced in Congress the Campus Sexual Assault Bill of Rights Act

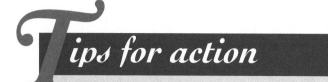

Tips for action

To diminish the odds for date rape:

- Develop clear lines of communication with the person you are dating. Communicate and clearly understand what each of you wants and expects from the date.
- Do not use psychoactive substances, including alcohol, in dating situations.
- Do not give clues or display body language that is flirtatious or indicates you are interested in having sex when you are not. For example, allowing a date to visit your bedroom may send a clue that you are interested in becoming intimate.
- Do not be coerced into unwanted sexual activities.

If you are the victim of date rape, don't blame yourself. Seek medical treatment and counseling.

Tips for action

Dos and Don'ts After A Sexual Assault

DO:

* Seek medical help as soon as possible.
* Bring a change of clothes to the emergency room.
* Get tested for sexually transmitted disease.
* Inquire about emergency contraception.
* Remember what you say to medical personnel could be used in court.

DO NOT:

* Shower or bathe
* Douche
* Change clothes until after the exam.
* Hesitate to call the police.

---

of 1991. He stated that more than 25% of college females have been raped by their date. In more than 70% of date rape cases, alcohol use — by either or both the sexual abuser and the victim — has been a contributing factor. Jealousy is the other major cause.

The concept of date rape is complex. Frequently individuals who come from homes where violence occurs between family members view violence as a normal part of relationships. Other date rape may be a result of miscommunication or differences in the way males and females interpret information concerning sex and invitations to participate.

Victimizing Behaviors

Rape

The crime of **forcible rape** is better defined than date rape. Unlike date rape, which in some cases may have a component of misunderstanding or be triggered by overconsumption of alcohol, the underlying motivation in forcible rape is a pathological need for power, induced by feelings of inferiority or insecurity. Legally, forcible rape is defined as the carnal knowledge of another person forcibly and against her will. (In contrast is statutory rape, which does not have the element of force. It often is applied to the case of an adult having sex with a person who has not reached the age of consent.)

Sexual assaults against women on college campuses are reported to be widespread.

Estimates of the number of women raped or sexually assaulted during their college years range from one in seven to one in twenty-five, according to the Congressional Research Service of the Library of Congress. Of college rape victims, 57% are victims of date rape. Under recent legislation, college campuses are required to collect statistics on campus crimes, including sex crimes, and to develop, publish, and distribute information regarding campus security policies and law enforcement.

The National Crime Victim Survey conducted by the U. S. Department of Justice shows that Hispanic, African American, and Anglo American women experience equivalent rates of violence committed by intimates.

Sexual Harassment/Stalking

Sexual harassment is the sexual pressuring of someone in a vulnerable or dependent position—a student or an employee, for example. A key component is that the overture must be unsolicited and unwanted. Harassers are people in positions of power—for example, a professor or an employer — to control or influence grades or jobs or salaries in exchange for sexual favors. They also might

KEY TERMS

Date rape sex without the consent of both partners
Forcible rape forced sex; assault
Sexual harassment unwanted sexual pressuring of someone in a vulnerable or dependent position by another in a position of power

punish the person for not complying. For example, a student may have a grade lowered, or an employee may be refused a raise or even fired. New federal laws make it easier for victims of sexual harassment to sue employers. Men are the more typical harassers because more men are in positions of power. Harassment, however, is gender-blind. The operative word is power. In Michael Crichton's novel and movie *Disclosure,* the harasser is a woman.

A person can commit harassment by **stalking**, a relatively recent social concern. Stalking is the intent to harass, annoy, or alarm another person. According to the law, it can consist of:

> *Before you marry, keep both eyes open. After you marry, shut one eye.*
> — Jamaican proverb

— repeated communications at inconvenient hours that invade the privacy of another and interfere in the use and enjoyment of another's home or private residence or other private property; or

— repeated insults, taunts, challenges, or communications in offensively coarse language to another in a manner likely to provoke a violent or disorderly response.

MARRIAGE AND ITS VARIATIONS

The traditional nuclear family (married mother, father, and their children under one roof) is not as common as it was 30 years ago. Now, 76% of families consist of the biological parents and their children.

Cohabitation

One popular adaptation of the traditional family unit is **cohabitation**, defined as the formation of a household unit by a couple living together as spouses (having sex) without being married. People who cohabit form what the U.S. Census Bureau terms the "unmarried-couple household." Its 1992 report indicated 3.3 million unmarried-couple households in the United States, double the number reported in 1980. This is in comparison to 53.5 million married couples. The married-couple household obviously is much more common than the unmarried-couple household. Even so, the trend toward living together is rising.

Cohabitation has assumed celebrity status, glamorized by couples such as the Atlanta Falcons' Andre Riser and rapper Lisa "Left Eye" Lopez, actors Ryan O'Neal and Farrah Fawcett, actors Kurt Russell and Goldie Hawn, and Maurice Templesman and the late Jacqueline Kennedy Onassis. Others, such as Eddie Murphy and Nichole Mitchell, and Donald Trump and Marla Maples, lived together for quite some time and started a family before deciding to marry. Among the reasons given for cohabitation is the need for freedom to dissolve the relationship without legal constraints if it does not work out. Some couples say their mutual love transcends the need for legal sanction.

In dissolving a cohabitative relationship, problems do arise. Because the couple was not legally married, state laws that govern spousal and child support and the division of property usually are not applicable to these unions. In the last 15 years many state courts and legislatures have had to make legal decisions that are comprehensive enough to cover this family arrangement. One of the first states to set this legal precedent was California, with the palimony case of actor Lee Marvin and his live-in companion, who sued him for financial support after their cohabitation ended. Even though public opinion about living together is more relaxed today than in the past, some family members and friends may pressure the cohabiting couple to marry.

Types of Marriage

Marriage is a legal and social institution whose criteria involve dedication, sharing, involvement, communication, and commitment. In the Western culture, only two individuals of the opposite sex are allowed to marry. Known as **monogamy**, this is the only legal type of marriage in the United States. A marriage in which one partner grants the other permission to have sexual intimacy with one or more others outside the marriage is called an **open-ended marriage**. An arrangement whereby both marriage partners agree to include others in sexual experimentation and variety is termed **swinging**.

What Does "Happily Married" Mean?

Seven characteristics of a happy marriage are:

1. The partners find their prime source of joy in each other but maintain separate identities.

2. They are generous and giving out of love, not because they expect repayment or are keeping score.

3. The partners enjoy a healthy and vigorous sexual relationship.

4. The partners "fight" in a constructive way, airing feelings and frustrations without attacking or blaming the other.

5. The partners communicate with each other openly and honestly.

6. The partners trust each other.

7. Both talk about their future together. They have mutual goals.

Source: *Positive Living and Health: The Complete Guide to Brain/Body Healing and Mental Empowerment,* by the Editors of Prevention Magazine (Emmaus, PA: Rodale Press, 1990). Reprinted by permission.

Another marital arrangement is **polygamy**, a general term to describe a marriage in which a person has more than one spouse simultaneously. **Polyandry** is a form of polygamy in which one woman has more than one husband simultaneously. **Polygyny** denotes one man with two or more wives simultaneously. Some cultures permit **group marriage** or **communal marriage**. In this configuration all familial activities and responsibilities are shared by a union of three or more individuals.

Contrary to what may appear to be otherwise in the media, men and women tend to marry people of their same race and ethnic background. Even though interracial marriage is more common today than ever before, at least 95% of the 53.5 million married couples in the United States in 1992 were married to a member of their own race. In 1992 the number of African American and Anglo American married couples was 21% of the interracial couples but only .5% of all married couples, according to the U.S. Census report.

In 1992 the estimated median age at first marriage was 26.5 years for men and 24.4 years for women, significantly higher than in recent years. Since the mid-1950s, when the median age at first marriage was at an all-time low, adults have been waiting longer and longer to marry.

The best marriages tend to be ones in which the partners are similar in:

— ethnicity
— locality (geography; urban or rural)
— maturity (emotional and social)
— goals and ideals
— intelligence levels
— amount of education
— economic level and financial resources
— social strata
— value system
— religious beliefs.

Sexual Intimacy in Marriage

Married couples in their 20s are more sexually active than older ones. The former have sexual relations an average of three to four times a week. As couples become older, their frequency of sexual intimacy usually declines.

Married couples engage in a wide variety of sexual behaviors. In addition to intercourse, sexual activity includes oral-genital stimulation, nongenital oral stimulation, mutual manual stimulation, and mutual masturbation.

In the 1993 *Janus Report on Sexual Behavior* at least 35% of married males and approximately

KEY TERMS

Stalking intent to harass, annoy, or alarm another person by repeated communications or actions

Cohabitation living together as spouses without being married

Marriage a legally and socially sanctioned union between a man and a woman

Monogamy marriage of a man and a woman

Open-ended marriage one in which one partner gives the other permission to have sexual relations outside the marriage

Swinging agreement by both partners in a marriage to engage in sexual experimentation outside the marriage

Polygamy a marriage of more than two people

Polyandry a marriage in which one woman has more than one husband simultaneously

Polygyny a marriage in which one man has more than one wife simultaneously

Group or communal marriage a marriage of three or more individuals who share all family functions

26% of married females admitted that they had been nonmonogamous. An earlier survey by Blumstein and Schwartz found that 57% of married females and 71% of married males had engaged in extramarital sexual activity. In most cases nonmonogamous activity is casual or "recreational adultery." It has a low level of emotional involvement.

Among the many reasons given for nonmonogamous relationships are the illness of one partner, one partner's lack of interest in sex, diminished passion, lack of love or respect, and boredom within the marriage. Conflicting interests and careers also can cause problems that may damage an otherwise stable relationship. Ultimately, the main reasons for infidelity are lack of love and commitment and unrealistic expectations of a partner.

In mature and responsible relationships, sexual intimacy is exclusive of others. It does not involve just a sexual act. It also includes showing appreciation for, sharing feelings with, showing respect for, sacrificing for, and being loyal to the partner. Sexual intimacy is an important part of marriage. It can enhance and enrich a marital relationship through mutual enjoyment, love, companionship, commitment, and procreation.

Extramarital relationships can be devastating. A mate who finds out about the infidelity of a formerly trusted partner feels a strong sense of betrayal. The resulting emotions can run the gamut of pain, anger, and depression, as well as fear of HIV/AIDS and other sexually transmissible diseases, to fear and anxiety about emotional, physical, and financial abandonment.

Love without esteem cannot go far or reach high. It is an angel with only one wing.
— Alexander Dumas

Marriage and Health

The National Center for Health Statistics has reported that married people have fewer health problems than unmarried people. They are less likely to have high blood pressure, cancer, and heart problems. Research verifies that happy marriage dramatically increases life expectancy. Death rates for single, divorced, and widowed individuals are significantly higher than the rates for married people. One postulated reason is that happy marriage helps keep the immune system strong.

But what about unhappily married people? They may be the worst off in terms of good health and a long life. They have poorer health than their single counterparts, including divorced people. Dissatisfaction with one's marriage can lead to depression, high blood pressure, and reduced immune system functioning. After careful consideration, divorce may be the best solution in some circumstances.

DIVORCE

In "Fairy Tales," Anita Baker sings of a relationship that has gone sour with the "knight in shining armor" bringing his love a "poison apple." The partners' expectations of marriage do not always mesh. Half of all marriages end in divorce. According to U.S. Census figures for 1992, 11% (16.3 million) of all adults age 15 years and older who had ever been married were divorced.

Even though the National Center for Health Statistics reports a decline in the divorce rate, the number of divorced persons compared to the number of married persons is increasing. In 1992 the ratio was 152 per 1,000 people in intact marriages. The figures by racial group are given in Table 4.4. Marriages dissolve for many reasons, including infidelity, lack of financial support, sexual, social, or educational incompatibility, physical or emotional abuse, and disagreements about childbearing and childrearing.

Table 4.4
Rates of Divorce for Selected Racial Groups, by Gender

Race and Gender	Divorces Per 1000
African American women	391
African American men	232
White women	164
White men	120
Hispanic women	161
Hispanic men	110

Source: U.S. Bureau of the Census, 1992.

Tips for action

Twelve Ways to Build Strong Family Values

1. Eat together as a family as often as possible, certainly several full family dinners a week. Involve everyone (for example, younger children can set the table and older ones can clear up).

2. Hold weekly gatherings to plan family activities, trips, and vacations, and discuss immediate and persistent problems.

3. Schedule daily stress-reduction periods when the entire household is quiet — no TV or CDs. According to your family values, read, meditate, pray, exercise, or whatever works for your family.

4. Volunteer time and talent to worthy causes in the church or community.

5. Participate in school. Become involved with teachers and administrators. Help with after-school and summer programs.

6. Do recreational activities as a family. Take walks, bike rides together.

7. Make or build things together. Share creative activities, and let children take the lead in some of these. Go for accomplishment, not perfection.

8. Take organized trips to sporting events, concerts, local fairs. Include everyone.

9. Bring children to work on occasion to let them see their parents' life away from home.

10. At least once a year travel away from home. Discuss vacation ideas with children.

11. Limit TV watching. Watch TV with children, monitor what they watch, and discuss what they see.

12. Stay involved. Keep informed about community and national issues that concern you and your children. Let children know your concerns and opinions, and listen to theirs.

Copyright by Dr. Benjamin Spock, in *A Better World for Children* (New York: National Press Books, 1994); excerpted from the *Denver Post*.

PARENTING

Most children in the United States are reared by both parents, a single parent, or grandparents. These adults serve as young children's primary role models, conveying and directing most of the formative information the children receive. A child's behavior, attitudes, beliefs, and ideas — about responsibility, expectations, love, respect, commitment, and sex — are byproducts of the adults who have reared them. Whether these attitudes, beliefs, and ideals are constructive or destructive, children most likely will utilize them. In most cases, these formative directives will serve as a roadmap for their children as they become adults, form relationships, and become parents or guardians.

Parenting is a continuous process. It demands that the caregivers expend considerable emotional and physical energies to create an environment for a child that is socially, emotionally, spiritually, and economically conducive to constructive growth and development. Parenting skills can be strengthened by utilizing resources such as community groups, churches, and private organizations. Some local community agencies, schools, colleges, and universities offer classes on parenting.

Single Parents

Single parents have a set of issues quite different from two-parent families. They are not able to divide the responsibilities of the household between

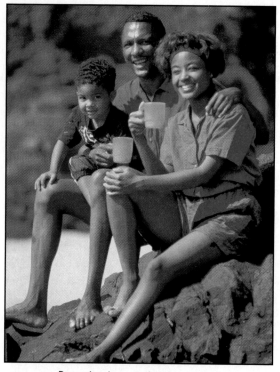
Parenting is a continuous process.

adults. The single parent often has greater financial pressures. In addition, a single parent often wishes to develop a romantic relationship with someone, which can be more difficult when children are part of the mix.

Most single parents are mothers. Currently, 45% of African American children live in female-headed households, according to the *Journal of Pediatric Nursing*. Overall, though, the number of single fathers is increasing. According to the 1992 Census, fathers now head 11% to 14% of single-parent household. James Levine, director of the Fatherhood Project at the Families and Work Institute in New York, says judges are increasingly awarding custody to fathers, turning away from the "tender years doctrine" that decreed that young children should stay with their mothers. Those who study the American family are beginning to conclude that absence of fathers in their children's lives deprives them of good male role models and is responsible for much of the increase in violence, crime, and gang memberships.

Tips for action

For Single Parents:

✳ Establish who has the power in the family. It's more difficult for one parent than two to have control — and it should not be the children.

✳ Set fair ground rules, and discipline with love.

✳ Be positive. Reward your child for good behavior.

✳ Be practical. Inform the child that money to buy and do things will not be plentiful, if that is the case.

✳ Give the child responsibility commensurate with his or her maturational level. Tell the child that he or she is part of the team. This will make the child feel wanted and needed.

✳ In cases of divorce, don't "badmouth" the opposite parent or sabotage the child's time with the other parent. The child feels responsible for the divorce anyway, and jeopardizing the child's relationship with the absent parent further conflicts the child.

✳ Be selfish! Don't put your life on hold or become a martyr. Maintain a social life and keep your hobbies and interests. A happy parent is a better parent.

✳ Enjoy your children. Children can be fun. If you're having a good time, they'll have a good time too.

✳ Be a good role model for your child.

✳ Stay physically fit. Exercise and eat right. The amount of energy you need as a single parent requires good nutrition and health.

✳ Set goals that are realistic, yet flexible. Work as a family unit toward those goals, and revise them as necessary. Elicit the child's input, and listen.

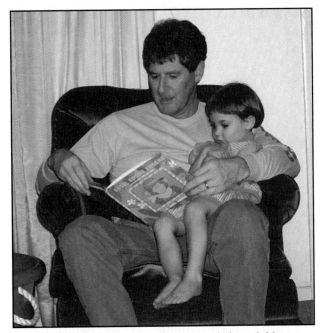

Parents should spend quality time with their children.

William Raspberry, syndicated columnist with the *Washington Post*, wrote in 1993:

> We have never doubted that children need fathers. Until now. We pay little attention to fathers as fathers, even less to the fact that many of the men absent from their children's lives have been shoved aside, not just by mothers of those children but by the courts and social agencies, buttressed by the growing cultural notion of the superfluous father.

Step-Parents

Another family unit that is becoming more prevalent is the blended family. In these families, previously divorced partners, one or both of which has children, combine to form another family unit. Being a step-parent is quite a challenge for many. The children retain loyalties to the absent biological parent. They also may consider a parent's new relationship a threat to their own relationship with that parent.

Counselors usually suggest that the step-parent not try to assume the role of parent or become the child's primary disciplinarian. The biological parent must have the primary parental role. Step-parents cannot expect their step-children to love them immediately. Love must be earned, and it grows gradually over time. A step-parent can, however, listen to the step-child and become a confidant, engendering rapport and, eventually, trust.

PROBLEMS IN FAMILIES

Not all families are functional. Many have serious internal problems. Some families become dysfunctional because of behaviors associated with alcohol and drug abuse (the topics of Chapters 12 and 13). Behavior patterns that are part of children's lives, unfortunately, tend to be perpetuated from generation to generation unless the cycle is broken. Nowhere is this pattern more obvious than in family violence and abuse. Studies have not uncovered differences between races or ethnic groups in abuse statistics. The National Crime Victim Survey, conducted by the U. S. Department of Justice, shows that African American, Hispanic, and Anglo American women experience equivalent rates of violence committed by intimates. Social status and its indicators (education, income, occupation) may be more significant in that people of lower socioeconomic status (SES) are associated with higher numbers.

Domestic Violence

Mate Abuse

The country was mesmerized by coverage of the Lorena and John Bobbitt and the O. J. Simpson cases. Although these are extreme and highly publicized examples of mate abuse, they are not isolated cases. Physical and emotional assault is a fact of life for all too many victims. Almost a third (30%) of the women murdered in 1990 were killed by husbands or boyfriends, according to the FBI. The National Clearinghouse on Domestic Violence has estimated that 3 to 4 million American women are battered each year by their husbands or partners. Between 25% and 45% of all battered women are abused during pregnancy. This increases the risk for birth defects and low birthweight babies. At highest risk of all are separated and recently divorced women.

Mate or spousal abuse is a potent and poisonous means of using force to control a victim. A complex phenomenon psychologically, Constance Dunlap, a Washington, DC psychiatrist, says the primary problem is denial. Often both the woman and the man who is abusing her have grown up in homes where they have witnessed abuse or have been abused themselves. Consequently, they have a hard time seeing this behavior as abnormal. These

Warning: This Relationship May be Dangerous to Your Health

What you see:	What he says:
Blaming:	"I love you, but you make me hit you."
Hypermasculine behavior:	"I make all the decisions in this family."
Emotional abuse:	"You are so stupid. I don't know why I married you."
Isolation:	"I don't like your friend Marva, and I don't want you going to the mall with her."
Intimidation:	"Just like I kicked that dog, I can kick you."
Coercion and threats:	"If you don't do what I say, I'll leave you. You can't make it without me."
Economic abuse:	"You don't need to make any more money. I can give you what you need when you ask me for it."

environments also do not nurture self-image or develop social skills. Further, most abuse occurs in a context of abuse of alcohol or other psychoactive substances, which lessens inhibitions and distorts judgment.

Although domestic violence is predominately male-perpetrated, the Bobbitt case illustrates that men can be victims, too. Women who assault men quickly discover that the partner is even more hesitant to report the abuse than women tend to be, often because of a "macho" orientation and also because the man does not tend to be believed. In some cases a man reporting abuse by a mate has been arrested and jailed himself.

Another complicating consideration arises from the differing values and practices of immigrants to the United States. For example, in many countries, women still are considered the property of men, as evidenced by dowries and arranged marriages. In many Asian countries, wives are expected to obey the

☎ Call for information

Family Violence Prevention Fund
800-777-1960

National Victim Center
800-FYI-CALL

husband as a duty to him. Women who do not are sometimes subject to beatings, many of which go unreported. In some South American countries, too, wives are considered as property or chattel.

Child Abuse

Abuse of children in families is a serious and widespread problem. Abused children often perpetuate the abuse or turn to other dysfunctional lifestyles to cope with it. In 1992 an estimated 1,261 children were confirmed victims of fatal maltreatment, according to the Child Welfare League of America. Between 1985 and 1992, child abuse fatality rates rose 49%. Of the total victims, 87% were under 1 year of age. In the states that included data on parental substance abuse, it was linked to 19% of the child maltreatment fatalities. The breakdown for child abuse mortality is:

physical abuse:	58%
physical neglect:	36%
both physical abuse and neglect:	6%

Some of the childhood deaths for which the recorded causes are sudden infant death syndrome (SIDS), and natural causes actually may be the result of abuse.

The mortality figures do not reveal the total amount of child abuse. Although reliable statistics are difficult to obtain, the most comprehensive and methodologically sound report to date was by the U. S. Department of Health and Human Services. Reported in 1990, DHHS found that approximately

On March 30, 1989, a Brooklyn Supreme Court Judge sentenced a batterer to 5 years probation for second-degree manslaughter in the hammer-beating death of his wife. Relying on the "cultural defense," the man's lawyer argued successfully that traditional Chinese values accounted for his extreme reaction to his wife's alleged infidelity. The ruling sent shock waves through the Asian community, along with a simple but clear message: The law will not protect Asian women from domestic violence, even unto death.

Source: National Clearinghouse for the Defense of Battered Women, Philadelphia, February , 1994 packet.

1 in 150 girls and approximately 1 in 500 boys are sexually abused. The report also indicated that one in every two reported cases is unfounded.

Irrespective of problems in accurate reporting, abuse is a serious problem, and most occurs in a family context. Child abuse may be physical, sexual, or psychological/emotional. Some forms of **physical abuse** are hitting any part of the body with an instrument or object, scalding with hot water or caustic liquids, and burning a child's body with cigarettes. **Sexual abuse** is defined as violation of a child's genitalia or sexually motivated acts perpetrated on a child. It can include fondling, massaging, genital contact, intercourse, oral sex (fellatio and cunnilingus), and similar acts.

As long as little children are allowed to suffer, there is no true love in this world.

— Isadora Duncan

Psychological/emotional abuse is negative and hostile verbal or nonverbal treatment of a child. It might take the form of swearing loudly at a child: "You're no good." "You're dumb." "You're stupid." "You'll never amount to anything." Nonverbal abuse might consist of ignoring a child or neglecting the child's physical and emotional needs. Some children never are told that they are doing well or that they are special. They are not hugged or touched—powerful means of making a child feel loved and secure.

Whether the abuse is physical, sexual, or emotional, the emotional pain is lasting and can do considerable and long-lasting harm to a child. Depending on the severity of physical abuse, long-term effects can include:

— a higher rate of perceptual-motor deficiencies
— lower scores on general intelligence tests
— poorer academic achievement rates
— more social and behavior problems and adjustment difficulties
— either extreme aggression or extreme withdrawal continuum
— defiance; nonconformity
— drug use (when older)
— delinquency

Long-term effects of child sexual abuse might include:

— compulsive masturbation, excessive curiosity about sex, "adult" behaviors, detailed information about sexual activity
— bedwetting and soiling the bed

— compulsive behavior
— disturbed sleep patterns
— disturbances in eating patterns
— learning difficulties
— artwork that reveals the sexual activity
— stomach aches
— skin disorders

As a cautionary note, these are mere indicators and should not be taken as conclusive evidence of abuse. Some children who have not been abused may display the same symptoms.

Older children tend to cope by escaping. The escape can be entering into an early marriage, becoming pregnant, running away from home, or committing suicide, as examples. Long-term consequences of childhood abuse in older children include:

— aggressive and violent behavior
— conduct disorders
— alcohol and drug use and abuse
— emotional problems such as anxiety, depression, hostility, and schizoid disorders
— suicide attempts and suicides
— problems with interpersonal relationships
— social incompetency
— difficulties in the workplace
— perpetuation of familial violence.

Abuse tends to revolve in a vicious cycle from generation to generation. About a third of abused children go on to abuse their own children. Children who grow up in an atmosphere of family violence are apt to think it is something to be expected, normal, and okay. As abused children become adults, they are more likely to engage in physical violence toward their family. Women who have been victims of child abuse are at greater risk for aggressive or defiant behavior from their mates than those who were not exposed to abuse. These females are more likely to socialize with, date, and marry men who

KEY TERMS

Physical abuse an act of physical harm intentionally inflicted on another

Child sexual abuse violation of a child's genitalia or sexually motivated acts toward child

Psychological/emotional abuse negative and hostile verbal or nonverbal treatment of another

have abusive backgrounds themselves. A large percentage of prostitutes are victims of abuse. Males who have lived in an environment of family violence are more apt to batter their mates than those who did not grow up in abusive homes.

FAMILY PLANNING

Most, but not all, couples eventually desire children. In today's world, when both men and women tend to work outside the home and financial needs are greater, couples are more likely to plan just when to have children. Many are opting to have children later in life, when they are more established. Nowadays, having a baby over age 40 is not the unusual occurrence it was in the past.

Contraceptives

Contraceptives encompass drugs, artificial devices, and surgical procedures used to prevent fertilization, prevent ovulation, or prevent implantation. Periodic abstinence also is considered a method of birth control.

When considering each method, variables include safety (health risks), effectiveness, cost, ease of use, availability, maintenance, and convenience. No contraceptive is 100% effective or 100% safe. Each has advantages and disadvantages (see Table 4.5). The user or prospective user should be knowledgeable of pros and cons. Sound judgment and personal responsibility are vital. Choice of contraceptives as a birth control method is an extremely

Table 4.5
Summary of Birth Control/Contraceptives

Type	Male Condom	Female Condom	Spermicides Used Alone	Sponge	Diaphragm with Spermicide	Cervical Cap with Spermicide
Estimated Effectiveness	About 85%	An estimated 74%–79%	70%–80%	72%–82%	82%–94%	At least 82%
Risks	Rarely, irritation and allergic reactions	Rarely, irritation and allergic reactions	Rarely, irritation and allergic reactions	Rarely, irritation and allergic reactions; difficulty in removal; very rarely, toxic shock syndrome	Rarely, irritation and allergic reactions; bladder infection; very rarely, toxic shock syndrome	Abnormal Pap test; vaginal or cervical infections; very rarely, toxic shock syndrome
Protection Against Sexually Transmitted Diseases	Latex condoms help protect against sexually transmitted diseases, including herpes and AIDS	May give some protection against sexually transmitted diseases including herpes and AIDS; not as effective as male latex condom	Unknown	None	None	None
Convenience	Applied immediately before intercourse; used only once and discarded	Applied immediately before intercourse; used only once and discarded	Applied no more than 1 hour before intercourse	Can be inserted hours before intercourse and left in place up to 24 hours; used only once and discarded	Inserted before intercourse; can be left in place 24 hours, but additional spermicide must be used if intercourse is repeated	Can remain in place 48 hours; not necessary to reapply spermicide upon repeated intercourse; may be difficult to insert
Availability	Nonprescription	Nonprescription	Nonprescription	Nonprescription	Prescription	Prescription

personal decision, which should be based on a medical profile, personal preference, and lifestyle.

Barrier methods place physical barriers between the sperm and egg. They prohibit the sperm from entering the cervix. These methods include the male and female condom, diaphragm, cervical cap, vaginal spermicide, and contraceptive sponge.

Male Condom

The **condom**, also termed a prophylactic, and informally called a "rubber," is a thin latex or sheep membrane sheath designed to cover the penis. The latex rubber condom is the most effective (Figure 4.1). When placed over the erect penis, the condom prevents semen from entering the vagina.

When using a condom without a reservoir, 1/2" should be left at the tip to capture semen and prevent the condom from tearing at ejaculation.

The condom is placed over an erect penis before any vaginal contact and insertion, and it is removed immediately from the vagina after the male orgasm and ejaculation. A reliable way of removing a condom is to hold the rim of the

KEY TERMS

Contraceptive any device, drug, or practice that prevents ovulation, fertilization, or implantation
Condom thin sheath placed over the penis that prevents semen from entering the vagina

Oral Contraceptive Pill	Implant Norplant	Injection Depo-Provera)	IUD	Periodic Abstinence (NFP)	Surgical Sterilization
97%–99%	99%	99%	95%–96%	Highly variable, perhaps 53%–85%	Over 99%
Blood clots, heart attacks and strokes, gallbladder disease, liver tumors, water retention, hypertension, mood changes, dizziness and nausea; not for smokers	Menstrual cycle irregularity; headaches, nervousness, depression, nausea, dizziness, change of appetite, breast tenderness, weight gain, enlargement of ovaries and/or fallopian tubes, excessive growth of body and facial hair; may subside after first year	Amenorrhea, weight gain, and other side effects similar to those with Norplant	Cramps, bleeding, pelvic inflammatory disease, infertility; rarely, perforation of the uterus	None	Pain, infection, and, for female tubal ligation, possible surgical complications
None	None	None	None	None	None
Pill must be taken on daily schedule, regardless of frequency of intercourse	Effective 24 hours after implantation for approximately 5 years; can be removed by physician at any time	One injection every 3 months	After insertion, stays in place until physician removes it	Requires frequent monitoring of body functions and periods of abstinence	Vasectomy is a one-time procedure usually performed in a doctor's office. Tubal ligation is a one-time procedure performed in an operating room
Prescription	Prescription; minor outpatient surgical procedure	Prescription	Prescription	Instructions from physician or clinic	Surgery

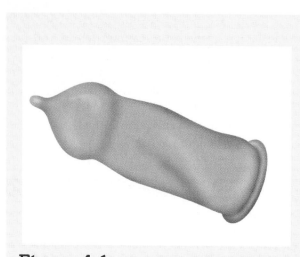

Figure 4.1 Male condom with reservoir tip

condom against the base of the penis. This allows the penis to be removed from the vagina without spilling sperm into the vagina.

When used properly and consistently, condoms coupled with vaginal spermicide (discussed later) can be quite effective as a birth control method. The latex condom also is the only contraceptive proven to be effective — though not totally — in protecting against pathogens that cause sexually transmitted diseases (STDs) such as HIV infection, gonorrhea, nonspecific urethritis (NGU), and oral or genital herpes (discussed in Chapter 6).

Condoms, some of which are lubricated or treated with a chemical spermicide, may be purchased in stores without a prescription. They are relatively inexpensive and cause no serious adverse side effects to either sexual partner. The most widely reported disadvantage is that condoms reduce male sensitivity. Also, when spermicide (non-oxynol-9) is added to condoms, it can cause vaginal irritation in some women.

Female Condom

In August of 1994 the **female condom** went on sale nationwide for the first time. It looks like a male condom but with soft plastic rings. It is said to be effective in preventing sexually transmitted diseases as well as pregnancy, though not as effective as the male condom.

Each female condom costs nearly four times as much as a male condom and can be used only once. Another disadvantage is that it remains visible even

after insertion, covering the outside of the vagina. The female condom and the male condom should not be used at the same time. Figure 4.2 illustrates how to insert a female condom.

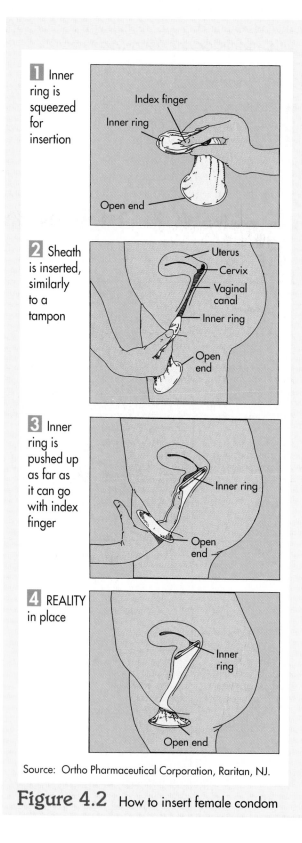

1 Inner ring is squeezed for insertion

Index finger
Inner ring
Open end

2 Sheath is inserted, similarly to a tampon

Uterus
Cervix
Vaginal canal
Inner ring
Open end

3 Inner ring is pushed up as far as it can go with index finger

Inner ring
Open end

4 REALITY in place

Inner ring
Open end

Source: Ortho Pharmaceutical Corporation, Raritan, NJ.

Figure 4.2 How to insert female condom

Diaphragm

The **diaphragm** is a round rubber or plastic cup with a flexible spring rim that fits inside the vagina near the cervix. After applying a chemical spermicide containing nonoxynol-9 around the rim and inside the dome of the cup, it is inserted into the vagina and placed over the cervical opening. The diaphragm is designed to prevent semen from entering the uterus and fallopian tubes.

Diaphragms are available after medical evaluation, including gynecological fitting and prescription. A health practitioner instructs the woman on how the diaphragm is to be inserted and removed. It is inserted no longer than an hour before intercourse. Before each act of intercourse the woman must feel the diaphragm to determine whether it covers the cervical opening properly. The diaphragm must be left in place at least 6 hours after intercourse. If intercourse is repeated during this 6-hour period, more spermicide must be added before each act of intercourse while the diaphragm is left in place.

Once the diaphragm is removed, it must be cleaned immediately with mild soap and warm water. After drying the device thoroughly and carefully, it should be placed in its container and stored in a cool, safe place.

Although the diaphragm may be difficult to insert at first, it is quite effective when used properly. It is even more effective when used in combination with the condom. In cases of weight gain, weight loss, and childbirth, a diaphragm has to be refitted. Some women have reported occasional irritation and bladder infections when using the diaphragm. With normal use a diaphragm should be replaced every 2 years.

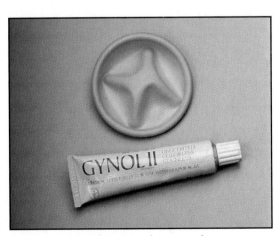

Diaphragm and spermicide.

Cervical Cap

The **cervical cap** is a small, thimble-shaped plastic or rubber cap that fits firmly around the neck of the cervix. Like the diaphragm, it must be prescribed by a health practitioner. Prior to insertion a chemical spermicide is placed in the cervical cap. An advantage of the cervical cap is that it may be inserted prior to intercourse and left in place 2 days (48 hours). Disadvantages of the cervical cap are that it may be difficult to insert and remove, some women have problems with proper fitting, and some women have reported discharges and unpleasant odors. Irregular Pap tests have been reported during the first 6 months of use of the cervical cap.

Vaginal Sponge

The **vaginal sponge** is constructed of a soft, white polyurethane foam containing the chemical spermicide nonoxynol–9. Once the sponge is removed from the airtight package, it is wet thoroughly with clean tap water. The water activates the spermicide. After squeezing the sponge to remove excess water, it is inserted high in the vagina to cover the cervix.

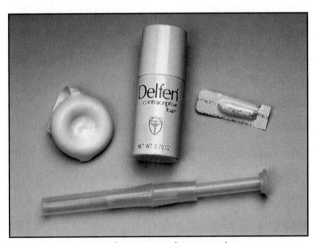

Vaginal sponge and spermicides.

KEY TERMS

Female condom sheath inserted into the vagina to prevent fertilization and sexually transmitted diseases

Diaphragm rubber cup that fits over the cervix and prevents semen from entering the uterus and fallopian tubes; available only by prescription

Cervical cap small rubber cap that fits over the cervix and is used with a spermicide to prevent fertilization

Vaginal sponge foam sponge containing a spermicide, inserted in the vagina to prevent fertilization

The sponge is effective up to 24 hours. During this time the sponge traps and absorbs sperm, and the spermicide kills the sperm. The sponge is removed by reaching high into the vagina and gently pulling the string loop that is attached to it. The sponge can be used only once and then is discarded. When the sponge is used consistently, according to printed instructions, its rate of effectiveness is 72% to 82%.

The sponge has some reported disadvantages. An individual who has had toxic shock syndrome (TSS) or TSS warning signs, such as dizziness, diarrhea, fever, or vomiting, should not use the sponge. Women with cervical or vaginal problems should not use the sponge. It should not be used after childbirth or after spontaneous or induced abortions. Some females have developed allergic reactions to the ingredients in the sponge. The sponge is available in stores without a prescription.

Chemical (Vaginal) Spermicide

Chemical **spermicide** kills sperm before they enter the uterus. Spermicides have many different forms, including foams, creams, vaginal suppositories, jellies, and vaginal contraceptive film. The chemicals must be placed close to the cervix less than one-half hour before intercourse. Intercourse must take place within the hour. Chemical spermicides should be applied before each act of intercourse. The chemicals lose their effectiveness after one use and after an hour.

Chemical spermicides are readily available; they may be purchased in stores without a prescription. The chemical spermicide may kill some of the pathogens that cause STDs, but the best protection is the latex condom. Therefore, chemical spermicide always should be used with a condom for better protection against pathogens that cause STDs.

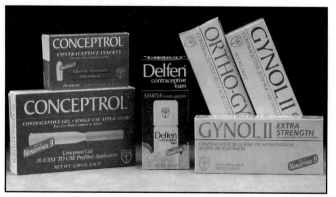
Chemical spermicides.

Chemical spermicide may cause irritation to genital tissue in females and males. Symptoms include burning, a fine rash, and inflammation of genital tissue.

Oral Contraception

Oral contraceptives, or birth control pills, are of two types: the combination pill and the progestin-only or minipill. All oral contraceptives are available to the female only after a gynecological examination and prescription. The examining health practitioner decides which type is best for the patient. The most common and effective, the combination pill, contains two hormones, synthetic estrogen and progesterone (progestin). Oral contraceptives are taken for 21 consecutive days, preferably at the same time each day. When taken as directed, the combination pill prevents ovulation.

The minipill contains a small amount of progesterone and no estrogen and is taken daily without fail. When the minipill is taken as directed, it alters the mucus in the cervix (makes it thick and tacky, thus blocking sperm) and does not allow the endometrium to thicken. This prevents implantation of a fertilized egg.

The multiphasic pill is a different formulation of the combination pill that is designed to release variable doses rather than constant doses of estrogen and progesterone. This cycle is more similar to that occurring naturally in the menstrual cycle. Like the other oral contraceptives, the multiphasic pill is taken for 21 consecutive days.

Some oral contraceptives are packaged with 28 tablets instead of 21. The last seven tablets in a 28-day pack are inert or inactive and do not contain any hormones. The purpose of those tablets is to remind the woman to stay on schedule.

A major advantage of oral contraception is that it is highly effective in preventing ovulation. Also, the pill does not interfere with sexual activities. Combination oral contraceptives offer protection against nondeficiency anemia, endometrial cancer, ovarian cancer, fibrocystic breast disease, and pelvic inflammatory disease (PID). A major disadvantage of oral contraception is that it provides no protection against the deadly HIV virus that causes AIDS or other pathogens that cause sexually transmitted diseases. Other problems that may be associated with "the pill" are candida (yeast) infections, weight gain, morning sickness (nausea), "breakthrough" bleeding

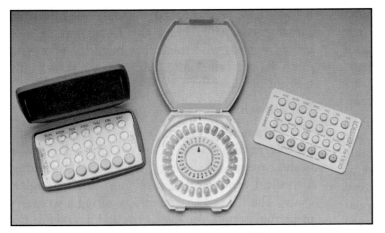

Oral contraceptives ("The Pill").

between periods, irritability, headaches, vaginal discharge, and depression.

Women who smoke cigarettes should not take oral contraceptives. Women with any medical condition should discuss this with the health professional so a safe decision can be made concerning their use of oral contraceptives. Many females interested in "the pill" will not be able to use it. The following medical conditions may prohibit use of oral contraceptives:

hypertension
stroke
diseases of the heart
gall bladder diseases
cancers of breast, cervix, vagina, and uterus
blood clots (history of blood clots in the leg)
severe headaches
diseases of the kidney and liver
family history of heart attack
diabetes
depression
epilepsy

Several medications may interfere with oral contraceptives' effectiveness. These may include various barbiturates (downers) and antibiotics.

Norplant®

Norplant® is a contraceptive consisting of six flexible, progestin-filled silicone tubes or capsules. The capsules, each about the size of a matchstick, are inserted surgically just underneath the skin of the upper arm. Norplant is a long-lasting contraceptive that secretes progestin

into the body slowly. While in place, it prevents pregnancy up to 5 years. If a woman wishes to become pregnant while the Norplant is in place, her health care provider can remove the capsules at any time.

Although Norplant is quite reliable and effective for women who weigh less than 150 pounds, the pregnancy rate increases in women who weigh more than 150 pounds. When using Norplant, women may have some side effects, especially within the first year. Some known side effects are weight gain, irritability, depression, headache, nausea, dermatological disorders (skin rash and acne), and breast tenderness. Additional side effects include irregular menstrual bleeding, enlargement of the ovaries and fallopian tubes, and excessive growth of facial and body hair. Infections at the site where Norplant is implanted may occur. This might cause excessive scar tissue or keloid formation in some African American women.

A study reported in the November 4, 1994, issue of the *New England Journal of Medicine* found that inner-city teen mothers who chose Norplant were 19 times better protected from a repeat pregnancy than girls who chose birth control pills.

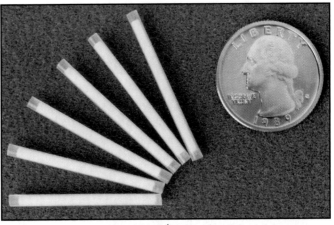

Norplant®.

KEY TERMS

Spermicide chemicals in the form of creams, foams, or jellies that kill live sperm

Oral contraceptives hormonal tablets taken by women to prevent ovulation

Norplant® long-lasting hormonal contraceptive implanted under the skin by a health care practitioner to prevent ovulation

On the flip side is the creation of new life that is anticipated with eagerness, reflecting to the bright side of human sexuality.

The sociological and psychological aspects of sexuality are covered in Chapter 4. This chapter addresses its physical facets, with the anticipation that awareness and understanding of the physiology of sex will contribute to its rational and satisfying expression.

We begin with the physiological differences between men and women — how one's sex is determined biologically. This is followed by a discussion of the male and female reproductive systems, common disorders and dysfunctions in these systems, and sexual arousal and response. We trace the reproductive cycle, beginning with conception and culminating in childbirth. Infant and maternal mortality rates are given. The chapter concludes with a discussion of infertility and adoption.

MALE AND FEMALE SEXUAL ANATOMY

Sex is the quality of being male or female. During prenatal development hormones and chromosomes are responsible for the formation of genitals that determine whether a person is male or female. The human sex organs serve two major functions: reproduction (procreation) and pleasure, including intimate personal communication.

Both males and females have a pair of **gonads**, or sex glands. The male gonads are called **testes**, and the female gonads are called **ovaries**. Gonads are responsible for the production of sex hormones and **gametes**, or sex cells. The male gametes are called **sperm** and the female gametes are called **ova**, or eggs.

When a sperm and an ovum unite, as a result of sexual intercourse, conception occurs, creating new life. About 8 weeks after conception the sex organs of this new life differentiate. How they do this depends upon genetic instructions dictated by the sex chromosomes X and Y. The father determines the sex, because some of his sperm carry the X chromosome and some carry the Y chromosome. The mother's eggs are all Xs. If a sperm carrying an X chromosome fertilizes an egg, the combined XX will produce a female. If a sperm carrying a Y chromosome fertilizes an egg, the resulting child will be a male with the identifying XY chromosome. This concept is illustrated in Figure 5.1.

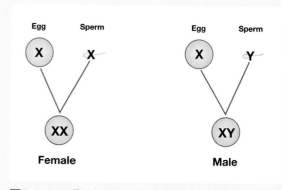

Figure 5.1 Sex determination

The Male Reproductive System

External Genitals

The external genitals include the penis, urethra, scrotum, testes, epididymis, and vas deferens, as illustrated in Figure 5.2. The **penis** is the male organ of sexual activity through which **semen**, the thick, milky fluid containing the sperm, is expelled and urine is eliminated from the body. The penis is constructed of spongy erectile tissue and many small nerves and blood vessels. At its tip is the

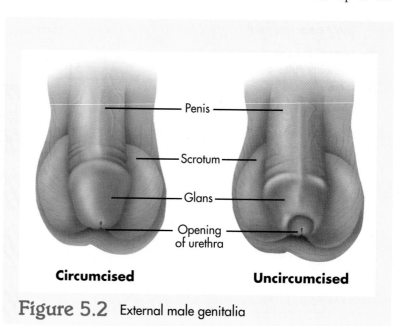

Figure 5.2 External male genitalia

glans, a sensitive part that is important in sexual arousal. During sexual arousal the spongy tissue becomes engorged with blood, causing the penis to become erect. **Erection** is necessary for sexual intercourse. Usually after **ejaculation**, the sudden discharge of seminal fluid, the penis returns to a flaccid position. The **urethra** is the long duct connected to the bladder, which runs through the center of the penis, carrying and releasing urine and semen from the body. These two processes cannot be accomplished at the same time, as they are controlled by muscular sphincters.

The **scrotum** is the loose pouch of skin that contains the testes, the epididymis, and the lower portion of the vas deferens. The major purpose of the scrotal sac is to protect the testes and to keep the testes at a stable temperature of at least 4° to 5° Fahrenheit below that of the body's normal 98.6° F. This means that the temperature of the testes should be around 93.6° F., so **spermatogenesis** (sperm cell production) can take place.

Internal Genitals

As shown in Figure 5.3, the two **testes** (testicles) are the almond-shaped glands that produce the male gametes (sperm) and the male hormone **testosterone**. Each testicle is composed of **seminiferous tubules** within which the sperm is produced. The production of testosterone, which begins in adolescence, stimulates the functioning of the male reproductive system and the development of secondary masculine characteristics. These characteristics include development of body hair, facial hair (beard and mustache), the formation of more defined muscles, and a deepening voice (Table 5.1).

The **epididymis** is the long, coiled, storage structure along the back of each testicle in which sperm cells mature until they are released. The **vas deferens** are the sperm-carrying tubes that take the sperm from the epididymis up the ejaculatory duct.

Table 5.1
Sex Changes Beginning at Puberty

Males	Females
Growth spurt begins	Growth spurt begins
Oil and sweat glands become more active (if clogged, acne may develop)	Oil and sweat glands become more active (if clogged, acne may develop
Testes start to grow	Breasts start to develop
Penis starts to grow	Menstruation begins
Body and facial hair starts to grow; stimulated by androgen	Secondary hair starts to grow, (pubic region, under arms, etc.) arrested by estrogen and progesterone
Genitalia produce mature sperm; often released during nocturnal emissions	Pregnancy becomes possible
Muscles become defined	Body becomes more "curved"
Skeletal system matures	Skeletal system matures

KEY TERMS

Sex the quality of being male or female

Gonads sex glands; the primary reproductive organs

Ovaries almond-shaped female sex glands that produce eggs, or ova, and the hormones estrogen and progesterone

Gametes sex cells

Sperm male gametes

Ova female gametes

Penis male organ of sexual activity

Semen fluid containing sperm

Glans sensitive tip of the penis

Erection the engorged, rigid state of the penis during sexual arousal

Ejaculation sudden discharge of semen from the penis as part of the sexual response

Urethra long duct running through center of penis, which carries and releases the urine and also the semen

Scrotum loose pouch of skin containing the testes

Spermatogenesis sperm cell production

Testes almond-shaped male sex glands that produce sperm and testosterone

Testosterone hormone that regulates male sexual development

Seminiferous tubules hollow, cylindrical structures that make up most of the testes and produce sperm

Epididymis storage structure along the top of each testicle where sperm cells mature

Vas deferens tubes that carry the sperm from the epididymis up the ejaculatory duct

Human Sexuality and Reproduction   ✳

Male Circumcision

The medical procedure of **circumcision** — surgical removal of the foreskin of the penis — has a cultural as well as a physical connotation. Actually, worldwide, circumcised males are in the minority; only about 15% of the population practices circumcision — most prominently Jewish and Muslim peoples, for religious reasons. Most Europeans, Asians, Central and South Americans, do not. Many Africans are Muslims or practice circumcision as a "rite of manhood."

From the early 1940s to the mid-1970s, most parents in the United States had their newborn sons circumcised. In 1971, however, the American Academy of Pediatrics (AAP) came out against the procedure as being unnecessary, and this was followed by a drop in rate of circumcision from 85% in 1974 to 60% by 1990.

Benefits of circumcision are cleanliness and prevention of infection resulting from bacteria being trapped under the foreskin. Recent research has further shown that uncircumcised infants have more urinary tract infections, which can lead to kidney damage. Circumcision also may reduce the spread of sexually transmitted diseases and cancer of the penis, the latter of which develops almost exclusively in uncircumcised men.

Drawbacks include pain to the infant (some compare it to female genital mutilation), and the risk of complications and surgical errors. Although the AAP now has taken a neutral stand, opponents of circumcision claim it is the leading unnecessary surgery in the United States.

The fluid-producing glands include the seminal vesicles, the prostate gland, and the Cowper's glands. The **seminal vesicles** are the glands that produce and secrete an alkaline fluid suitable for sperm mobility. The **prostate gland,** located directly below the bladder, produces the largest amount of seminal fluid released during ejaculation. The **Cowper's glands** (bulbourethral glands) are two pea-sized glands located alongside the base of the urethra. These glands produce an alkaline pre-ejaculatory fluid into the urethra during sexual excitement. Combined, the secretions from the testes, seminal vesicles, prostate gland, and Cowper's glands produce semen containing the sperm cells discharged from the urethra upon ejaculation.

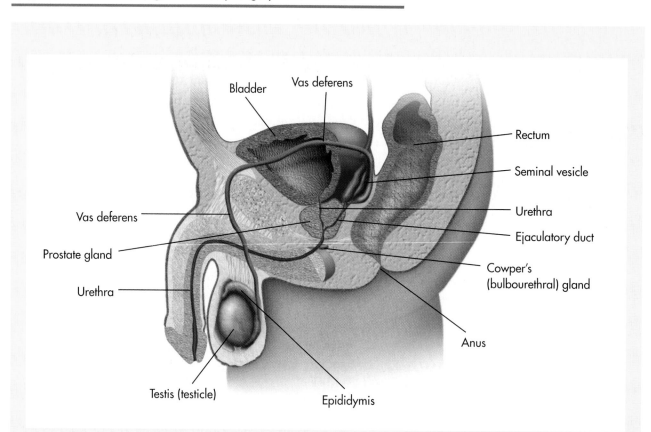

Figure 5.3 Internal male genitalia

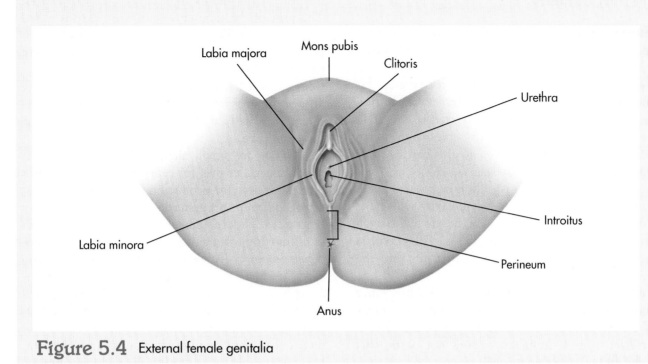

Figure 5.4 External female genitalia

The Female Reproductive System

External Genitals

The vulva is the outer covering of the genital area, which includes the mons pubis, labia majora, labia minora, urethra, vaginal opening (introitus), clitoris, and perineum, as identified in Figure 5.4. The **mons pubis** is the mound of fatty tissue covering the pubic bone. During puberty, pubic hair begins to grow on and eventually covers this tissue. The **labia majora** are the two large outer folds of spongy tissue covering the labia minora, clitoris, urethral opening, and vaginal opening. The **labia minora** are the two folds of skin within the labia majora, including a single fold of skin over the clitoris known as the **prepuce** or clitoral hood. The **urethra,** is the duct through which urine from the bladder is released from the body. Unlike the male urethra, the female urethra is not part of the genitals.

The vaginal opening, or **introitus,** is the passage leading from the vulva to the internal genitals and the uterus. The **hymen** is a membrane that may cover the vaginal opening partially at birth. In some cases it is not intact. The **clitoris** is a small, extremely sensitive, pea-shaped organ located at the upper end of the vulva above the urethral opening. When the female is sexually stimulated, the clitoris becomes engorged with blood. The perineum is the area between the vaginal opening and the anus.

KEY TERMS

Circumcision surgical removal of foreskin of penis

Seminal vesicles Glands that produce a fluid suitable for sperm mobility

Prostate gland organ that produces the most seminal fluid

Cowper's glands two pea-sized organs that produce pre-ejaculatory fluid

Mons pubis mound of fatty tissue covering the pubic bone

Labia majora two outer folds of tissue covering vaginal opening

Labia minora two folds of skin within labia majora

Prepuce single fold of skin that covers the clitoris and the glans of uncircumcised penis

Urethra duct through which urine from the bladder is released from the body

Introitus vaginal opening

Hymen membrane partially covering the vaginal opening at birth; may or may not be intact

Clitoris sensitive female sex organ, which becomes erect when sexually excited

Internal Genitals

Internal genitals of the female include the vagina, uterus and cervix, fallopian tubes, and ovaries (Figure 5.5) The **vagina** is a 3" to 5" tubular passage leading to the internal reproductive area. As one of the structures responsive to sexual arousal, the vagina is elastic enough to receive the erect penis and its ejaculate and to serve as the birth canal during vaginal delivery. It also carries menstrual blood outside the body.

The **uterus** (womb) is a hollow, pear-shaped, muscular organ within the pelvic cavity where the fetus gestates and develops. The uterus will stretch to accommodate the growing fetus. The **cervix** is the lower portion of the uterus that juts into the back of the vagina and sometimes is called the "neck" of the womb. The endometrium, the inner lining of the uterus, builds during the early stages of the menstrual cycle so it may accommodate a fertilized egg. If fertilization does not occur, this lining is shed monthly through menstruation.

The **fallopian tubes,** or oviducts, are small tubular passages about 4" long that lead from the upper portion of the uterus to each of the two ovaries. The part of the tube closest to the ovary is called the fimbriae. The **fimbriae** are responsible for pulling the egg cell into the fallopian tube. Lining the walls of the fallopian tubes are hairlike projections called **cilia**, which are responsible for moving an egg down the fallopian tube to the uterus. Fertilization usually occurs in the lower third of the fallopian tube.

Ovaries are small, almond-shaped gonads that produce eggs, or ova, for reproduction. The ovaries are responsible for producing the female hormones estrogen and progesterone. **Estrogen** controls female sexual development. It promotes the growth and function of the female sex organs and the development of female secondary sexual characteristics, such as breast development. This development begins at puberty (see Table 5.1). Estrogen is synthesized mainly by the ovaries. **Progesterone** promotes growth and maintenance of the uterine endometrium (lining), mammary glands, and placenta. It is responsible for preparing the endometrium for pregnancy. If fertilization occurs, it sustains the endometrium throughout pregnancy and prevents

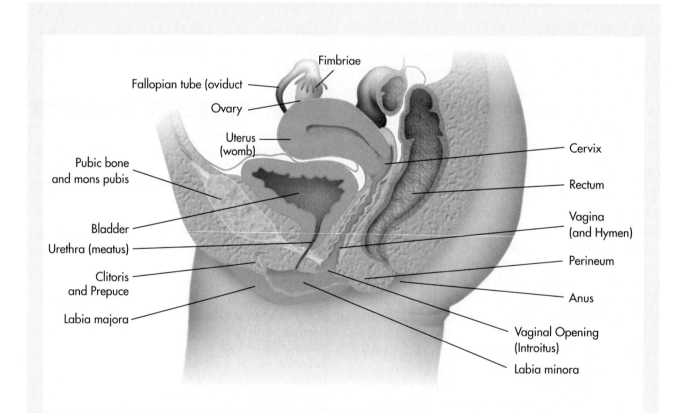

Figure 5.5 Internal female genitalia

the further release of eggs from the ovary. At puberty, these eggs start to mature, and usually one bursts from its **follicle,** or sac, each month. In later life hormone production decreases, eggs are no longer released, and the woman enters menopause (see Chapter 14).

COMMON DISORDERS OF THE REPRODUCTIVE SYSTEM

Male Disorders

Disorders of the male reproductive system most often involve the prostate gland. Aside from cancer, discussed in Chapter 7, the most common prostate condition is enlargement of the gland, called **benign prostatic enlargement (BPH).** "Benign" means that it is not cancerous. BPH rarely causes symptoms before age 40, but more than half of men in their 60s and as many as 90% of men in their 70s and 80s have this condition. Over time BPH can lead to urinary tract infections, bladder and kidney damage, and **incontinence** (inability to control urination voluntarily).

Symptoms of BPH vary, but the man typically has problems with or changes in urination, such as a hesitant, interrupted, weak stream; urgency and leaking or dribbling; and more frequent urination, especially at night. In some cases a man may find himself unable to urinate at all. This problem can be triggered by taking a decongestant drug. Urinary retention also can be brought on by alcohol, cold temperatures, or a long period of immobility.

Diagnosis involves, first, a rectal exam. If any suspicion is aroused, an ultrasound test may be done, displaying an image of the prostate gland on a screen. Sometimes the doctor will ask the patient to urinate into a special device that measures how quickly the urine is flowing; reduced flow often suggests BPH.

Another test used to diagnose conditions of the urogenital tract is the *intravenous pyelogram* (IVP). A dye is injected into a vein, followed by an x-ray. The dye reveals any obstruction or blockage in the urinary tract.

A third test procedure is the *cystoscopy,* in which, after numbing the penis with a solution, the doctor inserts a small tube through the opening of the urethra. The tube contains a lens and a light

system, which help the physician see the inside of the urethra and bladder.

A number of recent studies have questioned the need for early treatment when the gland is barely enlarged. The condition clears up without treatment in up to a third of all mild cases. Regular check-ups are suggested, however. *Alpha blocker drugs* may be prescribed to help relax muscles in the prostate; however, they do not cure the condition or reduce the need for future surgery. In a new drug treatment, *finasteride* (Proscar) is taken by mouth once a day. It can cause the prostate to shrink. This drug does not reduce the need for future surgery either. Finally, *balloon dilation* may be done as a temporary measure to stretch the urethra and allow urine to flow more readily. This is a fairly new treatment; therefore, the long-term benefits and risks are unknown.

When treatment is necessary, most doctors recommend removing the enlarged part of the prostate. In *transurethral surgery* no external incision is needed. It is done through the urethra, most often using a *resectoscope* inserted through the penis. If this procedure cannot be used, as is the case when the gland is greatly enlarged, an external incision may be the method of choice. Finally, *laser surgery* is being researched as a method of vaporizing the offending tissue.

Other disorders of the male reproductive system are listed in Table 5.2. Cancers of the male reproductive system are covered in Chapter 7.

KEY TERMS

Vagina tubular passage leading to internal reproductive area that connects with the uterus

Uterus (womb) pear-shaped, muscular organ where fetus develops

Cervix lower portion of uterus that connects with vagina

Fallopian tubes tubular passages leading from upper portion of uterus to each of the two ovaries

Fimbriae fingerlike projections; part of fallopian tube

Cilia hairlike projections lining wall of fallopian tubes

Estrogen hormone that controls female sexual development

Progesterone hormone that prepares uterus for pregnancy

Follicle egg sac in ovary

Benign prostatic enlargement (BPH) enlargement of prostate gland, not related to cancer

Incontinence inability to control urination voluntarily

Table 5.2
Selected Disorders of the Male Reproductive System

Disorder	Description
Gynecomastia	Excessive development of the male breasts
Hydrocele	Abnormal collection of fluid around the testes
Prostatitis	Infection or inflammation of the prostate gland
Urethritis	Infection or inflammation of the urethra

Female Disorders

The most common disorders involving the female reproductive system are endometriosis, uterine fibroid tumors, vaginitis, and premenstrual syndrome (PMS). Others are briefly outlined in Table 5.3.

Endometriosis

The lining of the uterus, the **endometrium**, is supposed to stay in the uterus until it is shed monthly in the form of menstrual blood. In some women pieces of the endometrium migrate to the fallopian tubes, the ovaries, or even the abdominal cavity. This condition, called **endometriosis**, affects more than 5 million women in the United States, 10%–15% of all women of childbearing age. Although the cause is unknown, it seems to be related to estrogen, as it rarely occurs before puberty and tends to disappear after menopause.

As the endometrium in the uterus responds to the hormones of the menstrual cycle by getting thicker and then bleeding, so does the endometrial tissue that is sticking to the other reproductive structures. These pieces of endometrium, or **implants**, bleed, may form cysts that can rupture, and cause scar tissue or adhesions to form in the pelvic cavity.

Signs and Symptoms The symptoms vary from woman to woman, but sharp pain and cramps and heavy bleeding during the menstrual period are common. Some women have chronic pelvic pain or pressure during coitus, or sexual intercourse. If the implants have migrated to the bladder or the intestines, the woman may have pain when she urinates or has a bowel movement, especially during the menstrual period. The urine or stool may even contain blood. Those affected also may have fatigue and lower-back pain.

Diagnosis Endometriosis should be diagnosed as soon as possible so it can be treated in the early stages of development. The notion that this condition is not common in African American women and teenagers is not accurate. Undiagnosed, endometriosis becomes progressively worse and may lead to fertility problems. Infertility affects about 30% to 40% of women with endometriosis. Women of any age should not ignore severe menstrual cramps — one of the first symptoms.

Table 5.3
Selected Disorders of the Female Reproductive System

Disorder	Description
Amenorrhea	Absence of menstruation
Cystocele	Protrusion into the vagina of a portion of the urinary bladder
Dysmenorrhea	Painful menstruation
Dyspareunia	Pain during intercourse
Fibrocystic disease of the breast	Benign (noncancerous) lumps in the breast
Leukorrhagia	Abnormal discharge from the vagina caused by any of several conditions
Menorrhagia	Abnormally long (more than 7 days) or heavy menstrual flow
Ovarian cyst	Abnormal swelling or saclike growth on an ovary
Pelvic Inflammatory Disease (PID)	Inflammation the uterus and fallopian tubes
Polycystic ovarian disease (PCOD)	A set of conditions in which the ovarian function is disturbed; ovary may enlarge and produce many small cysts
Prolapse of the uterus	Collapse, descent, or other change in position of the uterus
Rectocele	A condition in which part of the rectum protrudes into the vagina as a result of a hernia
Vaginitis	Inflammation of the vagina

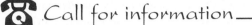

Call for information

Endometriosis Association
800-992-ENDO (3636)

Definitive diagnosis of endometriosis is made by **laparoscopy**. In this minor surgical procedure the abdomen is distended with carbon dioxide gas and the laparoscope (a flexible tube with a light) is inserted through a tiny incision in the abdomen near the navel. Looking through the laparoscope, the physician can see the exact location of the endometrial implants and check the condition of the other organs in the abdomen.

Treatment Objectives of the treatment are not only to relieve pain and stop more implants from growing but also to preserve reproductive functioning. The treatment for endometriosis varies. The woman may be advised to use one of several hormone or drug therapies (tablets, nasal spray, injection) that temporarily halt ovulation and the menstrual cycle. During this time the implants are supposed to shrink and the other symptoms disappear. A newer drug treatment uses gonadotrophin-releasing hormone analogs (**GnRH analogs**). This 6-month therapy medically induces menopause, sometimes with its attendant symptoms (hot flashes, vaginal dryness, bone loss). Other drugs being investigated are RU-486 (the "abortion pill"), steroids, and drugs that affect the immune system.

The alternative treatment for endometriosis is some form of surgery. In conservative surgical treatment laparoscopic surgery is used to remove or destroy the endometrial implants and scar tissue. In the most nonconservative surgery the uterus, ovaries, and fallopian tubes are removed.

Uterine Fibroid Tumors

You may have heard your grandmother refer to fibroid tumors as "fireball tumors." Uterine fibroids are one of the most common noncancerous gynecological conditions appearing in women of reproductive age. Estimates are that more than one in every four or five women over age 50 is affected. African-American women are more than three times as likely as Anglo-American women to develop fibroids. Fibroid tumors account for 30% of the hysterectomies performed annually in the United States.

Signs and Symptoms A **fibroid tumor**, or myoma, is a mass of muscle and connective tissue growing in the uterus. Fibroids vary in size (smaller than a jelly bean to larger than a cantaloupe), and their growth is believed to be stimulated by the hormone estrogen. Small fibroids usually do not cause problems. As they grow larger, however, they typically produce unusually heavy menstrual bleeding and pressure or pain in the abdomen. In some cases the fibroid can grow so large that it presses against the bladder and uterus, causing frequent urination and other problems with the urinary tract. Medium to large fibroid tumors may cause a woman's abdomen to protrude to the point at which she looks like she is in the third month of pregnancy.

Fibroids are classified by their position in the uterus. A *submucous fibroid* grows inward from the uterine wall, taking up space within the uterus. This type of fibroid is more likely to cause heavy and prolonged menstrual flow, which can result in anemia (deficiency of hemoglobin in the blood). The *pedunculated fibroid* grows on a stalk or a stem. This type can cause severe pain if the stalk becomes twisted and cuts off blood supply to the fibroid.

Diagnosis and Treatment Fibroids may be diagnosed in a number of ways, including the standard pelvic exam, ultrasound, computerized tomography, magnetic resonance imaging (MRI), x-ray, and laparoscopy. Options for treatment have to weigh the relief of symptoms against the need to preserve reproductive functioning. If the woman wants to have a baby, **hysterectomy**, surgical removal of the uterus, will be delayed. In some cases the fibroid is removed surgically; this is called a **myomectomy**. In

KEY TERMS

Endometrium inner lining of the uterus

Endometriosis a condition in which pieces of the endometrium migrate to fallopian tubes, ovaries, or abdominal cavity

Implants pieces of endometrium that have migrated to other areas

Coitus sexual intercourse

Laparoscopy a procedure that uses an optical device to view the abdominal cavity

GnRH analogs drug treatment for endometriosis

Fibroid tumor a mass of muscle and connective tissue growing in the uterus

Hysterectomy surgical removal of uterus

Myomectomy surgical removal of uterine fibroid tumor

extreme cases complications of heavy blood loss and scarring may prevent the woman from being able to bear children, and in some instances the fibroid will grow back.

Because fibroids tend to grow more slowly and may shrink in menopause, drug therapy options that stimulate menopause temporarily are available. Many gynecologists are prescribing GnRH analogs (as in endometriosis), which block the production of estrogen, which in turn causes the fibroids to shrink. These medications produce the side effects of menopause such as hot flashes, vaginal dryness, and bone loss. The other drawback is that when the medication is stopped, the fibroids begin to grow again.

Premenstrual Syndrome

Premenstrual syndrome (PMS) is a condition characterized by nervousness, irritability, emotional disturbance, headache, and depression in some combination, which affects some women for up to about 10 days before menstruation. The condition is associated with the accumulation of fluid in the tissues and usually disappears after menstruation begins. The female hormone progesterone is believed to be part of the cause, and a deficiency of essential fatty acids also has been observed.

Once a month, about 2 weeks before the menstrual period, estrogen and progesterone begin to amass and come into conflict. Estrogen levels may soar for one woman, making her anxious and irritable; or progesterone may predominate, dragging her into depression and fatigue. She might feel bloated and gain weight, have a headache, backache, acne, allergies, or tenderness in the breasts. Her mood may swing erratically from euphoria to depression. When the period finally arrives, symptoms leave.

PMS is believed to affect between a third and half of all American women between ages 20 and 50, says Dr. Susan Lark, director of the PMS Self-Help Center in Los Altos, California. Certain factors, such as bearing several children, seem to promote PMS, says Dr. Guy Abraham, a former professor of obstetrics and gynecologic endocrinology at the University of California, Los Angeles, School of Medicine. The problem may be inherited, according to Dr. Edward Portman, a PMS consultant, researcher, and director of the Portman Clinic in Madison, Wisconsin.

Not all PMS sufferers have the same symptoms and the same intensity of discomfort. And PMS sufferers do not necessarily respond to the same treatments. Finding the best way to handle PMS may require some trial and error.

SEXUAL AROUSAL AND RESPONSE

Sexual excitement is derived from stimuli such as touching, masturbation, intercourse, oral sex, and other sexual acts. It is often said that "90% of sex is in the mind" — indicating the powerful role of psychological factors in sexual arousal and function. The physiological mechanisms involved are:

* **Vasocongestion,** the increased supply of blood into the genitals during sexual excitement.

* **Myotonia,** which causes increased muscular contractions during orgasm.

Response Cycle

The human sexual response cycle has four phases:

1. *Excitement phase.* In this phase the male's penis becomes erect. The testes begin to expand, and the scrotal skin tenses and thickens. In females the vagina increases in size and a natural lubricant prepares the vagina to receive the penis. The uterus increases in size and elevates into the pelvic cavity, and the breasts swell. In both sexes the nipples become erect.

2. *Plateau phase.* The plateau phase is more intense and extended than the excitement phase. In men the penis becomes larger and harder and the testes enlarge. The Cowper's glands secrete a pre-ejaculatory fluid, and the testes become completely engorged with blood and fully elevated. In females the lower portion of the vagina enlarges, and lubrication of the vaginal

KEY TERMS

Premenstrual syndrome (PMS) a condition occurring about 10 days before menstruation, characterized by all or some of the following: nervousness, irritability, emotional disturbance, headache, or depression

Vasocongestion increased supply of blood to genitals during sexual excitement

Myotonia increased muscular contractions during orgasm

Tips for action

If You Have PMS:

* **Don't worry — be happy.** A positive, confident attitude can help you cope and maybe even prevent future episodes of PMS. Recite some positive affirmations (for example, "I can handle stress").

* **Eat a little a lot.** Poor nutrition doesn't cause PMS, but certain dietary factors can accentuate the problem. Eat small meals low in sugar several times a day.

* **Avoid empty calories.** Stay away from low-nutrient foods such as soft drinks and sweets containing refined sugar.

* **Decrease dairy foods.** Eat no more than one or two portions per day of skim or low-fat milk, cottage cheese, or yogurt. The lactose in dairy products can block the body's absorption of magnesium, which helps regulate the estrogen level and increases its excretion.

* **Ferret out fats.** Replace animal fats such as butter and shortening with polyunsaturated oils such as corn and safflower oils. Animal fats contribute to the high estrogen levels that may intensify PMS.

* **Take a nutritional supplement every day** containing vitamins B_6, A, C, D, E, calcium, magnesium, and L-tyrosine.

* **Restrict salt.** Go on a low-sodium diet for 7 to 10 days before the onset of your period, to offset water retention.

* **Eat a lot of fiber.** Fiber helps the body clear out excess estrogens. Eat plenty of vegetables, beans, and whole grains.

* **Cut down on caffeine.** Consume limited quantities of coffee, tea, chocolate, and other caffeine-containing substances.

* **Abstain from alcohol.** Alcohol is a depressant. It also can worsen PMS headaches and fatigue and cause sugar cravings.

* **Do not take diuretics.** Some over-the-counter diuretics draw valuable minerals out of the body along with water. Instead, stay away from substances such as salt and alcohol, which cause water retention.

* **Exercise.** Walk at a fast pace in fresh air, swim, jog, take up ballet or karate. Increase your level of activity for the week or two before PMS symptoms set in.

* **De-stress your environment.** Surround yourself with soothing colors and soft music.

* **Breathe deeply.** Shallow breathing, which many of us do unconsciously, decreases your energy level and leaves you feeling tense. Practice inhaling and exhaling slowly and deeply.

* **Soak in a tub.** Indulge yourself in a mineral bath to relax muscles from head to toe, at least 20 minutes.

* **Get extra sleep.** Go to bed earlier for a few days before PMS tends to set in.

* **Adhere to a schedule.** Set reasonable goals and schedules for each day to avoid feeling overwhelmed, even if this means cutting back in your routine.

* **Decline social obligations temporarily.** Postpone big plans like holding a dinner party until a time when you feel you can handle it better.

* **Talk.** Discuss your PMS problems with your mate, friends, or co-workers. This can be beneficial.

Sources:

Guy Abraham, M.D., former professor of obstetrics and gynecologic endocrinology, University of California, Los Angeles, UCLA School of Medicine

Penny Wise Budoff, M.D., director of Women's Medical Center, Bethpage, New York

Susan Lark, M. D., director of PMS Self-Help Center, Los Altos, California

Edward Portman, M.D., PMS consultant, researcher and director of Portman Clinic, Madison, Wisconsin

Peter Vash, M.D., endocrinologist and internist on clinical faculty of UCLA Medical Center

From *The Doctor's Book of Home Remedies*, by the editors of *Prevention Magazine* (Emmaus, PA: Rodale Press, 1990). Adapted by permission.

wall increases beyond that of the excitement phase. The uterus continues to increase in size and is elevated completely into the pelvic cavity. In both sexes the heart rate doubles and breathing becomes more rapid.

3. *Orgasmic phase.* The orgasmic phase is characterized in males by intense rhythmical contractions in the pelvic region, penis, seminal vesicles, prostate glands, and urethra. At this point orgasm and ejaculation of semen occur. In females rhythmical contractions occur in the vagina, uterus, and entire pelvic region. Not all women experience rhythmical contractions with penile insertion; some have clitoral orgasm a result of stimulation of the clitoris.

4. *Resolution phase.* The resolution phase is the resting, relaxation, or reversal stage. All changes beginning with excitement in male and female are reversed. The male's erection is lost because blood rushes out of the spongy, erectile penile tissue, the muscles relax, and the genital organs return to their original nonstimulated sizes and positions. At this point the male enters a **refractory period**, the time immediately following orgasm when he cannot be stimulated to orgasm again. Depending upon a man's age and health, the refractory period may last several minutes to several days. Women do not have a physical refractory period.

Sexual Problems

The sexual response can be influenced by a variety of physical and psychological factors that usually are interrelated. The physical problems discussed next may be caused by anxiety, worry, fatigue, alcohol or other drug consumption, relationship conflicts, lack of interest, and other physical or emotional sources.

Problems in the Female

Vaginal dryness During sexual arousal a clear fluid emerges in the vaginal wall. One function of this fluid is to facilitate entry of the penis into the vagina. In some women lubrication is insufficient, and during intercourse this problem may cause pain, irritation, and tearing of the vaginal tissue. Vaginal dryness can result from anxiety, hormonal

imbalance, aging, and the use of oral contraceptives, antihistamines, and other medications.

Remedies include more precoital stimulation (foreplay) and commercial vaginal lubricants (lubricating jelly) developed specifically to alleviate vaginal dryness temporarily. Vaginal lubricants are not contraceptives, so they do not afford protection from pregnancy. Petroleum jelly should not be used as a substitute for a lubricating jelly as it can cause vaginal irritation in some women. Also, when a condom is being used, petroleum jelly can cause the condom to weaken and tear.

The sexual response can be influenced by a variety of physical and psychological factors.

Vaginismus **Vaginismus** is a condition characterized by strong, involuntary contractions in the muscles of the lower third of the vagina. Depending on the extent of the contractions, penile insertion is difficult, if not impossible. A woman with vaginismus may have contractions during pelvic exams and may even feel extreme discomfort with the insertion of one finger. The fundamental cause of vaginismus usually is **dyspareunia** (painful intercourse) induced by fear, sexual conflict, or unpleasant sexual feelings. Women with this condition should consult a gynecologist.

Problems in the Male

Impotence Erectile dysfunction or **impotence** is the inability to obtain an erection or to maintain an erection for coitus. This problem may be caused by diseases, by medication, by the use of alcohol and drugs, and by other psychological and physiological disorders.

After age 40 impotence is more common than previously thought. In a survey of nearly 1,300 men aged 40 to 70 in Boston, 52% reported some degree of impotence. Contributing factors were high blood pressure, heart disease, smoking, diabetes, some medications, and extreme anger or depression.

Premature ejaculation **Premature ejaculation** is a sexual problem in which men reach orgasm and ejaculation consistently too quickly or within 30 seconds to 2 minutes of beginning coitus. This understandably can be frustrating to both partners. Any man who has long-term problems with premature ejaculation or impotency should consult a urologist.

REPRODUCTION

The Menstrual Cycle

A healthy female's reproductive organs begin to function at an average age of about 11 to 12 years, and the trend has been toward earlier onset; age 9 is no longer a rarity. The reproductive structures discussed earlier in the chapter are intended to enlarge, mature, and become functional so the female can reproduce. One of the first signs that these processes are occurring is the onset of the first **menstruation** or menarche. During menstruation, the lining of the uterus or the endometrium is shed in the form of blood through the vagina (the menstrual period). When a female menstruates, she is not pregnant and the reproductive organs are presumed to be working normally. If a female has not reached menarche by her 16th birthday, a gynecologist should be consulted to confirm that the reproductive system is developing normally.

The average length of each menstrual cycle is 28 to 32 days, although the cycle ranges from 25 to 32 days in the female population. During this time a variety of events are happening. Some can be seen; others are taking place behind the scene in the brain, the ovary, and the bloodstream. For the purpose of the discussion here, the length of this cycle will be considered to be 28 days, divided into four 7 day-segments: menses, estrogenic, ovulation, progestational (see Figure 5.6).

During the first 7-day segment of the menstrual cycle, the menstrual period, the lining of the uterus is shed in the form of blood. The first day of bleeding marks the first day of the menstrual cycle and the menstrual period, which ranges from 3 to 7 days. The endometrium is shed because hormone levels in the bloodstream have dropped. The hormone levels have dropped because implantation has not occurred.

At the end of the second 7-day segment of the menstrual cycle, another vital process — **ovulation**

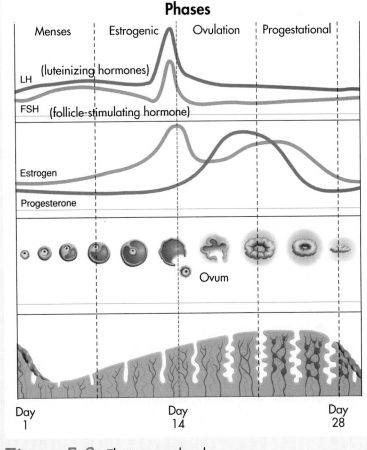

Phases

Menses | Estrogenic | Ovulation | Progestational

LH (luteinizing hormones)

FSH (follicle-stimulating hormone)

Estrogen

Progesterone

Ovum

Day 1 | Day 14 | Day 28

Figure 5.6 The menstrual cycle

— occurs. It marks the middle of the 28-day menstrual cycle, occurring about the 14th day. The ovaries contain between 200,000 and 400,000 egg cells (ova), each housed in a tiny follicle. Upon

KEY TERMS

Refractory period the time immediately following orgasm when a male cannot be sexually stimulated

Vaginismus strong, involuntary contractions in the muscles of the lower part of the vagina

Dyspareunia painful intercourse

Impotence inability to obtain or maintain an erection for coitus

Premature ejaculation emission of semen and loss of erection within 30 seconds to 2 minutes of beginning coitus

Menstruation (menarche) the discharge of blood from the uterus through the vagina

Ovulation the release of a mature egg from the ovary in the middle of the menstrual cycle

chemical signals from the **pituitary gland** in the brain, **follicle-stimulating hormone (FSH)** and **luteinizing hormone (LH)** are activated. Usually only one egg cell matures and is released from the ovary during a menstrual cycle. The follicle secretes estrogen, which causes the pituitary to continue sending its signal of LH. The increase of LH and estrogen production causes the ovary to release from the activated follicle the egg cell or ovum that now is mature. The fimbria of the fallopian tube or oviduct grab the egg and ferry it through the tube to the uterus. If no sperm are present, the egg degenerates after about 24 to 48 hours, and the menstrual cycle continues.

In the third 7-day segment of the menstrual cycle, the follicle from which ovulation originated becomes enlarged and is called the **corpus luteum,** Latin for "yellow body." This corpus luteum continues to make estrogen and secrete progesterone, another female hormone. Progesterone is the hormone that sustains the lining of the uterus in preparation for implantation of an anticipated fertilized ovum.

If the ovum does not implant, the fourth 7-day segment of the menstrual cycle ensues. In response to the high levels of estrogen and progesterone in the bloodstream, the pituitary gland stops producing FSH and LH. At this point the corpus luteum degenerates, estrogen and progesterone levels plummet, and the thickened layer of the endometrium is discharged through the vagina. Menstrual flow consists of blood, mucus, and endometrial tissue.

These four 7-day segments are supposed to occur in a continuous pattern. When the female menstruates again, this marks the first day of the next menstrual cycle. The process repeats itself again and again until the female reaches menopause, which usually occurs between ages 45 and 50 or so. Menopause, the cessation of menstruation, is discussed in Chapter 14.

Conception

When healthy spermatozoa are present in the fallopian tube at the time of ovulation, one of them may be successful in penetrating the egg cell. This union of egg and sperm cells is called **fertilization,** which is supposed to take place in the fallopian

tube. The product of this process is called a **zygote,** or fertilized egg. **Conception** has occurred.

Usually one sperm and one egg unite to produce one baby. Two different scenarios, however, are possible:

1. The women's ovaries may produce two or more eggs upon ovulation. Each egg that is fertilized by a male sperm will develop into a separate embryo — and eventually into the birth of twins, triplets, or more babies — termed a **multiple birth**. Twins who develop from this process are termed **fraternal twins**. They may be both boys, both girls, or one of each.

2. Another type of twins derives from a single fertilized egg dividing into two cells that develop separately. Because the genetic material is the same, they are **identical twins**.

At fertilization the zygote moves in the tube toward the uterus. This journey takes about a week. Cell division and differentiation of the zygote occur during the trip. By the time this product of conception reaches the cavity of the uterus, it is referred to as an **embryo**. The embryo then sinks into the plush layer of the endometrial lining that has been prepared for it. This is called **implantation**. The implanted embryo continues to differentiate, and its developing placenta sends a hormone signal called the **human chorionic gonadotrophin (HCG)** through the mother's bloodstream to the pituitary gland. FSH and LH are not released, and the hormones from the corpus luteum continue to secrete so the blood and mucous layer of the endometrium will remain intact to sustain the pregnancy.

Pregnancy

Pregnancy is defined as a condition of having a developing embryo or fetus in the uterus. How does a woman know she is pregnant? To hear some guests on popular talk shows tell stories of not knowing they were pregnant until they went into labor is amazing! Generally a woman experiences several symptoms that indicate life is growing inside her uterus. These signs vary from woman to woman, as anyone who has discussed pregnancy in "girlfriend sessions" will tell you.

Confirmation of pregnancy is by fetal movement, fetal heart sounds, and ultrasound.

The first signs typically are:

* Missed menstrual period
* Nausea and vomiting (morning sickness)
* Enlargement and tenderness of breasts and abdomen
* Frequent urination
* Sleepiness and fatigue
* Mood swings (resulting from hormonal changes)
* Increased secretions and discharge from vagina

A woman with any combination of these symptoms might suspect pregnancy. The usual course of action is to confirm these suspicions through a pregnancy test. The woman may have the test done at a health practitioner's office or may purchase one of the over-the-counter (OTC) pregnancy test kits available at most pharmacies or retail outlets that sell feminine products. These tests all are designed to confirm the presence of the hormone HCG, which is present in the urine and the bloodstream of the woman if she is pregnant. HCG can be detected in the blood before it is detectable in the urine. Laboratory tests for pregnancy are more accurate (about 98%) than OTC home pregnancy tests. Following the manufacturer's instructions exactly will reduce the chances of false positive or false negative results.

The more definite signs of pregnancy begin to appear in the second trimester of pregnancy. When they do, there is no doubt that the woman has a fetus in her uterus. Confirmation is by:

1. Fetal movement
2. Fetal heart sounds
3. Discovery of fetus by ultrasound or x-ray.

Because radiation can damage the fetus, a pregnant woman should avoid x-rays and notify any health practitioner of her suspected or confirmed pregnancy if she is scheduled to be exposed to radioactive materials.

Prenatal Care

Regular medical visits should be scheduled as soon as the pregnancy is confirmed. This scheduled maintenance of the mother and the expected baby is vital to the health of the mother and the fetus as well. During these regular medical examinations the health of the mother and fetus is monitored. If any problems arise, they can be taken care of before they become too serious and threaten the life of the mother, the survival of the fetus, or the health of the baby after delivery.

The National Center for Health Statistics in 1992 surveyed medical risk factors by race of the mother and found that major risks were higher for American Indian mothers than for any other racial or ethnic group. For example, the incidence of pregnancy-related hypertension was four times as high as that for Chinese mothers (the lowest-incidence group for hypertension).

In prenatal care the mother receives periodic physical examinations, including blood and urine tests, to monitor her health status and development of the fetus. She also receives instructions and advice about nutrition and weight, exercise, and medications to enhance the chances of delivering a healthy baby.

Nutrition is particularly important for both the mother and the developing fetus. For example, if the mother's diet is low in iron or calcium, the fetus

KEY TERMS

Pituitary gland a pea-sized body in the brain, which releases hormones including FSH and LH

Follicle-stimulating hormone (FSH) a hormone that stimulates growth of the follicle in the ovary and spermatogenesis in the testes

Luteinizing hormone (LH) a hormone that stimulates ovulation in females and testosterone in males

Corpus luteum enlarged follicle from which ovulation that secretes progesterone originated

Fertilization union of egg and sperm cells; conception

Zygote fertilized egg

Conception the start of pregnancy, when a sperm cell fertilizes an egg cell

Multiple birth birth of twins, triplets, or more babies

Fraternal twins two babies conceived about the same time as the result of fertilization of two egg cells

Identical twins two babies conceived at the same time as the result of a single fertilized egg that divides into two cells that develop separately

Embryo product of conception from weeks 2 through 7

Implantation attachment of embryo to lining of the uterus

Human chorionic gonadotrophin (HCG) a hormone produced by the placenta that signals the pituitary gland is not to release FSH and LH

Pregnancy condition of having a developing embryo or fetus in the uterus

takes most of it, resulting in a deficiency in the mother. The old axiom, "You have to eat for two" should not imply that the woman should eat twice as much. She instead has to make sure that her diet contains all the nutrients needed for both. Needs for protein, calcium, vitamins A, B, C, D, and E, iodine, iron, magnesium, and zinc increase as the fetus develops. Intake of folic acid should be doubled during pregnancy. A sensible, well-rounded diet for pregnant women will provide these nutrients, with the possible exception of iron, which often is prescribed to be taken orally.

Various health practitioners can provide prenatal care. Foremost is the **obstetrician**, a medical doctor who specializes in the care of women during pregnancy, delivery, and the period immediately following birth. The other practitioner who has credentials to deliver prenatal care is the **certified nurse-midwife**. This practitioner is a registered nurse who has returned to school to learn to care for women during pregnancy and delivery. The nurse-midwife can administer medication and deliver prenatal care for uncomplicated pregnancies. If medical problems arise during the pregnancy, the nurse-midwife has been educated to identify them and turn over the care of the patient to an obstetrician.

Childbirth classes are offered in most communities. Prospective mothers and fathers alike attend sessions to prepare these soon-to-be parents, training them in what to expect, how to ease the mother's pain, and how to facilitate the birth process. The mother practices a variety of techniques while the father coaches and serves as a support person, helping her breathe and relax.

Prospective parents should recognize the effects on the fetus's health of smoking, drinking alcohol, and taking other drugs. Table 5.4 summarizes the possible effects on the fetus of tobacco, alcohol, and other drugs during pregnancy.

Fetal Tests

Various tests can be done during gestation to gain information about the fetus. These tests include:

1. *Ultrasound.* High-frequency soundwaves create a visual image (sonogram) of the fetus in the uterus, showing the position, size and gestational age, and possible anatomical problems. Sonograms sometimes can reveal the sex of the fetus.

Table 5.4
Effects of Tobacco, Alcohol, and Other Drugs During Pregnancy

Substance	Possible Effects
Tobacco	Spontaneous abortion
	Separation of placenta
	Bleeding during pregnancy
	Brain damage from reduced oxygen
	Abnormal breathing
	Sudden infant death syndrome (SIDS)
	Ear nose and throat infections
	Bronchitis
	Pneumonia
	Asthmatic attacks
	Decreased lung efficiency
Alcohol	Miscarriage
	Low birthweight
	Contaminated breast milk
	Fetal alcohol syndrome (FAS)
	Growth retardation
	Facial abnormalities
	Brain damage
	Heart defects
	Poor muscle coordination
	Hearing impairment
	Developmental delay (motor, social, language)
Other Drugs (cocaine, heroin)	Spontaneous abortion
	Separation of placenta
	Low birthweight
	Brain damage
	Learning disabilities
	Short attention span
	Severe behavioral problems
	Sudden infant death syndrome (SIDS)
	Neonatal abstinence syndrome (NAS)

2. *Alpha-fetoprotein (AFP) screening.* This test analyzes AFP levels in a sample of the mother's blood. High levels may indicate neural tube defects such as anencephaly (part or all of the brain is missing) and spina bifida. Low levels of AFP may indicate a chromosomal defect such as Down syndrome. This test usually is done between 15 and 20 weeks into the pregnancy.

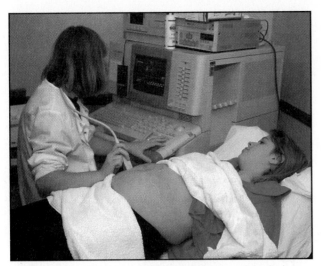
Ultrasound testing can determine position of the baby, any abnormalities, and often the sex.

3. *Amniocentesis.* In this test fluid is removed from the uterus through a long, thin needle inserted through the abdominal wall and the uterus into the amniotic sac. Genetic analysis of the fetal cells in the fluid can reveal possible birth defects and sex of the fetus. It usually is done about 16 weeks into gestation.

4. *Chorionic villus sampling (CVS).* As a newer alternative to amniocentesis, a tiny piece of chorionic villi, containing fetal cells, is removed through the cervix using a catheter. CVS can be performed between the 9th and 11th weeks of pregnancy.

Gestation

The period of **gestation** may be divided into 3-month periods called **trimesters**. A full-term pregnancy has three trimesters.

First Trimester After fertilization, the egg divides in half within about 30 hours, the first of many divisions. On about the fourth day the cluster of cells reaches the uterus, and on the sixth or seventh day is attached to the lining of the uterus. Just one week after conception the little mass of cells is considered an embryo. Between the second and ninth weeks all the major body structures are formed, and some — the heart, liver, testes — begin to function. This is a particularly vulnerable time for damage if the mother has an infection or uses drugs (discussed in Chapters 6, 12, and 13). By the end of the second month the embryo is considered a fetus

and at the end of the first trimester is about 4" long and weighs about an ounce.

The three structures that are vital to survival of the fetus are the placenta (afterbirth), the amniotic sac, and the umbilical cord (navel cord). These structures must develop at the beginning of the first trimester.

1. The **placenta** is a structure about the size of a pie pan, attached directly to the endometrium. Through this structure nutrients, gases, and waste materials are exchanged from mother to fetus and fetus to mother. The placenta is not necessary for the fetus to survive after delivery; therefore it is expelled. Its other name, afterbirth, is certainly appropriate.

2. The **amniotic sac**, or amnion, is a transparent but tough membrane that surrounds the fetus like a balloon. This sac is filled with amniotic fluid and serves as a climate-controlled environment for the developing fetus. It cushions the fetus and protects it from external bumps and jars. Cells that have sloughed from the skin of the fetus float in this amniotic fluid. To prevent the fetus from becoming waterlogged, mucus plugs the nose and throat, and the skin is covered by a substance called vernix.

3. The **umbilical cord** is a bundle of blood vessels that tethers the fetus, which floats freely in the amniotic sac, to the placenta. One end of the umbilical cord is attached to the placenta and the other to the fetus's abdomen. Materials from the placenta pass back and forth through the cord from the mother to the developing

KEY TERMS

Obstetrician medical doctor who specializes in the care of women during pregnancy, delivery, and the period immediately following birth

Certified nurse-midwife registered nurse who specializes in caring for women during pregnancy and delivery

Gestation period from conception to birth (259–287 days)

Trimesters the three 3-month periods of pregnancy

Placenta organ through which fetus receives nourishment and empties waste via mother's circulatory system; the afterbirth

Amniotic sac (amnion) tough, transparent membrane that surrounds the fetus like a balloon

Umbilical cord strand of tissue connecting the fetus to the placenta, through which fetus receives nourishment

fetus. After the child is born, the umbilical cord is tied, severed, and discarded along with the placenta, to which most of it still is attached.

Second Trimester   At the beginning of the second trimester, the mother's abdomen is obviously distended, and she usually can feel the fetus's movements between the 16th and 18th weeks. The fetus's hair is starting to appear, along with eyelashes and eyebrows, and the eyes are open. The fetus makes sucking movements. During this period of major growth, the fetus must receive adequate food, oxygen, and water through the placenta.

Third Trimester   The fetus gains the most weight during the last 3 months, and in rare cases fetuses born at the beginning of this trimester have survived. By the 34th week the fetus probably would survive outside the uterus, with proper care. The fetus's food intake must include calcium, iron, and nitrogen, derived from the food the mother eats. Mainly, the fetus is acquiring a fat layer and refining its respiratory and digestive organs, as well as gaining immunity from certain communicable diseases for a period after birth. Figure 5.7 traces fetal development.

Changes in the Mother's Body   Figure 5.8 illustrates the changes that transform the mother's body during pregnancy. These can be summarized as:

❋ Enlarged pituitary gland because of increased hormonal secretions

❋ Patches of pigmentation on the face

❋ Enlarged thyroid gland

❋ Slightly enlarged heart

❋ Raised diaphragm to allow the developing fetus more room

❋ Enlarged breasts and pigmented streaks on breast; darkened areola and enlarged nipples

❋ Enlarged cortex of adrenal glands

❋ "Stretch marks" on abdomen and breasts

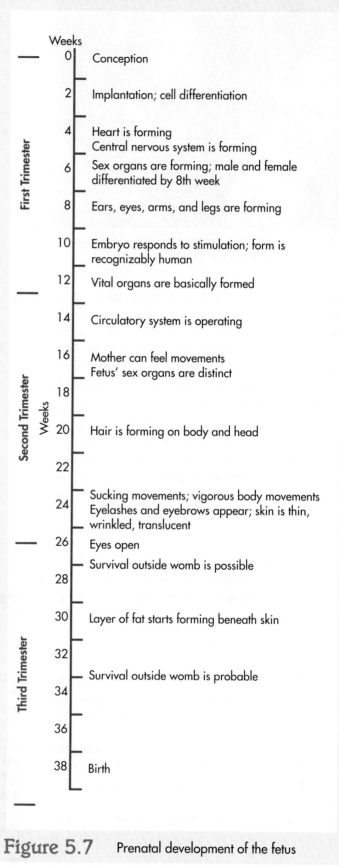

Figure 5.7   Prenatal development of the fetus

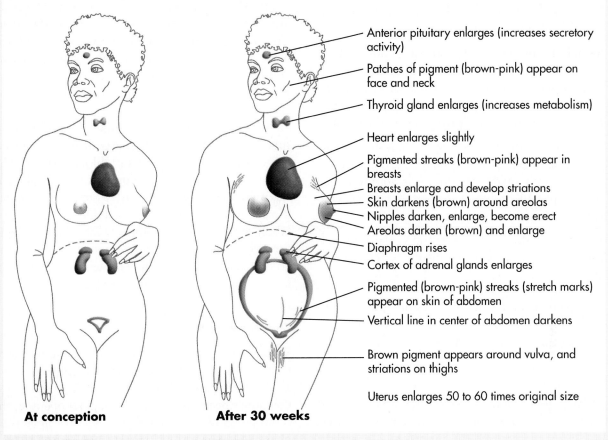

Labels in figure:

At conception

After 30 weeks

Anterior pituitary enlarges (increases secretory activity)

Patches of pigment (brown-pink) appear on face and neck

Thyroid gland enlarges (increases metabolism)

Heart enlarges slightly

Pigmented streaks (brown-pink) appear in breasts

Breasts enlarge and develop striations

Skin darkens (brown) around areolas

Nipples darken, enlarge, become erect

Areolas darken (brown) and enlarge

Diaphragm rises

Cortex of adrenal glands enlarges

Pigmented (brown-pink) streaks (stretch marks) appear on skin of abdomen

Vertical line in center of abdomen darkens

Brown pigment appears around vulva, and striations on thighs

Uterus enlarges 50 to 60 times original size

Figure 5.8   Changes in mother's body during pregnancy

* Vertical brown line down the center of abdomen
* Uterus enlarged to 50–60 times its original size

Throughout pregnancy the uterus contracts periodically, known as **Braxton-Hicks contractions**. At the end of pregnancy these may be confused with labor pains.

Birth

When a pregnancy terminates or ends by a live birth, it is known as **parturition**. This is accomplished through the process of labor — certainly an appropriate term for the work involved! **Labor** is defined as regular contraction of the uterus and dilation of the cervix for the purpose of expelling the fetus and the placenta. No matter how long this process takes, labor is divided into three stages: dilation, delivery of the fetus, and delivery of the placenta. Decisions regarding anesthesia must be made.

Anesthesia

General anesthesia, once the norm, now is used rarely during childbirth. It slows contractions, causes sluggishness, and may precipitate respiratory problems in the baby. The common forms of anesthesia used today are:

1. **Pudendal block.** A local anesthetic is injected through the wall of the vagina or the skin of the buttock to desensitize the pudendal nerve. This

KEY TERMS

Braxton-Hicks contractions normal uterine contractions that occur periodically throughout pregnancy

Parturition live birth at end of pregnancy

Labor regular contraction of the uterus and dilation of the cervix to expel the fetus

Pudendal block a local anesthetic that eliminates feeling from the lower vagina

eliminates pain and feeling from the lower vagina.

2. **Paracervical block.** A local anesthetic is injected around the opening of the uterus.

3. **Spinal anesthesia.** A solution containing a local anesthetic is injected between the fourth and fifth vertebrae of the lower back into the fluid-filled sac surrounding the spinal cord. This blocks the pain messages from below the waist.

4. **Epidural anesthesia.** The anesthetic is injected at the same place as the spinal anesthetic, but, rather than a single injection, it is administered over a period of hours through a tiny plastic tube.

5. **Caudal anesthesia.** This method is the same as the epidural except that the tube is inserted at the tip of the spine.

Both caudal and epidural anesthesia can slow labor if administered too soon, so they are not given until the woman is in active labor.

Dilation

The first stage of labor is the longest. Anyone who has delivered a baby will attest that it is not the easiest. During this time the uterus is contracting and the opening to the cervix of the uterus also is getting wider to allow the fetus to emerge (Figure 5.9). This process is called **dilation** or **dilatation**. The cervix has to dilate (open) 10 centimeters, or about 4", for the fetus to pass through. The cervix also becomes thinner, a process termed **effacement**. The transition phase of this first stage of labor is most painful, and the mother may be nauseous and vomit. During transition the cervix dilates most rapidly, from about 7 centimeters until it reaches complete dilation.

Another event that may take place during the first stage of labor is a discharge from the widened cervix of a mucous plug or "bloody show" that serves as a stopper. This plug was held in place by the undilated cervix. In most women the amniotic sac or "bag of waters" ruptures during this stage of labor. Some first-time mothers mistake this liquid for urine. If the rupture occurs too soon before labor begins, the fetus is exposed to microorganisms in the vagina that may cause an infection.

Delivery of the Fetus

When the cervix is fully dilated, the fetus moves from the uterus into the vagina, which now serves as the birth canal (Figure 5.10). When the top of the baby's head appears at the vaginal opening, this is aptly known as **crowning**. At this time some physicians perform an **episiotomy**, a surgical procedure in which they make an incision from the bottom of the vaginal opening toward the anus (the

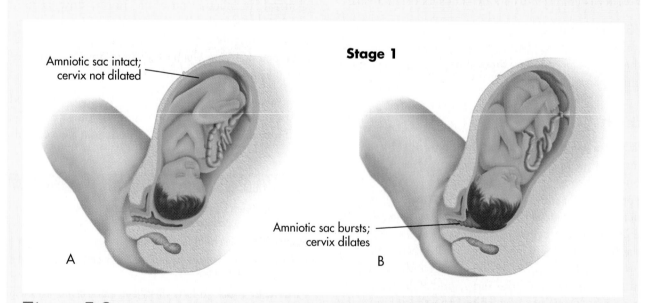

Amniotic sac intact; cervix not dilated

Stage 1

Amniotic sac bursts; cervix dilates

A

B

Figure 5.9 (A) Position of fetus in uterus before delivery; (B) First stage of labor

Stage 2

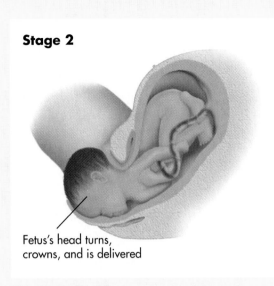

Fetus's head turns, crowns, and is delivered

Figure 5.10   Delivery of the fetus

perineal area) to prevent the vagina from tearing during the second stage of labor. Other medical professionals believe this procedure need not be standard for every delivery. Before the delivery the woman should discuss with her physician the need for an episiotomy.

During this second stage of labor, muscular contractions of the uterus should continue at regular intervals, and the mother is asked to push with each contraction. Strong contractions force the baby to be delivered, usually head-first. After the head emerges, the baby's body rotates, and a continuing wave of strong contractions allows the shoulders and upper body to emerge. Additional contractions deliver the legs and feet. When the baby is out of the vagina, the mother's contractions subside for several minutes. The umbilical cord is tied and cut during this time.

The baby is wet and covered with a waxy substance called **vernix**. The head usually is misshapen because of the narrow passageway it has traversed. The bones are flexible enough at this time to resume a normal appearance within a day or so. The birth process squeezes air out of the baby's lungs, but once the baby is born, the chest can expand and fill with air for the first time. The baby announces this event by crying loudly. Between 1 and 5 minutes after birth, the baby's condition is assessed for heart rate, respiration, color, reflexes, and muscle tone. The resulting **Apgar score** provides a quick indication as to the infant's physical status.

Delivery of the Placenta

Because the baby now has made "other living arrangements," the fetal materials left behind are no longer needed by either the baby or the mother. The placenta (afterbirth) is a flat structure about 8" in diameter and weighing approximately a pound. Contractions of the uterus are necessary to dislodge the placenta from the uterus. As it separates or peels itself from the uterus where it was attached, contractions push it and the umbilical cord attached to it out of the vagina (Figure 5.11). When this occurs, the final or third stage of labor is complete.

Stage 3

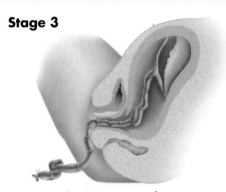

Placenta separates from uterus and is delivered

Figure 5.11   Delivery of the placenta

KEY TERMS

Paracervical block a local anesthetic injected around opening of the uterus

Spinal anesthesia solution containing local anesthetic to block pain

Epidural anesthesia spinal anesthesia administered over a period of hours

Caudal anesthesia similar to an epidural, but injected at tip of the spine

Dilation (dilatation) opening of the cervix to 10 centimeters; occurs during first stage of labor

Effacement thinning of cervix during labor

Crowning the top of the fetus's head appearing at the vaginal opening

Episiotomy procedure in which an incision is made from the bottom of the vaginal opening toward the anus to prevent tearing of vagina

Vernix waxy coating on skin of a fetus and newborn

Apgar score an evaluation of baby's health at birth based on heart rate, respiration, color, reflexes, and muscle tone; maximum score is 10

The uterus must stay contracted after the third stage of labor to prevent **hemorrhage** (excessive blood loss). This can be accomplished by massaging the mother's abdomen after delivery of the placenta. A natural way to stimulate uterine contractions is to allow the newborn to suck the mother's nipples. Either method encourages the uterus to contract and become firm so the mother will not have complications from excessive bleeding after delivery. Failure of the placenta to be expelled completely can cause the mother to hemorrhage. Therefore, the delivered placenta is inspected carefully. If any piece from it is left behind, it has to be removed.

Postpartum Period

With reference to the mother, the period of approximately 3 months after childbirth is called **postpartum**. The pre-birth to post-birth transition often is difficult physically and psychologically. The uterus continues to contract for several days after the birth as it returns to its normal size. The woman's reproductive system requires about 6 to 8 weeks to assume its prebirth condition. A bloody discharge called **lochia** may last several weeks after the birth. The psychological adjustment is more difficult to define, and it is specific to each woman and her circumstances. Nevertheless, it is real and merits attention. If the woman falls into a deep or persistent depression, medical attention should be sought.

The production of milk, **lactation**, begins about 3 days following childbirth. Before that the breasts secrete a yellowish liquid called **colostrum**, which contains antibodies that help the newborn ward off infectious diseases; it also is a source of protein. Breast-feeding is recommended over bottle feeding nowadays because breast milk is most suited to the baby's nutritional and digestive needs. Breast-feeding also stimulates contractions that help the uterus return to normal and may contribute to weight loss after pregnancy.

Complications of Pregnancy and Birth

Although most pregnancies are normal and progress to full term and delivery, a variety of complications can develop at any time. Some of these problems are Rh incompatibility, eclampsia,

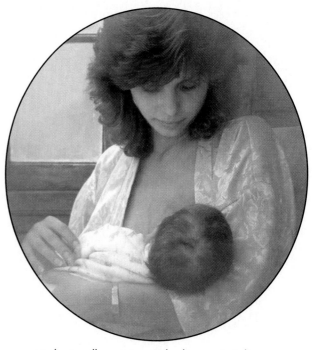

Mother's milk contains antibodies against disease.

toxoplasmosis, ectopic pregnancy, spontaneous abortion, breech presentation, and cesarean section, among others.

Rh Incompatibility

Among the traits inherited from the mother and father is blood type, as well as the presence or absence of a chemical in the bloodstream called the rhesus factor or **Rh factor**. About 85% of the population has inherited this chemical, and these individuals are designated Rh$^+$. The remaining 15%, who do not have this chemical, are designated Rh$^-$.

If the mother is Rh$^-$ and the fetus she carries is Rh$^+$, a problem could develop. Even though the circulatory systems of the mother and fetus are completely separate, small amounts of blood from the fetus may leak into the mother's circulatory system during the third trimester. The Rh$^-$ mother does not have this chemical, so her body responds by producing antibodies to protect her from the Rh$^+$ chemical invasion. These antibodies, which protect the mother, pass through the placenta to her fetus. What protects the mother now becomes a health hazard to the fetus. The antibodies can destroy the fetus's red blood cells, causing jaundice, severe anemia, and other complications, which may lead to death.

The Rh factor usually is not a problem in the first pregnancy because the mother does not produce enough antibodies to harm the fetus. If a subsequent fetus is Rh$^+$, however, the mother's system is alerted to invading chemicals and quickly activates the antibodies, which can pose a serious threat to the health of the new fetus.

Today a vaccine called **RhoGAM** has made most complications of Rh incompatibility preventable. A dose of RhoGAM is administered to the Rh$^-$ mother between weeks 28 and 32 of pregnancy. Another dose is given within 72 hours after delivery. This vaccine eliminates any Rh$^+$ chemical of the fetus from maternal circulation before the mother becomes sensitized and makes Rh$^+$ antibodies that would harm the fetus.

The poet Carl Sandburg wrote:
"The first cry of a newborn baby
in Chicago, or Zamboango,
in Amsterdam, or Rangoon,
each has the same pitch
and key, each saying 'I am,
I have come through! I belong!
I am a member of the family.'"

Eclampsia

High blood pressure can result from pregnancy for unknown reasons. Known as **eclampsia**, it occurs during the last trimester. The first indicators, termed preeclampsia, are elevated blood pressure, sudden weight gain, protein in the urine, and edema (swelling from water retention), especially in the face, hands, and feet. If uncontrolled, this condition may become more serious and progress to eclampsia. In eclampsia convulsions accompany the symptoms of preeclampsia.

Risks to the pregnant woman include cerebral hemorrhage (burst blood vessel in the brain), damage to the liver or kidneys, and possible death. In addition, the obvious risk to the fetus is premature labor and delivery. Women at greatest risk for developing preeclampsia are:

— teens
— women over 35 years old
— women with blood relatives who had the condition
— women with inadequate diets (malnourished)
— women who had hypertension before pregnancy

Preeclampsia usually can be treated by adjusting the diet. African American women are at greater risk for this complication of pregnancy.

Complications From Maternal Heart Disease

If a woman has a known heart condition before pregnancy, both mother and baby are at higher risk. Diet becomes particularly important, as well as abstention from smoking and drinking alcohol. Any medications should be approved by a physician.

A woman who has congenital (present at her birth) heart disease has a greater risk of having a baby with a heart defect. A fetal ultrasound test may detect such an abnormality.

Gestational Diabetes

A unique form of diabetes is called **gestational diabetes**, diagnosed in about 3% to 5% of pregnant women in the United States. It differs from the other forms (discussed in Chapter 7) because it begins during pregnancy and disappears after delivery. Risk factors for gestational diabetes are:

— obesity
— family history of diabetes
— previous birth of a large baby, a stillbirth, or a child with a birth defect
— too much amniotic fluid
— women older than 25 years

A major problem affects the baby through an abnormality known as **macrosomia**, which means

KEY TERMS

Postpartum the first 3 months after childbirth

Lochia discharge of blood and mucus that may last several weeks after childbirth

Lactation milk secretion from the breasts

Colostrum yellowish liquid secreted from the breasts; contains antibodies and protein

Rh factor chemical in bloodstream of most people that can cause complications during pregnancy when a mother who is Rh$^-$ (no Rh chemical) carries an Rh$^+$ fetus

RhoGAM vaccine to counteract complications of Rh incompatibility

Eclampsia high blood pressure during pregnancy

Gestational diabetes form of diabetes (a metabolic disorder) that occurs only during pregnancy

Macrosomia literally, "large body," referring to a condition in which fetus converts extra glucose from mother to fat

"large body." The fetus converts extra glucose received from the mother to fat. The resulting high blood glucose and high insulin levels result in large deposits of fat in the fetus. Sometimes the baby grows too large to be delivered vaginally, and a cesarean section becomes necessary. In addition, gestational diabetes increases the risk of hypoglycemia (low blood sugar) in the fetus immediately after delivery, when it no longer receives sugar input from the mother but retains the high insulin level. Other complications include congenital defects and stillbirth. African American diabetic women, for some reason, are more likely than other diabetic women to lose their babies during and after birth.

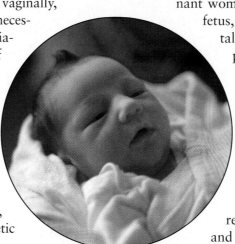

A mother's proper self-care will help promote a healthy baby.

The Council on Diabetes in Pregnancy (American Diabetes Foundation) strongly recommends that all pregnant women be screened for gestational diabetes. The most common of the several tests is the 50-gram glucose test. Complications of gestational diabetes are manageable and preventable. The key is to control blood sugar through a diet prescribed by a qualified practitioner. The woman should use salt in moderation, cut down on caffeine intake, avoid sugars and fats in the diet and emphasize complex carbohydrates, dietary fibers, iron, calcium, and protein. She also should avoid smoking and drinking alcohol.

German Measles

German measles, officially termed **rubella,** formerly was a common concern during pregnancy. Immunization at least 3 months prior to pregnancy can rule out this disease as a risk factor to the baby (it is relatively innocuous in adults). If a pregnant women has rubella during the first 3 months of pregnancy, the fetus has a 20% to 30% risk of damage to the eyes, ears, brain, or heart. This virus also can cause spontaneous abortion, low birthweight, or stillbirth. The best course of action is to become immunized before contemplating pregnancy.

Toxoplasmosis

Toxoplasmosis, resulting from exposure to a parasite when preparing or eating uncooked meat or handling a cat's litter box, presents another risk. This disease is caused by an organism that lives in the intestines of many mammals and birds. Toxoplasmosis tends to be mild in adults, but if a pregnant woman transmits the organism to her fetus, it may produce blindness or mental retardation. Precautions are simple: Thoroughly cook all meat, and wash your hands after handling pets. Do not handle the cat's litter box.

Sexually Transmitted Diseases

Sexually transmitted diseases, discussed in Chapter 6, pose a real threat to developing fetuses and can leave lingering problems. Syphilis carries increased risk for miscarriage, and infected infants have greater risk for premature death, low birthweight, mental retardation, and chronic health problems. Untreated gonorrhea reduces a woman's chances of becoming pregnant, and if she does, it increases the risk for miscarriage. A woman who has active herpes at the time of delivery should have a cesarean section so the newborn will not be exposed to the virus in the birth canal. Infection in a newborn can cause blindness, mental retardation, neurological problems, and even death. Children born to HIV/AIDS-infected mothers tragically may have the disease also. Their symptoms and prognosis, like those of adults, paint a bleak picture for these children.

Ectopic Pregnancy

Implantation outside of the uterus is termed **ectopic pregnancy.** This usually occurs in some portion of the fallopian tube, although the fertilized egg may attach itself to the ovary or within the abdominal cavity. At highest risk for this dangerous condition are women who have had a prior ectopic pregnancy, women who have had pelvic inflammatory disease (PID) as a result of gonorrhea or chlamydia, and women who use the intrauterine device (IUD) contraceptive. The rates of ectopic pregnancy are increasing and may range from one in 65 to one in 200 normal pregnancies.

Signals of ectopic pregnancy include sweating, faintness and dizziness, rapid pulse, falling blood

Tips for action

To reduce complications during pregnancy, at delivery, and after delivery:

1. Begin prenatal care as soon as you know you are pregnant. If you cannot afford prenatal care from a private physician, it is available through your local public health department. Prenatal care is important for:

   a. consistent monitoring of the status of the mother and fetus.

   b. consistent monitoring of the mother's weight gain.

   c. consistent monitoring of the mother's nutritional needs.

2. Do not use any psychoactive substances, including tobacco and alcohol, during pregnancy. Drug use may cause problems in the pregnancy and damage the unborn baby.

3. Do not become pregnant without being certain that you have been inoculated against German measles.

4. If indicated, have any of the fetal tests defined in this chapter.

---

pressure, and abdominal pain. Because hormone production to prevent shedding of the endometrium is reduced, another symptom of ectopic pregnancy is vaginal bleeding in the form of spotting. The greatest risk to the pregnant woman is internal hemorrhage. A woman who suspects an ectopic pregnancy should seek medical attention immediately. The problem can be corrected by removing the contents of the affected fallopian tube surgically (possible in early diagnosis), by removing the entire fallopian tube, or, if necessary, by removing the uterus.

Spontaneous Abortion

A pregnancy that terminates itself prior to the 20th week is known as **spontaneous abortion,** or **miscarriage,** as it is commonly called. Most spontaneous abortions occur during the first trimester. The causes of spontaneous abortions are variable and may be related to a genetic defect of the fetus, infection, hormonal disturbances, alcohol intake, and even cigarette smoking. An estimated 10% to 40% of all pregnancies end this way. About 60% are attributed to chromosomal abnormalities in the fetus.

The signals for impending spontaneous abortion are vaginal bleeding and abdominal cramps. If the cervix continues to dilate, fetal and placental

tissue pass into the vagina. Vaginal bleeding should be reported immediately to the health care provider. Bed rest and refraining from intercourse are the tried-and-true recommendations to stop an impending spontaneous abortion. If tissue is being passed, the process cannot be reversed. When the pregnant woman reports to the hospital, dilation and curettage (D&C) is done to remove from the uterus all fetal membranes that were not expelled if the spontaneous abortion was incomplete. This is done to prevent further complications.

Breech Presentation

In a normal delivery the top of the baby's head emerges first. If the fetus is positioned so the buttocks are seen or touched first, it is termed **breech presentation.** About 3% of full-term

KEY TERMS

German measles (rubella) viral infection that can damage eyes, ears, brain, or heart of the fetus during pregnancy if the mother contracts the disease

Toxoplasmosis parasitic disease resulting from exposure to uncooked meat or cat litter; can produce blindness or mental retardation in fetus

Ectopic pregnancy implantation outside of the uterus

Spontaneous abortion (miscarriage) termination of pregnancy prior to 20th week; contents of uterus are expelled

pregnancies are breech. Breech presentations are more likely if the fetus is premature or if the mother is carrying more than one fetus in her uterus. To avoid complications for the mother and the fetus, a medical decision has to be made quickly whether to deliver the fetus in the breech position or perform a cesarean section.

Cesarean Section

Occasionally the mother cannot deliver her baby through the vagina. When this situation arises, the fetus is removed through an opening created by a surgical incision through the mother's abdomen and uterus. This procedure is called a **cesarean section** or **C-section**. Typically, cesarean delivery is performed under local anesthesia. Because this procedure involves surgery, it is more complicated than vaginal delivery.

Cesareans typically are performed when the fetus's head is larger than the mother's pelvic girdle or if the fetus is in an unusual position. If the mother has health problems such as heart disease, diabetes, high blood pressure, or eclampsia, a C-section may ease the strain of a long labor and delivery. If the baby is in some sort of distress, such as having the umbilical cord pinched, or is subject to infection through vaginal delivery, a C-section may be indicated.

Critics of the growing reliance and possible overuse of cesarean section believe that many of these surgeries are done unnecessarily. Estimates of C-sections range from one in ten of all births to as many as one in four. The risk for maternal death is higher than that for vaginal delivery. Healthy People 2000 has a goal of reducing C-sections to no more than 15% of births by the year 2000.

MATERNAL AND INFANT MORTALITY

In 1991, 323 women died of maternal causes. This number does not include all deaths occurring to pregnant women but only to deaths from complications of pregnancy, childbirth, and the puerperium (the 42-day period following childbirth). Minority women have a higher risk for maternal death than Anglo-American women do. The rate for African American women is highest of all — three times the rate for Anglo-American women.

The infant mortality rate (IMR) in 1991 was the lowest ever recorded in the United States (see Figure 5.12). IMR is defined as the number of babies in every 1,000 born who die within the first year of life. Neonatal (newborn) mortality rates historically have declined for all racial and ethnic groups, although the declines have been more rapid for the Anglo-American population. Figure 5.13 gives the leading causes of infant mortality.

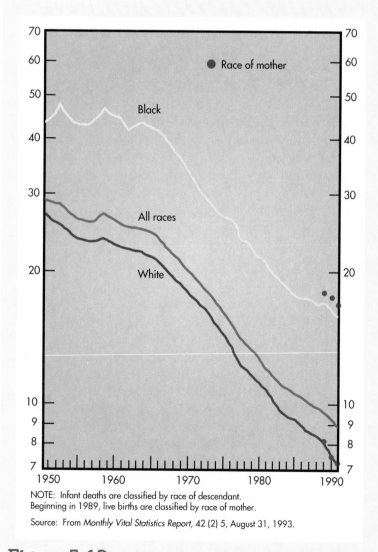

NOTE: Infant deaths are classified by race of descendant.
Beginning in 1989, live births are classified by race of mother.

Source: From *Monthly Vital Statistics Report*, 42 (2) 5, August 31, 1993.

Figure 5.12 Trends in infant mortality rates in United States

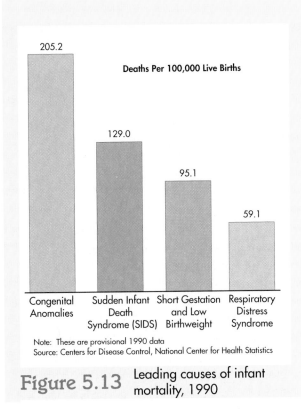

Deaths Per 100,000 Live Births

205.2 — Congenital Anomalies

129.0 — Sudden Infant Death Syndrome (SIDS)

95.1 — Short Gestation and Low Birthweight

59.1 — Respiratory Distress Syndrome

Note: These are provisional 1990 data
Source: Centers for Disease Control, National Center for Health Statistics

Figure 5.13 Leading causes of infant mortality, 1990

The leading cause of infant mortaility is a group of defects called **congenital anomalies,** a wide range of conditions that are present in the infant at birth. Some of these are inherited. For example, **Tay Sachs disease,** a fatal enzyme deficiency, occurs almost exclusively among children of Eastern European Jewish ancestry and relates to a genetic defect. Other congenital anomalies are induced by the mother's behavior during pregnancy (for example, smoking cigarettes, drinking alcohol, having nutritional deficiencies).

Ranking second in the IMR statistics are babies who die from **sudden infant death syndrome,** widely known as **SIDS.** Asian-American babies seem to have the lowest risk, and African-American and American Indian babies have the highest risk. This tragic and mysterious disease may not have one single cause. We do know that boys die from SIDS more often than girls do. SIDS tends to occur more than once in families. Some possible causes may be viral infections and allergies. Cigarette smoking by the mother during pregnancy seems to be one of the biggest risk factors for SIDS. Other risk factors are the use of psychoactive drugs such

as cocaine and heroin. Interestingly, more SIDS deaths occur in winter than in summer.

The Office of Minority Health Resource Center (OMH–RC) reports that the infant mortality rate (death rate of babies from birth to age 1) of African-American babies is approximately twice that of Anglo-American babies (coincidentally, pregnant African American women are twice as likely as pregnant Anglo-American women to receive absolutely no prenatal care or care beginning in the last trimester of the pregnancy, and three times as likely to have babies born with defects. Social and economic factors contribute to the alarming disparity in the infant mortality rate between minority groups and Anglo-Americans. Some of these factors are:

— low income and limited medical insurance

— preexisting medical problems

— poor nutrition

— problems with transportation and child care that impede the use of services

— lack of maternal education.

A significant cause of infant mortality is **low birthweight** (defined as weighing less than 5½ pounds at birth). Low birthweight often is attributable to premature birth (about 6 months or less). Many low birthweight babies, however, are born at full term.

The major risk factors for having a low birthweight baby are drinking alcohol during pregnancy, an absence of health care, and teen pregnancy. Of recent concern is the alarming rise in the teen birth rate. From 1986 through 1991 the rate skyrocketed 27%. In 1994, however, the rate

KEY TERMS

Breech presentation positioning of fetus so buttocks are seen first at birth

Cesarean section (C-Section) delivery of fetus through opening in abdomen and uterus created by a surgical incision

Congenital anomalies defects that are present in a baby at birth

Tay-Sachs disease An enzyme deficiency occurring almost exclusively among children of Eastern European Jewish ancestry.

Sudden infant death syndrome (SIDS) death of a baby by an undetermined cause, usually while sleeping at night

Low birthweight weighing less than 5½ pounds at birth

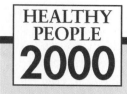

OBJECTIVES FOR PREGNANCY AND BIRTH

❋ Reduce to no more than 30% the proportion of all pregnancies that are unintended.

❋ Reduce infant mortality to a new low of 7 deaths per 1,000 live births.

❋ Reduce the percentage of low-birthweight babies to no more than 5%.

❋ Reduce percentage of cesarean section deliveries to no more than 15% of all deliveries.

dropped 2%, giving a ray of optimism that the pattern may begin to reverse. The Healthy People 2000 objective is to reduce the percentage of babies born at low birthweight to no more than 5%.

INFERTILITY

Amidst rising birth rates and concern about overpopulation, the plight of one group may be overlooked. Many couples — approximately 15% of couples trying to become pregnant — are frustrated and disappointed because they cannot conceive. Approximately one in every seven to twelve American couples that tries to have a baby fails.

According to the American Fertility Society, in 40% of the couples who fail to conceive, the male is the sole contributing cause. In about a fourth of the cases, more than one factor is at work.

Of the many different factors that can cause male infertility, most of the problems relate to sperm production. In most cases the underlying cause is unknown, but some known causes are:

❋ *Testicular disease*, which can result in *azoospermia,* or the complete absence of sperm in the semen

❋ Having *mumps* after puberty

❋ *Hormone deficiencies*

❋ *Varicoceles,* or varicose veins above one or both testicles

❋ An obstruction of the vas deferens (because of infection by sexually transmitted disease, injury, or surgery).

Treatments for male infertility include antibiotic therapy for infection, surgery to correct varicose

veins in the scrotum or obstruction of ducts, and hormones to improve sperm production.

Female contributors to infertility include uterine abnormalities. About 10% to 15% of women with recurrent miscarriages have an abnormality in the structure of the uterus.

❋ *Incompetent cervix.* The cervix cannot support a pregnancy without surgical correction (which usually is successful).

❋ *Septate uterus.* The septum (ridge) protrudes into the uterine cavity. About 3% of the entire female population has this condition, but it does not cause a problem in half of these women.

A hysteroscopy or a special x-ray called a hysterosalpinogram (HSG) can identify abnormalities within the uterus. It also is used to determine if the fallopian tubes are open.

Another cause of female infertility is:

❋ PCOD, *polycystic ovarian disease* (also called Stein-Leventhal syndrome or hyperandrogenism). Basically, this condition involves overproduction of androgen and estrogen, which prevents ovulation and may result in ovarian cysts. The diagnosis is confirmed by measuring blood hormone levels, and an ultrasound may reveal the cysts. Some causes of PCOD are thought to be obesity (fatty tissue produces an excess of estrogen), diabetes, and dysfunctional adrenal glands.

The treatment generally involves weight loss (if overweight), induction of ovulation through

☎ Call for information

American Society for Reproductive Medicine
205-978-5000

injections of HMG drugs, and hormone treatments (low-dose oral contraceptives). In rare cases surgery is done.

Hormonal dysfunctions also may cause a woman to be infertile.

✳ *Luteal phase inadequacy.* The luteal phase of menstruation is crucial to implantation. If progesterone levels are low during this phase, infertility or miscarriage can result because the lining does not develop adequately for the embryo to implant securely. An endometrial biopsy can be used to assess problems related to the luteal phase, and disorders usually are treated by medical prescription.

✳ *Underactive or overactive thyroid gland,* for which diagnosis is made through a simple blood test. Thyroid disorders usually can be treated with medication.

In addition:

✳ *Genetic defects.* The embryo or fetus is found to be defective in an estimated 50% to 60% of first-trimester miscarriages. The most common genetic defect is an abnormal number of chromosomes. If the placenta or the fetus of a woman having her first miscarriage has the normal number of chromosomes, the second pregnancy has only a 50% chance of being abnormal, but if the first pregnancy is genetically abnormal, the chance for an abnormal second pregnancy is greater.

Genetic cause may be diagnosed by a **karyotype** on the fetal tissue and on blood from both parents. A chromosomal analysis usually is recommended for all couples with a history of two or more early pregnancy losses. In about 5%, an abnormality in one parent explains the recurrent miscarriage.

✳ *Infections:* No evidence exists to support the assertion that infections are a cause of pregnancy loss. Chlamydia has been linked to miscarriage, but it is associated more clearly with infertility and tubal infection.

Finally:

✳ *Immunologic causes.* The mother may have antibodies that cause blood clotting, which poses serious risks to pregnant women and inhibits fetal development. This usually leads to miscarriage.

Fertility in men and women alike declines with age, even though the man has the potential to father a child longer than a woman can conceive. Unfortunately, some women delay pregnancy during the time in their life when they are most fertile, only to have problems later. The infertility problem for other couples is really a timing problem. They are not having intercourse during the ovulation phase of the woman's menstrual cycle.

Charting basal body temperature (BBT) throughout the woman's menstrual cycle reveals when ovulation occurs and, thus, when she has the best chance to conceive. The only equipment required is a thermometer. The woman takes her temperature upon waking every morning. If the basal body temperature has gone up for several days, ovulation has occurred. Figure 5.14 presents a BBT chart. The spaces with Xs indicate days of menstruation. Couples wishing to conceive should have intercourse at the time of ovulation.

Some possible solutions to infertility are:

1. *Boxer shorts.* Men wearing jockey shorts may keep the groin area too warm and reduce the activity of the sperm. Boxer shorts are an attested remedy for many.

2. *Fertility drugs.* Clomid and Serophene act on the hypothalamus, and Pergonal acts on the pituitary gland to ultimately stimulate egg or sperm production. Fertility drugs may be prescribed if one or both partners has a hormone imbalance, but these drugs do have side effects, and some increase the probability for multiple births.

3. *Surgery.* In some cases microsurgery may be done to remove scar tissue that is blocking the fallopian tubes in the female or the vas deferens in the male.

4. *Tubal ovum transfer.* In **tubal ovum transfer** the woman's eggs are retrieved and placed into the end of the fallopian tube that opens to the uterus. The couple has intercourse or the woman is artificially inseminated.

KEY TERMS

Karyotype photograph of a cell during cell division; shows chromosomes in order of size from largest to smallest; used to detect chromosome defects

Tubal ovum transfer retrieval and placement of a woman's eggs into the end of fallopian tube

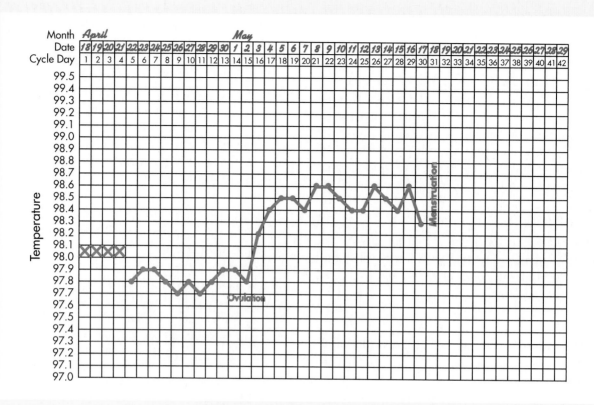

Figure 5.14   Basal body temperature (BBT) chart

5. *Artificial insemination.* Using the technique of **artificial insemination**, sperm from the artificial insemination-husband (AIH) or the artificial insemination-donor (AID) are introduced into the woman's uterus via a catheter (a hollow tube) when the woman is ovulating. Ovulation may be natural, or it may be induced by a fertility drug.

   a. **Gamete intrafallopian transfer (GIFT).** Sperm and eggs are collected, mixed, and inserted immediately into the fallopian tube. To complete this procedure, the fallopian tube must be healthy.

   b. **In vitro fertilization.** Several egg cells are harvested from the woman and placed into a glass dish, where they are incubated with donor sperm. The fertilized eggs are implanted into the woman's uterus. In 1978 Louise Joy Brown from England became the first "test tube baby." Many more have been born since that time. Assisted reproductive technology has raised ethical and moral questions that are being debated by

ethicists, scientists, theologians, and legislators worldwide.

ADOPTION

A final option for those who want children is adoption. Each agency has different requirements concerning age, religion, race, and so on, so a couple sometimes has to check with several to find one that is compatible with their needs. Some variations on adoption are:

1. *Closed versus open.* In the past, **closed adoption** was the standard. This means that the biological

KEY TERMS

Artificial insemination medical procedure in which sperm are placed into uterus via a catheter

Gamete intrafallopian transfer (GIFT) eggs and sperm are collected and inserted into fallopian tube

In vitro fertilization procedure in which a woman's eggs are placed in a glass dish and incubated with donor sperm

Closed adoption adoption in which exchange of parental information is not allowed

☎ Call for information

National Council on Adoption
202-328-1200

North American Council on Adoptable Children
(NACAC)
612-644-3036

parents and the adoptive parents had little or no knowledge of each other and in no circumstances were the biological parents allowed contact with their biological child. The adoption records were closed to all the parties involved. More recently, **open adoption** is gaining acceptance with legal underpinnings. This usually means limited exchange of information and contact between the birth parents and the adoptive parents. Some agencies allow the birth parents to choose the adoptive couple from preselected prospects.

2. *Infant and older child adoption.* To adopt an infant usually requires that the adoptive adult be under a certain age, usually 35 to 45. Older couples are encouraged to adopt older children. Many agencies require at least 15 years between the age of the adoptive parents and the age of the child.

3. *Interractial adoption.* Agencies differ in their requirements regarding adopting a child of a race different from the prospective parents'. The rationale is that different races have different value systems, customs, and traditions and will encounter difficulties that would not be present in same-race adoption.

4. *Special needs adoption.* "Special needs" refers to a child who is not totally physically or emotionally healthy. Adopting a special needs child requires a tremendous commitment of time and energy.

KEY TERMS

Open adoption adoption in which some parental information is exchanged and some contact is allowed between the birth parents and the adoptive parents

Summary

1 Males have an X and Y chromosome, and females have two Xs; the male, therefore, determines the offspring's sex.

2 Three common disorders of the female reproductive system are endometriosis, uterine fibroid tumors, and premenstrual syndrome (PMS).

3 The sexual response has four phases: excitement, plateau, orgasmic, and resolution.

4 Sexual problems include vaginal dryness and vaginismus in the female and impotence and premature ejaculation in the male.

5 The typical menstrual cycle is 28 days, with four segments: menses, estrogenic, ovulation, and progestational.

6 Various tests to gain information about the fetus include ultrasound, alpha-fetoprotein (AFP) screening, amniocentesis, and chorionic villus sampling (CVS).

7 Types of anesthetic used during delivery are the pudendal block, paracervical block, spinal anesthesia, epidural anesthesia, and caudal anesthesia.

8 Complications during birth and delivery include Rh incompatibility, ecalmpsia, complications from maternal heart disease, gestational diabetes, German measles, toxoplasmosis, sexually transmitted diseases (to baby), ectopic pregnancy, spontaneous abortion (miscarriage), breech presentation, and other conditions that may necessitate a cesarean section.

9 Infant mortality is most often the result of congenital anomalies, sudden infant death syndrome (SIDS), and low birthweight.

10 Measures to correct infertility include fertility drugs, surgery, tubal ovum transfer, and artificial insemination.

11 Adoptions can be closed, open, interracial, older children, and children with special needs.

Select Bibliography

Arriaga, E. E. "Changing Trends in Mortality Decline During the Last Decades," edited by L. Ruzicka, G. Wunsch, and P. Kane, editors. *Differential Mortality: Methodological Issues and Biosocial Factors.* Oxford: Clarendon Press, 1989.

Dixon, Barbara. *Good Health for African Americans.* New York: Crown, 1994.

Editors of Consumer Guide. *Family Medical & Prescription Guide.* Lincolnwood, IL: Publications International, 1993.

Editors of Market House Books Ltd. *The Bantam Medical Dictionary* (rev). New York: Bantam, 1990.

Editors of *Prevention* Magazine. *The Doctors Book of Home Remedies.* Emmaus, PA: Rodale Press, 1990. (Bantam edition 1991)

Endometriosis Association. *What is Endometriosis?* Milwaukee, WI: The Association, 1991.

Farley, Dixie. "Endometriosis Painful, but Treatable." *FDA Consumer,* May, 1993.

MacDorman, M. F., and Rosenberg, H. M. "Trends in Infant Mortality by Cause of Death and Other Characteristics, 1960–1988." *Vital and Health Statistics,* 20 (20), 1993.

Mayfield, Eleanor. "Choosing a Treatment for Uterine Fibroids." *FDA Consumer Special Report,* January, 1994.

Monthly Vital Statistics Report, 42:5 (August 31, 1993).

Randal, Judith. "Trying to Outsmart Infertility." *FDA Consumer,* May, 1993.

TAP Pharmaceuticals. *Endometriosis, the Disease and Its Treatment.* Deerfield, IL: TAP, 1991.

U. S. Department of Health and Human Services. "Pregnancy and Minorities." *Closing the Gap.* Washington, DC: Office of Minority Health, 1991.

✓ Self-Assessment

Test Your Knowledge of the Male Reproductive Anatomy

NAME _____ DATE _____

COURSE _____ SECTION _____

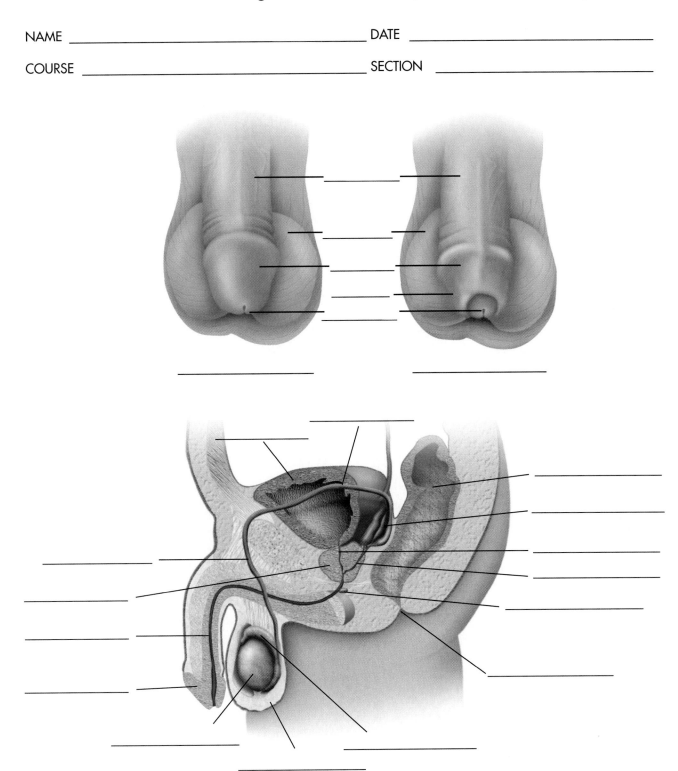

✔ Self-Assessment

Test Your Knowledge of the Female Reproductive Anatomy

NAME _____ DATE _____

COURSE _____ SECTION _____

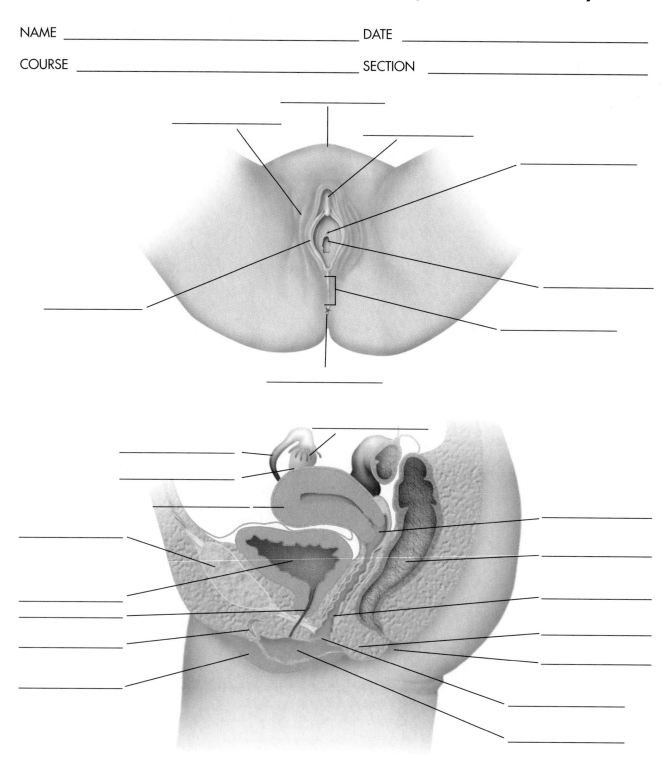

Communicable Diseases

6

OBJECTIVES

* Define infectious or communicable disease.

* Name the classifications of the pathogens.

* Describe the methods of pathogen transmission.

* Explain the course of infection.

* Describe the mechanism involved in the immune response.

* Name the communicable diseases for which immunizations are available.

* List the better known communicable diseases.

* Describe the symptoms and effects of common sexually transmitted diseases.

* Describe the demographics of HIV/AIDS.

*M*any life forms exist that are unseen without the aid of magnification. These creatures inhabit the planet along with us. Some are beneficial; some are not. The latter invade our bodies, make us ill, and sometimes even cause death. These sinister creatures are called pathogens, disease-causing organisms. Their mission is to invade the body and then silently move to the next victim.

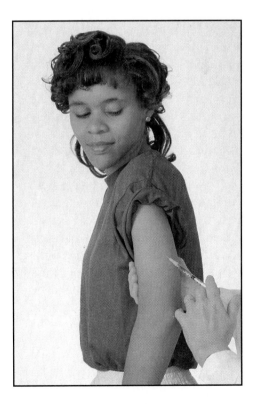

Pathogens are the causative agents of **infectious diseases**, conditions in which the pathogen can be spread from person to person, contaminated object (**fomite**) to person, or animal to person. These conditions also are called *communicable* or *contagious* diseases.

CLASSES OF PATHOGENS

Many pathogens surround us, causing a variety of illnesses. These organisms can be grouped into the following categories for the purpose of this discussion:

❋ Viruses

❋ Bacteria

❋ Fungi

❋ Protozoa

❋ Metazoa

Figure 6.1 depicts these classes of pathogens.

Viruses are microorganisms that do not have an independent metabolism and must reproduce or replicate within the living cells of the person they invade. Viruses consist of genetic material protected by a protein shell. Examples of infectious conditions caused by viruses are the common cold, influenza (flu), and chicken pox. When comparing pathogens by size, the viruses are the smallest of the pathogenic organisms and are often air-borne.

Bacteria probably are the most familiar of the pathogens, because they seem to be named as the culprit when people get sick. These infamous microorganisms come in three basic shapes: the spherical-shaped coccus, the rod- or club-shaped bacillus, and the spiral-shaped spirillum or spirochete. Tuberculosis, strep throat, and syphilis are among the diseases caused by bacteria. Some bacteria are carried in body wastes — a good reason for washing your hands, particularly before eating.

Rickettsiae once were believed to be closely allied with viruses but now are

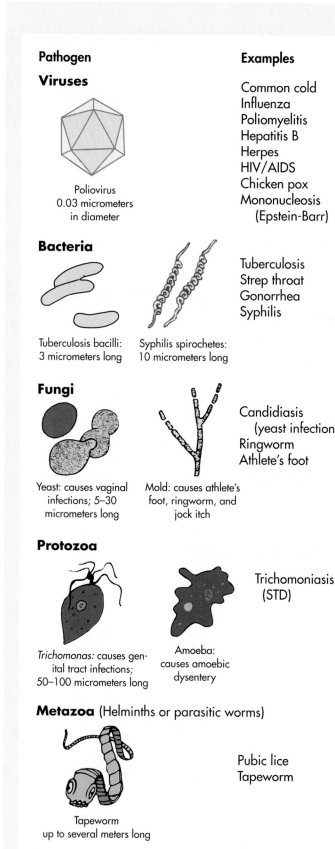

Figure 6.1 Classes of pathogens with examples of each

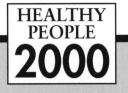

HEALTHY PEOPLE 2000

OBJECTIVES FOR COMMUNICABLE DISEASES

❋ Reduce the indigenous cases of the following vaccine-preventable diseases:

    Diphtheria among people age 25 and younger

    Tetanus among people age 25 and younger

    Polio

    Rubeola

    Rubella

    Congenital rubella syndrome

    Mumps

    Pertussis

believed to be a small form of bacteria. Rickettsiae are transmitted by vectors. Two examples of Rickettsiae diseases are Rocky Mountain spotted fever, carried by a tick, and typhus, carried by lice, fleas, and ticks.

Fungi are plant-like organisms that lack chlorophyll. They include mushrooms, molds, and yeast. Fungi like to grow in warm, dark, and moist environments. Common infectious diseases caused by fungi include athlete's foot, ringworm of the scalp ("tetter"), and yeast infection. Human yeast infections are different from the yeasts used for making bread or beer.

Protozoa are microscopic, one-celled (or unicellular) animals capable of living as parasites in humans. Some infectious illnesses caused by protozoa require a vector, or insect carrier, for transmission to humans. Malaria, African sleeping sickness, and the sexually transmitted disease (STD) trichomoniasis are caused by protozoa.

Metazoa are multicellular animals with differentiated cells. The metazoa, largest of the pathogens, can be seen without magnification. They live as parasites in and on humans and animals. Intestinal roundworms and lice are examples of conditions caused by metazoa. Tapeworms, for example, can be several feet long. Worm infections usually come from contaminated food or drink and their spread is controlled by good hygiene.

THE COURSE OF INFECTIOUS DISEASE

For an infectious illness to occur, a pathogen and a victim must be present. In most cases the pathogen invades the person's body, multiplies, causes illness, and then dies. Death of the pathogen may result from the work of the immune system of the infected person or from some medication the person takes to fight the condition. The course of most infectious diseases is fairly predictable, beginning with exposure and infection, followed by an incubation period, a prodomal period, the actual illness, then recovery or relapse, and termination.

Exposure and Infection

First the person comes in contact with pathogens because of exposure to infected persons, animals,

KEY TERMS

Pathogens disease-causing organisms

Infectious diseases conditions in which a pathogen can be spread from person to person; also called communicable or contagious diseases

Fomite an object contaminated with a pathogen

Viruses microorganisms without their own metabolism that reproduce within the living cells of the person they invade

Bacteria a type of disease-causing microorganism

Rickettsiae type of pathogen transmitted to humans through insect bites

Fungi plantlike organisms that lack chlorophyll; some are pathogens

Protozoa one-celled animals that can live as parasites in humans

Metazoa multicellular animals, the largest pathogens, that live as parasites in and on humans and animals

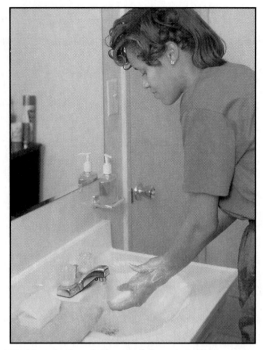

Washing the hands is one of the most effective means of preventing infectious diseases.

or fomites. Upon exposure these pathogens invade the body through natural openings, breaks in the skin, or mucous membrane, such as in the nose. Once inside the body, the pathogens multiply and begin their destruction, which manifests itself as an infection. In some cases the infection may remain in one region of the body (surrounding tissue or organs). This is called a **local infection**. If the pathogen moves to the circulatory and lymphatic systems and spreads to other regions or body systems, the condition is called a **systemic infection**. Systemic infections usually are more difficult to treat than local infections.

Incubation Period

Upon exposure to pathogenic organisms, the symptoms of an infectious illness do not appear immediately. If this were the case, treatment would ensue immediately and responsible people would not expose others knowingly. This lag time or **incubation period** is the time between the infection and the appearance of signs of illness. During the incubation period the pathogens are working quietly but effectively and without the infected person's knowledge. The person is **asymptomatic**. Although he or she has no signs or symptoms of illness, the infected person is able to expose others to the

pathogens he or she is carrying. The incubation period varies from one infectious disease to another — from a few days to a few weeks to several years.

Prodromal Period

The **prodromal period** is one of high communicability. During this stage the person becomes sick with nonspecific signs or warnings of illness that may include irritability, a slight fever, or general aches and pains. Some type of treatment might help alleviate the symptoms during this phase of the disease.

Actual Illness

At this point the specific symptoms of the illness manifest themselves. An accurate diagnosis usually can be made during the actual illness. In most cases the person is still contagious.

Recovery

In the recovery stage the body's defenses or the medication overcome the pathogen, the symptoms disappear, and the person becomes well again. Or the person may have a relapse, during which time the symptoms reappear, returning the person to the stage of actual illness.

Termination

The termination phase denotes victory. Because of the person's level of wellness or medical advances, he or she becomes well and may advance to one of three states of being:

1. After an attack by certain pathogens, the person becomes protected for a lifetime and will not be able to contract the disease even if he or she is exposed to the pathogen again. Examples of this type of protection are found in the childhood diseases, such as measles (rubeola), (discussed later).

2. After having certain infectious diseases, the infected person does get well but may become ill again if reexposed to the pathogens. This is termed **resusceptibility**. German measles is an example.

3. Some individuals recover completely from an infectious illness but retain vestiges of the illness, which they can transmit to others. These people show no signs of illness but shed the pathogens

of the disease that continue to take refuge in their bodies. They are *asymptomatic carriers.* An example of an infectious disease in which pathogens can be transmitted by an asymptomatic person or carrier is genital herpes.

ROUTES OF INVASION AND SOURCES OF CONTAMINATION

Pathogens can enter the body by four common routes and sources:

1. *Skin or other body surfaces.* Pathogens may enter directly through breaks caused by cuts, abrasions, burns, or punctures in the skin or other body surfaces. Some pathogens can be absorbed through mucous membrane where no break exists. Other pathogens have the ability to penetrate intact skin.

2. *Inhalation.* Some pathogens are air-borne and may enter through the mucous membranes of the nasal passages or via the lungs.

3. *Contaminated food or water.* People may expose themselves to pathogens by inadvertently eating or drinking something in which pathogens are living.

4. *Fomites.* Under certain conditions exposure to objects such as used hypodermic needles and syringes or bed linen contaminated with pathogens can introduce the pathogen into the body.

THE BODY'S DEFENSE MECHANISMS

The Defenders — The First Response

The human body is designed to defend itself from the marauding pathogens that assault it daily. On the front line of the defense is the top layer of skin, the **epidermis**. Without this protective covering humans would not survive long. By acting as a shield or cover, the epidermis stops most pathogens from invading the more vulnerable interior surfaces of the body. Often pathogens can be removed by washing with soap and water before they have the opportunity to enter through breaks in the skin.

Mucous membranes are tissues that, although not as strong as epidermis, help protect the interior surfaces from pathogenic invasion. The tissue is bathed with mucous secretions that trap particles and pathogens before they are able to establish infection. These secretions contain enzymes that inactivate pathogens. Mucous membranes line the digestive, respiratory, urinary, and reproductive tracts. Other "first-response" defenders are tears and saliva, which contain antibacterial substances that dilute organisms or particles so they are rendered ineffective. Cilia, specialized hairlike projections that line the bronchial tubes, sweep particles and pathogens from the lungs into the digestive tract, where they are killed by gastric secretions.

The Defenders — The Second Response

If the pathogenic raiders overwhelm the systems that protect people initially, a second response comes from the body's immune system. The **lymphatic system** (Figure 6.2) includes a specialized group of vessels that network throughout the body. At various sites in this system are situated larger lymph structures called **lymph nodes**. Familiar locations of the lymph nodes include regions of the head and neck, the armpits, the small of the back, and the groin. The lymphatic system functions to bathe the body tissue.

KEY TERMS

Local infection an infection that remains in the area of the body where the invasion of the pathogen occurred

Systemic infection an infection that spreads throughout the body

Incubation period the time between infection and appearance of signs of illness

Asymptomatic without signs of illness

Prodomal period time during which an infectious disease is most communicable; characterized by nonspecific symptoms

Resusceptibility vulnerability to reinfection with a disease after having recovered from it

Epidermis top layer of skin

Mucous membranes tissues that help protect the interior surfaces of the body from invasion by pathogens

Lymphatic system specialized groups of vessels that network throughout the body and cleanse body tissues

Lymph nodes larger glands of the lymph system found in the head, neck, armpits, small of the back, and groin

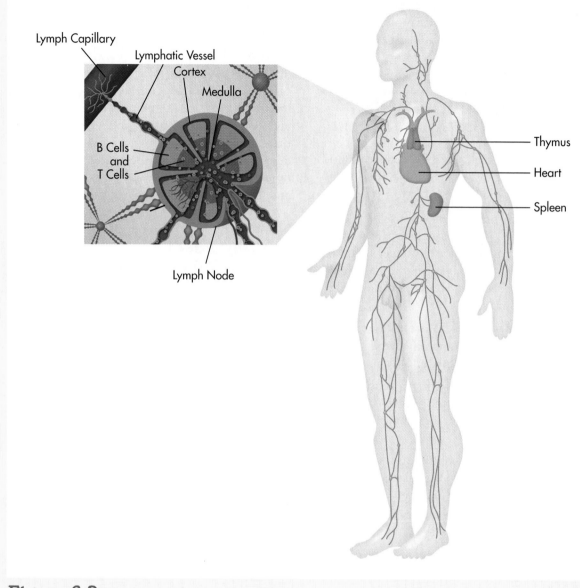

Figure 6.2 The lymphatic system

Specialized blood cells called **macrophages** (phagocytes) and **lymphocytes** together fight pathogens. Macrophages are the "Pac Man" cells of the immune system. They seek invading bacteria and foreign substances, engulf and destroy them. This process is called **phagocytosis**.

Lymphocytes are made by bone marrow. These specialized cells work with the macrophages. Some lymphocytes stimulate the body to produce more lymphocytes as well as stimulate the production of antibodies.

When the body is invaded by pathogens, phagocytosis alone is not enough protection in some instances. A more elaborate mechanism of the immune system must be activated. The immune system senses the pathogen as a foreign substance, which now acts as an antigen in the body. An **antigen** is a substance that triggers or stimulates a specific immune response. At this point the lymphocytes come to the body's rescue to fight the infection. The **B-cells** (a type of lymphocyte) produce **antibodies** that are able to deactivate the

To keep your immune system healthy . . .

✳ Eat a balanced diet including lots of fresh fruits and vegetables for vitamin C and beta carotene, and meat, milk, and eggs for vitamin E.

✳ Exercise moderately and often (but not when you're ill, as that can prolong recovery). Brisk walking at least four times a week for 45 minutes will benefit most people.

✳ Develop close personal relationships, those in which you trust and can readily confide and vent frustrations. Stress is hard on the immune system.

✳ Be sure to get enough sleep — 6 to 8 hours a night — as lack of sleep leaves a person more vulnerable to infections and illness, and sleep bolsters the immune system.

✳ Don't smoke, as smoking lowers the level of some immune cells; and drink only in moderation, if at all.

✳ Wash your hands with soap and water, as most viral diseases are spread by hand-to-hand contact.

✳ Avoid contact with people who have airborne diseases such as flu, chicken pox, and tuberculosis.

invading pathogens so other body defenses can rid the body of these organisms. What is amazing about this process is that the antibodies produced are specific to the particular antigen for which they were created. People have many pathogen-specific antibodies in their immune systems.

The other lymphocytes, the **T-cells**, function to activate additional B-cells, suppress the activity of B-cells when the attack on the pathogen is completed, and destroy normal cells that have mutated and have become cancerous. T-cells also can attack pathogens. Once activated by the antigen, the T-cells target the cells of the pathogen or the cells of the infected person that the invading pathogens actually have penetrated. The T-cells then destroy these cells to protect the person.

The first exposure to the pathogen triggers the **immune response** (Figure 6.3). It may not have been strong enough to prevent the person from becoming ill at the first attack. If the person is reexposed to the same pathogen at a later time, however, the memory T-cells and B-cells "remember" the specific antigen from the initial exposure. They then spring into action to protect the person from becoming ill from this new attack. The immune response on this occasion is much faster and stronger than it was on the first exposure.

The memory T-cells and B-cells do not leave the body; they remain in the person's lymphatic and circulatory system for many years, even for life in some instances. The type of **immunity** conferred by these memory cells, called **acquired immunity**, is diagrammed in Figure 6.4.

KEY TERMS

Macrophages specialized cells (phagocytes) that destroy pathogens

Lymphocytes specialized white blood cells produced in the bone marrow that identify pathogens and help macrophages fight pathogens

Phagocytosis the destruction of pathogens by macrophages (phagocytes)

Antigen a substance that triggers the immune response

B-cells a type of lymphocyte that produces antibodies capable of deactivating invading pathogens

Antibody a protein substance that interacts with an antigen and forms the basis of immunity

T-cells lymphocytes that activate additional B-cells, stop B-cell activity when the pathogen is destroyed, kill normal cells that have become cancerous, and attack pathogens

Immune response body's reaction to first exposure to a pathogen

Immunity resistance to disease; may be natural or acquired

Acquired immunity protection from reacquiring an infectious disease because the first occurrence triggered antibodies against it.

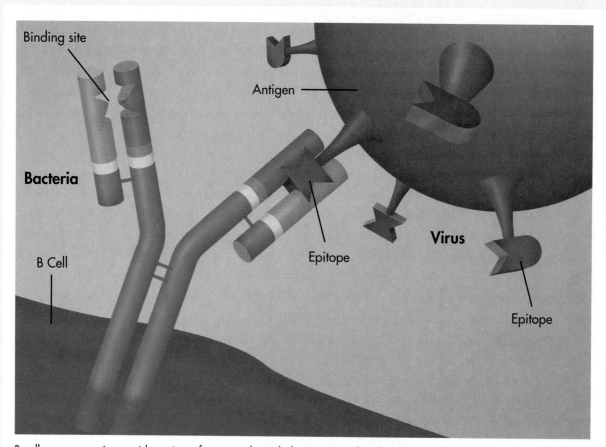

Binding site

Antigen

Bacteria

B Cell

Epitope

Virus

Epitope

B cells can recognize a wide variety of enemies through the *receptors* that dot their outer membrane. When a receptor encounters a foreign substance, it examines the shape of *epitopes* — molecular appendages — protruding from the invader's surface. If an epitope's "key" matches the receptor's "lock," the two will form a bond. Once a receptor has locked onto an epitope, it triggers a chain reaction of sorts in the B cell that culminates in the mass production of antibodies. Virtually identical to the B cell receptor itself, the antibodies travel through the blood vessels and the lymphatic system, locking onto any antigens that match the first.

Figure 6.3 The immune response

Acquired immunity is possible and usually permanent in many of the so-called childhood diseases. Exposure to some other pathogens, however, does stimulate antibody production but does not confer protection to the person after subsequent reexposure and reinfection. This means that the person is resusceptible and may become ill with the same disease many times throughout the lifespan. This is true of many sexually transmitted diseases (discussed later in the chapter).

Also, because the various infectious diseases are caused by different and distinct pathogens, immunity to one does not confer immunity to another. A person can be infected with more than one communicable disease at one time.

Immunodeficiency

Cancer, HIV infection, some congenital (inborn) disorders, and a miscellany of other conditions are associated with **immunodeficiencies**, failure of the immune system to react to pathogens. A unique disorder of the immune system is **autoimmunity**, in which the immune system attacks the body's own cells and tissues. Strictly speaking HIV infection is not an autoimmune disease, although it does leave the body susceptible to many diseases. To the best of our knowledge, autoimmune disorders such as rheumatoid arthritis are noncommunicable. These are included in Chapter 7.

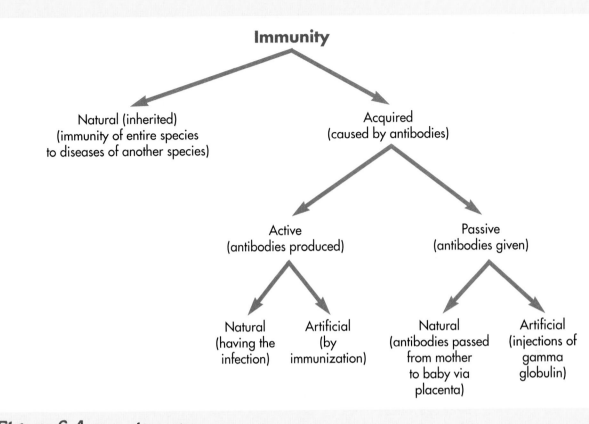

Immunity

Natural (inherited)
(immunity of entire species
to diseases of another species)

Acquired
(caused by antibodies)

Active
(antibodies produced)

Passive
(antibodies given)

Natural
(having the
infection)

Artificial
(by
immunization)

Natural
(antibodies passed
from mother
to baby via
placenta)

Artificial
(injections of
gamma
globulin)

Figure 6.4 Types of immunity

IMMUNIZATION

One of the success stories of modern times is the development of vaccines that have virtually eliminated many of the highly contagious diseases that formerly left their mark on many people, particularly children. For example, four decades after polio vaccines were first developed, the disease has been vanquished in the western hemisphere. The last case was in Peru in 1991.

Today, however, the health status of many Americans is being compromised by the return of some infectious diseases that were perceived as being no longer threats to health. Tuberculosis is on the rise. Public health departments are reporting more cases of measles (rubeola) and other childhood diseases. With the exception of chicken pox, effective immunizations have been developed to prevent these childhood illnesses (listed in Table 6.1). Reported cases are on the rise not because the vaccines are ineffective but, rather, because of parents' failure to immunize their children.

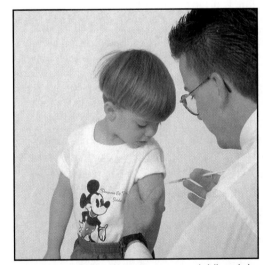

Immunization is the best protection against childhood diseases.

KEY TERMS

Immunodeficiency failure of the immune system to react to pathogens

Autoimmunity a disorder of the immune system in which the immune system attacks the body's own cells and tissues

Table 6.1

Communicable Childhood Diseases

Disease	Characteristics	Dangers
Diphtheria	Bacterial disease usually affecting the throat and sometimes other mucous membranes and the skin. Sore throat, fever, and chills are the main manifestations.	Can make a child choke so badly that all breathing stops. Sometimes causes heart failure or pneumonia.
Hepatitis B	Disease of the liver passed from mother to infant during birth.	Greatest danger is meningitis and also can cause pneumonia.
Hib disease or H-flu	Form of influenza. Children between 6 months and 1 year old are particularly susceptible.	Serious potential complication is meningitis.
Mumps	Swelling of salivary glands on one or both sides of the face, preceded by fever, headache, and vomiting.	Can cause deafness, diabetes, meningitis, encephalitis and brain damage. In adult men can cause sterility.
Rubella (German Measles)	Tends to be mild in children; greatest threat is to fetus of pregnant women in early pregnancy, when risk of deformed baby is up to 80%; miscarriage also common. Children usually receive vaccination together with rubeola and mumps (MMR).	In a pregnant woman can cause a miscarriage or lead to birth defects in the baby.
Rubeola (Red Measles)	Symptoms similar to cold plus fever; affects respiratory system, skin, and eyes. Overt indication is the characteristic "rash" — small, red spots on the body.	Can lead to pneumonia, blindness, ear infections and deafness, encephalitis, and brain damage.
Pertussis (Whooping Cough)	Bacterial disease affecting mucous membranes lining the air passages. Cough for which it is named is a persistent, paroxysmal whooping that is the primary characteristic.	Pneumonia is a common complication. Can cause convulsions and brain damage.
Polio	Virus affecting central nervous system. Depending on the form, symptoms are flulike, affect respiration, involve muscle stiffness, weakness and in one variation, paralysis. No treatment is available, but development of vaccine in 1955 reduced incidence to near zero.	Often cripples and sometimes kills. If a child gets polio, little can be done.
Tetanus (Lockjaw)	Enters the body when something sharp like a nail punctures or cuts the skin, or from abrasions or insect stings. Main characteristic is spasmodic contraction of muscles, first in the jaw and neck and later at other sites throughout the body.	High fever, convulsions, and pain are common. Can kill.

Adapted from *Medical Self-Care* by Brent Q. Hafen (Englewood, CO: Morton Publishing, 1983), p. 298, and updated by *Parents Guide to Childhood Immunization*, by U. S. Department of Health and Human Services, 1994.

Most school districts require that children be immunized before they enter school. These regulations, however, do not protect children who are under 5 years old and not enrolled in an away-from-home educational program. More than half of U.S. infants are not getting all their recommended immunizations, according to *American Health* magazine. In 1990, more than 27,000 cases of rubeola were reported to the Centers for Disease Control and Prevention (CDC) in Atlanta. Nearly half of those cases were children under age 5. In addition, the CDC reported that minority children under age 5 in poor inner cities have a much higher risk for measles than other children do.

A study at the University of Washington, Seattle, reported that, in their first 8 months, only 42% of Anglo American infants and 29% of African American babies received all their immunizations. Immunizations for preventable childhood diseases are available to everyone, regardless of ability to pay, at local branches of county public health departments. Table 6.2 presents a schedule of the childhood diseases for which immunizations have been developed, along with selected immunizations for adults in various situations.

☎ Call for information _____

National Immunization Information Hotline
1-800-232-2522
1-800-232-0233 (Spanish-speaking)

COMMON INFECTIOUS DISEASES

With the rise in living standards, sanitation methods, access to medical care, and immunizations, many infectious conditions are no longer considered

✺ Table 6.2
Recommended Immunization Against Infectious Diseases

Immunization	Children*	Adults
Diphtheria/pertussis tetanus combination (DPT)	2, 4, 6, and 15–18 months and at 4–6 years (before or at school entry)	
Diphtheria/tetanus booster	14–16 years	Every 10 years
Poliomyelitis	2, 4, and 15–18 months and at 4–6 years	Those who might be exposed (those in health and sanitation occupations, travelers); normally no booster needed
Measles (rubeola)/ mumps/rubella combination (MMR)	12–15 months and just before entering school	Adults under age 32 who received only one measles shot at 1 year of age or after. Adults whose initial dose was given along with immune globulin — as routinely occurred from 1963 to 1975 — should get two doses at least 1 month apart
HIB (Hemophilus influenza type B)	2, 4, and 15–18 months	Effective against meningitis
Influenza		Yearly, because of the changeability of viral strains
Tuberculosis	Those exposed to individuals with active tuberculosis	Those exposed to individuals with active tuberculosis
Hepatitis B	Those exposed to infected individuals or to contaminated food and water. At birth for infants whose mothers have tested positive for Hepatitis B	Those who may be exposed (health workers who ingested contaminated food or water; travelers)
Rabies	Only those bitten by rabid animal. Series of vaccinations	

*Recommended by American Academy of Pediatrics

threats to the public's health. Others, however, still undermine the health of our citizens, particularly minority groups. And diseases thought to be eradicated have reemerged in some instances as health concerns. A discussion of the more common of these follows.

The Common Cold

Of all human disease conditions, the cold, depicted in Figure 6.5, is truly the most common. Most people have at least one cold a year, and as many as four may not be unusual. The **common cold** has eluded a cure in part because it can be caused by more than 200 different viruses. A common cold is an inflammation of the upper respiratory tract — the nose, throat, and sinuses. Colds are spread by droplet. The virus enters the body through the mouth or nose. What differentiates a cold from other viral infections is the lack of high fever.

Symptoms of a cold appear 1 to 3 days after being infected. The first clues may be a scratchy throat or tickle in the throat, cough, tightness or dryness in the nose or throat, loss of appetite, and an "out-of-sorts" feeling. This is followed by additional symptoms such as a stuffy nose and sneezing. The illness usually is full-blown within 48–72 hours with teary eyes, runny nose, husky voice, difficult breathing, and dulled taste and smell. Colds sometimes are accompanied by headache.

A cold typically lasts a week or two. Like many other viral conditions, the cold still has neither a cure nor an effective immunization for prevention. Megadoses of vitamin C have been touted as a preventive measure, but many studies have shown no measurable effect. Antibiotics are not effective against colds.

Cold sufferers tend to rely on tried-and-true methods for relief from symptoms, the foremost of which are to get adequate rest, avoid chilling and extreme temperature changes, drink a lot of fluids (including juices), and eat nourishing foods. Commercial cold remedies on the market include:

✳ *Decongestants:* shrink nasal blood vessels, relieving swelling and congestion, but may dry mucous membranes in the throat and worsen the condition.

✳ *Antihistamines:* decrease nasal secretions, although they are most useful in treating allergies; may dry out mucous membranes in the throat and intensify a cough.

✳ *Expectorants:* stimulate the formation of respiratory secretions (phlegm), resulting in more but less viscous sputum. The Food and Drug Administration does not endorse expectorants, because they are ineffective.

✳ *Antitussives:* suppress coughing through codeine or other drugs that block the cough centers in the brain. Their use may lead to failure to clear the lungs of phlegm and pathogens. Most appropriate for dry coughs.

✳ *Local anesthetics:* suppress coughing; these throat lozenges and similar painkillers help relieve sore throats but are short-acting.

✳ *Analgesics* (aspirin, Tylenol®, acetaminophen): help relieve muscle aches but may prolong the life of the cold; aspirin also is associated with the development of Reyes syndrome in children. Even though **Reyes syndrome** is rare and is becoming even more uncommon, aspirin should not be administered to children who have colds or flulike symptoms or fever. Excessive long-

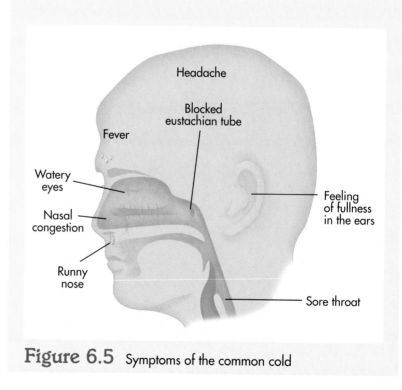

Figure 6.5 Symptoms of the common cold

Headache

Blocked eustachian tube

Fever

Watery eyes

Nasal congestion

Runny nose

Feeling of fullness in the ears

Sore throat

Tips for action

To cope with a cold:

* **Drink a lot of fluids** (at least 8 ounces every 2 hours). Fluids, especially if hot, soothe the throat and help relieve congestion. Avoid alcoholic beverages because they tend to dehydrate the body.

* **Gargle with salt water.** One teaspoon of salt in warm water every 4 hours is recommended. This helps to reduce swelling in the throat.

* **Get plenty of rest.** Rest helps heal and restore.

* **Use disposable tissues instead of handkerchiefs.** Handkerchiefs can harbor germs for up to several hours.

* **Inhale warm, moist air (steam).** A vaporizer or humidifier, or pan of water on the stove, can be used. Take moderately warm to hot showers. These practices soothe inflamed mucous membranes.

* **Take medications only to relieve symptoms, and follow the advice on the label.** Consult a physician if cold symptoms persist beyond a week.

Source: *Medical Self-Care and Assessment* by Brent Q. Hafen (Englewood, CO: Morton Publishing, 1983), p. 202; originally printed by American College Health Association.

term consumption of acetaminophen leads to kidney failure.

Influenza

Influenza, or flu, can be mistaken for the common cold. Usually, however, it has more pronounced symptoms and more severe complications. Contrary to popular belief, flu viruses do not cause the nausea, vomiting, and diarrhea of the so-called stomach flu or intestinal flu. Those diseases are caused by other pathogens. Flu is an infection of the nose, throat, bronchial tubes, and lungs caused by specific influenza viruses. The disease is spread by droplets from sneezing and coughing.

Flu is caused primarily by two main types of virus, the A virus and the B virus. Each has several strains named for their place of origin, such as the Hong Kong flu virus. Flu viruses are unique in that once a strain has spread in a population, its structure changes and it then is capable of causing a new form of flu because the antibodies produced to combat the original virus are not effective against the new form. An entirely new strain appears about every 10 years. Flu viruses may be particularly

virulent because they are air-borne viruses, which are easily transmittable.

Flu symptoms include high fever, chills, headache, muscle aches, and fatigue. Those infected also may have a dry cough and inflamed nasal passages.

Flu usually has to run its course and is treated only by relieving the symptoms. Treatment is the same, in general, as that for colds. Some forms of flu are treated by aspirin substitutes, particularly amantadine hydrochloride.

By way of prevention, the vaccines developed in anticipation of the disease are administered to those who seek it, mainly aging people and those with chronic diseases. Vaccines are said to be 67% to 92% effective.

KEY TERMS

Common cold inflammation of the upper respiratory tract caused by a virus

Reye's syndrome a disease that affects children from 2 to 16, which can be fatal

Influenza (flu) a viral infection of the nose, throat, bronchial tubes, and lungs

Strep Throat

A sore throat may be a symptom of a cold or flu, or it may signal a more serious streptococcal infection, particularly if the sore throat is accompanied by fever, aching, and fatigue. To be on the safe side, the affected person should see a health professional. The only way to diagnose **strep throat** is to have a throat culture taken, the results of which can be obtained in minutes. Strep throat infection is extremely contagious. Because it is caused by bacteria, it is treated by antibiotics to halt progression of the disease to possible rheumatic fever.

Mononucleosis

Infectious **mononucleosis**, better known as "mono," is a contagious viral illness that attacks the lymph nodes in the neck and the throat, resulting in prolonged weakness, sore throat, swelling of the nodes, headache, fever, and nausea. Mono is caused by the Epstein-Barr virus and is spread by contact with moisture from the mouth and throat of a person infected with the virus. Through the years it has come to be known as the "kissing disease." Kissing, or sharing drinking glasses and eating utensils or toothbrushes, or touching something that has been in contact with the mouth of an infected person, may transmit the virus.

Teenagers and young adults are the most susceptible to mono, although cases have been found in children less than a year old. It is rare in individuals over age 35.

Most cases simply run a course over 6 to 8 weeks, but sometimes it lasts as long as 6 months. Occasionally the infection spreads to the liver, causing jaundice (yellow-appearing skin and whites of the eyes), or the spleen, which could burst.

Diagnosis is obtained from blood samples. The best treatment is to rest and drink plenty of liquids. Viruses do not respond to antibiotics. If mono is accompanied by strep throat, the antibiotic is prescribed to treat that condition. In severe cases corticosteroid drugs are prescribed.

Chronic Fatigue Syndrome

The cause of **chronic fatigue syndrome (CFS)** is still unknown to the medical community. Some professionals consider it to be a recurring form of mononucleosis and link it to the Epstein-Barr virus. The defining characteristic is found in its name — fatigue — and other symptoms are similar to mono, including aches and pains, swollen lymph glands, and low-grade fever. The symptoms may last from 6 months to several years, off and on.

According to one group of professionals, the Chronic Fatigue Immune Dysfunction Syndrome (CFIDS) Foundation in San Francisco, chronic fatigue syndrome seems to combine both autoimmune and immunodeficiency disorders. The immune cells act as if they are constantly battling a viral infection. The CFIDS Foundation says the disease affects about 1 million Americans, 70% to 85% of them women. Other estimates of incidence are as high as 3 million.

The British and Canadians call this disease *myalgic encephalomyelitis;* the Japanese call it

Is It Strep? Is It A Cold?

	STREP	COLD
Onset of symptoms	Rapid	Slower
Soreness	Marked	Less marked
Fever, aches, malaise	Marked	Mild
Respiratory symptoms	Present in half of cases	Present in most cases
Lymph nodes	Large and tender	No enlargement or tenderness
Complications	Rheumatic-fever, streptococcal pneumonia, middle-ear infection, mastoiditis, nephritis	Bacterial sinusitis middle-ear infection
Treatment	Antibiotics	OTC medications or gargling with salt water

> **Any sore throat that lasts longer than 10 days or seems especially severe should be treated by a doctor.**

Source: American Pharmaceutical Association and Dr. Jack Gwaltney, a cold expert at the University of Virginia School of Medicine in Charlottesville. Originally printed in *American Health,* December, 1994.

Call for information

Chronic Fatigue and Immune Dysfunction Syndrome (CFIDS)
900-896-2343

low-natural-killer-cell syndrome; and some patients' groups call it *chronic-fatigue-immune-dysfunction syndrome*. No procedure is available yet to diagnose this condition. Although analgesics, antidepressants, and complete rest have been tried, no specific treatment has been found to be effective for all patients. This mysterious disease continues to baffle the medical community.

Hepatitis

Several types of the viral disease **hepatitis**, an inflammation of the liver, have been identified. **Hepatitis A** is transmitted by food or water contaminated with feces. An injection of gamma globulin can protect against or lessen the symptoms of infection. Sometimes the symptoms are so mild that the presence of the disease is not apparent but the disease still can be transmitted to others. A more serious form, Hepatitis B, is included under the discussion of sexually transmitted diseases.

Pneumonia

Pneumonia is an inflammation of the bronchial tubes and alveoli (tiny air sacs) in the lungs. It can be caused either by bacteria or by viruses and even by environmental chemicals. This infection typically follows a cold or the flu but may be a primary infection.

The four major symptoms are chest pain, abrupt rise in body temperature, coughing, and difficulty breathing. In one type, called "walking pneumonia," the only symptom at first may be the cough. Eventual diagnosis by x-ray will reveal the presence of pneumonia. Additional diagnostic measures include analysis of the sputum and listening to the chest with a stethoscope to detect any fluid present in the lungs.

Viral pneumonia is generally treated by bed rest, a high fluid intake, a light diet, and painkillers as necessary. Bacterial pneumonia is treated with antibiotics such as penicillin, plus rest. Conditions that make a person more vulnerable to pneumonia include poor nutrition, chronic bronchitis, emphysema, cancer, alcoholism, sickle cell anemia, and AIDS. People in these risk groups should get a one-time vaccination for pneumococcal pneumonia, which provides protection against most pneumonias. Over-the-counter pain relievers, antihistamines, and decongestants can relieve the symptoms. Pneumonia, however, should be treated by a medical professional.

Tuberculosis

One of the leading causes of death at the turn of the century was **tuberculosis (TB)**. During the 1950s TB was virtually put in check by the development of effective antibiotics to treat the infection. Now TB seems to be defying modern medicine and coming back to haunt us. In 1985 the reported number of cases in the United States was 22,201. By 1992 that number had reached 26,673. It is the leading cause of death by acute infectious diseases other than pneumonia. According to the World Health Organization and the Centers for Disease Control and Prevention, an estimated 90 million new cases of TB may cause up to 30 million deaths worldwide in the next 5 years.

Why are the numbers of TB cases on the rise? One reason is the rise in number of cases of HIV infection. HIV-infected individuals are susceptible to other infections including TB because the immune system has been weakened by HIV. Another reason for the rising rates of TB is that some TB microbes have become strong enough to withstand the drugs that formerly wiped them out. Still,

---

KEY TERMS

Strep throat an extremely contagious infection caused by a bacteria and treated with antibiotics

Mononucleosis ("mono") a contagious viral illness that attacks the lymph nodes in the neck and throat

Chronic fatigue syndrome (CFS) a viral illness that produces extreme fatigue and other symptoms similar to mononucleosis

Hepatitis an inflammation of the liver caused by a virus

Hepatitis A a mild form of hepatitis transmitted by food or water contaminated with feces

Pneumonia an inflammation of the bronchial tubes and air sacs of the lungs

Tuberculosis (TB) a bacterial infection in the lungs characterized by coughing blood, pain in the chest, fever, and fatigue

according to Dr. Lee Reichman of the National Tuberculosis Center in Newark, New Jersey, almost all TB is preventable and treatable.

Tuberculosis is caused by the rod-shaped bacterium *Mycobacterium tuberculosis*. The pathogens are spread from person to person through nasal, throat, and lung discharges emitted into the air when an infected persons sneezes, coughs, or laughs. Typically, the TB bacteria cause infection in the lungs, but the brain, spine, and other parts of the body, too, may be affected.

A person who has been exposed to the TB bacteria may have the TB infection for years but not be aware of it because of the absence of symptoms. If this person is exposed to HIV and becomes infected, the virus weakens the person's immune system and the symptoms of TB appear, first as the prodomal symptoms of fatigue, weight loss, fever, and night sweats. As the condition worsens, symptoms of TB of the lung include a long-term cough, pain in the chest, and coughing blood. These symptoms also apply to several other communicable diseases, so an accurate diagnosis is essential. Also, an early diagnosis is advantageous because TB infection now can be treated by medication before it progresses to TB disease.

The diagnosis for TB infection is the **tuberculin test**, or the TB skin test. Individuals who have a positive reaction are advised to have a follow-up chest x-ray. If the person is found to have TB, he or she is advised and treated appropriately.

Tuberculosis, once virtually eliminated, is on the rise worldwide.

Some people with concurrent HIV and TB infections do not react to the TB skin test. Individuals who are HIV-infected and have a negative skin test for TB but have the symptoms of TB infection should have other diagnostic tests to make certain they do not have TB. Untreated TB progressively damages the lungs and can be fatal.

Lyme Disease

Lyme disease is a bacterial infection carried by a tick that lives on deer, mice, and other small mammals (see Figure 6.6). The deaths of some people in the late 1980s brought this infectious disease into national prominence. Outbreaks occurred predominantly along the Atlantic coast, and in Minnesota, Wisconsin, California, and Oregon. The incidence dropped 15% nationwide from 1992 to 1993, but increased in some states.

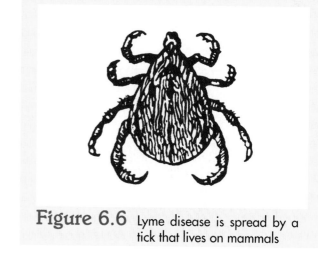

Figure 6.6 Lyme disease is spread by a tick that lives on mammals

The disease progresses in stages. The first symptom usually is a rash that erupts 2 days to 5 weeks after a tick bite, sometimes accompanied by flulike symptoms. During the second stage, which occurs weeks to months later in 10%–20% of untreated individuals, the infected person may develop an abnormal heart rhythm, impaired coordination, partial facial paralysis, severe headaches, and memory lapses. These symptoms usually disappear in a few weeks. About half of untreated people have chronic or recurring inflammation of the joints, which may be related to a hereditary factor. The disease also can cause miscarriages and birth defects.

Antibiotics are used to treat Lyme disease in its early stages, but preventive measures, of course, are best. Two vaccines being tested could someday halt the disease by killing the Lyme spirochete inside the tick's body as soon as it bites. Precautions include wearing long pants rather than shorts when walking through woods or high grass, using insect repellents containing DEET or a clothing spray containing the insecticide permethrin, and knowing how to identify and remove a tick, using tweezers. If a tick is on a person less than 24 hours, he or she stands a good chance of not contracting the disease. Also, domestic animals can bring the tick indoors with them and can be infected with the disease also. Before allowing pets in the house after they have been outdoors they should be checked for ticks.

SEXUALLY TRANSMITTED DISEASES

Much has been written about the **sexually transmitted diseases (STDs)**, some of it accurate and some not. STDs are like other communicable diseases in that they are caused and spread by identifiable pathogens, have definite courses of development, and can be treated. Most are curable. Pathogens thrive on warm, moist, body surfaces or in body fluids. The pathogens can be exchanged during sexual acts or close physical contact with reproductive structures, and no one has or can develop immunity to any STD. Consequently, having an STD does not protect a person from acquiring it again in the future. Anyone who is sexually active may be exposed to the pathogens causing STDs. Statistically, the number of reported cases is highest for 18- to 35-year-olds.

Risks for STDs

Various risk factors for STDs have been identified. Upon examining these carefully, two factors emerge as the primary contributors to risk:

1. Sex acts without using prophylactics (latex condoms and spermicides containing nonoxynol-9).

2. Unprotected sex acts with multiple partners or with individuals who have multiple partners.

Most of the common STDs may be grouped as:

— being blood-borne (HIV/AIDS, syphilis, hepatitis B). These STDs can damage many body systems after primary invasion of the circulatory system by their causative agents.
— causing vaginitis or urethritis.
— producing lesions.
— caused by insect parasites.

Some of the STDs fall into more than one category because of multiple symptoms that appear during the course of the disease. Table 6.3 gives examples from each category.

HIV Infection and AIDS

Much media attention has been given to HIV and AIDS during the past decade since its appearance on the North American scene in the early 1980s. Rock Hudson was the first well-known person to announce that he had AIDS; he died from the disease in 1985. Because AIDS still does not have a cure and the number of cases continues to rise, it remains of prime concern. When Earvin "Magic" Johnson announced to the world in November of 1992 that he was retiring from professional basketball because he was infected with HIV, the public was shocked and saddened. When tennis icon Arthur Ashe succumbed to AIDS, people grieved the loss of a fine human being and role model. These incidents, it was hoped, would give credence to the slogan "AIDS does not discriminate."

Despite the publicity surrounding AIDS, the essentials have not changed. HIV infection still is incurable and deadly. Scientists know how HIV is and is not transmitted and how people can protect themselves. The safety of the blood supply is better than it has ever been thanks to effective screening techniques. Reducing the risk of infection with HIV depends on education, behavior changes, and social supports for these changes.

Table 6.3
Classifications of Common Sexually Transmitted Diseases

Type	Examples of STDs
Blood-borne	HIV/AIDS Syphilis Hepatitis B
Causing vaginitis cervicitis, or urethritis	Chlamydia Gonorrhea Trichomonas Candida
Producing lesions	Herpes Genital warts
Caused by insect parasites	Pubic lice Scabies

KEY TERMS

Tuberculin test a skin test that diagnoses TB
Lyme disease a bacterial infection transmitted by a tick bite
Sexually transmitted diseases illnesses caused by pathogens that are transmitted during sexual acts

Myths About AIDS

If you've heard one or more of these statements, they're all untrue:

❋ You can get AIDS by donating blood.

❋ You can get AIDS through casual contact, such as shaking hands with or hugging an infected person.

❋ You can catch AIDS if an infected person coughs or sneezes on you.

❋ You can get AIDS from a mosquito.

❋ AIDS could spread rapidly through the general population.

❋ If you're not gay and don't shoot drugs, you're safe.

❋ If you don't have symptoms, you're not contagious.

❋ If you're HIV-positive, you'll know it from the symptoms.

❋ If you test positive for HIV, you have AIDS.

❋ Abstinence is the only way to protect yourself against AIDS.

Acquired immune deficiency syndrome or **AIDS** was first recognized as a communicable condition in the United States in 1981. Even though much about AIDS remains unknown, enough is known to help people greatly reduce their risk for acquiring the pathogen that causes the condition. The pathogen that causes AIDS, and how it spreads, is no mystery. Unfortunately, the media, in early reporting, led many people to believe that if they were not members of one of the "high-risk" groups, they were safe from AIDS. Today we know that no safety resides in ignorance and that anyone who is sexually active can be at risk for acquiring AIDS and other STDs as well. Behavior, not social grouping, is what puts a person at risk for HIV infection and AIDS.

HIV/AIDS is caused by a virus known as **human immunodeficiency virus** or **HIV**. HIV is fragile. It does not live on surfaces outside the body for long periods. It cannot survive in extremely cold or hot temperature, and it can be killed by chlorine bleach. This virus invades the body and circulates freely in the bloodstream. The highest concentrations of HIV are found in blood, semen, vaginal secretions, and breast milk. HIV is *not* spread through casual contact such as kissing, handshaking, and other forms of causal contact. The virus is *not* spread by vectors such as mosquitoes, or by contact with the toilet seat. Trace amounts of HIV found in tears, saliva, and other body fluids have not been found to cause infection. Today, the risk of contracting HIV from blood transfusions is low. Since 1985, the Food and Drug Administration (FDA) requires that donated blood, blood products, tissue, and organs be screened for HIV.

After 13 years of study of HIV infection and AIDS, new information continues to be revealed about various aspects of these conditions. The modes of transmission of the virus that were first reported, however, have not changed. The virus is spread largely through vaginal, anal, or oral sex, sharing needles to inject drugs or pierce the skin, mother-to-child/fetus transmission, and exposure to infected blood.

AIDS seems to draw all the attention from the condition that *precedes* it, HIV infection. A person does *not* develop AIDS without being infected with HIV first. The incubation period for HIV infection is much shorter than that for AIDS. Antibodies for HIV infection may be detected in a person's blood as early as 8 weeks after exposure to the virus. Most people, however, convert to seropositive (test positive on a blood test) within 3 to 6 months after exposure to HIV.

Physiology of HIV Infection and AIDS

Infection with HIV can occur when blood, semen, vaginal secretions, or breast milk of an infected person comes into direct contact with the bloodstream or mucous membranes of another person. HIV can be transmitted sexually during unprotected vaginal, oral, or anal intercourse with an infected person. People who have been exposed to HIV may or may not become infected. Some people who have been exposed only once have become infected, while others with multiple exposures remain uninfected.

From the moment HIV enters the body, however, a person is infected for life, can be infectious to others, and is considered **HIV-positive**. Although the virus is present and begins multiplying immediately upon entering the body, infection cannot be detected clinically until antibodies have developed, usually 8 weeks to 6 months after the initial infection. Physically, a person may have symptoms similar to flu or mono that go away after a couple of days or weeks (**acute HIV infection**), or they may have no symptoms at all. Feeling fine, most people have an HIV antibody test or develop symptoms of the disease.

Most people with HIV infection are completely asymptomatic for years. Some people with HIV have been infected for 10 or more years and remain symptom-free. Unfortunately, HIV attacks special white blood cells (CD4 lymphocytes) of the immune system that are essential in protecting a person from disease. Eventually this results in a depressed immune system, which makes a person susceptible to other infections and causes the first noticeable symptoms of HIV disease.

Typical early signs of symptomatic HIV disease include persistent:

— fatigue
— dry cough
— fever
— night sweats
— diarrhea
— skin rashes
— swollen lymph nodes
— vaginal yeast infections
— unexplained weight loss

People with HIV can live in this symptomatic phase of HIV disease for months or years and may, with treatment, have symptom-free periods. Over time, however, the immune system may become so weakened that a person with HIV disease becomes seriously ill, developing **opportunistic infections**, diseases and cancers that generally would not affect a person with an intact immune system. At this point a person is diagnosed with AIDS, the most serious and life-threatening phase of HIV disease.

The 1993 AIDS Surveillance Case Definition, as defined by the Centers for Disease Control and Prevention (CDC), includes 26 opportunistic infections that, in an HIV-positive person, lead to an AIDS diagnosis. This list includes:

✳ *Pneumocystis carinii pneumonia* (PCP), a deadly lung infection caused by a parasitic protozoan.

✳ *Kaposi's sarcoma* (KS), a rare type of cancer that produces purple/blue skin lesions as well as lesions on the internal organs.

✳ *Candidiasis*, persistent yeast infection of bronchi, trachea, lungs, esophagus, or vagina.

✳ *Cytomegalovirus* (CMV), a viral disease that often infects the retina, leading to blindness.

✳ *Herpes virus infections*, including chronic ulcers of the mouth, esophagus, or genitals, and shingles.

✳ *Pulmonary tuberculosis* (TB), a communicable infection caused by bacteria that damage the lungs.

✳ *Invasive cervical cancer.*

The case definition of AIDS also includes all people with HIV who have a CD4 lymphocyte count less than 200/mm^3, whether they do or do not have an opportunistic infection. Because of damage HIV can cause in the central nervous system, some people with AIDS develop a condition known as **AIDS dementia**, in which they have deteriorated mental and motor capacity. Symptoms range from inability to concentrate and remember to loss of ability to walk or talk to incontinence (loss of bladder and bowel control).

The average time from the point of infection with HIV to developing serious enough symptoms for an AIDS diagnosis is more than 10 years. Although some people progress to AIDS much more quickly than that, it is not yet known if everyone who is infected with HIV will go on to develop AIDS. Some people with AIDS regain their health and live without symptoms for many years; others suffer recurrent bouts of opportunistic infections, often living with more than one at a time; others die soon after, or even before, an AIDS diagnosis.

Evidence is mounting that some strains of HIV are weaker than others. In an Australian study of 25 people infected by blood transfusions, recipients of blood from donors who developed AIDS 10 or more years after infection were more than twice as likely to be alive 10 years later than recipients of blood from donors who developed AIDS sooner.

KEY TERMS

Acquired immune deficiency syndrome (AIDS) an incurable, sexually transmitted viral disease

Human immunodeficiency virus (HIV) a fragile virus spread through the exchange of blood and semen that circulates freely in the bloodstream and always precedes the onset of AIDS

HIV-positive determined to have HIV infection by testing

Acute HIV infection having symptoms similar to flu or mono, which disappear within days or a few weeks

Opportunistic infections illnesses that normally would not be serious but take hold in a person's body because of a weakened immune system caused by HIV

AIDS dementia deteriorated mental and motor capacity

The Demographics of HIV/AIDS

Worldwide some 4.5 million people have developed AIDS since the beginning of the epidemic. Since the mid-1970s HIV has infected more than 17 million people. The heaviest toll has been in Africa. At present, HIV infections are increasing most rapidly in Asia, according to Dr. Michael Merson of the World Health Organization (WHO). Figure 6.7 gives a breakdown of current numbers of HIV cases worldwide.

The Centers for Disease Control and Prevention estimate that at least 1 million Americans are infected with HIV — one in every 250 people. AIDS is the leading cause of death of U.S. men between the ages of 25 and 44. It is the fourth leading cause of death of women in the same age group.

At the time AIDS was first recognized as a disease in the United States, most of the people identified with symptoms were urban, Anglo gay men, so researchers understandably turned their attention to that segment of the population to try to find answers to this mysterious and deadly phenomenon. As the rest of the population was lulled into false comfort, the virus was making its way into all segments of the American community through unprotected sexual activity, injectable drug use, and the blood supply. People of all ages, races, sexual orientations, geographic locations, and both genders have become infected, though in different numbers. The CDC indicates that African American men are almost five times as likely as Anglo men to have AIDS and that African-American women are nearly 15 times as likely as Anglo women to have the disease. Figure 6.8 shows the trends in HIV/AIDS infection for various groups of Americans.

Until recently, limited attention was given to the way HIV/AIDS affects women. Women usually acquire HIV through injectable drug use and unprotected intercourse with an infected partner. Women are more likely than their male partners to become infected with HIV during heterosexual sex, because the concentration of HIV is higher in semen than in vaginal secretions. Woman to woman transmission seems to be rare.

Additional kinds of diseases and opportunistic infections are being connected to HIV/AIDS in women. The CDC added invasive cancer of the cervix to the list of opportunistic infections that lead to an AIDS diagnosis. Other conditions of which a woman should be aware that may signal HIV infection include:

— gonorrhea, chlamydia, and pelvic inflammatory disease (PID) that will not go away when treated by a physician.

— frequent yeast infections that cannot be explained by other risk factors

Sub-Saharan Africa — 10 Million

South and Southeast Asia — 2–3 Million

North Africa and Middle East — 100,000

South America — 2 Million

Eastern Europe and Central Asia — 50,000

North America — 1 Million

East Asia and Pacific — 50,000

Western Europe — 500,000

Australia — 25,000

250,000 HIV-infected adults

Source: World Health Organization.

Figure 6.7 Current HIV cases worldwide

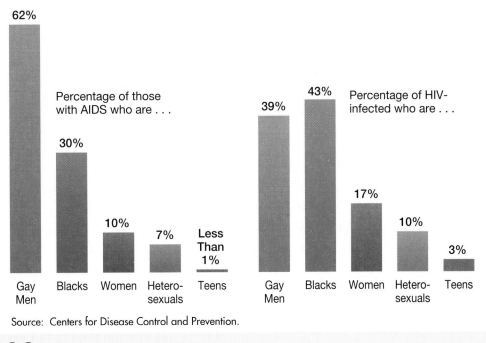

62%

Percentage of those
with AIDS who are . . .

30%

10%

7%

Less
Than
1%

Gay
Men

Blacks

Women

Hetero-
sexuals

Teens

39%

43%

Percentage of HIV-
infected who are . . .

17%

10%

3%

Gay
Men

Blacks

Women

Hetero-
sexuals

Teens

Source: Centers for Disease Control and Prevention.

Figure 6.8 Trends in HIV and AIDS cases for various groups

— abnormal Pap smears (Class II or III dysplasia).

A woman with any of the above conditions who has engaged in unprotected sex should ask her gynecologist to test for HIV antibodies.

A pregnant woman can pass the virus to the fetus. The virus can be passed before or during birth and through breast-feeding. In the past the risk of transmission to the fetus was thought to be 100%. Now we know that the risk is somewhere between 25% and 35%. This will have to be studied further to determine why HIV is not transmitted to the fetus in every case. According to a study by Michael St. Louis reported in the *Journal of the American Medical Association,* the baby is more likely to become infected if the mother is in the earliest stage of infection, when more HIV is present in the circulatory system, when she has AIDS, or if the placental membrane is inflamed. Infected fetuses might be born with congenital health problems or become ill with AIDS. In many cases, because of the mother's drug use, the baby is born not only HIV-infected but also drug-exposed. The risk to fetuses can be reduced if the mother takes the drug zidovudine (**AZT**) during the final trimester of pregnancy.

HIV infection has affected the U. S. African American and Hispanic communities disproportionally. Approximately 12% of the U. S. population is African American, yet 27% of all people with AIDS are African American. Similarly, 8% of the U. S. population is Hispanic, but Hispanic Americans account for 15% of all AIDS cases. Figure 6.9 highlights these statistics. As of June 1994,

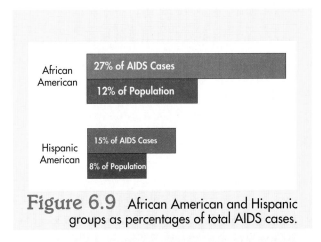

African
American

27% of AIDS Cases

12% of Population

Hispanic
American

15% of AIDS Cases

8% of Population

Figure 6.9 African American and Hispanic groups as percentages of total AIDS cases.

KEY TERMS

AZT a drug used to treat AIDS

Should You Take an AIDS Test?

The question about whether to get tested for HIV has concerned many individuals. When HIV infection and AIDS are concerned, clouds of fear, suspicion, and misunderstanding still loom large in many communities. Fears of being ostracized by family and friends, being kicked out of school, or losing a job have kept many people who suspect exposure to HIV from being tested. In some cases people simply cannot face the possibility of a positive test and do not want to know. If you are considering having a screening test for HIV:

❋ Take your test anonymously in an alternative-site facility where you will be given a number and your name will not be used (some facilities do confidential, not anonymous testing).

❋ Make sure the testing site does counseling before and after the test.

according to the Centers for Disease Control, 130,382 African Americans and 68,903 Hispanic Americans have been diagnosed with AIDS.

According to the CDC, 38% of those who have AIDS are heterosexual men and women who are intravenous drug users. Another 38% of the cases are related to either homosexual or bisexual contact among males; and 7% of African Americans with AIDS are homosexual or bisexual men who also inject drugs.

In the Hispanic community the reported AIDS cases are related to homosexual or bisexual contact among males (42%) and IV drug use among females and heterosexual males (40%). Males reporting homosexual or bisexual contact who also inject drugs account for 7% of the AIDS cases in the U. S. Hispanic community.

The rates for AIDS among women and children in the African American and Hispanic communities are devastating. Among all women diagnosed with AIDS, 54% are African American and 25% are Hispanic. Among all pediatric cases, 56% are African American and 21% are Hispanic.

Diagnosis and Treatment

In 1985 a reliable blood test was developed to screen blood and blood products for HIV antibodies. HIV infection can be diagnosed by a blood test called **ELISA** or **EIA** (enzyme-linked immunoassay). This screening test is done to check for antibodies to HIV that a person will develop after being exposed to the virus. ELISA does not test for the presence of the virus in the bloodstream, only antibodies to it.

If a person tests positive on the ELISA, the test is performed a second time. If that test is positive also, another blood test called the **Western Blot** is done to confirm the presence of HIV antibodies. AIDS is diagnosed by the presence of HIV antibodies *and* one or more of the opportunistic infections or conditions mentioned earlier.

Again, AIDS has no cure, nor is an immunization available to prevent or cure HIV infection. Effective drug therapies have been developed to prevent or treat specific opportunistic infections, but most of these drugs are toxic and have significant side effects. Several antiviral medications, including AZT (zidovudine), DDI (didanosine), and DDC (dideoxycytidine), are used to slow the progress of the HIV infection and improve quality of life, but they have not been shown to prolong survival.

The ability of HIV to adapt and evolve has frustrated efforts to significantly prolong life. A new class of potential anti-AIDS drugs known as **protease inhibitors** shows some promise. These are different from the existing drugs in that protease inhibitors target a later point in the viral life cycle. Still, progress against AIDS is slow. Dr. Dani Bolognesi of Duke University predicted, at the Tenth International Conference on AIDS in Japan in the summer of 1994, that an AIDS vaccine will not be available for widespread testing for at least 1-3 years.

Prevention

In the United States the CDC estimates that by 1995, 40,000 to 50,000 AIDS cases will be reported yearly. As of June, 1994, 401,749 cases of AIDS and 243,423 deaths had been reported in the United States since 1981. Roughly 40,000 people are dying of AIDS in the United States each year.

A particularly vulnerable group in the United States is the adolescent population. Experimentation with sex and drugs, in combination with alcohol use and a sense of indestructibility, makes young people especially vulnerable to HIV infection. Most adolescents know the facts about HIV/AIDS and risk reduction but find it difficult to *do* what they *know*. More than 45% of people diagnosed with AIDS were infected with HIV during their teens and 20s.

The number of AIDS cases attributed to heterosexual contact grows each year, especially among young people. According to *AIDS Weekly*, March 21, 1994, the number of people who acquired AIDS heterosexually jumped 130% from 1992 to 1993.

Transmission rates among young gay and bisexual men are very high as the changes the older gay community have made have not yet reached younger men. According to a study directed by Dr. Gary Remafedi of the Youth and AIDS Projects at the University of Minnesota and published in the August, 1994, issue of *Pediatrics*, 63% of the gay and bisexual young men surveyed were at "extreme risk."

How to reach this group, any group that engages in at-risk behaviors, remains a challenge. Several studies suggest renewed focus on prevention efforts among older youth and young adults.

Because HIV/AIDS has no cure or way to achieve immunity, we must look to education and behavior change to slow its progression. Former U.S. Surgeon General C. Everett Koop was very direct when he announced to the nation the ways individuals could reduce their risk for HIV infection. He stated that if a person did not choose sexual abstinence, reducing the risk of HIV infection would depend on the following conditions:

❋ A mutually monogamous sexual relationship with a noninfected partner.

❋ Use of a latex condom with *each* sexual act that exposes either sex partner to semen, vaginal secretions, or blood.

❋ Use of the spermicide nonoxynol-9, which kills HIV.

❋ No sharing of hypodermic needles, syringes, and other "works" by persons using any injectable drug including anabolic steroids.

☎ Call for information

CDC National AIDS Hotline
800-342-AIDS
   (24 hours daily)
(in Spanish): 800-344-7432
   (8:00 a.m. – 2:00 p.m. 7 days a week)

Shanti Project
(counseling and assistance for persons with AIDS)
415-864-2273

AIDS in drug (clinical) studies
800-874-2572

❋ No sex acts with persons known to use or suspected of using injectable drugs.

The methods for preventing HIV/AIDS espoused by Dr. Koop have not changed. Sexually active people must alter their behavior to reduce their risk or thousands more will become infected with HIV before an immunization is discovered. HIV does not discriminate by race, creed, color, occupation, sexual orientation, religious affiliation, or country club membership. Anyone who is engaging in unprotected sex can be exposed to HIV. Therefore, sexually active people must become informed and eliminate risky behavior to reduce their personal risk.

Syphilis

As one of the oldest known STDs, **syphilis** has been researched and documented for centuries. One of the more successful tests for this condition (the Hinton-Davies test for syphilis) was developed by an African American, William Hinton. Another event linking the African American community with this disease was the unethical experiment (the "Tuskegee Study") conducted by the U. S. Public

KEY TERMS

ELISA (EIA) a blood test that diagnoses HIV by exposing the presence of HIV antibodies

Western Blot a blood test performed after ELISA comes back positive twice and used to confirm the results of the ELISA tests

Protease inhibitors new class of potential anti-AIDS drugs that target a later point in the viral life cycle

Syphilis a sexually transmitted disease caused by a spirochete bacterium

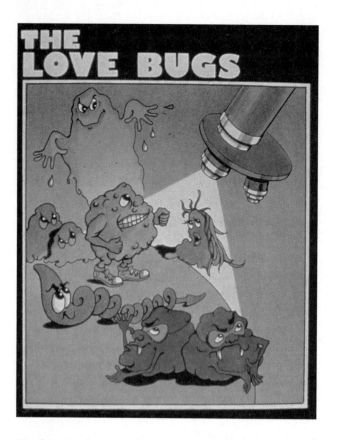

THE LOVE BUGS

Health Service on African Americans from 1932 to the early 1970s in Macon County, Alabama. With the knowledge and direction of the Public Health Service, African American men who were exposed to syphilis were medically supervised but were not treated. As the disease ran its course, clinical evidence was gathered at the expense of the health of these unwitting victims.

Syphilis is caused by a spiral-shaped (spirochete) bacterium called *Treponema pallidum,* which has the ability to penetrate the outer layer of skin, the epidermis. Spirochetes can enter the body at virtually any site and invade the circulatory system. Once in the bloodstream, the bacteria move freely through the body systems and leave destruction in their wake. The body systems especially vulnerable to this damage are the cardiovascular system, the central nervous system, and the musculoskeletal system.

The course of syphilis, which takes many years, can be discussed in four separate stages. Each stage has a separate set of symptoms, distinct from the others. If discovered in time, syphilis can be treated and cured so the person will not progress from one stage to the next.

In the first stage, *primary syphilis,* the symptoms appear from 10 to 90 days after the spirochetes invade the body. Usually the symptoms

appear within 3 to 5 weeks after exposure to the pathogen. A **chancre,** or lesion, appears at the exact place the bacteria entered the person's body. The chancre is painless and vanishes without treatment. These circumstances may lull the infected person into a false sense that the problem has gone away so diagnosis and treatment are unnecessary. A person who is not familiar with the symptoms of primary syphilis will not connect the appearance of a lesion to a sexual or close physical encounter of several weeks past.

The chancre is the vehicle by which the person passes the syphilis spirochete. Even if not treated, the chancre disappears in a few weeks. The person has no other symptoms and seems to be healthy. Meanwhile the spirochetes continue to circulate through the bloodstream and produce a different set of symptoms later.

The stage of *secondary syphilis* usually begins weeks to months after the symptoms of primary syphilis leave. In this second stage of syphilis, the symptoms seem totally unrelated to those of primary syphilis. They include low-grade fever, general malaise, swollen glands, and white patches on the mucous membranes of the throat. In addition, a body rash may appear on the torso and even the palms and soles, and the person may lose hair temporarily.

During this stage the person continues to be contagious and, as in primary syphilis, will test positive on a blood test for this condition. Within 3 to 6 weeks the symptoms of secondary syphilis disappear as mysteriously as they appeared. If the person is treated during this stage, the pathogens are killed and the progression of this disease ends. If it is not treated, however, the spirochetes continue to circulate freely within the bloodstream and work silently toward the destruction of many body systems.

The stage of *latent syphilis* disease may begin 2 to 4 years after the signs and systems of secondary syphilis have disappeared. Unfortunately, latent syphilis has no outward signs. This asymptomatic state presents a two-part problem.

1. The person continues to be contagious during the early part of this phase and is capable of passing the pathogens during intimate contact.

2. The person feels fine and is unaware of the damage to certain systems of the body.

Latent syphilis in people is like termite infestation in a house. The termites begin their silent

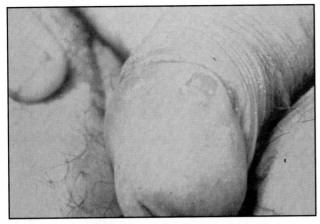
Chancre on head of penis

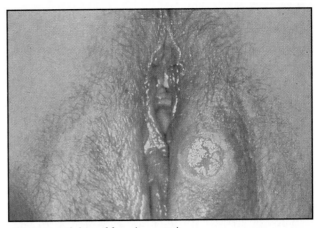
Chancre on labia of female genitalia

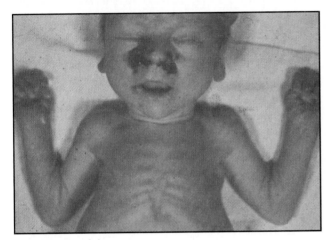
Congenital syphilis

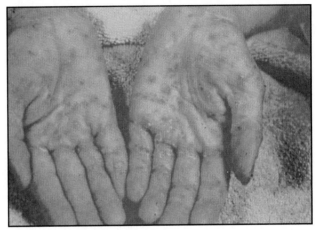
The rash of secondary syphilis

destruction of the wood structures of the home, and the owner is not aware of the extent of the infestation and the damage until a wooden support gives way.

During the early phases of latent syphilis, the person will test positive on a blood test. As this phase continues, the person no longer is able to infect others during sexual contact, but a woman still can pass along the disease to offspring. If latent syphilis is not treated, damage to the cardiovascular and other body systems continues.

Late syphilis may appear 10 to 20 years after latency. During late syphilis the person's immune system has killed the bacteria, but widespread tissue damage is permanent. Health problems that may arise as a result of untreated syphilis are:

❋ *central nervous system damage*
    dementia and insanity
    blindness
    deafness
    partial paralysis

❋ *cardiovascular system damage*
    heart disease
    damage to the aorta

❋ *musculoskeletal system damage*
    syphilitic arthritis

In late syphilis this damage to the body cannot be reversed by medication, and death usually results from heart failure.

Syphilis is diagnosed through a physical examination and a blood test. Treatment consists of administering penicillin or other antibiotics. Some advanced cases of late syphilis cannot be treated.

Women who are infected with the bacteria of syphilis during pregnancy should seek medical

KEY TERMS

Chancre a painless ulcer that develops at the site where infection enters the body and is the primary symptom of syphilis attention immediately. The spirochetes move freely in the mother's bloodstream, so they can and do cross the placenta and invade the circulatory system of the developing fetus. If this situation does occur and is not treated, the fetus will be delivered with a condition known as **congenital syphilis**. The fetus has gross birth defects or may have no outward signs of infection but may develop neurological and other health problems later in life. To avoid the possibility of genital syphilis, a woman receiving prenatal care and who suspects that she has been exposed to syphilis during her pregnancy should report this to her physician or health care provider.

Hepatitis B and C

Hepatitis B, or serum hepatitis, is caused by a virus that lives in the bloodstream but also is found in semen and vaginal secretion. It causes inflammation of the liver. In the past the risk of acquiring hepatitis B was linked to receiving contaminated blood through transfusions and exposure to contaminated blood in a hospital and to heroin addicts who inject. Today, many of the 240,000 reported cases annually stem from injectable drug use and sexual contact.

Hepatitis B is the most common cause of liver cancer worldwide.

The incubation period for hepatitis B ranges from 15 to 180 days. The condition is characterized first by flulike symptoms (low-grade fever, fatigue, joint and muscle nausea, vomiting, and diarrhea). As the liver enlarges, symptoms include jaundice (yellowing of the skin), dark urine, and abdominal pain.

If hepatitis B is not treated, it may persist many years, even a lifetime. It is the most common cause of liver cancer worldwide, and 5,000 people die each year from hepatitis-related cirrhosis of the liver. The virus eventually destroys the liver and results in death.

Diagnosed by a blood test and other laboratory analyses, hepatitis B usually is treated by injection of immunoglobulin (antibodies for hepatitis B), special diet, and rest. It cannot be cured, and the virus can be passed from an infected mother to her baby during birth, in which case a shot is recommended 12 hours after birth. Hepatitis B vaccination is recommended as a routine childhood immunization.

A **hepatitis C** virus has been identified. Its mode of transmission, symptoms, and treatment are similar to those of hepatitis B. Hepatitis C is found more commonly in those who inject drugs and those who have received blood from countries where the blood supply is not screened properly (as it is in the United States).

STDs That Cause Vaginitis, Cervicitis, and Urethritis

Vaginitis means inflammation of the vagina. **Cervicitis** denotes inflammation of the cervix. Symptoms of these conditions include pain or discomfort, redness of the tissue, and a vaginal discharge. Both vaginitis and cervicitis sometimes are caused by pathogens that have been transported to the vagina during coitus. Trichomoniasis causes vaginitis. Gonorrhea and chlamydia cause vaginitis and cervicitis.

When men have symptoms of an STD, they generally appear in the urogenital tract. **Urethritis** is an inflammation of the urethra. It is the most common condition affecting the male reproductive system. Symptoms of urethritis may include pain or discomfort in the urethra, especially during urination. The STDs associated with urethritis in males are gonorrhea, chlamydia, and trichomoniasis. Women, too, may experience urethritis when they are affected by the STDs that produce vaginal inflammation.

Urethritis is diagnosed by medical examination, sometimes including a bacterial culture. It is treated with antibiotics.

Chlamydia

Chlamydia has been called the "silent epidemic," but it is now the most common STD in the United States (see Figure 6.10), affecting more than 4 million people each year, according to the CDC. It is caused by a bacteria called *Chlamydia trachomatis*. In females the signs and symptoms may not appear until several months after exposure. In some cases they are so mild that the woman does not notice them or may even ignore them. Symptoms include inflammation of the cervix and whitish discharge

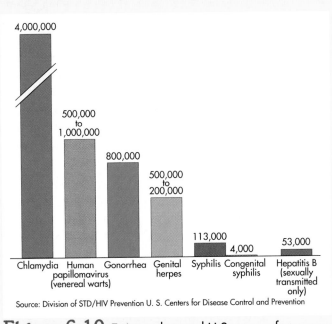

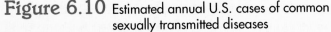

Source: Division of STD/HIV Prevention U. S. Centers for Disease Control and Prevention

Figure 6.10 Estimated annual U.S. cases of common sexually transmitted diseases

from the vagina, bleeding between menstrual periods, and abdominal pain. Some women have discomfort during urination. The discharge, whether it comes from the cervix or the urethra, contains the chlamydia organism. It can be passed during coitus and other sex acts.

Unfortunately, chlamydia infection may go undetected in women for months or even years as the organism moves to the upper reproductive tract. If untreated, the woman may develop inflammation of the uterus, fallopian tubes, and ovaries. Inflammation of the upper reproductive organs is known as **pelvic inflammatory disease (PID)**. It is not one specific disease. Complications of PID include lower back pain, scarring of the fallopian tubes, and possible sterility.

If a woman has a chlamydia infection, the organisms may be passed to the fetus during vaginal delivery, causing complications such as eye infection (conjunctivitis) and pneumonia in the fetus. More than 30,000 babies are born with chlamydia each year. The risk for spontaneous abortion and stillbirth is high.

The signs and symptoms of chlamydia are more likely to appear sooner in men. Still they may not become apparent until several weeks after exposure. Symptoms usually include urethritis, with a characteristic fluid and mucous discharge from the penis and discomfort during urination.

Chlamydia trachomatis can infect the urethra of men, causing a seemingly innocuous infection called **nongonococcal urethritis (NGU)**. Symptoms include discharge from the penis and burning during urination. For the purpose of effective treatment, NGU should be considered an STD infection and not a simple urinary tract infection. Untreated NGU can become serious. The organisms can move to the prostate gland, vas deferens, and epididymis, causing complications in the urogenital tract.

Diagnosis of chlamydia can be done within half an hour by taking a sample of secretions. Treatment for chlamydia is with an antibiotic such as tetracycline. Neither penicillin nor any OTC medication is effective in treating chlamydia. Antibiotic treatment usually is complete within 2 to 3 weeks. Individuals being treated for chlamydia who choose to have intercourse should use a latex condom to prevent the spread of the pathogens to the other sex partner.

Gonorrhea

Gonorrhea is one of the most common STDs, with the highest incidence among 20–24 years olds, in

KEY TERMS

Congenital syphilis a condition in which a baby is born with syphilis transmitted by the mother

Hepatitis B a form of hepatitis caused by a virus that lives in the bloodstream, in semen, and in vaginal secretions; transmitted through sexual contact or contaminated hypodermic needles

Hepatitis C a form of hepatitis caused by a virus similar to hepatitis B; commonly found among IV drug users and those who have received improperly screened blood

Vaginitis inflammation of the vagina

Cervicitis inflammation of the cervix

Urethritis inflammation of the urethra

Chlamydia a common STD caused by the bacteria *Chlamydia trachomatis*

Pelvic inflammatory disease (PID) inflammation of the uterus, fallopian tubes, and ovaries

Nongonococcal urethritis (NGU) infection in the urethra of men, usually caused by the chlamydia bacteria

the United States according to the Centers for Disease Control. One of the "fortunate" aspects of gonorrhea infection is that, at least in men, it is not easily ignored. **Gonorrhea**, sometimes called the "clap," is caused by the bacteria *Neisseria gonorrheae*. Like most pathogens that produce STDs, it thrives on warm, dark, and moist body surfaces. It can survive in the reproductive tract for years. The gonococcus is passed during coitus and produces urethritis in men and cervicitis in women. If individuals engage in oral or anal sex, the bacteria living in the pus discharge can invade the mucous lining of the throat or anus and cause infection at those sites.

In men the incubation period usually is about 2 to 10 days after exposure. Symptoms in men include pus discharge from the urethra in the penis and burning during urination. This discomfort usually is enough to send men to a physician for prompt treatment. Because the incubation period is so brief, men generally are aware of their infection within a week. As with any STD, the advantage of a short incubation period is that the infected person will notice the symptoms and seek treatment promptly. Again, any partner should be advised to seek treatment.

Untreated gonorrhea infection in men can have serious consequences. The gonococcus can spread, infecting the urinary tract, vas deferens, and testes. Scar tissue that forms in the urogenital tract as a result of the infection can cause problems with urination and lead to sterility.

The signs of early gonorrhea infection in women are not detected easily. Generally, women are asymptomatic. Some have a pus discharge from the vagina and burning during urination. In any case, the bacteria continue to live in the reproductive tract, infecting the uterus, fallopian tubes, and ovaries. Untreated gonorrhea in women may lead to pelvic inflammatory disease and infertility.

Gonorrheal infection of the female poses a threat to the newborn in vaginal delivery. The gonococcus may invade the eyes of the fetus while passing through the vagina during delivery. This may cause inflammation of the eyes, which can produce blindness. Today this complication is averted by routinely placing silver nitrate or penicillin drops in the eyes of newborns immediately after delivery to prevent infection.

Gonorrhea produces urethritis in men and cervicitis in women.

The most reliable test to diagnose gonorrhea is analysis of bacteria cultured from discharges of the urethra, vagina, throat, or anus of the person seeking treatment. Penicillin (or some other antibiotic if a person is allergic to penicillin or has a case of penicillin-resistant gonorrhea) is the most effective treatment. Gonorrhea cannot be cured with over-the-counter preparations. People who have been exposed and are with or without symptoms should seek treatment by appropriate health care professionals.

Trichomoniasis

A form of vaginitis known as **trichomoniasis**, "trich," or TV is caused by a one-celled organism or protozoan called *Trichomonas vaginalis*. As with other pathogens that cause STDs, the trichomonad of TV thrives in warm, dark, and moist environments. The reproductive structures of men and women alike are perfect environments for these protozoa to survive. They emerge when the body defense mechanisms are weakened.

Men usually are asymptomatic while the TV organisms are living in their urogenital tracts. During coitus a man can transmit the protozoa to the female vagina, where they multiply. Signs and symptoms of trichomoniasis in women are itching of the vagina, labia, and perineal area, and a translucent discharge from the vagina that is bubbly or foamy, green-yellow in color, and malodorous.

This discharge contains the trichomonad and therefore is contagious. If exchanged during sexual intercourse, the male partner could become infected and have symptoms of urethritis (discomfort of the urethra and frequent urination). In some cases men may remain asymptomatic and simply pass on the trichomonad to another sexual partner.

The TV organism does not limit its invasion to the vagina or urethra of men. It moves to the upper regions of the reproductive tracts of both women and men, where topical medications cannot reach it. To reduce the risk of continuous or recurring infections, TV should be treated as soon as symptoms appear. Trichomoniasis is diagnosed easily by a gynecologist or urologist, who can identify the trichomonad in the discharge from the vagina or the urethra. TV *cannot* be treated with OTC

OBJECTIVES FOR SEXUALLY TRANSMITTED DISEASES

✳ Decrease the annual incidence of diagnosed AIDS cases and the prevalence of HIV infection.

✳ Increase the proportion of sexually active, unmarried people who used a condom at last sexual intercourse.

✳ Reduce the incidence of gonorrhea, chlamydia, and syphilis.

✳ Reduce the incidence of congenital syphilis.

✳ Reduce the incidence of sexually transmitted hepatitis B infection.

medications. The effective treatment is an oral prescription medicine called Flagyl, which should be taken as directed.

To reduce the risk of "ping-pong" infection, both partners should be treated simultaneously even if one is asymptomatic. If the couple is to engage in coitus during treatment, the man should wear a latex condom to protect both partners from exchange of body secretions that may contain the trichomonad that has yet to be killed by the medication.

Candida

As a result of advertisements on television and in women's magazines, **candida** is getting unprecedented coverage. This common condition, affecting at least half a million American women a year, also is known as candidiasis, moniliasis, and yeast infection. It is caused by one of four varieties of the candida fungus, of which *Candida albicans* is the most common. These fungi inhabit the vagina normally but will multiply and cause problems if certain agents and conditions are present. Diabetes, lowered immunity, birth control pills, pregnancy, and antibiotics all can decrease the acidity of the vagina and render it a fertile arena for excessive growth of the fungi.

Symptoms of yeast infection include itching or burning of the vagina and labia, redness of the vagina and labia, and lumpy or curdlike discharge from the vagina that clings to the vaginal walls and labia.

The white discharge contains the fungi and can be passed during sex acts. A woman usually avoids coitus during the time of infection because the vagina is irritated and intercourse is uncomfortable. Men usually are asymptomatic for candida even though they may be carriers of the fungi.

Until 1990 the most effective treatments for candida were the prescription fungicides clotrimazole and miconazole nitrate. Now these medications are available to women in over-the-counter (OTC) medications as preparations to be inserted into the vagina and rubbed on the labia. Any woman with a first-time vaginal yeast infection should consult a gynecologist for a diagnosis before using an OTC medication. If her self-diagnosis is not correct, the medication will not kill the pathogens causing the symptoms, the condition will worsen, and the woman can expose her sex partner. If she is advised to use an OTC medication, the woman should follow the manufacturer's instructions and use the medicine as directed to be sure that all of the fungi present will be killed. If the woman chooses to have vaginal intercourse during the course of treatment, her partner should wear a condom to reduce the risk of "ping-pong infection."

No matter if the fungi of candidiasis were transmitted sexually or multiplied for some other reason, the condition can recur if it is not treated properly. Because no one is immune to candida, a person can be reinfected.

KEY TERMS

Gonorrhea bacterial STD; also called "clap"

Trichomoniasis STD caused by protozoan; also known as trich or TV

Candida common STD caused by a fungus; also known as candidiasis, moniliasis, and yeast infection

Herpes

Herpes is an STD that produces distinctive lesions. The culprit is a family of viruses called the *Herpes simplex* virus (HSV). Approximately a half million new cases are reported to the CDC each year, and CDC estimates the total prevalence at 20 million Americans. Other herpes viruses are *Herpes zoster* or varicella, which causes chicken pox and shingles, and the Epstein-Barr virus, which causes mononucleosis (discussed earlier in the chapter).

The herpes virus is capable of producing lesions in the form of blisters on the epidermis (skin) as well as on mucous tissue. *HSV Type 1* produces oral lesions, called "fever blisters" or "cold sores," on the lips, in the mouth, and sometimes in the nose. *HSV Type 2* produces lesions or blisters on the genitalia. HSV Type 2 is transmitted sexually and is referred to as *genital herpes*. Oral-genital contact can introduce HSV Type 1 to the genital area and HSV Type 2 to the mouth and face.

The signs and symptoms of genital and oral herpes are similar for both sexes. Usually within 2 weeks after exposure, painful clusters of blisters appear on the genitals (penis, scrotum, vagina, cervix), on the thighs, buttocks, anal area, lips, or mouth of the infected person. These fluid-filled lesions contain the virus and make the person contagious. The blisters remain for several days, then disappear without treatment. Generally the first outbreak of herpes is the most painful.

Infection with HSV Types 1 and 2 are permanent. The virus never leaves the person; it lies dormant in nerve endings in the cheek and lower back, respectively. During times of physiological or psychological stress, or any condition that suppresses the immune system, the virus can activate in recurring outbreaks weeks, months, or even years after the first one. Before the outbreak some people have vague signs (prodromal period) such as irritability, fever, and a tingling or burning sensation in the area where the blisters will appear. Some people learn to recognize the prodromal signs and prepare for subsequent outbreaks.

A common complication of herpes is **autoinnoculation**, spreading the virus to other parts of one's own body, such as the mouth and eyes. Women who are infected with herpes have a higher risk for cervical cancer. If a woman with active herpes lesions delivers a baby vaginally, the baby has a one-in-four chance of becoming infected. If infected, the baby can become blind, incur damage to internal organs, have mental retardation, and die. A caesarean section delivery lowers the risk of infecting the baby.

Herpes is diagnosed by microscopic examination and culture of the fluid contained in the blisters. It has no cure, although it can be treated with topical over-the-counter preparations that ease the pain and dry the blisters. A more effective treatment is the prescription medicine Zovirax (acyclovir), an ointment that can be applied directly to the lesion or taken orally in capsule form. The oral medication, taken daily, tends to reduce the number of recurring outbreaks but should be taken only under medical supervision.

Individuals applying ointment or otherwise handling the lesions should wash their hands thoroughly before touching other parts of the body so they will not introduce HSV to other body sites (self-inoculation). Because a person may be

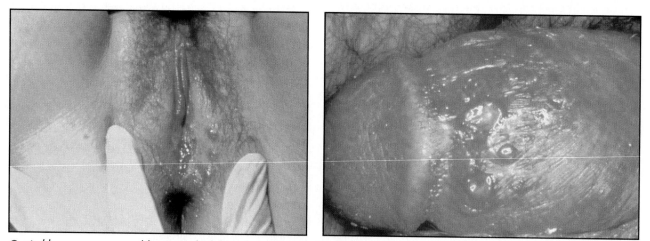

Genital herpes appears as blisters on the labia of a woman and on the male penis.

contagious prior to the appearance of active lesions, honesty with sex partners about this condition is important so the partner can make an informed decision about sexual activity.

Genital Warts

HPV or human papilloma virus is another sexually transmissible virus that produces recognizable lesions. These are called *condyloma acuminatum* **genital** or **venereal warts**. This STD, one of the most prevalent STDs in the United States, infects up to a million Americans each year. It is the most common STD for which students seek medical attention at college clinics, and is most prevalent in ages 16–25.

About 60% of those exposed to HPV develop genital warts (those with a weak immune system are more susceptible), some people never develop symptoms, and some women reveal symptoms only under internal medical examination by **colposcopy** or a new photographic procedure using a cerviscope or a DNA probe.

When asymptomatic, the first and only sign of HPV infection in women is the appearance of painless cauliflowerlike warts on the labia, in the vagina, on the cervix, or near the anus. These areas are warm and moist and thus are ideal environments for the warts to thrive. The warts are unsightly in appearance and occasionally can block the entrance to the vagina or cervix or obstruct the urethra. They may grow faster during pregnancy and shrink after the baby is born. The virus can be transmitted from mother to child during birth, sometimes causing the baby to develop warts in the throat, which obstruct breathing. Researchers are studying the possible link to cervical cancer, and genital warts may play a role in other genital cancers as well, including cancer of the penis.

In men, genital warts may form on the glans or shaft of the penis, on or near the anal opening, or in the rectum. Genital warts are found more often in uncircumcised than circumcised males.

Because the warts are so distinctive, they usually can be diagnosed by a simple physical exam. As with the other STDs caused by viruses, HPV has no cure. The warts (not the virus) may be removed by surgery (including laser surgery), cauterization, freezing (cryosurgery), or applying chemicals to the affected areas.

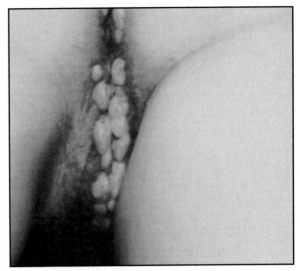

Genital warts

Pubic Lice

Often called crab lice or crabs, **pubic lice** infest the pubic hair of their host. The condition is caused by a metazoan named *Phthirius pubis*. Crab lice are transmitted when the pubic hair of the partners rubs together during sexual activity. Further, crabs can be contracted from contaminated clothing, towels, or linen that have had contact with the carrier's pubic area. Even though crab lice are associated with pubic hair, they may infest the facial hair (beards, mustaches, eyebrows) of partners if oral-genital contact has occurred. The incubation period is brief, 24 to 48 hours.

To ensure continuous infestation, the female lice lay eggs, called nits, that are attached to the hair shaft. After several days these eggs hatch and another generation of crabs emerges. Signs and symptoms of **pediculosis** or louse infestation are:

— intense itching of the pubic and perineal areas

KEY TERMS

Herpes an STD caused by the herpes simplex virus (HSV), which produces distinctive lesions

Autoinnoculation spreading a virus to other parts of one's own body

Genital (venereal) warts an STD caused by a virus that produces lesions on the genitals

Colposcopy an internal medical examination performed to detect the presence of genital warts in women who are asymptomatic

Pubic lice small insects that infest the host's pubic hair

Pediculosis infection with lice

— skin irritation (even sores, from scratching)

— visual identification of lice in hair and nits on hair shafts.

The advantage of the short incubation period is that an infested person is likely to seek treatment promptly and can identify the source of the infection. To prevent reinfestation, the treatment for lice (pubic, head, or body) must include a method for both killing the lice and removing the nits. Several OTC preparations (R.I.D.) come in the form of special shampoos. Kwell is available by prescription in most states. The instructions should be followed, and the treatment should be repeated in 7 days to kill any lice that hatched from eggs that were not removed during the initial treatment. Contaminated clothing and linen need not be destroyed, but these items should be washed and dried or dry-cleaned.

Scabies

Like pubic lice, **scabies** is caused by a multicellular parasite (a mite). This microscopic pest, *Sarcoptes scabiei*, burrows under the skin of the infected person and lays eggs. The signs and symptoms of scabies are:

— intense itching of infected areas.

— skin lesions that appear in the pubic area, on the genitals, legs, and abdomen.

Treatment for scabies is similar to that for infestation of lice. If these parasites do not respond to treatment or the lesions do not heal, however, a physician should be consulted. As with crab lice, scabies can be transmitted by towels, linens, and clothing. This infestation does not have dire consequences, though it certainly is not pleasant.

Other STDs

Lymphogranuloma Venereum (LGV)

Caused by one of several strains of chlamydia, *Lymphogranuloma venereum (LGV)* is a system-wide STD. After a short incubation period, the first symptom is a small, painless pimplelike lesion that usually appears on or near the genital region. In the secondary stage of LGV, symptoms include fever, chills, and headaches stemming from the systemic involvement. The lymph nodes in the groin enlarge, become firm, and then soften and rupture. Late complications, because of blockage of the vessels of the lymphatic system, are swollen limbs and genitals (elephantiasis).

LGV is treated with antibiotics. Although it is more common in tropical climates, the number of reported cases has been increasing in the United States.

Chancroid

Sometimes known as soft chancre, chancroid is caused by the bacteria *Haemophilus ducreyi*. The incubation period ranges from 2 to 14 days; the average is about 2 to 5 days. Symptoms of chancroid are small bumps or papules appearing on the genitals or in the perineal area. These lesions erode and become soft, painful ulcers that produce a discharge. Lymph nodes in the groin also may be affected. Treatment for chancroid includes keeping the affected areas clean of discharge so surrounding tissue will not be infected, plus the use of antibiotics.

Granuloma Inguinale

Granuloma inguinale, sometimes referred to as Donovanosis, is caused by the bacterium *Calymmatobacterium granulomatis*. This condition is most common in tropical and subtropical areas of the world. Few cases are reported in the United States. The incubation period is 8 to 80 days.

Granuloma inguinale is recognized by the appearance of hard, painless nodules (bumps) on the genitals. These lesions erode and create larger beefy-red lesions on adjacent areas, including the area near the anus. This condition is treated with antibiotics.

Reducing the Risk for STDs

Abstaining from sexual acts that include a partner will eliminate the chances of acquiring an STD. Some people have chosen abstinence and masturbation as a means of reducing their risk. If abstinence is not a viable alternative, other measures can be taken to sharply reduce the risk of acquiring STDs, although they do not eliminate the risk completely. Each person must take responsibility for reducing his or her own risks. Figure 6.11 presents the risks for contracting various STDs by gender.

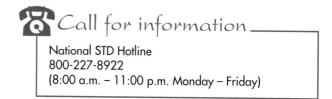

☎ Call for information

National STD Hotline
800-227-8922
(8:00 a.m. – 11:00 p.m. Monday – Friday)

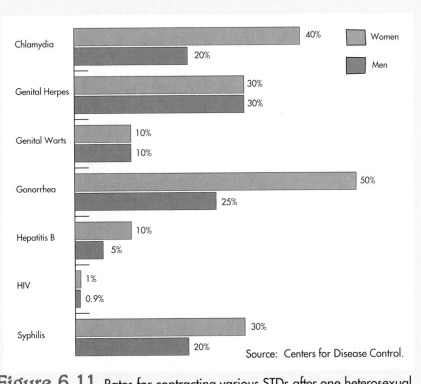

Figure 6.11 Rates for contracting various STDs after one heterosexual unprotected intercourse

DIAGNOSIS, TREATMENT, AND OTHER CONCERNS

Prompt, effective treatment, and education about safer sex are necessary to reduce the spread of STDs. If a private practitioner is not available or affordable, a person can be diagnosed and treated for STDs at the city or county public health department STD clinic. Because this service is supported by taxes, individuals are treated regardless of their ability to pay. The telephone number of the clinic usually can be found in the Blue Pages of the local telephone directory under the listing of Department of Health, Infectious Disease, or Specialty Clinics.

Diagnosis and treatment are the first steps in controlling STDs. People reporting to the clinic are examined, and any tests necessary are performed to diagnose or discover which STD is the cause of the problem. Administration of appropriate medication should follow the diagnosis. Patients will be instructed on proper use of the medication and appropriate follow-up. Medications must be used as directed so the symptoms do not come back. Even during treatment individuals may be contagious and should take precautions not to infect partners if sexual activities continue during treatment.

Because they have been exposed to the pathogen, sexual partners of infected individuals also should be contacted so they can be treated. Assistance in notifying partners and in investigating cases are important functions of public health departments in controlling the spread of STDs in the community. Individual rights and privacy are protected by confidentiality and anonymity.

Before leaving a public STD clinic, those reporting for treatment should be counseled about their health, the risk of infecting others, and ways to reduce the risk of exposure and new infection. There is no immunity to any STD. Educating the client about the risk reduction is a vital function of the public health department. Table 6.4 lists relevant information pertaining to selected sexually transmitted diseases.

KEY TERMS

Scabies condition caused by parasite that burrows under the skin and lays eggs

Table 6.4
Summary of Common Sexually Transmitted Diseases

Name	Pathogen Type	Distinguishing Sign or Symptom	Diagnosis	Treatment
Candidiasis (yeast infection)	fungus	female: cottage cheese-like discharge, strawberry-red color of vagina and labia, pain in genital area; male: usually asymptomatic	identification of discharge	prescription or OTC fungicide (miconazole) (cure)
Chlamydia	bacterium	male: watery discharge from urethra; female: usually asymptomatic; sometimes a similar discharge; leading cause of PID*; can cause prostatitis in men	culture of discharge	antibiotics other than penicillin (cure)
Genital herpes	virus	blisters in genital and rectal areas	presence of blisters and laboratory identification of virus in fluid of blister	Zovirax (acyclovir) (not a cure)
Genital warts (venereal warts)	virus (HPV)	cauliflowerlike growths in genital and rectal areas	presence of lesions	removal of lesions by surgery or chemicals (not a cure)
Gonorrhea (clap)	bacterium	male: pus discharge from urethra, burning during urination; female: usually asymptomatic; can lead to PID*; sterility (in both)	culture of discharge	ceftriaxone sodium (cure)
HIV/AIDS	virus	asymptomatic at first; opportunistic infections	blood test; usually none in initial stages	AZT (now called ZDV) and ddI (not a cure)
Pubic lice (crabs)	metazoan	intense itching of areas covered with pubic hair	presence of lice and nits (eggs) on pubic hair	prescription or OTC pediculocide shampoo (cure)
Syphilis	bacterium (spirochete)	primary: chancre secondary: rash latent: asymptomatic late: irreversible damage to central nervous system, cardiovascular system	blood test	penicillin or other antibiotic (cure)
Trichomoniasis	protozoan	female: frothy, foul odor, vaginal discharge, itching of genital area; male: usually asymptomatic	identification of trichomonad in discharge	Flagyl (metronidazole) (cure)

*PID = Pelvic inflammatory disease, a generic term describing inflammation of upper reproductive tract of females

Tips for action

To reduce your chances of acquiring a sexually transmitted disease:

✳ Know what you want sexually, and communicate with your partner about choices and strategies for making sex safer and pleasurable.

✳ Do not overuse alcohol and drugs. They blur judgment about risks.

✳ Limit sexual activity to a relationship in which both partners are not infected with any STD and agree to be sexually active with only each other (keep in mind that mutual monogamy cannot be verified).

✳ Use latex condoms, water-based lubricants, and spermicides (if allergies are not a problem) every time you have intercourse.

✳ Use latex condoms for oral sex on a male partner (fellatio). For oral sex on a female (cunnilingus) or oral-anal contact, use a latex barrier such as a split condom or dental dam.

✳ Urinate before and after intercourse or oral sex to cleanse the urethral opening.

✳ Wash hands and genitals before and after sex. Do not douche after sex.

✳ Clean "sex toys" with soap and water. Do not share them without cleaning thoroughly or covering with condoms.

✳ Recognize the signs of STDs, and inform your partner if any appear. (Almost all STDs often are present without symptoms of any kind.)

✳ Know when self-diagnosis and treatment are appropriate and when they are not.

✳ Know where to get medical care if it becomes necessary. Women should get annual Pap tests.

✳ If you are sexually active, get tested for STDs if:

— you know or suspect your partner is infected.

— you have had unsafe sex with a partner whose health status you do not know.

— there are signs of:

  ✳ a vaginal or penile discharge ("the drip").
  ✳ rash, warty growths, pimple, itchiness, or sore on genitals.
  ✳ persistent lower abdominal pain.
  ✳ pain when urinating.
  ✳ women: changes in menstrual flow, unusual bleeding.

✳ Get tested for HIV if:

— you have had unprotected vaginal, anal, or oral sex with an infected person.

— you have shared needles to inject drugs or steroids.

— you have had a blood transfusion or received blood products before April, 1985.

— you have had unprotected sex with an injectable drug user.

Summary

1 Pathogens have been classified in this chapter as viruses, bacteria, fungi, protozoa, and metazoa.

2 The course of infectious disease begins with exposure and infection, followed by an incubation period, then a prodomal period, the actual illness, recovery (or relapse to an earlier stage), and finally, termination.

3 A person can become infected through the skin or other body surface, by inhaling an air-borne pathogen, by eating contaminated food or drinking contaminated water, or through fomites such as contaminated hypodermic needles or bed linen.

4 The first defenders against disease are the skin and the mucous membranes.

5 Immunity may be either natural (inherited) or acquired (conferred by antibodies in the immune response).

6 Immunodeficiencies result from failure of the immune system to react to pathogens. In autoimmune diseases the immune system attacks the body's own cells and tissues.

7 Infectious childhood diseases for which immunizations are recommended include polio, diphtheria, pertussis (whopping cough), tetanus (lockjaw), rubeola (red measles), rubella (German measles), mumps, hepatitis B, and Hib disease, or H-flu.

8 Of all human diseases the cold is the most common and it still has no cure. Types of cold viruses number in the hundreds.

9 Tuberculosis, once one of the leading causes of death, is on the rise again, often in connection with HIV/AIDS.

10 Of the sexually transmissible diseases, HIV/AIDS is the most devastating, because a cure or vaccination has not been found and the number of cases continues to rise worldwide. It leaves the body vulnerable to attack by opportunistic diseases.

11 Two other blood-borne STDs are syphilis and hepatitis B.

12 STDs that cause vaginitis or urethritis are candida, trichomonas, chlamydia, and gonorrhea.

13 Herpes and genital warts are lesion-producing STDs.

14 Parasites produce pubic lice and scabies.

15 Prompt diagnosis and treatment can reduce the spread of most STDs. Risk reduction through abstinence or use of latex condoms and spermicides is imperative.

Select Bibliography

Ashe, Arthur. *Days of Grace: A Memoir*. New York: Alfred A. Knopf, 1993.

Baxter, R. "Uncommon Facts About the Common Cold." *Healthline*, October, 1988.

Bruess, Clint, and Glenn Richardson. *Decisions for Health*, 3d edition. Dubuque, IA: Wm. C. Brown, 1992.

"[The] Common Cold." *Mayo Clinic Health Letter*, September, 1992.

Hahn, Dale, and Wayne Payne. *Focus on Health*, 2d edition. St. Louis: Mosby–Year Book, 1994.

Editors of Consumer Guide. *Family Medical & Prescription Drug Guide*. Lincolnwood, IL: Publications International, 1993.

Editors of Time-Life Books. *The Defending Army*. Alexandria, VA: Time-Life Books, 1994.

Hafen, Brent Q., and Werner W. K. Hoeger. *Wellness: Guidelines for a Healthy Lifestyle*. Englewood, CO: Morton Publishing, 1994.

Johnson, Earvin (Magic). *What You Can Do to Avoid AIDS*. New York: Random House, 1991.

Jones, James H. *Bad Blood: The Tuskegee Syphilis Experiment*. New York: Free Press, 1981.

Mullen, Kathleen, Robert Gold, Philip Belcastro, and Robert McDermott. *Connections for Health*. Dubuque, IA: Wm. C. Brown, 1993.

St. Louis, Michael, et al. "Risk for Perinatal HIV-I Transmission According to Maternal, Immunologic, Virologic, and Placental Factors." *Journal of the American Medical Association*, June 9, 1993.

Segal, Maria. "Women and AIDS." *FDA Consumer Special Report*, January, 1994.

Shilts, Randy. *And the Band Played On — Politics, People, and the AIDS Epidemic*. New York: Penguin Books, 1988.

Are You Up-to-Date on Your Immunizations?

NAME _____ DATE _____

COURSE _____ SECTION _____

Table 6.2 shows the immunization schedule recommended for all children from the time of birth until the 16th birthday. Place a checkmark (✔) in the box for each immunization you have received.

VACCINE	MONTHS					YEARS	
	2	4	6	12–15	15	4–6	14–16
Diphtheria, tetanus, pertussis (DTP)							
Oral polio vaccine (OPV)							
Measles, mumps, rubella (MMR)							
Haemophilus influenzae type b (Hib)							
Td — contains tetanus and diphtheria vaccines (for children 7 years and older)							
	Birth	1–2 Mos.	4 Mos.	6–18 Mos		(or other)	
Hepatitis B (Hep B)							

How Much Do You Know About AIDS?

NAME _____ DATE _____

COURSE _____ SECTION _____

	Yes	No
1. AIDS is the end stage of infection caused by HIV.	_____	_____
2. HIV is a chronic infectious disease that spreads among individuals who engage in risky behaviors such as unprotected sex or the sharing of hypodermic needles.	_____	_____
3. AIDS now has a cure.	_____	_____
4. Abstaining from sex is the only 100% sure way to protect yourself from HIV infection.	_____	_____
5. Condoms are 100% effective in protecting you against HIV infection.	_____	_____
6. If you're sexually active, latex condoms provide the best protection against HIV infection.	_____	_____
7. Each year more and more teens are getting infected with HIV.	_____	_____
8. You can become HIV-infected by donating blood.	_____	_____
9. You can tell by looking at someone if he or she is HIV-infected.	_____	_____
10. The only means to determine whether someone has HIV is through an HIV antibody test.	_____	_____
11. HIV can completely destroy the immune system.	_____	_____
12. The HIV virus may live in the body 10 years or longer before AIDS symptoms develop.	_____	_____
13. People infected with HIV have AIDS.	_____	_____
14. Once infected with HIV, a person never becomes uninfected.	_____	_____
15. HIV infection is preventable.	_____	_____

Adapted from *Test Your Survival Smarts: Self-Quiz on Drugs and AIDS*, National Institute on Drug Abuse, U. S. Department of Health & Human Services; and *Principles and Labs for Physical Fitness and Wellness*, 3d edition, by Werner W. K. Hoeger and Sharon A. Hoeger (Englewood, CO: Morton Publishing, 1994), pp. 375–376.

Answers:

1. Yes. AIDS is the term used to define the manifestation of opportunistic diseases and cancers that occur as a result of HIV infection (also referred to as HIV disease).

2. Yes. People do not get HIV because of who they are but, rather, because of what they do. Almost all of the people who get HIV do so because they choose to engage in risky behaviors.

3. No. AIDS has no cure, and none seems likely soon.

4. No. Abstinence does protect a person from getting HIV infection from sex, but it can still be contracted by sharing hypodermic needles.

5. No. Only abstaining from sex gives you 100% protection, but condoms are effective in protecting against HIV infection if they're used correctly.

6. Yes. Proper use, however, is necessary to minimize the risk of infection.

7. Yes. In the early 1990s, the number of infected teens increased by 96% over a short span of 2 years. Probably about 20% of the AIDS patients today were infected as teenagers.

8. No. A myth regarding HIV is that it can be transmitted by donating blood. People cannot get HIV from giving blood. Health professionals use a new needle every time they draw blood. These needles are used only once and are destroyed and thrown away immediately after each individual has donated blood.

9. No. The symptoms of AIDS often are not noticeable until several years after a person has been infected with HIV.

10. Yes. Nobody can tell if an HIV infection exists unless an HIV antibody test is done. Upon HIV infection, the immune system's line of defense against the virus is to form antibodies that bind to the virus. On the average the body takes 3 months to manufacture enough antibodies to show up positive in an HIV antibody test. Sometimes it may take 6 months or longer.

11. Yes. The virus multiplies, attacks, and destroys white blood cells. These cells are part of the immune system, and their function is to fight off infections and diseases in the body. As the number of white blood cells killed increases, the body's immune system gradually breaks down and may be completely destroyed.

12. Yes. Up to 10 years may go by before the person develops AIDS.

13. No. Being HIV-positive does not necessarily mean the person has AIDS. On the average, it takes 7 to 8 years following infection before the individual develops the symptoms that fit the case definition of AIDS. From that point on, the person may live another 2 to 3 years. In essence, from the point of infection, the individual may have the chronic disease 8 to 10 years.

14. Yes. There is no second chance.

15. Yes. The best prevention technique is to abstain from sex until the time comes for a mutually monogamous sexual relationship. In the absence of sharing needles, that one behavior, according to Dr. James Mason, director of the Centers for Disease Control in Atlanta, will almost completely remove the risk of contracting HIV or developing any other sexually transmitted disease.

Noncommunicable Diseases

OBJECTIVES

✳ Explain the mechanism by which cancer develops.

✳ List the seven warning signs of cancer.

✳ List the cancer sites and possible preventive measures for each.

✳ Define COPD and describe its manifestations.

✳ Identify blood-borne diseases and the defining characteristics of each.

✳ Differentiate Type I and Type II diabetes.

✳ Define rheumatic diseases and give examples.

✳ Identify three skin conditions related to ethnicity.

✳ Give examples of diseases of the digestive tract.

✳ Define neurological disorders and give examples.

*A*t the beginning of the century, the top killers in the United States were communicable diseases such as tuberculosis, diphtheria, polio, and other highly infectious diseases that ravaged communities and sometimes wiped out entire families. Today, the leading causes of death in the United States are all noncommunicable diseases, those that cannot be transmitted from one person to another. The top three killers of Americans are cardiovascular conditions, cancer, and chronic obstructive pulmonary disease (primarily bronchitis and emphysema). The number-one killer, cardiovascular disease, is covered in Chapter 8.

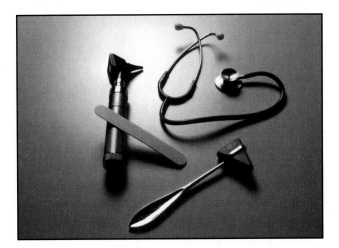

Cancer — actually a number of diseases rather than a single condition — is the second leading cause of death in the United States. The cancers are discussed here by the body site affected. The discussion then turns to diseases of the respiratory system. The anemias are discussed next, then the two types of diabetes.

A growing number of conditions fall into the category of autoimmune diseases, those in which the body's immune system turns on itself. These diseases include the many forms of arthritis and several skin disorders, along with some of the allergies, such as hay fever. The chapter concludes with sections on disorders of the digestive tract and on the neurological disorders of epilepsy and the several types of headaches.

CANCER

Just the mention of the word "cancer" continues to arouse fear and elicit an emotional response. In some circles the taboo surrounding discussion of cancer is just as strong as that surrounding sexuality and STDs. The reluctance to discuss this health problem — the second leading cause of death of adults in the United States (23.5%) next to heart disease — is part of the problem, as many cancers now are preventable and curable.

How It Begins

Normally, as cells become worn-out, they reproduce themselves in an orderly way. Each of the body's approximately 100 trillion cells has a nucleus containing **ribonucleic acid (RNA)** and **deoxyribonucleic acid (DNA)**, the latter of which contains the body's genetic code. DNA contains **oncogenes**, which prompt cell division (up to 100 times each), and tumor suppressor genes, which stop the action. During cell division the DNA molecule is supposed to be duplicated exactly. Sometimes, however, a **mutation**, a change in the genetic material, occurs. An enzyme called **telomerase** allows the cells to reproduce indefinitely, forming a **tumor**. If it remains self-contained and does not spread, it is termed **benign**. Most benign tumors have little effect on body functioning and are harmless.

The disease we often call **cancer** is actually a group of diseases characterized by uncontrolled growth and the spread of abnormal cells. In its wake normal cells are overcome and eventually die. A cancer, or **malignancy**, begins as a localized tumor, confined to one area. If, however, the tumor continues to grow and begins to invade surrounding tissues and organs, it is called an **invasive tumor**. Cancer can be found in any body tissue. When cells break off from a malignant tumor, migrate to other parts of the body through the circulatory or lymphatic system, and form new cancers, **metastasis** has occurred.

Most adults have precancerous or cancerous cells in their bodies. If the immune system is healthy, it can keep these cells in check. Just one errant cell, however, can produce cancer, of which some types take years to develop and others mobilize rapidly. Figure 7.1 depicts the process.

Research has uncovered a variety of agents, both internal and external, that can instigate cancer. These cancer-causing agents, known as **carcinogens**, include:
— occupational hazards and pollutants
— chemicals in food and water
— certain viruses
— radiation (including the natural radiation from the sun).

Other factors that contribute to the development of cancer include a genetic predisposition and psychological factors.

Some misconceptions regarding cancer have been passed from one generation to the next. One popular notion is that cancer is one disease that ravages the human body. Some people have resigned themselves to the mistaken idea that cancer just happens and a person can do little to avoid it. One of the most disturbing consequences of these misconceptions is that some people are paralyzed into inaction when they notice a symptom or sign that a health professional should investigate.

Actually, the news about cancer is much better than one might think. Many forms of cancer that account for the highest incidence and mortality rates are related to lifestyle factors that a person can alter or even eliminate to reduce the risk of cancer. Further, the most successful treatment of cancer comes in the early stage. If people would be proactive against cancer, much of it could be halted. Attitude also plays a role in cancer. Many people underestimate their ability to reduce their risk and turn the prognosis in their favor. Figure 7.2 shows the estimated role of major cancer-causing agents.

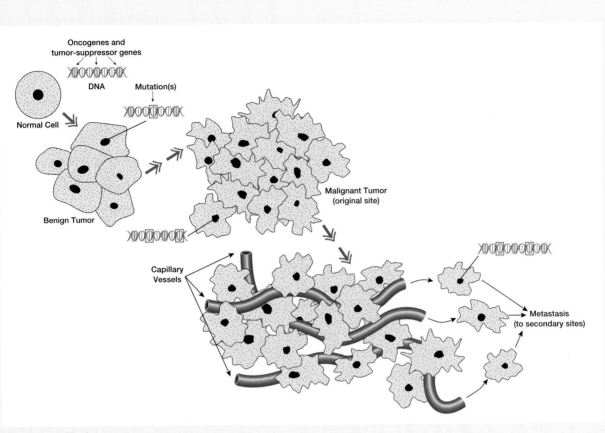

Figure 7.1 How cancer starts and grows

Labels in figure:
- Oncogenes and tumor-suppressor genes
- DNA
- Mutation(s)
- Normal Cell
- Benign Tumor
- Malignant Tumor (original site)
- Capillary Vessels
- Metastasis (to secondary sites)

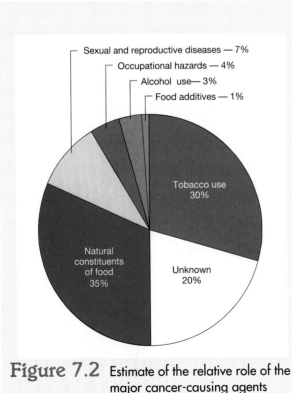

Figure 7.2 Estimate of the relative role of the major cancer-causing agents

Labels in pie chart:
- Sexual and reproductive diseases — 7%
- Occupational hazards — 4%
- Alcohol use — 3%
- Food additives — 1%
- Tobacco use 30%
- Unknown 20%
- Natural constituents of food 35%

KEY TERMS

Ribonucleic Acid (RNA) nucleic acid found in the nucleus of cells that controls protein synthesis

Deoxyribonucleic acid (DNA) found in the nucleus of cells and contains the body's genetic code

Oncogenes genes that prompt uncontrolled cell division

Mutation change in genetic material; variation in genetic structure

Telomerase enzyme that allows the cells to reproduce indefinitely, forming a tumor

Tumor an abnormal growth of tissue that grows independently of surrounding tissue and serves no useful function; neoplasm

Benign tumor that remains self-contained; noncancerous

Cancer group of diseases characterized by uncontrolled growth and spread of abnormal cells that kill normal cells

Malignancy a tumor that is cancerous

Invasive tumor a tumor that continues to grow and encroach upon surrounding tissues and organs

Metastasis new cancers formed when cells from a malignant tumor break off, travel to other parts of the body, and form new cancers

Carcinogen cancer-causing agent or substance

Incidence and Mortality

Even though anyone can develop cancer, incidence and death rates from cancer are generally higher in African Americans than Anglo Americans. In 1990 the incidence for African Americans was 423 per 100,000, in comparison to 393 per 100,000 for Anglo Americans. For that same year the death rates were 230 per 100,000 for African Americans and 170 per 100,000 for Anglos. African Americans have higher incidence of death rates for cancers of the esophagus, stomach, liver, larynx, prostate, and cervix. African American women are more than twice as likely to die of breast cancer within 5 years of diagnosis than Anglo American women are. The reason given by Dr. William Eley of the Emory University School of Public Health,

Atlanta, is that the diseases in African Americans were diagnosed in later stages. According to the American Cancer Society, more than 90% of women whose breast cancer is diagnosed before it spreads survive at least 5 years, whereas survival drops to as low as 18% in women whose cancer has spread before it is diagnosed.

Table 7.1 lists the numbers of cancer deaths by site of the cancer and ethnic group. These numbers do not give incidence rates within each group. Nevertheless, they do indicate relative incidence among selected subpopulations.

Cultural differences cannot be discounted. Florence Bonner, a sociology professor at Howard University and principal investigator for the National Black Leadership Initiative on Cancer, commented that the African American community

Table 7.1
Number of Cancer Deaths for Selected Ethnic Groups in United States

Cancer Site	Black Males	Black Females	American Indian	Chinese	Japanese	Hispanic*
All sites	31,995	25,082	1,275	1,527	1,122	14,003
Oral cavity	1,000	311	23	60	23	232
Esophagus	1,433	541	19	45	32	233
Stomach	1,341	917	67	117	132	811
Colon & rectum	2,898	3,169	117	166	168	1,414
Liver & other biliary	757	615	68	168	66	769
Pancreas	1,442	1,581	52	65	77	795
Lung (male)	10,632	—	205	238	148	1,824
Lung (female)	—	4,512	117	145	75	787
Melanoma of skin	51	55	9	2	3	89
Breast (female)	—	4,659	89	88	79	1,246
Cervix uteri	—	972	47	22	12	296
Other uterus	—	899	12	15	14	168
Ovary	—	975	34	29	22	385
Prostate	5,181	—	59	42	56	728
Bladder	466	381	9	21	12	210
Kidney	563	382	39	12	14	355
Brain & central nervous system	372	319	21	35	14	376
Lymphoma	747	573	50	47	42	688
Leukemia	854	737	52	47	27	735
Multiple myeloma	745	708	39	15	6	273

* Persons classified as of Hispanic origin on death certificates may be of any race. Hispanic origin reporting, however, may be incomplete on death certificates in some states. These numbers are believed to include over 90% of cancer deaths in Hispanics in 1990.

Source: American Cancer Society, 1990.

historically has viewed good health as a privilege and remains reactive rather than proactive toward health care. In regard to cancer, Bonner commented that people of lower economic status within the African American community are more fatalistic about being diagnosed ("once you're diagnosed, you're dead").

Linda Burhansstipanov of the Native American Research Consortium in Denver reported that language barriers and different communication patterns in the Native American community may be a barrier when non-Native health care professionals are serving Native Americans. Most indigenous languages have no word for cancer. In the Hispanic-Latino community, too, language differences may present problems.

In addition to the socioeconomic and cultural differences that may erect barriers to patient care, misunderstanding of medical jargon or directions on how to take medications may be problematic. Chapter 15 provides practical information on how minorities can access the health care system.

Symptoms, Diagnosis, and Treatment of Cancer

The American Cancer Society has developed a list of symptoms that individuals should be aware of so early diagnosis and treatment can be possible. These are given in Table 7.2.

Because cancer is not a single condition but instead encompasses a group of conditions, no one diagnostic test can be used to determine if cancer is present. Some of the general procedures are:

※ **Biopsy.** A small piece of tissue is removed through a special hollow needle and examined

New Cancer Test

A new test, based on recent advances in molecular biology, can detect several kinds of cancerous human cells earlier than standard tests. As reported late in 1994 by scientists from the Johns Hopkins School of Medicine, the test scans the DNA sequence of cells for signs of aberrant cells. This test holds promise for refining the diagnosis and recognition of the stages of cancer, detecting the spread of malignant cells in the body, and monitoring the effects of drugs and other anti-cancer therapies. The test recently confirmed the presence of bladder cancer from frozen tissue taken from the late Hubert Humphrey, an uncertain diagnosis at that time.

microscopically to determine if a tumor is benign or malignant.

※ **Magnetic resonance imagery (MRI).** Magnetic fields and radio waves produce a computer image of body tissue that may reveal abnormalities. The newer models can scan the full body in 18 seconds instead of the usual 45 minutes.

※ **Computerized axial tomography (CAT scan).** Radiation allows the viewing of internal organs that usually are not visible by x-ray.

Table 7.3 lists some of the screening measures for various cancer sites and how often they should be done.

Treatment, too, varies. The following are the most widely utilized methods of treatment:

※ **Surgery.** The tumor and its surrounding tissue are removed by excising them.

※ **Radiation.** Often combined with surgery, x-rays are aimed at the site of the tumor to destroy or

Table 7.2
Cautions for Cancer

Acronym	Warning Signal
C	Change in bowel or bladder habits
A	A sore that does not go away
U	Unusual bleeding or discharge
T	Thickening or lump in the breast or elsewhere
I	Indigestion or difficulty in swallowing
O	Obvious change in a wart or a mole
N	Nagging hoarseness or cough

KEY TERMS

Biopsy microscopic examination of a small piece of tissue that has been removed with a special needle

Magnetic resonance imagery (MRI) use of radio waves and magnetic fields that produce a computer image of the body to locate abnormalities

Computerized axial tomography (CAT scan) use of radiation to view internal organs that do not show up on x-ray

Surgery removal of tumor and surrounding tissue

Radiation emission of rays from a common center that can destroy cancerous cells

Table 7.3
Medical Screening Tests

Cancer	Detection Procedure	Who	When
Prostate	DRE (digital rectal exam) PSA (prostate-specific antigen blood test)	Men after age 50	Annually
Breast	Breast physical examination	All women over age 20	Every 3 years for women age 40 and under; yearly thereafter
Breast	Mammography (breast x-ray)	All women over age 35	*Baseline between ages 35 and 40; every 1 to 2 years between ages 40 and 49; yearly after age 50
Reproductive system cancers in women	Pelvic examination	All women over age 20	Every 3 years for women age 40 and under; yearly thereafter
Cervical	Pap test (microscopic examination of cells)	Women ages 20 to 65; younger women who are sexually active	After two negative exams 1 year apart, perform at least every 3 years.
Uterine	Endometrial (uterine) tissue sample	**Women at high risk	At menopause
Colorectal	Test for blood in stools	Everyone over age 50	Annually
Rectal	Digital rectal examination	Everyone over age 40	Annually
Colorectal	Sigmoidoscopy (examination of colon/rectum)	Everyone over age 50	After two negative exams 1 year apart, perform every 3 to 5 years

* American Cancer Society guidelines. National Cancer Institute says screening need not begin until after age 50. American College of Obstetrics and Gynecology recommends a *yearly* pap test.
**High-risk women have histories of infertility, obesity, failure to ovulate, abnormal uterine bleeding, or estrogen therapy.

Source: American Cancer Society.

stop the growth of cancerous cells. A **radiologist** determines how much radiation is necessary. A drawback of radiation therapy is that it destroys some healthy cells at the same time.

* **Chemotherapy.** Any or a combination of more than fifty drugs is administered intravenously to kill cancerous cells. Chemotherapy is a systemic treatment used when cancer cells have spread throughout the body. A promising new drug, **Taxol,** is obtained from the bark and needles of the pacific yew tree.

* **Immunotherapy.** The body's own immune system is activated to fight cancer cells within it by injecting the person with **interferon,** a protein produced by the body naturally to counteract invasion by viruses.

The treatment plan for cancer must be tailored to the individual. The form of treatment depends on variables such as the type of cancer, site of the malignancy, how early it was diagnosed, and the patient's general health. The physician who specializes in treating cancer is called an **oncologist.**

Representative Cancers: An Overview

The following is an overview of the most common cancers. American Cancer Society estimates of cancer incidence and deaths by site and sex are shown in Figure 7.3. The highest incidence for men is prostate cancer, and for women, breast cancer. The highest death rate from cancer for both men and women is lung cancer.

📞 Call for information

Cancer Information Service
800-4-CANCER (422-6237)

Lung

Lung cancer continues on the rise and now is the leading cause of death in men and women alike. Since 1987, more women have died from lung cancer than breast cancer. What is most disturbing is that lung cancer is one of the most preventable forms of cancer because the greatest risk factor for this condition is cigarette smoking. The death rate for lung cancer could be cut in half if people did not smoke cigarettes. Because African American males tend to smoke cigarettes with a higher tar and nicotine content, they are at greater risk for developing lung cancer than other groups. African American females do not smoke as much as other groups. Other risk factors for lung cancer include exposure to asbestos, radiation and certain chemicals, and secondhand smoke (discussed in Chapter 12).

KEY TERMS

Radiologist physician specializing in the use of radiation

Chemotherapy drugs taken intravenously to kill cancer cells

Taxol new drug used in chemotherapy, obtained from the bark and needles of the Pacific yew tree

Immunotherapy use of the body's own immune system to fight cancer

Interferon a protein produced by the body to fight viruses, injected to stimulate the body's own immune system to fight cancer

Oncologist physician who specializes in treating cancer

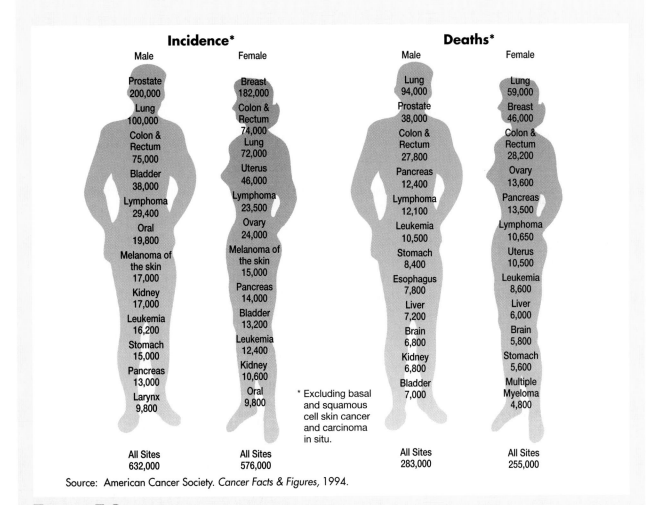

Source: American Cancer Society. *Cancer Facts & Figures*, 1994.

Figure 7.3 Leading sites of cancer incidence and death, 1994 estimates

Fighting Cancer with What You Eat

To protect yourself from cancer:

❋ Cut dietary fats to no more than 30% of your total calories by:
 — trimming all fat from meat and removing skin from poultry before cooking
 — cutting down on the amount of fat and oil used in cooking
 — substituting low-fat for high-fat dairy products
 — limiting intake of meat to no more than 3 to 6 ounces a day
 — using less fat and oil in cooking

❋ Eat more fruits and vegetables — at least two or three a day. Include cabbage, yellow vegetables, onions, garlic, potatoes, peas, green leafy vegetables, citrus fruits.

❋ Eat vegetables raw or cook them by steaming or stir-frying. Eat fruits raw, as canned and preserved fruits lose nutrients.

❋ Eat a lot of fiber — in whole-grain cereals and breads — and use whole-wheat flour in baking.

❋ Substitute fruit and vegetable juices for coffee, tea, and soda.

❋ Drink two to four glasses of low-fat milk each day.

❋ Eat fish two or three times a week.

❋ Cook by baking, broiling, steaming, poaching, and roasting rather than frying or barbecuing.

❋ Drink alcohol only in moderation.

Signals that should be reported to a physician as soon as they appear are a nagging or persistent cough, blood in the sputum (phlegm coming from the lungs), pain in the chest, shortness of breath, hoarseness, weight loss, loss of appetite, anemia, and recurring lung infections such as bronchitis. Early detection of lung cancer is difficult, though, because some of the symptoms that people are taught to look for do not appear until the lung cancer is advanced.

If lung cancer is diagnosed early, the person has a 33% chance of surviving 10 to 16 months and an overall chance of surviving 2 years. If the tumor can be removed surgically, the person has a 40%–80% chance of surviving 5 years. Treatments other than or in addition to surgery include radiation and chemotherapy.

Colon and Rectum

Cancer of the colon and rectum is the second leading cancer site in women and the third leading cancer site in men. A major risk factor for colorectal cancer is a family history of colorectal cancer or **polyps**, small growths on the wall of the colon or rectum. Diets high in fat and low in fiber have been linked to increased risk.

Signals of colorectal cancer include bleeding from the rectum, blood in the stool (the bowel movement), and changes in bowel habits or characteristics such as recurring constipation or diarrhea.

A physician can detect colorectal cancer in its early stages (even if the person reports no symptoms) by performing a digital rectal examination, a stool blood test, and a proctoscopic examination in some combination. If problems are discovered, the physician can use more extensive diagnostic tests. The most common treatment is surgery, sometimes followed by radiation. Chemotherapy also is used in some cases.

Breast

The American Cancer Society estimated that 182,000 new cases of breast cancer in women and 1,000 new cases of breast cancer in men would be diagnosed in the United States in 1994. One in every nine women develop cancer of the breast. It is the second leading cause of cancer death in women. A woman's age (over 40) is a risk factor for breast cancer, and the incidence of breast cancer increases with age. Women with a family history or personal history of breast cancer, early onset of menstruation, and late age at menopause are at risk. Other

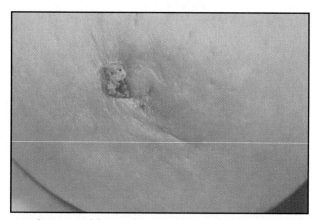

Dimpling around the nipple is one of the signs of breast cancer.

risk factors include never having a child and having a first birth at a late age.

The American Cancer Society recommends that women 20 years of age and older should do a breast self-examination (BSE) once a month (see Figure 7.4) to spot any irregularity or unusual lump. Signs and symptoms that should be reported to a physician immediately include a persistent lump, swelling, thickening, or distortion of the breast, persistent pain, tenderness of the nipple, and discharge of blood or other fluid from the nipple. Figure 7.5 illustrates different sizes of lumps in the breast and their detection. **Mammography** is the newest diagnostic method. It does not seem to reduce breast cancer mortality for premenopausal women. For women age 50 and older, however, this screening reduces deaths from breast cancer 26%. Mammography may be more effective with older women because their breasts have a higher fat content, increasing the test's sensitivity in detecting small tumors.

> Women with diets rich in beta-carotene who have breast-cancer surgery do 12 times better.

If breast cancer is diagnosed early, the woman has at least a 92% chance of surviving 5 years. If the cancer has not spread, the survival rate is 100% with treatment. Chemotherapy or hormonal therapy is used in early stages, sometimes in conjunction with surgery to remove the lump only (lumpectomy) or all of the breast (mastectomy).

KEY TERMS

Mammography an x-ray used to detect breast cancer

Polyps small growths on the wall of the colon or rectum

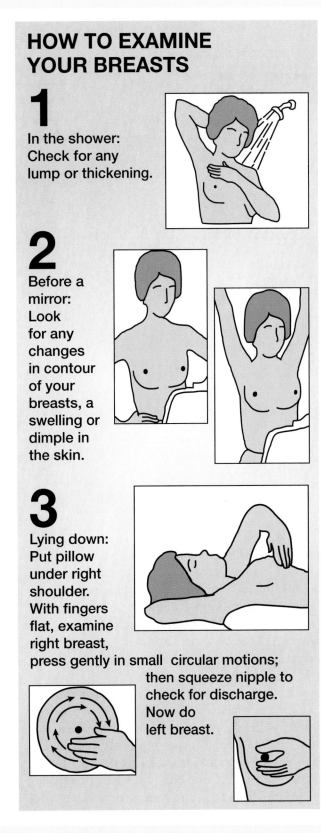

HOW TO EXAMINE YOUR BREASTS

1 In the shower: Check for any lump or thickening.

2 Before a mirror: Look for any changes in contour of your breasts, a swelling or dimple in the skin.

3 Lying down: Put pillow under right shoulder. With fingers flat, examine right breast, press gently in small circular motions; then squeeze nipple to check for discharge. Now do left breast.

Figure 7.4 Breast self-examination (BSE)

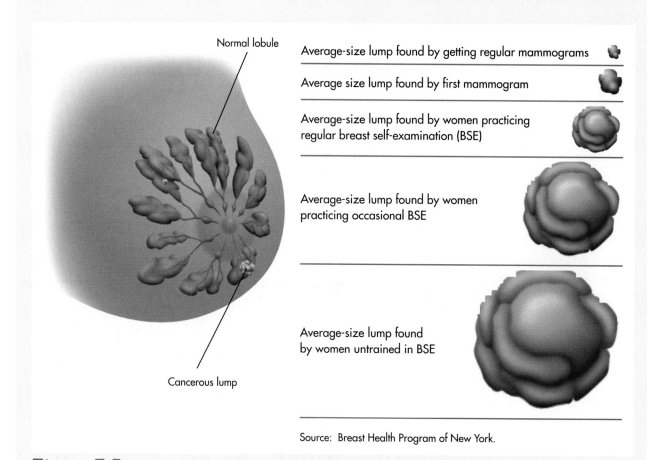

Normal lobule

Average-size lump found by getting regular mammograms

Average size lump found by first mammogram

Average-size lump found by women practicing regular breast self-examination (BSE)

Average-size lump found by women practicing occasional BSE

Average-size lump found by women untrained in BSE

Cancerous lump

Source: Breast Health Program of New York.

Figure 7.5 Size of tumors found by mammography and breast self-exam

Prostate

Like breast cancer, prostate cancer has a higher incidence rate in older individuals. Prostate cancer is the second leading cause of death in men. The greatest risk factors for cancer of the prostate, unfortunately, are two that cannot be controlled: being over age 65 and being African American. One in nine African American males will get prostate cancer. This rate, the highest in the world, is 30% higher than for Anglo men.

Symptoms of prostate cancer are similar to those of other problems of the prostate and urogenital tract. Therefore, a man with any of these symptoms should report to a physician for an examination and diagnostic tests. Signs of a problem include weak or interrupted urine stream; inability to urinate or difficulty starting or stopping urination; frequent urination, especially at night; blood in the urine; pain or burning during urination; continuing lower back pain or pelvic pain;

fatigue; anemia. The American Cancer Society recommends that men age 50 and over have a digital rectal examination (DRE) and the prostate-specific antigen (PSA) blood test every year.

If prostate cancer is diagnosed early, the person has a high chance of recovery. Because half of the men diagnosed with this form of cancer are 70 or older, however, many who develop this type of

To Prevent Prostate Cancer

A low-fat diet seems to play a role in preventing prostate cancer. *The Harvard Health Letter,* 1994, noted that the lowest rate of prostate cancer in the world is among Chinese men in San Francisco. Perhaps a diet containing, steamed carrots, spinach salad with olive oil and vinegar dressing, and tofu burgers has something to do with it.

cancer will die of other diseases. A recent controversy has arisen as to the advisability of surgery for this slow-growing cancer.

Testicles

Testicular cancer is one of the most common cancers in males at early adulthood, with the highest risk between ages 15 and 34. Probable causes have not been identified, except that males who had undescended testicles during childhood seem to have the greatest risk. Testicular cancer may run in families. Also, men who have had mumps have a higher rate of testicular cancer.

In early stages this cancer is painless. Because the first symptom is an enlargement or thickening of the testis, a regular testicular self-examination is advised. The procedure, which takes only 3 minutes and is best done after a warm bath or shower, is simple:

1. Roll each testicle gently between the thumb and fingers of both hands.

2. If you find any hard lumps or changes in the normal configuration, see your doctor. Although you can spot the symptoms, only a physician can make a definite diagnosis.

Uterus: Cervix and Endometrium

Cancer of the cervix of the uterus is the more common of the two forms of uterine cancer. When it is found in its early or precancerous stage (**carcinoma in situ**), it is highly curable. Warning signs of cervical cancer are abnormal uterine bleeding or spotting and abnormal discharge from the vagina. The risk factors for cervical cancer are early age at first intercourse, multiple sex partners, infection with STDs, genital herpes, or the human papaloma virus. Because the risk factors for cervical cancer are related to behavioral factors, teens and young women should know them so they can reduce their risk.

Females also should have regular **Pap tests** for early detection. Every woman should have an annual Pap test in conjunction with the pelvic examination. In the Pap test (named for the

---

Exercise Cuts Cancer Risk

Breast Cancer:

A study by the University of Southern California's Norris Comprehensive Cancer Center in 1994 found that women of childbearing age who spent more than 4 hours a week exercising cut their risk of breast cancer by almost 60%. Even though older women are more likely to get breast cancer, this study points to the value of prevention and lifestyle factors in lowering the risk for breast cancer.

Colon Cancer:

A sedentary lifestyle contributes to the risk for colon cancer, a disease that killed more than 50,000 Americans in 1991. Studies in America, Europe, and China have indicated a link between regular exercise and significantly lower rates of colon cancer. Exercise may help to prevent colon cancer by speeding waste through the bowel, reducing the amount of time cancer-causing agents remain in contact with the lining of the large intestine. Further protection comes from eating vegetables and fruits that are high in fiber and rich in vitamin C and beta-carotene (which the body uses to make vitamin A).

Greek physician George Papanicolaou) a sample of cells is taken from the cervix for microscopic examination. The mortality rate for cervical cancer is more than twice as high for African American women as Anglo American women, suggesting that the former should be more proactive in getting an annual Pap test. Again, early detection is the key to recovery.

Cancer of the endometrium or the lining of the uterus occurs more frequently in women over age 50. Any women who is experiencing abnormal bleeding should see a physician. This is important for women who have gone through menopause. Early detection of endometrial cancer is through an annual pelvic examination. Treatment consists of surgery in the early stages and radiation in later stages.

Ovaries

Ovarian cancer is difficult to detect. As a result, by the time the most noticeable symptoms appear, the cancer is in its advanced stage. When a woman reports to her physician with symptoms such as

KEY TERMS

Carcinoma in situ an early cancer that does not extend beyond the surface layer

Pap test diagnostic test for cancer of the cervix performed by taking a sample of cells from the cervix for examination under a microscope

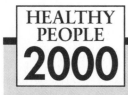

HEALTHY PEOPLE 2000

OBJECTIVES FOR CANCER

❋ Slow the rise in lung cancer deaths.

❋ Reduce deaths from breast cancer, cancer of the cervix, and colorectal cancer.

❋ Increase the proportion of black women age 40 and older who have ever received a clinical breast examination and a mammogram, and those age 50 and older who have received them within the preceding 1 to 2 years.

❋ Increase the proportion of women aged 18 and older with uterine cervix who have ever received a Pap test, and those who received a Pap test within the preceding 1 to 3 years.

bloating, abdominal pain, and gas, these may be considered as indications of a gastrointestinal problem such as an ulcer. More than 13,000 women died in 1994 of cancer of the ovary. Risk factors are higher with a family history of the disease and for women who have never had children.

Women should have thorough pelvic examinations regularly to detect ovarian problems. Tests used to diagnosis ovarian cancer include the pelvic ultrasound and a blood test called the CA–125. The effectiveness of these methods in identifying ovarian cancer, however, is questionable. A biopsy of the ovary is used to confirm a diagnosis. The Pap test, by the way, cannot be used to detect cancer of the ovaries. The drug Taxol holds promise as a treatment.

Skin

Almost anyone can develop skin cancers. They are more common, however, in light-skinned people. The two types of skin cancer that have the highest incidence and can be treated successfully if found in time are **basal cell carcinoma** and **squamous cell carcinoma**. Another form of skin cancer that is not as common but is much more serious is **malignant melanoma**. Other than having light skin pigmentation, the main risk factor for developing skin cancer is too much exposure to the **ultraviolet (UV) rays** of the sun. Of all skin cancers, 90% occur on parts of the body not usually covered with clothing — the face, hands, forearms, and ears.

Symptoms vary depending on the type of cancer. Suspicious signs are skin lesions or bumps that "bleed-heal-bleed" or become scaly, tender, or painful. In the case of a melanoma, the person may notice that a mole has gotten larger and darker and the border around it has become irregular. Changes in moles and other skin lesions should be brought to a physician's attention as soon as they are found. Skin cancers are curable, especially if they are treated early. If not treated, however, skin cancer can spread to other parts of the body.

To reduce the risk of skin cancers, people should avoid unnecessary exposure to the sun or ultraviolet rays for long periods. Individuals with light skin pigmentation are more at risk. When outdoors, people should wear protective clothing, such as a hat with a brim, and use sunscreen. The American Academy of Dermatology recommends a sunscreen product with a **sun protection factor (SPF)** of 15 or higher. The SPF number can be found on the label of the product. Tanning salons and sunlamps should be avoided.

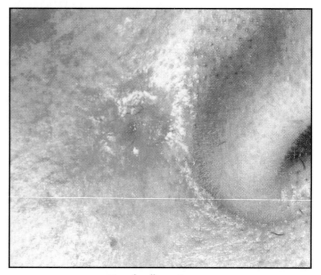

Basal cell carcinoma.

Tips for action

To help prevent skin cancer:

❋ Avoid the sun. Try to stay out of the sun from 10 a.m. to 3 p.m., when sun rays are strongest.

❋ Cover up. When you're out in the sun, wear wide-brimmed hats, long-sleeved shirts, and pants. Keep your neck covered.

❋ Use a sunscreen with a sun protection factor (SPF) of 15. Sunscreen keeps out the ultraviolet rays. Apply it at least 15–30 minutes before going in the sun. Put on more after swimming or sweating.

❋ Beware of cloudy days. You still can get burned then.

❋ The sun's rays can reach through 3 feet of water, so even though you may feel cool in the water, the sun can still burn you.

❋ Watch out for the sun in wintertime. Snow reflects sunlight, which can burn you.

❋ Don't use sunlamps, tanning parlors, or tanning pills. They can be just as harmful to your body as the sun.

❋ Look at your skin. Check moles, spots, and birthmarks monthly. If they change in appearance or grow, consult a doctor.

Oral Cavity

The major risk factors for cancer of the oral cavity are combustible and smokeless tobacco products and excessive use of alcohol (also see Chapter 12). If one form of cancer is related directly to a person's behavior, this is it. Anyone who smokes (cigarettes, cigars, pipe) or uses chewing tobacco or snuff should examine the mouth regularly, including the lips and tongue, for lesions.

Signs to be alerted to are sores that bleed or will not heal and a red or white lesion (patch) that will not go away. These may appear on the area of the lip where the cigarette or cigar rests or inside the lip where the chewing tobacco or snuff is placed. Other symptoms, such a persistent sore throat, should be reported to a physician or dentist. Oral cancer is easy to detect but not easy to cure.

DISEASES OF THE RESPIRATORY SYSTEM

Following cardiovascular diseases and cancer on the list of leading causes of death in the United States is the category of **chronic obstructive pulmonary disease (COPD),** also called chronic obstructive lung disease (COLD). The major lung diseases, aside from cancer, are chronic bronchitis and emphysema. Most are caused by cigarette smoking (discussed in Chapter 12). Environmental pollution (discussed in Chapter 15) is a contributing factor.

The respiratory system consists of the nose, throat, larynx, trachea, bronchi, and lungs (see Figure 7.6). Its function is to supply the blood with oxygen and relieve it of carbon dioxide. This

KEY TERMS

Basal cell carcinoma common type of skin cancer that usually does not metastasize

Squamous cell carcinoma common type of skin cancer that affects the squamous layer of the epidermis

Malignant melanoma a more serious type of skin cancer in the form of a pigmented mole or tumor

Ultraviolet (UV) rays rays from the sun that contribute to the development of skin cancer when a person is exposed to them

Sun protection factor (SPF) the rating by number given to a product that tells the consumer how effectively the product protects from the sun's ultraviolet rays

Chronic obstructive pulmonary disease (COPD) lung diseases characterized by decreased breathing functions that include chronic bronchitis and emphysema

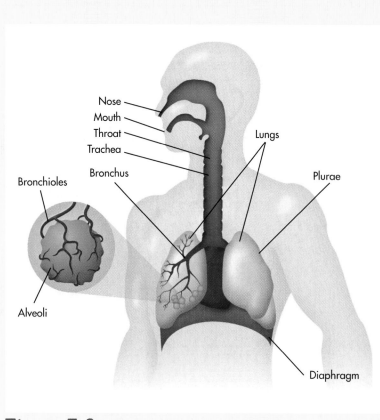

Figure 7.6 Respiratory system

mucous secretion further clogs the bronchi and has to be coughed up to keep the breathing tubes free. Symptoms of bronchitis include a cough, wheezing, and shortness of breath, persisting for several weeks. Over time, chronic bronchitis may cause the bronchial tubes to become severely obstructed. The heart enlarges because it has to pump harder than usual to deliver oxygen to the rest of the body.

Diagnosis is by chest x-ray and special machines that measure the amount of air flowing in and out of the lungs. Treatment consists of drinking plenty of water, being in humid surroundings, and taking bronchodilator drugs.

Emphysema

Emphysema is a progressive lung disease that eventually destroys the alveoli so that people who are affected have more and more difficulty breathing. The alveoli become nonfunctional and stiff rather than elastic. As the disease progresses, the oxygen supply in the blood is diminished, which overburdens the cardiovascular system and damages the heart.

Tobacco smoke and air pollutants are the most common causes of emphysema. The main symptom is shortness of breath, accompanied by a cough and difficulty breathing. Advanced-stage patients tire easily because of the large effort involved in merely breathing. Overinflation of the lungs produces the barrel-shaped chest often identified with people who have emphysema. The lack of oxygen may cause the lips, ear lobes, skin, and fingernails to be tinged blue.

Except for the few cases caused by a genetic disorder, no one test can be used to diagnose emphysema. Blood tests and chest x-rays do not uncover emphysema in its early stages. Only through a series of tests can it be diagnosed. Unfortunately, effects of the disease cannot be reversed, and the person's life is shortened.

The disease can be slowed, however, by removing the irritants that led to it, and those affected

exchange of oxygen and carbon dioxide takes place in the lungs. Air enters the lungs through the nose, where it is warmed, moistened, and filtered before it goes into the throat and **trachea** (windpipe). The trachea divides into two main **bronchi**, which connect to each of the two lungs.

In the lung the bronchi divide and subdivide, forming smaller passageways called bronchioles, and ending in air sacs called **alveoli**. The exchange of gases takes place in the alveoli, through tiny capillaries. During inhalation and exhalation the lungs expand and contract by movements of the rib cage and the diaphragm. The **pleurae**, membranes that line the chest cavity, allow the surfaces of the lungs and chest cavity to move past each other smoothly.

Bronchitis

Chronic **bronchitis** is more than a bad case of the common cold. It can be a serious, even life-threatening respiratory disorder. It is characterized by inflammation and swelling of the bronchi, which impair normal respiratory function. The increased

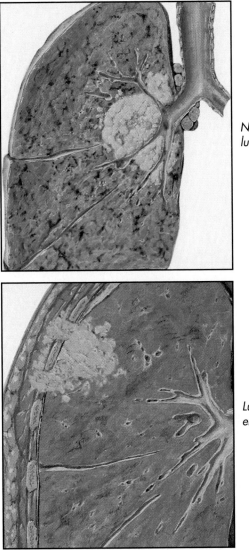

Normal lung.

Lung with emphysema.

immune system is what precipitates the allergic reaction. Medical relief usually is found in the form of antihistamines. Hay fever, though not considered serious in itself (although the discomfort is not denied), sometimes leads to asthma.

Asthma

Asthma is a respiratory disease characterized by acute attacks of wheezing and difficulty breathing, caused by obstruction (or narrowing) of the bronchioles. It is most common in children and often disappears with the passing of time. Three distinctly different causes are (a) allergens, (b) nonallergen, stress-related causes (discussed in Chapter 3), and (c) exercise-induced asthma. The latter type is most common in athletes. It is brought on by overexertion, particularly in cold weather, which dries out the bronchi. It is easily treated and usually can be prevented by warming up 10 minutes before vigorous exercise.

In the first type, agents such as pollen, dust, animal fur, bee venom, or specific foods bring on the asthma attack. It can be prevented or treated by **immunotherapy**, in which the person is desensitized through injections of weakened allergens. Antihistamines and corticosteroid drugs also are successful in reducing inflammation. Once an attack has begun, bronchodilator drugs are taken through an inhaler. This usually restores breathing to normal.

The number of people who have asthma has risen markedly since 1982, especially in women and minorities. Death rates from asthma are highest among people who are at least 55 years old. Even though overall death rates still are relatively

can be made more comfortable by drinking large amounts of fluids, getting adequate rest, eating a balanced diet, and, upon the advice of a physician, exercising moderately. Vaporizers and humidifiers may be helpful. In addition, several drugs act to loosen mucus (an indication of chronic bronchitis) and expand the air passages. Oxygen therapy may be necessary.

Hay Fever

Hay fever is considered a mild respiratory ailment related most often to agents in the environment that induce the production of histamines in the body. It often is seasonal, evoked by buds on trees in spring and the pollens from various plants in autumn. Characterized by sneezing and itchy, watery eyes and nose, hay fever seems to run in families. An overly active

KEY TERMS

Trachea windpipe; tube that connects the larynx to the lungs

Bronchi two main passageways that connect to each lung from the trachea

Alveoli air sacs in the lungs where the exchange of gases takes place

Pleurae membranes that line the chest cavity

Bronchitis inflammation of the bronchial tubes in the lungs

Emphysema progressive lung disease that eventually destroys the alveoli and greatly reduces lung functioning

Hay fever mild respiratory ailment caused by environmental agents that provoke the body to produce histamines

Asthma respiratory disease characterized by attacks of wheezing and difficulty breathing caused by narrowing of the bronchi

Immunotherapy desensitization to allergen through periodic injections of weakened allergens

The Possible Role of Allergy in Asthma

Symptoms	Probable Cause
❋ Is your asthma worse in certain months? If so, are there symptoms at the same time of allergic rhinitis — sneezing, itching, runny and obstructed nose?	pollens and outdoor molds
❋ Do symptoms appear when visiting a house that has indoor pets?	animal dander
❋ Do eyes itch and become red after handling a pet? If the pet licks you, does a red, itchy welt develop?	animal dander
❋ Do symptoms appear in a room where carpets are being vacuumed?	animal dander, mites, dust
❋ Does making a bed cause symptoms?	mites
❋ Do symptoms develop when you go into a damp basement or a vacation cottage that has been closed up for some time?	molds
❋ Do symptoms develop related to certain job activities, either at work or after leaving work?	environmental agents; indoor pollution
❋ If symptoms develop at work, do they improve when away from work for a few days?	indoor pollution

Source: Public Health Service, National Institutes of Health, U.S. Department of Health and Human Services, 1994.

low (about five per million), the death rate for urban African Americans in the age range 15–44 years is five times higher than that for Anglos. Hispanics also have higher asthma-related death rates.

A study conducted by researchers at Hahnemann University Hospital in Philadelphia concluded that metropolitan air pollution apparently is not the cause, as outdoor pollution declined during the period when the death rates from asthma went up. Other suspected reasons are indoor air pollution and secondhand smoke.

A long-term study of nearly 2,500 asthma patients in Rochester, Minnesota, concluded that the survival rate of asthmatics is no different from people who do not have asthma. The exception is the patients who were at least 35 years old when their asthma was diagnosed and people who had additional lung diseases.

BLOOD DISORDERS

The blood disorders that most often come to mind are the anemias — iron-deficiency anemia and pernicious anemia. An inherited form of anemia, sickle cell anemia, is generally associated largely with African Americans. A brief overview of the anemias follows.

Anemia

Anemia is a condition in which a person has an insufficient quantity or quality of red blood cells. The function of these cells is to carry oxygen to the tissues and organs so the bodily systems can function normally. Oxygen is carried in the red blood cells by the chemical **hemoglobin**, which also is responsible for the cell's red color. Individuals with anemia may experience fatigue and other symptoms. If the anemia becomes too severe, the person is susceptible to infection and may have trouble healing.

In many cases anemia is the result of inadequate amounts of iron in the diet. Called **iron-deficiency anemia**, it can be corrected by an iron supplement. Chapter 9 contains additional information on iron in the diet. Sometimes health conditions such as cancer or heavy menstrual flow may cause a person to be anemic. The cause has to be diagnosed so the proper treatment can follow.

Another type of anemia, which stems from a nutritional deficiency, is called **pernicious anemia.** In this condition the person has a deficiency in vitamin B_{12} because the body is not able to absorb it. Pernicious anemia is treated by vitamin B_{12} injections.

Sickle Cell Disease

Some forms of anemia are attributable to an inherited trait. One type of genetic-based anemia, or **hemoglobinopathy**, is called **sickle cell disease**. Approximately 72,000 African Americans have sickle cell disease. The sickle cell gene also is carried by people whose ancestors come from countries around the Mediterranean Sea, the Arabian Peninsula, and portions of India. According to the March of Dimes, one in every 1,000 to 1,500 Latinos living in the United States has sickle cell disease. In addition, many people carry one sickle gene or have the sickle cell trait. This means that, although they do not have the disease itself, they can pass the gene on to their children.

Generations of Africans living in the "malaria belts" of the African continent were protected genetically from malaria when, over time, they developed a sickle gene that altered the composition of their red blood cells. Those who carried one sickle gene were more resistant to the blood-borne parasite that causes malaria. This inherited protection, the sickle cell gene, was passed to successive generations and was brought to the Americas with the slave trade. This is why one in 10 or 12 African Americans carries the sickle gene and has sickle cell trait. Sickle cell anemia is just one of several sickle cell diseases. Other common sickle cell diseases are *sickle hemoglobin C disease* (SC disease) and *sickle cell thalassemia disease* (S/Thal).

Normally, red blood cells are soft, round, doughnut-shaped cells that are able to pass through even the tiniest blood vessels. Sickle cells, in contrast, take on the sickle shape for which the disease is named (see Figure 7.7). Instead of passing through the blood vessels, these cells clump together and clog tiny vessels (impeding the flow of oxygen-carrying blood) which is painful. Most people with sickle cell disease have at least one or two crises, called *painful episodes*, each year, and 15% to 20% endure these crises more frequently.

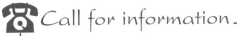Call for information

National Association for Sickle Cell Disease
800-421-8453

Sickle Cell Disease
800-358-9295

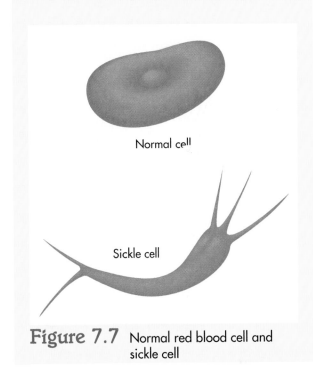

Figure 7.7 Normal red blood cell and sickle cell

Inheritance

Because sickle cell anemia is a recessive trait-inherited condition, two recessive genes (sickle genes) have to be present to produce sickle cell anemia in a child. One sickle cell gene has to come from the mother and the other from the father. Figure 7.8 illustrates the way the sickle cell gene is inherited. *A* designates the gene for normal hemoglobin, and *S* denotes the sickle cell gene. Because the child gets half of his/her genetic material from each parent, *AA* designates two inherited genes for normal hemoglobin. The child who inherits one gene for normal hemoglobin and one for sickle cell hemoglobin is designated *As* and has the sickle cell *trait*.

KEY TERMS

Anemia condition characterized by an insufficient quantity or quality of red blood cells

Hemoglobin a chemical in the blood that carries oxygen and is responsible for the blood's red color

Iron-deficiency anemia anemia caused by too little iron in the blood

Pernicious anemia anemia caused by a vitamin B$_{12}$ deficiency that occurs when the body is unable to absorb it

Hemoglobinopathy abnormal hemoglobin

Sickle cell disease an inherited form of anemia that produces sickle-shaped cells that clump together and clog tiny blood vessels

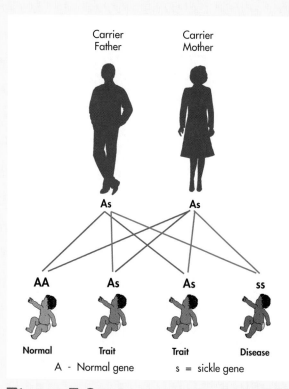

Carrier
Father

Carrier
Mother

As

As

AA

As

As

ss

Normal

Trait

Trait

Disease

A - Normal gene   s = sickle gene

Figure 7.8 How sickle cell anemia is inherited

The letters *ss* indicate that the child inherited two sickle genes, one from each parent, and has sickle cell anemia.

If both parents have normal hemoglobin (*AA*), any children they conceive will have normal hemoglobin as well. Conversely, if both parents have sickle cell anemia (*ss*), any children they conceive will have the disease like their parents. If, however, both parents have sickle trait (*As*), the probability or odds for *each* child to have the genes *AA*, *As*, or *ss* are as follows:

✳ 25% risk of inheriting two sickle genes and thus sickle cell anemia (*ss*)

✳ 25% chance of inheriting two normal genes and thus normal hemoglobin (*AA*)

✳ 50% chance of inheriting one normal and one sickle gene and thus sickle cell trait (*As*).

Symptoms, Diagnosis, and Treatment

Individuals with sickle cell trait generally have no apparent symptoms. Though healthy, the person carries an inherited sickle cell gene that can be passed on to any children conceived. Sometimes individuals with sickle cell trait become short of

breath temporarily or have some pain if they are in an environment in which the oxygen levels are lower than normal, such as at high altitudes while traveling in the mountains, when deep-sea diving, or after receiving general, inhalation-type anesthesia for surgery.

People with sickle cell anemia may develop symptoms as early as 6 months of age. One sign is pain and swelling in the hands or feet. Babies with sickle cell disease may stop making red blood cells for a short time, called an **aplastic crisis**. Symptoms include inactivity, pallor, and rapid breathing and heartbeat. As its name implies, aplastic crisis requires immediate medical attention.

A fever over 100°F may indicate an infection. A person with sickle cell anemia has a weakened immune system and thus is susceptible to infection. In the past, many people with sickle cell anemia died by age 20, and few survived past 40. Now infants and young children (under 6 years) are prescribed **prophylactic penicillin therapy** as a preventive measure against infections such as meningitis, hepatitis B, and pneumonia, which are major causes of complications and death. Penicillin, however does not cure sickle cell anemia.

In early 1995 the National Institutes of Health announced a new treatment for severe cases of sickle cell anemia. The cancer drug hydroxyurea proved to be so effective in alleviating the pain of sickle cell episodes that the NIH ended drug trials 4 months early and made the drug available to physicians. It seems to work by stimulating the body to produce a type of hemoglobin that resists sickle cell clumping. Although this drug is not a cure, it is a welcome advance in the treatment of sickle cell disease.

Still, the emphasis is shifting to prevention, through education and genetic counseling. The basic screening test used to determine if a person carries the sickle gene is a blood test called **hemoglobin electrophoresis**. With the aid of this test, couples who are considering conceiving a child are able to weigh their risk of having a child with sickle cell anemia.

A DISEASE OF THE METABOLISM: DIABETES

The **endocrine system** manufactures the body's hormones and secretes them directly into the bloodstream. The hormones are responsible for regulating body functions. The ductless glands include the pituitary, thyroid, parathyroid, adrenal, ovary, testis, and part of the pancreas. **Diabetes mellitus,** usually called "diabetes" or "sugar diabetes," is a chronic condition in which a person has excessive amounts of glucose or blood sugar in the circulatory system because of insufficient production of the hormone **insulin.** It affects nearly 14 million Americans and is the seventh leading cause of death in the United States. Insulin is produced by the *beta* cells of the pancreas in the **islets of Langerhans** and is secreted into the bloodstream. Insulin has two major functions:

1. To move glucose from the blood to the cells of the body where it is used as energy.

2. To convert excess glucose to glycogen, stored as an "energy reserve" in the liver and muscles.

Types of Diabetes

People with diabetes are unable to process glucose properly and, as a result, the glucose accumulates in the blood. The form of diabetes in which the pancreas is not producing insulin is called **Type I or insulin-dependent diabetes.** This form, the more serious of the two, requires regular insulin injections. Although it accounts for only about 5% or less of all diabetes in the United States, that figure represents as many as a half million cases.

Type I diabetes is unknown or rare in some ethnic groups, including the Japanese, Chinese, Polynesians, and South African Blacks. On the other hand, Scandinavians (specifically Swedish and Finnish peoples) have much higher rates than the U. S. population.

Recent evidence indicates that Type I diabetes may be triggered by a virus that infects only people whose genes make them vulnerable to the disease. According to Dr. Massimo Trucco of the University of Pittsburgh, if the virus can be identified, a vaccine might be devised to administer to newborns and thereby prevent them from contracting the diabetes.

In the more common form, **Type II or non-insulin-dependent diabetes,** the pancreas produces some insulin, but the body is not able to

Type II Diabetes

The ethnic group with the highest known incidence in the world of Type II diabetes is the Pima Indian tribe in the southwestern United States. Half of the tribe members over age 35 develop the disorder. Up until about 40 years ago, the Pimas did not have this high rate. Through about 1940 they survived mainly on desert foods — vegetables, grains, subsistence crops. As Western, high-fat, high-calorie foods became more and more available, obesity became more widespread. Combined with a possible genetic predisposition for insulin resistance, obesity triggered the high incidence of Type II diabetes in the Pimas.

Source: Robert Silverman, *Diabetes in Adults* (Washington DC: U.S. Department of Health and Human Services, 1990).

use it effectively. As many as 95% of diabetics over age 20 are of this type. Type II diabetes (also called adult-onset diabetes) usually occurs after age 40, and fully half do not know they have it!

Type II diabetes is about twice as prevalent in minority groups (except Asians) as in Anglos. In African Americans it is the fourth leading cause of death from disease. African American women are more than twice as likely as Anglo women to develop diabetes. About one in ten African Americans between ages 45 and 65 has diabetes, and the incidence increases with advancing age. One in four African American women over age 55 has diabetes. Figure 7.9 shows the proportional prevalence

KEY TERMS

Aplastic crisis interruption in the body's production of red blood cells; may occur in babies with sickle cell disease

Prophylactic penicillin therapy use of penicillin to prevent infections from occurring in infants and young children with sickle cell anemia

Hemoglobin electrophoresis screening test to identify sickle cell gene carriers

Endocrine system body system that manufactures and secretes hormones

Diabetes mellitus chronic condition characterized by excessive amounts of glucose in the blood

Insulin hormone essential for processing glucose in the body

Islets of Langerhans cells in the pancreas that produce insulin

Type I (insulin-dependent) diabetes form of diabetes in which the pancreas does not produce insulin

Type II (noninsulin-dependent) diabetes form of diabetes in which pancreas produces some insulin but the body is not able to use it well

Signs and Symptoms of Diabetes

The symptoms of Type I diabetes appear suddenly and dramatically. In some cases people develop ketoacidosis before they even think about seeing a physician. Symptoms of Type I diabetes include fatigue and irritability, abnormal hunger and thirst, frequent urination, and weight loss. Some of the same symptoms occur in Type II diabetes. The signals seem to be more subtle for Type II diabetes, and the person may not notice them until a blood test is done during a routine health examination. Other signs that may signal Type II diabetes are drowsiness, blurred vision, itching, slow-healing cuts, skin infections, and numbness of fingers or toes.

In Type I diabetes two life-threatening complications can arise if the person's blood sugar level becomes too high or too low because of an imbalance of insulin: diabetic coma and insulin reaction. In **diabetic coma** the amount of insulin the person has injected is not enough to process the glucose in the bloodstream. This causes hyperglycemia and leads to ketoacidosis. If this problem is not corrected, it can lead to coma and death. The person experiences the same symptoms as those when Type I diabetes was first diagnosed. Additional symptoms include dry skin and mouth, labored breathing, nausea and vomiting, a sweet or fruity breath odor, large amounts of ketones in the urine, and a blood sugar level of more than 300 mg/dl. Because diabetic coma develops slowly, the person usually can be transported to a hospital in time to receive insulin treatment.

If a person has injected too much insulin, skipped a meal, or engaged in excessive physical activity, the blood sugar level may drop below normal levels. The result is called **insulin reaction**, a form of **hypoglycemia** or low blood sugar. Unlike diabetic coma, the onset of insulin reaction is sudden. Some of the symptoms are a weak or faint feeling, hunger, trembling, moist skin, headache, confused or irritable behavior that may escalate to

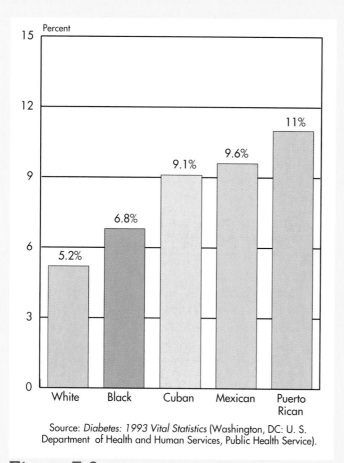

Source: *Diabetes: 1993 Vital Statistics* (Washington, DC: U. S. Department of Health and Human Services, Public Health Service).

Figure 7.9 Prevalence of diabetes in U.S. subpopulations

of diabetes by various ethnic minorities in the United States. Other risk factors for Type II diabetes include having a family history of the condition and being overweight.

In both Type I and Type II, when the diabetic person eats a meal, the glucose accumulates in the blood and produces a condition called **hyperglycemia,** or high blood sugar. Because the cells of the body cannot get glucose for energy from the blood and the body has no glycogen reserve, the cells burn protein and fat as their source of fuel. The burning of fat causes the formation of acid substances called ketones. The accumulation of these ketones leads to **ketoacidosis** or **ketosis,** which can result in coma and death.

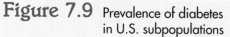

"Diabetes increases fourfold a woman's risk of developing heart disease."
— David M. Nathan, M.D., Massachusetts General Hospital, Boston

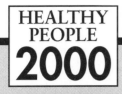
❋ Reduce diabetes-related deaths in general.

❋ Reduce diabetes-related deaths among American Indians and Alaska Natives.

❋ Reduce the most severe complications of diabetes:

   End-stage renal disease
   Blindness
   Lower extremity amputation
   Perinatal mortality
   Major congenital malformation

hostility, rapid heartbeat and shallow breathing, and loss of consciousness. An insulin reaction can be stopped by giving the person candy, orange juice, or anything sweet. Sometimes proper first aid is delayed or no aid is given because insulin reaction is mistaken for diabetic coma or alcohol intoxication.

Individuals with both types of diabetes should receive long-term medical care from of a physician so the condition can be controlled and serious health complications will not develop. Over time diabetes affects the cardiovascular system and the central nervous system severely. If diabetes is not controlled, the following chronic conditions can develop:

❋ *Diabetic retinopathy*, a disease of the retina, which can lead to blindness

❋ *Cardiovascular complications* such as atherosclerosis, heart attack (diabetics are twice as likely as nondiabetics to have a heart attack), hypertension, stroke, poor circulation to the legs and feet, gangrene and subsequent amputation.

❋ *Kidney (renal) diseases* such as kidney infections and kidney failure

☎ Call for information

American Diabetes Association
800-342-2383

Juvenile Diabetes Foundation International
800-223-1138

❋ *Diabetic neuropathy*, a disease of the nerves, which can lead to numbness of the hands and feet, muscle weakness, skin disorders, impaired bladder functioning, and sexual impotence.

In addition, the infant of a mother with Type I diabetes has a higher-than-average risk of birth defects, stillbirth, respiratory distress, and other problems at birth.

Control of Diabetes

Normal blood glucose levels range from 70 to 110 milligram/deciliter (mg/dl) of blood. Factors such as time of day, meals, illness, medicines, and stress can cause a person's glucose level to rise or fall. Regardless of the time the last meal was consumed, a blood sugar level of more than 200 mg/dl suggests a problem. A physician uses a blood test called the **glucose tolerance test** to diagnose diabetes.

For both types of diabetes, the diabetic person has to be able to balance blood sugar, food intake,

KEY TERMS

Hyperglycemia high blood sugar caused by the body's inability to process glucose from the blood

Ketoacidosis (ketosis) accumulation of acid substances (ketones) caused by the incomplete burning of fat for energy

Diabetic coma unconsciousness induced by ketoacidosis

Insulin reaction low blood sugar caused by too much insulin

Hypoglycemia low blood sugar

Glucose tolerance test blood test used to diagnose diabetes

and activities. Type I diabetics are able to achieve this balance in most cases by monitoring their blood glucose and adjusting the amounts of insulin they inject daily (or continuously infuse by a pump) based on food intake and daily activities meal-by-meal. Type I diabetes, then, is controlled by proper diet, exercise, and daily injections of the hormone insulin.

Type II diabetes can be controlled through diet and exercise. Oral medication might be required in some cases, but daily insulin injections are not. Individuals with diabetes should be under the care of a physician who has expertise in treating the disease. Often the diabetes can be controlled without medication if regular physical activity is combined with a weight-loss diet. Public health epidemiologist Susan Helmrich suggests that an increase in physical activity can be effective in *preventing* noninsulin-dependent diabetes in the first place.

ARTHRITIS AND RHEUMATIC DISEASES

The term **arthritis** is a layperson's term for more than 100 medical disorders called **rheumatic diseases**. Rheumatic diseases cover a wide spectrum, including rheumatoid arthritis, osteoarthritis, fibromyalgia, carpal tunnel syndrome, lupus, bursitis, gout, and scleroderma, among many others. What they all have in common is that they are characterized by inflammation and pain in tissues or joints.

Any place in the body where two bones meet is a joint. The ends of the bones are covered by **cartilage**, a tough, elastic tissue that acts as a shock absorber and keeps the bones from rubbing against each other. The entire joint is enclosed in a capsule lined by the inner skin called the **synovial membrane**, which releases a lubricating synovial fluid between the bones and facilitates movement. Surrounding the joint are muscles, tendons, and ligaments. Tendons are cordlike structures that attach muscles to bones. Ligaments connect bones to each other. Fluid-filled sacs called **bursae**, found among the muscles, bones, ligaments, and tendons, keep all these structures moving

☎ *Call for information*

Arthritis Foundation
800-283-7800

smoothly against each other when everything is functioning normally. Figure 7.10 contrasts a normal joint with an arthritic joint.

When the joints are traumatized or invaded by a foreign object, **inflammation** is the body's reaction, manifested by swelling, redness, and pain in the affected area. In arthritis the joint (arthro) is what becomes inflamed (itis). Onset can be slow or sudden. Once a person has arthritis, it usually is for life.

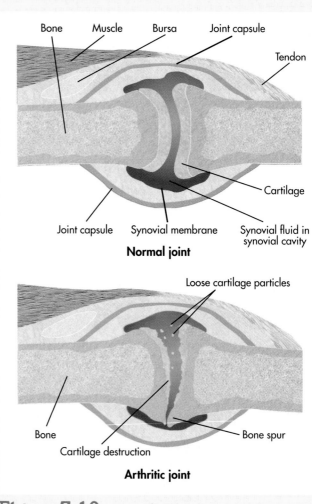

Bone   Muscle   Bursa   Joint capsule

Tendon

Cartilage

Joint capsule   Synovial membrane   Synovial fluid in synovial cavity

Normal joint

Loose cartilage particles

Bone   Bone spur

Cartilage destruction

Arthritic joint

Figure 7.10   Normal and arthritic joints

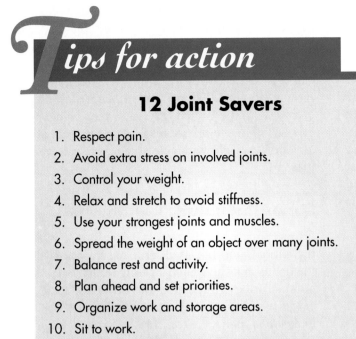

Tips for action

12 Joint Savers

1. Respect pain.
2. Avoid extra stress on involved joints.
3. Control your weight.
4. Relax and stretch to avoid stiffness.
5. Use your strongest joints and muscles.
6. Spread the weight of an object over many joints.
7. Balance rest and activity.
8. Plan ahead and set priorities.
9. Organize work and storage areas.
10. Sit to work.
11. Use labor-saving devices.
12. Ask for help.

Source: Arthritis Foundation, 1994.

Arthritis is the number-one disabling diseases in the United States, affecting an estimated 37 million people, about one in seven, according to the Arthritis Foundation. The prevalence of rheumatic conditions is higher in African Americans (53% of total cases) than Anglos (46%). Because we cannot cover all the rheumatic diseases here, we highlight lupus, which is also an autoimmune disorder, along with three prevalent types of arthritis. Osteoporosis, the most common form, is discussed in Chapter 14.

Lupus

Lupus erythematosus, more commonly called **lupus**, is a chronic disorder of the immune system that causes inflammation of tissues and vital organs of the body. The joints can be affected, complicating the disease. The normal function of the immune system is to protect healthy tissue and organs. People with lupus instead produce antibodies that attack normal cells, producing inflammation, cell injury, and

☎ Call for information

Lupus Foundation of America
800-558-0121

cell destruction. Although the cause of lupus is unknown, individuals may be genetically predisposed to lupus, and certain environmental factors, such as sunlight, may trigger it.

Lupus is an insidious condition in that it develops gradually and subtly. The symptoms come and go and mimic other illnesses, which makes diagnosis difficult. Lupus may be mild in some people, in that it affects just a few body organs. In others it may cause serious, even life-threatening, health problems.

More than half a million people in the United States have been diagnosed with lupus, with about 6,000 new cases each year. Lupus is most common in women ages 20-30. According to the Arthritis Foundation, lupus is more common in African Americans, Hispanics, American Indians, and Asian women than in other groups.

One of the two main types of lupus, *discoid lupus*, is confined to the skin. It is characterized by persistent flushing of the cheeks in disc-like lesions (a rash) that appear in the "butterfly" area of the face, on the neck, scalp, ears, arms, and other areas exposed to ultraviolet light. Discoid lupus is not life-threatening.

About 10% of these cases develop into *systemic lupus erythematosus (SLE)*, which affects a number of body systems. In some people this may mean only the skin and joints. In others it may affect the joints, kidneys, blood, and central nervous system, causing arthritis and nephritis. SLE is characterized

KEY TERMS

Arthritis general classification of numerous diseases that cause swelling and pain in the joints, muscles, and bones

Rheumatic diseases disorders that involve inflammation and swelling of the joints and restrict range of motion

Cartilage elastic tissue at ends of bones that acts as a shock absorber and buffer between bones

Synovial membrane lining of joint that releases a lubricating fluid

Bursae fluid-filled sacs found among muscles, bones, ligaments, and tendons

Inflammation body's reaction to pathogen or trauma, characterized by redness, pain, and swelling

Lupus chronic disorder of immune system accompanied by inflammation of various parts of the body

by periods of remission when the person has less severe symptoms and by "flare" periods during which the condition becomes highly active again.

A third, and rare, type of lupus is drug-induced. Certain prescribed medications create a lupuslike syndrome similar to SLE, but the nervous system is rarely affected. Two medications associated with drug-induced lupus are *hydralazine* (to treat hypertension) and *procainamide hydrochloride* (to treat irregular heart rhythm). Only a tiny fraction of those who take these drugs will develop lupus, and when the medication is discontinued, the symptoms of lupus fade in those who do.

The onset of lupus is gradual, with only vague signs of the disease. Until specific symptoms develop, the following symptoms are found commonly in people in the early stages of lupus:

fever	fatigue
loss of appetite	weight loss
aches and pains	swollen glands
nausea and vomiting	headache
depression	easy bruising
hair loss	edema and swelling

In addition to these generalized symptoms, the following are more suggestive of lupus:

❈ a rash over the cheeks and bridge of the nose (hence, the moniker "wolf disease")

❈ discoid lupus lesions

❈ development of rash after exposure to sun and fluorescent light

❈ bald spots

❈ ulcers inside the mouth

❈ swelling and pain of two or more joints

❈ pleurisy (pain in the chest on deep breathing)

❈ seizure

❈ Raynaud's phenomenon (fingers or toes turning white or blue in the cold).

Several tests have been developed to diagnose lupus. The two usually used to make an initial diagnosis are the *antinuclear antibody (ANA) test*, followed by the *fluorescent ANA test*. In conjunction with lab tests, the American College of Rheumatology has issued a list of symptoms to help differentiate lupus from other diseases.

Corticosteriod drug therapy often is prescribed to those diagnosed with lupus, and they are advised to get adequate rest. No cure has been found, but

the Fall 1994 issue of the Rocky Mountain Chapter of the *Arthritis Observer* reported on "exciting gains in lupus research," indicating progress in identifying a gene that may cause lupus. Most cases can be managed through proper treatment, although about 5,000 people die from this disease each year in the United States. Of those diagnosed, 80%–90% live more than 10 years after diagnosis, and most people with lupus can expect a normal lifespan.

Other Rheumatic Conditions

Osteoarthritis affects almost 16 million people in the United States. This disease occurs primarily in the hands and the weight-bearing joints — the knee and hip. It has been called the "wear and tear" disease. People who are born with slight defects that make their joints fit together incorrectly or move incorrectly may be more likely to develop osteoarthritis. In some families osteoarthritis possibly is the result of a hereditary defect in one of the genes responsible for a major protein component of cartilage called collagen.

African American women have higher rates of osteoarthritis than Anglo women do. This may be related in some part to a genetic predisposition and also to the greater propensity of African American women to be overweight (discussed in Chapter 10).

Studies have shown that people who carry extra weight in their 20s greatly increase their risk of developing arthritis of the knees and hips later in life. This is true for moderately overweight as well as obese individuals. Dr. Allan Gelber, a Johns Hopkins School of Medicine rheumatologist, said that each 20-pound increment of extra weight raises a person's chances of developing osteoarthritis by 50%. Research has indicated that vitamin E can be effective in reducing the pain somewhat.

Rheumatoid arthritis is similar to osteoarthritis, but it is more severe because it can affect all joints of the body. It is characterized by pain and joint inflammation that results in crippling deformities. It strikes most commonly between ages 20 and 45. Of all cases, an estimated 80% are women in their childbearing years. It is an autoimmune disorder. Table 7.3 compares rheumatoid arthritis with osteoarthritis.

Fibromyalgia, or fibromyositis, is the second most common rheumatic disease. The onset occurs most often in women between ages of 20 and 55.

This disease does not involve inflammation of tissues but, rather, unexplained pain (myalgia). People with fibromyalgia may feel deep muscular aching, throbbing, burning, or stabbing pain, along with total fatigue. Related symptoms include disturbances in deep-level sleep, headaches, chest pain, dizziness, and abdominal pain.

However painful, fibromyalgia does not seem to damage connective tissues or organs permanently, and it does not lead to deformity. The lack of objective physical evidence and absence of overt signs make diagnosis difficult. Because x-rays and typical blood tests are normal, this disease has been largely unrecognized and underreported until recently.

The search for a cause remains elusive. Proposed theories include trauma to the central nervous system, an infectious agent such as the flu virus, and changes in muscle metabolism, among others.

The most successful original treatment for arthritis, still used, is aspirin. Other available remedies encompass:

—various medications (nonsteroidal anti-inflammatory agents and cortisones)
— exercise
— rest/relaxation
— application of heat or cold
— joint protection (by brace or other device)
— surgery
— weight control (long-term).

SKIN CONDITIONS

Skin conditions cover a wide range from psoriasis to eczema to ringworm. Some conditions are particularly applicable to African Americans because of unique skin characteristics. Some African Americans' hair texture is like that of people of European ancestry. Typically, however, African Americans' hair is coarser and curlier than that of other ethnic groups. The curlier hair texture can cause a skin problem for African American men, known as *pseudofolliculitis barbae*, a condition that occurs when curved beard hairs are cut during shaving. Shaving gives the tips of the curled hair sharp points that penetrate the skin, causing a painful and irritating rash (razor bumps). The affected follicles may become inflamed, requiring antibiotics to treat the infection. Permanent scarring may result.

A logical solution is to stop shaving, and this may be a reason so many African American men have beards. Some men use a chemical depilatory (a shaving powder) to remove facial hair. Several studies have indicated that nearly 45% of African Americans in the military who shave develop razor bumps sooner or later.

Two other skin conditions that affect African Americans disproportionately are vitiligo and keloids.

Vitiligo

Vitiligo is an autoimmune skin disorder characterized by a gradual

Table 7.3
Comparison of Osteoarthritis and Rheumatoid

Osteoarthritis	Rheumatoid Arthritis
Usaually begins after age 40	Usually begins between ages 25 and 50
To age 45, more common in men; after age 54, more common in women	Women outnumber men three to one
Usually develops slowly, over many yearts	Often develops suddenly, within weeks or months
Often affects joins on only one side of the body	Usually affects same joint on both sides of the body (e.g., both knees)
Usually doesn't cause joint inflammation	Causes inflammation of the joint
Affects only certain joints; rarely affects elbows or shoulders	Affects many joints, including elbows and shoulders
Doesn't cause a general feeling of sickness	Often causes a general feeling of sickness, fatigue, weight loss, fever

Source: Arthritis Foundation, Atlanta, GA.

KEY TERMS

Osteoarthritis most common form of arthritis affecting primarily the hands and weight-bearing joints

Rheumatoid arthritis more severe form of arthritis that affects all joints of the body, causing inflammation

Fibromyalgia disease that causes unexplained muscular pain

Vitiligo an autoimmune skin disorder characterized by gradual destruction of the pigment-producing cells

Tips for action

To prevent razor bumps:

* Before shaving, lather the beard area thoroughly.

* Use only disposable razors, and throw them away after one use to prevent reintroducing bacteria to the affected area.

* Avoid electric razors; they produce a sharper hair tip.

* Don't stretch the skin. Once tension is released, the hairs retract and penetrate the follicle.

* Keep the skin scrupulously clean.

* Use a baby shampoo to prevent irritation to sensitive skin.

* Shave only every other day.

* If you spot an embedded hair, release it with a clean needle.

* Massage the beard area daily with a washcloth or coarse sponge.

If the condition doesn't clear up in a few weeks, an antibiotic ointment or oral antibiotics may be prescribed.

Source: Colonel Madison Patrick, M.D., U.S. Army Health Clinic, Oahu, Hawaii.

---

destruction of the **melanocytes** or pigment-producing cells. As a result of this destruction, the person with vitiligo begins to lose pigment in the skin and hair. Even though it can affect individuals of any race, it is particularly disfiguring and unsettling to people who have dark pigmentation. The cause of vitiligo is unknown, but a family history of the condition has been reported in at least 30% of the cases. It can appear at any age and seems to affect men and women equally. Vitiligo was thrust into the spotlight when pop star Michael Jackson reported that he was not bleaching his skin but, rather, had lost pigmentation because of this condition.

Vitiligo is of three types:

1. In *localized* or *patterned vitiligo*, the person may have one or several patches of "white spots," areas of depigmentation (macules), on one or two areas of the body.

2. *Generalized vitiligo* is characterized by large or small macules scattered on the body in no special pattern. These macules often are symmetrical. In one form of generalized vitiligo, the macules are confined to the tips of fingers and toes and the lips. In some cases the person loses all skin pigmentation (turns "white").

3. In *mixed vitiligo*, the loss of pigmentation can be widespread and localized.

Vitiligo is treated using PUVA photochemotherapy and corticosteriods. Even after treatment some areas of the body will not repigment. Some people with vitiligo use special cosmetic preparations to cover the white areas.

Keloids or Cicatrices

A **keloid,** or cicatrix, is a raised scar that results from an overgrowth of fibrous tissue following a trauma to the skin such as a cut or burn. Keloids may look like blisters filled with fluid, but they are not. The irregularly shaped scar becomes progressively larger because of excessive amounts of **collagen** (a fibrous protein found in connective tissue) that forms during the healing process. The scar that forms does not stop growing as it is supposed to.

A keloid can form on many surfaces of the body. The face, neck, and upper chest are the most common sites. The configuration or pattern of the

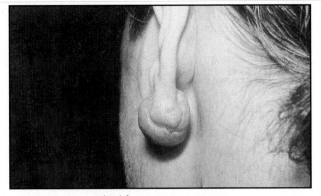

Keloid from earring piercing.

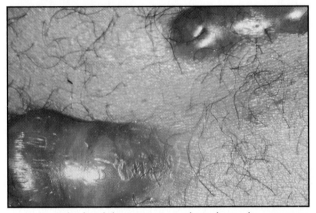

Keloid with hyperpigmented overlying skin.

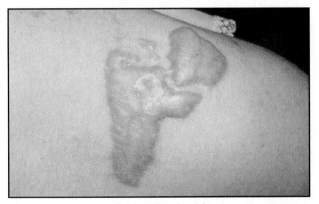

Keloid on the shoulder.

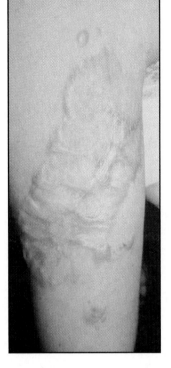

Keloid from burn.

keloid can be unusual, depending on the site and the type of trauma. You may have seen the Ω (Greek letter omega) in the form of a dark, raised scar on the upper arm or chest of a fraternity member. This scar is the result of trauma to the skin by a hot branding iron.

Although keloids can form on individuals of any ethnic group, they are more common in African Americans and people with a family history of keloid formation. People with a propensity for "keloid skin" should be careful when considering ear piercing, cosmetic surgery, or other forms of adornment that cause trauma to the skin.

Removing a keloid by cutting it away may seem like a simple proposition. Surgically removing the keloid however, would result in another scar that would heal as a keloid. Keloids should be treated by a dermatologist or a plastic surgeon with experience in skin disorders of African Americans. In treating a keloid, the physician has to consider the size and location of the keloid, as well as how long the person has had it. Nonsurgical treatments include massage, ultrasound, and corticosteroid creams and ointments that soften and shrink the scar. In some cases steroids are injected directly into the keloid. Some physicians use laser surgery to remove the keloid because it leaves a smaller scar. Silastic gel sheeting, or SGS, used to reduce scar tissue formation after burns, has been approved to treat keloids. This treatment makes the keloid flatter and reduces the symptoms of burning and itching.

KEY TERMS

Melanocytes pigment-producing cells of the skin

Keloid raised scar that results from overgrowth of fibrous tissue following a cut or burn to the skin

Collagen fibrous protein found in connective tissue

DISORDERS OF THE DIGESTIVE TRACT

As with the other body systems, the digestive tract can function abnormally from a number of different causes. Figure 7.11 illustrates the digestive tract and the organs that may be affected.

Peptic ulcers can form in the lining of the stomach or the small intestine as the result of the corrosive effect of digestive juices. These irritate the lining, reduce the protective mucus, and actually begin to digest the tissue itself. Because the exact cause is unknown, preventing peptic ulcers is difficult. The propensity for ulcers does seem to run in families. In addition, ulcers tend to develop in people who are under chronic stress, those whose diet is high in fat, and those who consume large amounts of alcohol.

The former standard recommendation to alleviate ulcers by drinking milk was found to be faulty because it causes the stomach to secrete more acid to digest the lactose and fat in milk. Currently, drugs that reduce stomach secretions or soothe irritated linings are prescribed. In addition, people with ulcers should avoid high-fat foods, alcohol, and other substances that irritate the stomach lining.

Colitis is a recurring inflammation of the large intestine. Because the cause is basically unknown,

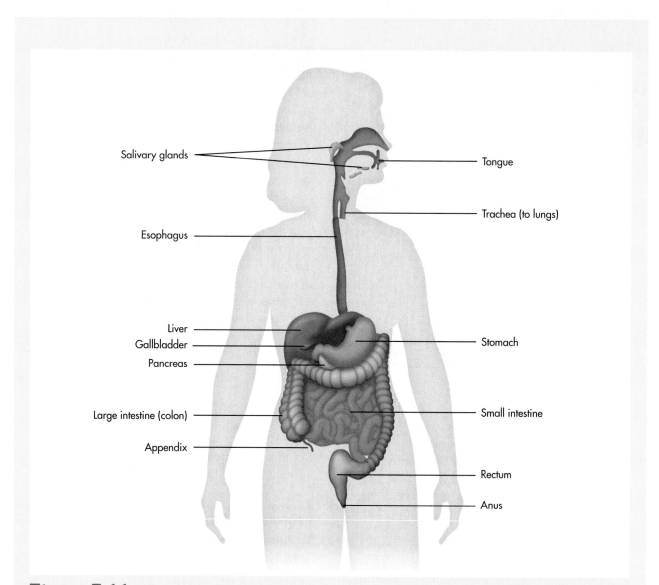

Figure 7.11 The digestive tract

treatment focuses on relieving the symptoms. Anti-inflammatory drugs and steroids are the main treatments, along with increasing dietary fiber intake.

Diverticulosis is a painful condition resulting when the intestinal wall, usually of the small intestine, becomes weakened. Small pouches develop. These fill with fecal matter passing through the intestine and become irritated. This disease is most prevalent at middle age or after, though it can develop at any age. If it persists, bleeding and chronic obstruction may occur, which can be life-threatening. In some cases a person may have an attack that seems like it could be appendicitis, but the discomfort of diverticulosis occurs on the left side of the body instead of the right because of the configuration of the intestine.

Lactose intolerance, resulting from a deficiency of the lactase enzyme in the stomach, is discussed in Chapter 9.

NEUROLOGICAL DISORDERS

The **central nervous system** consists of the brain and the spinal cord. The brain is the body's control center. It sends messages to and receives stimulation from all parts of the body via the nervous system. The brain, not surprisingly, is the most complex organ in the body. It is the receptacle of thoughts, feelings, behaviors, physical sensations, movements, and senses. The brain also controls involuntary functions such as breathing and swallowing. It houses an intricate network of nerve cells called **neurons**, which form the foundation of this complex electrochemical communication system.

Unlike most other cells in the body, neurons cannot be replaced if they die. Therefore, death of neurons has a severe impact on memory, cognition, and behavior. This is the case with Alzheimer's disease, discussed in Chapter 14. Representative brain disorders discussed here are headaches and epilepsy.

Headaches

The headache is the most common assault on the brain. More than 45 million Americans suffer from chronic, recurring headaches, a statistic that continues to grow every year, according to the National Headache Foundation. The three main categories of headache are:

1. Tension (ache in the area where the muscles of the head and neck meet).

📞 **Call for information**

National Headache Foundation
800-843-2256

2. Vascular (migraine, toxic, and cluster headaches).

3. Organically caused (tumors and diseases).

Tension Headaches

Most headaches, about 90%, are classified as **tension headaches**. The pain typically is generalized all over the head. Some people have headaches almost daily. They usually awaken in the morning with the headache and frequently have an accompanying sleep disorder. This type of headache is often caused by depression or other emotional problems.

Others have episodic headaches. As the name indicates, these headaches occur spasmodically and seem to have no pattern. If they continue over time, though, they are distressing.

Vascular Headaches — Migraines and Cluster Headaches

Migraine headaches usually have a hereditary component. If both parents have them, their children have a 75% chance of having them also. If one parent has migraines, each child has a 50% chance of getting them. African Americans seem to have a lower prevalence of migraines than Anglo Americans. This may be related to a higher platelet level of the tyramine-joining enzyme, which protects against migraine by metabolizing suspected dietary triggers. A comparison of migraine headaches in

KEY TERMS

Peptic ulcers irritations in the lining of the stomach or small intestine caused by the corrosive effect of digestive juices

Central nervous system the brain and the spinal cord

Colitis recurring inflammation of the large intestine

Diverticulosis painful condition caused by weakened places in the intestine that bulge, fill with fecal matter and become irritated

Tension headaches headaches characterized by generalized pain all over the head

Migraine headaches vascular form of headaches characterized by severe pain

Neurons the foundation for electrochemical communication system in the brain

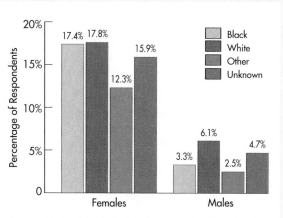

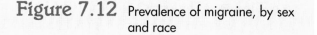

Source: *National Headache Foundation Newsletter,* Summer 1992.

Figure 7.12 Prevalence of migraine, by sex and race

African Americans and in Anglo Americans is shown in Figure 7.12.

Migraines can be brought on by stress, poor sleeping habits, and changes in altitude and temperature. In addition, foods and beverages including chocolate, red wine, and aged cheese can provoke a migraine, as can noise, certain odors, bright lights, and watching TV.

Some migraines are preceded by a warning signal known as an **aura**, tingling or numbness of limbs, speech impairment, or visual disturbances such as flashing spots in front of the eyes. This is followed by severe pain on one side of the head. The pain may be so extreme that it causes nausea and vomiting, cold hands, shaking, and sensitivity to light and sound. Attacks last several minutes to several days.

Drug treatments include ergotamine and preventive medications including beta blockers, NSAID, and antidepressants. Nondrug therapies include diet control, relaxation tapes, and biofeedback, to manage the muscle contractions and swelling of blood vessels.

As their names implies, **cluster headaches** come in groups, up to four headaches per day during a cluster period. A headache can last 15 minutes to several hours, and a cycle can last days, weeks, or months, eventually retreating into long periods of remission. The pain is intense. Excess smoking and alcohol consumption can trigger these headaches.

Prescription medications that have proven successful include special nose drops, ergotamine, and oxygen therapy (inhaling pure oxygen through a facial mask).

Organically Caused Headaches

Organic causes account for only 2% of all headaches. These, however, often are symptomatic of more serious disorders such as tumors.

Other Types of Headaches

Sinus An allergic reaction can produce a constant, gnawing pain in the sinuses. A fever may accompany the headache. Despite what most people believe, sinus headaches, are rare. Many people who think they have a sinus headache actually have a tension or migraine headache.

TMJ A dull ache in and around the ear that gets worse when a person chews, talks, or yawns may be a result of dysfunction of the temporomandibular joint (TMJ). Treatments may consist of heat, massage, painkillers, and a bite plate. Relaxation techniques also may be effective.

In general, behavioral management techniques have proven helpful in managing chronic headaches. These methods include:

✳ *Biofeedback and relaxation training.* Biofeedback techniques (introduced in Chapter 3) are used to measure physical activity that may be contributing to the headaches. The activity measured may be muscle tension, blood flow, skin resistance, or skin temperature. The patient learns to use this feedback to exert voluntary control over a physical function. Between a third and a half of individuals with vascular and tension headaches seem to benefit from these treatments.

✳ *Cognitive-behavioral psychotherapy.* The patient learns problem-solving and coping skills that can be used to manage stress and situations thought to increase the frequency and intensity of headaches. Cognitive therapies focus on the relationships among thoughts, feelings, and behaviors and how to replace dysfunctional patterns with functional ones.

✳ *Operant behavioral treatment.* Treatment consists of withdrawal from all medications with addictive potential, increasing physical activity, and developing positive reinforcements (rewards) for positive behaviors. Candidates for this technique are those with chronic headaches over at least a 3-month period who have not responded to medical treatment and who are functionally disabled by the headaches. These techniques usually are reserved for the most difficult and disabled patients.

In addition, headache sufferers are advised to avoid caffeine altogether.

Seizure Disorders

The more common term for seizure disorder is **epilepsy**. Approximately 1% of all Americans have some form of seizure-related disorder. Caused by abnormal electrical activity in the brain, they are characterized by muscular malfunctioning that ranges from minor twitching in the mildest form to convulsions and loss of consciousness in the extreme form. The most common forms of seizure are:

1. *Grand mal*: often preceded by an aura, major convulsions throughout the body culminating in a loss of consciousness from 30 seconds to several minutes or longer.

2. *Petit mal*: minor twitching of muscles with no convulsions; minor loss of consciousness that may not even be noticed.

3. *Psychomotor*: mental confusion and listlessness, accompanied by unusual repetitive movements and behaviors such as lip smacking.

4. *Jacksonian seizure*: begins in one part of the body and moves to the hand, arm, or other parts, usually on only one side of the body.

In about half of the cases of epilepsy, the cause is identified as head injury, congenital abnormality related to inflammation of the brain or spinal column, drug poisoning, tumors, nutritional deficiency, or hereditary factors. In the other half of cases, the cause is unknown.

Because of effective medications, most people with epilepsy can lead a normal life. The disease does not get progressively worse nor is it fatal.

KEY TERMS

Aura warning signals that may precede migraine headaches

Cluster headaches headaches that occur in groups and cycles; characterized by intense pain

Epilepsy a seizure disorder caused by abnormal electrical activity in the brain

---

Summary

1 Cancer, the second leading cause of death in the United States, results from a mutation of genetic material followed by uncontrolled growth of abnormal cells.

2 Chronic obstructive pulmonary disease (COPD) consists primarily of chronic bronchitis and emphysema.

3 Sickle cell disease is an inherited blood disease.

4 Diabetes has two forms — Type I, the more serious of the two, and Type II, or adult-onset — both involving deficient insulin production in the body.

5 Rheumatic diseases, commonly termed arthritis, consist of about 100 conditions involving inflammation of the joints and supporting tissues.

6 Skin conditions that are almost exclusively a problem of African Americans are *pseudofolliculitis barbae*, vitiligo, and keloids.

7 Representative digestive disorders are peptic (stomach) ulcers, colitis, and diverticulosis.

8 The major types of headache are: tension, vascular (migraine and cluster), and organically caused (from a brain tumor).

9 The most common forms of epileptic seizure are: grand mal, petit mal, psychomotor, and Jacksonian.

Select Bibliography

American Cancer Society. *Cancer Facts and Figures—1994*. Atlanta: ACS, 1994

American Cancer Society. *Guidelines on Diet, Nutrition, and Cancer*, 41:6 (1991), 334-338.

Carper, Jean *Food–Your Miracle Medicine*. New York: Harper Collins, 1994.

Caruana, Claudia. "Scar Wars." *Essence*, October, 1993.

"Diabetes and Minorities." *Universal Healthworld*, 1:5 (June 1990), 34-36.

Dixon, Barbara M. *Good Health for African Americans*. New York: Crown Publishing, 1994.

Dunkin, Mary Anne, "Fibromyalgia." *Arthritis Today*, September-October, 1993.

Eckhout, Kim. "Exciting Gains in Lupus Research." *Arthritis Observer*, 46:2 (Fall 1994), pp. 1-2.

Editors of *Consumer Guide Family Medical Guide & Prescription* Lincolnwood, IL: Publications International, 1993.

Facts About Lupus. Rockville, MD: Lupus Foundation of America.

Gatson, Marilyn, et al. "Oral Prophylaxis with penicillin in children with sickle cell anemia." *New England Journal of Medicine*, 314:25 (June 19, 1986).

Good Housekeeping. *Family Health & Medical Guide*. New York: Hearst Books, 1980.

Hoeger, Werner W. K., and Sharon A. Hoeger. *Lifetime Physical Fitness and Wellness*, Englewood, CO: Morton Publishing, 1994.

Henry, W. L., Jr., K. A. Johnson, and L. Villarosa. *Black Health Library Guide to Diabetes*. New York: Henry Holt & Co., 1993.

Huddleston, James. In *The Wellness Book*, edited by Herbert Benson and Eiken Stuart. New York: Birch Lane Press, 1992.

Needham, Catherine. "Cultural Differences Shape Cancer Care." *Journal of the National Cancer Institute*, 86:4. February 16, 1994.

Newborn Screening for Sickle Cell Disease and Other Hemoglobinopathies, 6:9 (April 6–8, 1987).

Sauer, Gordon C. *Manual of Skin Diseases*, 6th edition. Philadelphia: J. B. Lippincott Co., 1991.

"Still at Large: The Most Common Concerns." *Hippocrates*. January-February, 1989, p. 44.

University of California at Berkeley *Wellness Letter*, (Sept. 1994), p. 8.

"Vitiligo." *Update: Dermatology In General Medicine*. New York: McGraw-Hill Book Co., 1983.

Cancer: Assessing Your Risk

NAME _____ DATE _____

COURSE _____ SECTION _____

INTRODUCTION

You can reduce your risk of developing some types of cancer, such as lung cancer, by changing your lifestyle behaviors. For other types of cancer, such as breast and colorectal cancers, your chance for cure is greatly increased if the cancer is found at an early stage through periodic screening examinations.

This questionnaire has been designed by the American Cancer Society to help you learn about (1) your risk factors for certain types of cancer and (2) the chances that cancer would be found at an early stage when a cure is possible.

TESTING SCORING DIRECTIONS

Read each question concerning each site and its specific risk factors. Be honest in your responses. Circle the number in parenthesis next to your response.

For example, Question #2 on lung cancer, below: if you are 53 years old (50–59) then circle 5 as your score. Total your scores in each section.

Men: Complete the first three sections only. Women: Complete all sections unless otherwise noted.

ABOUT YOUR ANSWERS

You may check your own risks with the answers contained in this assessment.
You are advised to discuss this assessment with your physician if you are at higher risk.

IMPORTANT: REACT TO EACH STATEMENT

Individual numbers for specific questions are not to be interpreted as a precise measure of relative risk, but the totals for a given site should give a general indication of your risk.

LUNG CANCER

1. **SEX:** a. Male (2) b. Female (1)
2. **AGE:** a. 39 or less (1) b. 40–49 (2) c. 50–59 (5) d. 60+ (7)
3. **EXPOSURE TO ANY OF THESE:**
   a. Mining (3) b. Asbestos (7) c. Uranium & radioactive products (5) d. None (0)
4. **HABITS:** a. smoker (10)* b. Nonsmoker (0)*
5. **TYPE OF SMOKING:**
   a. Cigarettes or little cigars (10) b. Pipe and/or cigar, but not cigarettes (3) c. Nonsmoker (0)
6. **NUMBER OF CIGARETTES SMOKED PER DAY:**
   a. 0 (1) b. less than ½ pack per day (5) c. ½–1 pack (9) d. 1–2 packs (15) e. 2+ packs (20)

ENDOMETRIAL CANCER

(Body of Uterus) — These questions do not apply to a woman who has had a total hysterectomy.

1. **AGE GROUP:**   a. 39 or less (5)   b. 40-49 (20)   c. 50 and over (60)
2. **RACE:**   a. Oriental (10)   b. Black (20)   c. Hispanic (20)   d. White (20)
3. **BIRTHS:**   a. None (15)   b. 1 to 4 (7)   c. 5 or more (5)
4. **WEIGHT:**   a. 50 or more pounds overweight (50)   b. 20–49 pounds overweight (15)
   c. Normal or underweight for height (10)
5. **DIABETES** (elevated blood sugar):   a. Yes (3)   b. No (1)
6. **ESTROGEN HORMONE INTAKE*:**   a. Yes, regularly (15)   b. Yes, occasionally (12)   c. None (10)
7. **ABNORMAL UTERINE BLEEDING:**   a. Yes (40)   b. No (1)
8. **HYPERTENSION (HIGH BLOOD PRESSURE):**   a. Yes (40)   b. No (1)

Subtotal _____

DETECTING CANCER EARLY

9. I have had a negative pelvic examination and Pap smear or endometrial tissue sampling (endometrial biopsy) performed within the past year. (If yes, subtract 50 points.)

Yes   No

TOTAL _____

*NOTE: This excludes birth control pills.

Answers and Test Analysis

LUNG   Answers

1. Men have a higher risk of lung cancer than women. Since women are smoking more, their incidence of lung and upper respiratory tract (mouth, tongue and voice box) cancer is increasing.

2. The occurrence of lung and upper respiratory tract cancer increases with age.

3. Cigarette smokers may have 20 times or even greater risk than nonsmokers. However, **the rates of ex-smokers who have not smoked for ten years approach those of nonsmokers**.

4. Pipe and cigar smokers are at a higher risk for lung cancer than nonsmokers. Cigarette smokers are also at a much higher risk for lung cancer than nonsmokers or than pipe and cigar smokers. All forms of tobacco, including chewing or dipping, markedly increase the user's risk of developing cancer of the mouth.

5. Male smokers of less than ½ pack per day have a five time higher lung cancer rate than nonsmokers. Male smokers of 1–2 packs per day have a 15 times higher lung cancer rate than nonsmokers. Smokers of more than 2 packs per day are 20 times more likely to develop lung cancer than nonsmokers.

6. Smokers of low tar/nicotine cigarettes have slightly lower lung cancer rates. Please note however that smokers of low tar/nicotine cigarettes may unconsciously smoke in a manner that **increases** their exposure to these chemicals.

7. The frequency of lung and upper respiratory tract cancer increases with the duration of smoking.

8. Exposures to materials used in these and other industries have been shown to be associated with lung cancer, especially in smokers.

If your total is:

24 or less ....You have a low risk for lung cancer.

25–49 ....You may be a light smoker and would have a good chance of kicking the habit

50–74 ....As a moderate smoker, your risks for lung and upper respiratory tract cancer are increased. The time to stop is now!

75–over ......As a heavy cigarette smoker, your chances of getting lung cancer and cancer of the upper respiratory or digestive tract are greatly increased.

REDUCING YOUR RISK — Make a decision to quit today. Join a smoking cessation program. If you are a heavy drinker of alcohol, your risks for cancer of the head and neck and esophagus are further increased. Use of "spitting" tobacco increases your risks of cancer of the mouth. Your best bet is not to use tobacco in any form. See your doctor if you have a nagging cough, hoarseness, persistent pain or sore in the mouth or throat or lumps in the neck.

COLON RECTUM Answers

1. Colon cancer occurs more often after the age of 50.
2. Colon cancer is more common in families with a previous history of this disease.
3. Polyps and bowel diseases are associated with colon cancer. Cancer of the breast, ovaries, or stomach may also be associated with an increased risk of colon cancer.
4. Rectal bleeding may be a sign of colon/rectum cancer.

I. RISK FACTORS* — If your total is:

5 or less ....You are currently at low risk for colon and rectum cancer. Eat a diet high in fiber and low in fat and follow cancer checkup guidelines.

6–15 ....You are currently at moderate risk for colon and rectum cancer. Follow the American Cancer Society guidelines for early detection of colorectal cancer. These are: (1) a digital rectal exam ** every year after 40 and (2) a fecal occult blood test every year and sigmoidoscopic, preferably flexible, exam every 3–5 years after age 50.

16 or greater...You are in the high risk group for colon and rectum cancer. This rating requires a lifetime, on-going screening program that includes periodic evaluation of your entire colon. See your doctor for more information.

II. SYMPTOMS — The presence of rectal bleeding or a change in bowel habits may indicate colon/rectum cancer. See your physician right away if you have either of these symptoms.

III. REDUCING YOUR RISKS AND DETECTING CANCER EARLY — regular tests for hidden blood in the stool and appropriate examinations of the colon will increase the likelihood that colon polyps are discovered and removed early and that cancers are found in an early, curable state. Modifying your diet to include more fiber, cruiferous vegetables, and foods

---

* If your answers to any of these questions change, you should REASSESS YOUR RISK.

** This test has an additional advantage in that it is also an early detection method for cancer of the prostate in men.

rich in Vitamin A; and less fat and salt-cured foods may result in a reduction of cancer risk.

SKIN   Answers

1. The sun's rays are more intense the closer one lives to the equator.
2. Excessive ultraviolet light from the sun causes cancer of the skin.
3. These materials can cause cancer of the skin.
4. Persons with light complexions are at greater risk for skin cancer.
5. A severe sunburn while growing up may increase one's risk for melanoma.
6. A tendency to have pre-cancerous moles or melanomas may occur in certain families.
7. Persons with a previous skin cancer or melanoma are at increased risk for developing a skin cancer or melanoma.
8. Tanning beds use a type of ultraviolet ray which adds to skin damage by the sun, contributing to skin cancer formation.
9. Any change in a mole may be a sign of melanoma.

If you answered "yes" to any of the first nine questions, you need to use protective clothing and use a sun screen with an SPF rating of 15 or greater whenever you are out in the sun and check yourself monthly for any changes in warts or moles. An answer of "yes" to question 10, 11, and 12 can help reduce your risk of skin cancer or possibly detect skin cancer early.

REDUCING YOUR RISKS AND DETECTING CANCER EARLY — Numerical risks for skin cancer are difficult to state. For instance, a person with dark complexion can work longer in the sun and be less likely to develop cancer than a person with a light complexion. Furthermore, a person wearing a long-sleeved shirt and wide-brimmed hat may work in the sun and be at less risk than a person who wears a bathing suit for only a short time. The risk for skin cancer goes up greatly with age.

Melanoma, the most serious type of skin cancer, can be cured when it is detected and treated at a very early stage. Changes in warts or moles are important and should be checked by your doctor.

BREAST   Answers

If your total is:

Under 100 ......Low risk women (and all others). You should practice monthly Breast Self-Examination, have your breasts examined by a doctor as part of a regular cancer-related checkup, and have mammography in accordance with ACS guidelines.

100–199........Moderate risk women. You should practice monthly BSE and have your breasts examined by a doctor as part of a cancer-related checkup, and have periodic mammography in accordance with American Cancer Society guidelines, or more frequently as your physician advises.

200 or higher..High risk. You should practice monthly BSE and have your breasts examined by a doctor, and have mammography more often. See your doctor for the recommended frequency of breast physical examinations and mammography.

DETECTING CANCER EARLY — One in 9 American women will get breast cancer in her lifetime. Being a woman is a risk factor! Most women (75%) who get breast cancer don't have other risk factors. BSE and mammography may diagnose a breast cancer in its earliest stage with a greatly increased chance of cure. When detected at this stage, cure is more likely and breast-saving surgery may be an option.

CERVICAL Answers

1. The numbers represent the relative risks for invasive cancer in different age groups. The highest incidence of invasive cancer is among women over 40 years of age. However, abnormal changes and early noninvasive cancers occur more commonly in the 20s and 30s age groups. These early changes can be found with the Pap test.

2. Puerto Ricans, Blacks, and Mexican Americans have higher rates for cervical cancer.

3. Women who have delivered more children have a higher occurrence.

4. Viral infections of the cervix and vagina are associated with cervical cancer.

5. Women with earlier age at first intercourse and with more sexual partners are at a higher risk.

6. Irregular bleeding may be a sign of uterine cancer.

If your total is:

40–69.............This is a low risk group. Ask your doctor for a Pap test and advice about frequency of subsequent testing.

70–99.............In this moderate risk group, more frequent Pap tests may be required.

100 or more....You are in the high risk group and should have a Pap test (and pelvic exam) as advised by your doctor.

DETECTING CANCER EARLY — Early detection of this cancer by the Pap test has markedly improved the chance of cure. When this cancer is found at an early stage, the cure rate is extremely high and uterus-saving surgery and child-bearing potential may be preserved.

ENDOMETRIAL Answers

1. Endometrial cancer is seen among women in older age groups. Numbers in parentheses by the age groups represent approximate relative rates of endometrial cancer at different ages.

2. Caucasians have a high occurrence.

3. The fewer children one has delivered the greater the risk of endometrial cancer.

4. Women who are overweight are at greater risk.

5. Cancer of the endometrium is associated with diabetes.

6. Cancer of the endometrium may be associated with prolonged continuous estrogen hormone intake which occurs in only a small number of women. You should consult your physician before starting or stopping any estrogen medication. The medical use of estrogen in combination with progesterone does not appear to increase risk and may have other health benefits in this case.

7. Women who do not have cyclic regular menstrual periods are at greater risk. Any bleeding after menopause may be a sign of this cancer.

8. Cancer of the endometrium is associated with high blood pressure.

If your total is:

45-59 ....You are at very low risk for developing endometrial cancer.

60-99 ....Your risks are slightly higher. Report any abnormal bleeding immediately to your doctor. Tissue sampling at menopause is recommended.

100 and over ....Your risks are much greater. See your doctor for tests as appropriate.

DETECTING CANCER EARLY — Once again, early detection is a key to your chance of a cure for this cancer. Regular pelvic examinations may find other female cancers such as cancer of the ovary.

Are You At Risk For Diabetes?

NAME _____ DATE _____

COURSE _____ SECTION _____

Write in the points next to each statement that is true for you. Before each statement that is not true for you place a zero. Then add up your total score.

1. I have been experiencing one or more of the following symptoms regularly:

❋ excessive thirst	Yes 3	_____
❋ frequent urination	Yes 3	_____
❋ extreme fatigue	Yes 1	_____
❋ unexplained weight loss	Yes 3	_____
❋ blurry vision from time to time	Yes 2	_____

2. I am over 30 years old.   Yes 1 _____

3. I am more than 20% overweight.   Yes 2 _____

4. I am a woman who has had more than
    one baby weighing over 9 lbs. at birth   Yes 2 _____

5. I am of American Indian descent.   Yes 1 _____

6. I am of Hispanic or African American descent.   Yes 1 _____

7. I have a parent with diabetes.   Yes 1 _____

8. I have a brother or sister with diabetes.   Yes 2 _____

                                          Total _____

Scoring 3–5 points:
If you scored 3–5 points, you probably are at low risk for diabetes. Don't just forget about it, though, especially if you're 30, overweight, or of African American, Hispanic or American Indian descent.

Scoring over 5 points:
If you scored over 5 points, you may be at high risk for diabetes. You may even have diabetes already.

What to do about it:
See your doctor promptly. Find out if you have diabetes. Even if you don't have diabetes, know the symptoms. If you experience any of them in the future, you should see your doctor immediately.

Note: This test is meant to educate and make you aware of the serious risks of diabetes. Only a medical doctor can determine if you do have diabetes.

Source: American Diabetes Association.

Cardiovascular Diseases

8

Foremost of the noncommunicable diseases are those affecting the heart and the cardiovascular system. More than 900,000 people in the United States die of cardiovascular diseases each year, representing 43.8% of all deaths in the country. The cardiovascular diseases include atherosclerosis, heart attack, angina, stroke, rheumatic fever, and congenital defects. Of these, coronary heart disease (heart attacks and angina) are most common, and stroke is singled out as the third leading cause of death of adults in the United States. Although some of the risk factors for cardiovascular disease are immutable, many more

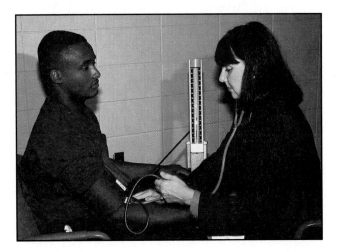

are related to diet, exercise, and other lifestyle habits and thus are preventable.

Figure 8.1 shows the death rates for the major cardiovascular diseases. People over age 40 are most at risk for heart disease, but many deaths occur before that time. According to the National Center for Health Statistics, the death rate from heart disease for African Americans exceeded the Anglo-American rate by 38%, and deaths from strokes was 82% higher for African Americans than Anglo-Americans. Figure 8.2 compares the death rate from cardiovascular disease between African Americans and Anglo-Americans. Comparable figures are not available for other ethnic minorities.

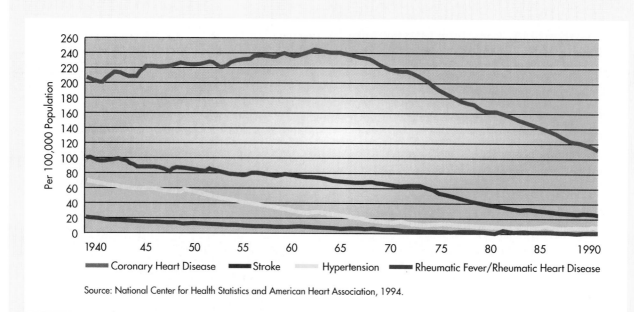

Source: National Center for Health Statistics and American Heart Association, 1994.

Figure 8.1 Age-adjusted U.S. death rates for major cardiovascular diseases

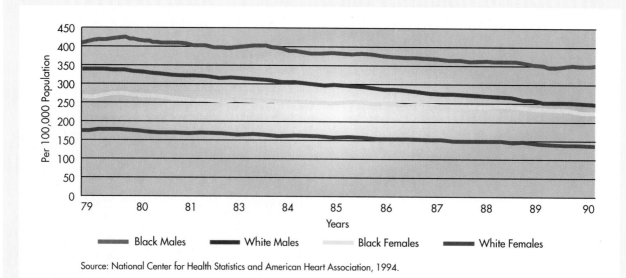

Source: National Center for Health Statistics and American Heart Association, 1994.

Figure 8.2 Age-adjusted U.S. death rates for cardiovascular disease by sex and race

THE CARDIOVASCULAR SYSTEM

The cardiovascular system consists of the heart and two main types of blood vessels — the arteries and the veins. This system is responsible for transporting blood throughout the body. The blood — about 5 or 6 quarts in the average human body — has numerous functions. It carries nutrients, waste products, hormones, and enzymes; regulates body temperature, water levels in the cells, and acidity levels; and helps the body defend against invading pathogens.

As the **arteries** that carry oxygen-rich blood leave the heart, they divide into smaller blood vessels called **arterioles** and then into even smaller vessels called **capillaries**. The capillary walls are so thin that they allow nutrients, oxygen, waste products, hormones, and enzymes to pass through. The **veins** and the smaller **venules** return to the heart the blood that carries waste products and carbon dioxide. This blood is pumped to the lungs, where it dispenses the impurities and picks up fresh oxygen. The entire cycle is repeated about once a minute. Figure 8.3 depicts the circulatory system.

The organ that makes blood circulation possible is the heart, illustrated in Figure 8.4. The heart is a muscular pumping organ situated slightly left of center of the chest and just behind the ribs. Even though the heart is only slightly larger than a fist, it is strong enough to pump 5 quarts per minute, 75 gallons per hour, and 2,000 gallons of blood per day. The heart beats (contracts and expands) approximately 100,000 times a day throughout a person's life. The contraction is called **systole**, and the relaxation between contractions is termed **diastole**.

The heart is bisected lengthwise by a wall called the **septum**, which separates the right side from the left so blood that has returned to the heart for oxygen (pulmonary circulation) will not mix with blood on the left side that has received oxygen and is on its way back to the body to nourish its systems (systemic circulation). The heart has four compartments or chambers. The two upper chambers, or "receivers," are called **atria**, and the two lower chambers, or "pumpers" are the **ventricles**. The right atrium receives blood through the largest vein in the body, the superior and inferior **vena cava**. The left atrium receives blood returning from the

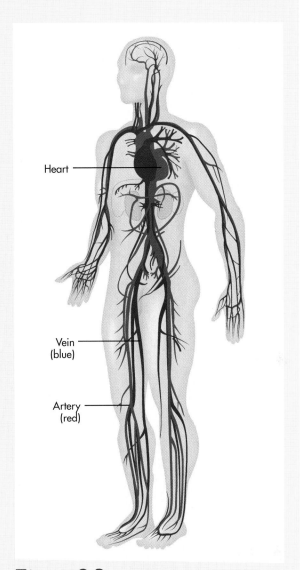

Heart

Vein (blue)

Artery (red)

Figure 8.3 Circulatory system

KEY TERMS

Arteries blood vessels leaving the heart with blood full of oxygen

Arterioles very small arteries

Capillaries extremely small blood vessels with thin walls that allows nutrients and oxygen to pass through

Veins blood vessels that return the blood with carbon dioxide to the heart

Venules very small veins

Systole contraction segment of heartbeat

Diastole relaxation of the heart between beats

Septum wall that bisects the heart lengthwise

Atria the two upper chambers of the heart that receive the blood (atrium is singular)

Ventricles the two lower chambers of the heart that pump the blood

Vena cava largest vein in the body; brings the blood back to the heart for more oxygen

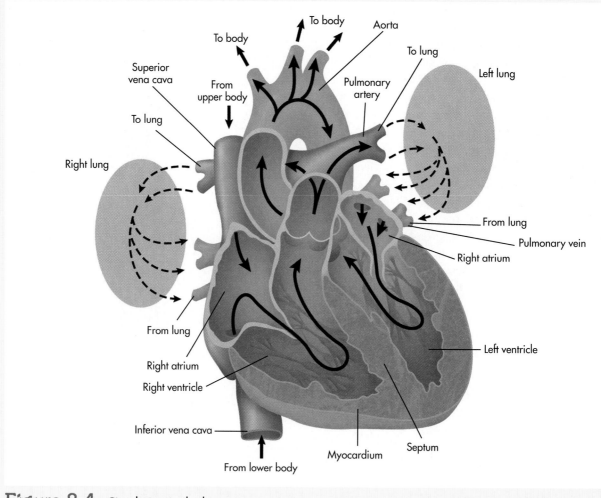

Figure 8.4 Circulation in the heart

lungs with oxygen that soon will be on its way back to the body. The right ventricle pumps blood in need of oxygen to the lungs, and the left ventricle pumps blood rich in oxygen through the **aorta** to arteries that nourish the body systems.

MAJOR RISK FACTORS FOR CARDIOVASCULAR DISEASE

Over the years certain conditions or risk factors for cardiovascular disease (CVD) have been identified. The major predisposing or unchangeable risk factors are:

✴ *Heredity*. You can choose your friends, but you cannot choose your family members. If the reverse were true, selecting parents with no

family history of circulatory problems would be wise. Tendencies toward various CVDs, particularly atherosclerosis and hypertension, run in families.

✴ *Age and sex*. Heart attacks occur across the age spectrum. About half of those who die from heart attacks are men in the 40–65 age group, in the prime of life. Although heart attacks in women have not been studied as extensively, recent statistics are showing that nearly as many women as men die from heart attacks. Heart disease is the number-one killer of men and women alike.

Although African Americans and Hispanics are at greater risk for CVDs than Anglo-Americans, the risk factors may be related more to lifestyle patterns. The major modifiable, behaviorally related risk factors include hypertension, high levels of blood lipids (as related to diet and obesity), cigarette smoking, and lack of exercise. Contributing risk factors also include diabetes and stress. Figure 8.5 shows the interrelationships of the risk factors discussed in the next few pages.

Hypertension

Blood pressure is the force of the blood against the walls of the arteries caused by the heart pumping. The pressure, greatest during the heart's contraction, is known as **systolic blood pressure.** The lower pressure during the heart's relaxation phase is termed the **diastolic blood pressure.**

Blood pressure is measured by an instrument called a **sphygmomanometer**, which displays a column of mercury that rises and falls with the blood pressure. Blood pressure readings are given as two numbers, the top one of which is the systolic pressure and the bottom of which is the diastolic pressure. Because normal blood pressure depends on a variety of factors, it is given in

KEY TERMS

Aorta artery through which oxygen-rich blood is transported from the heart to arteries that nourish the body systems

Systolic blood pressure force in the blood vessel during the heart's contraction

Diastolic blood pressure force in the blood vessel during the heart's relaxation phase

Sphygmomanometer instrument used to measure blood pressure

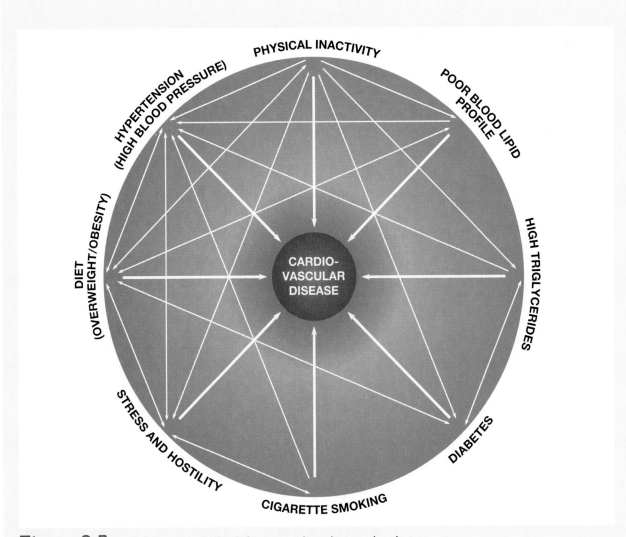

Figure 8.5 Interrelationship of risk factors and cardiovascular disease

ranges. A blood pressure slightly lower or higher than the "textbook" average of 120/80 mm Hg is no cause for alarm. A systolic pressure consistently above 140 and a diastolic pressure consistently above 90 are considered abnormal. Individuals with these readings should see a physician.

High blood pressure is a risk factor for several conditions, among them heart attack and stroke. When the blood pressure is constantly above normal ranges, it increases the workload of the heart, eventually enlarging it. High blood pressure strains the blood vessels, which can become scarred, hardened, and narrower, restricting the needed blood flow. Occasionally clots may form, obstructing the arteries. The American Heart Association estimates that one in four American adults has high blood pressure. African Americans, Puerto Ricans, Cubans, and Hispanics are more likely to have high blood pressure than Anglo Americans.

Unfortunately, hypertension usually has no symptoms or warning signs. The American Heart Association has estimated that about 35% of the people with high blood pressure are not aware of it. This is why hypertension is sometimes called the "silent killer."

Hypertension has no cure, but it can be treated and controlled. A major contributor is stress, discussed in Chapter 3. Home remedies should not be used to treat hypertension. Drinking vinegar, vinegar water, or lemon juice will not lower the blood pressure. High blood pressure has to be treated by a physician who will develop a treatment plan that includes some combination of diet, exercise, and medication. Medications used to lower blood pressure, listed in Table 8.1, are called **antihypertensives**. These are available only by prescription. In addition, people who have high blood pressure should look for ways to lower their stress levels.

Blood Lipids

The American Heart Association has named elevated levels of **blood lipids** or **lipoproteins** as one of the main causes of damage to the blood vessels that can lead to cardiovascular diseases. The culprits are cholesterol and triglycerides. Cholesterol is a soft, fatlike substance manufactured by the liver and needed in small amounts by the body. Unfortunately, most people consume too much additional cholesterol in animal foods such as meat, egg yolks, and dairy products. Foods from plants do not contain cholesterol.

Cholesterol cannot dissolve in blood, just as oil cannot dissolve in water. It is transported throughout the circulatory system by the cholesterol carrier **low density lipoprotein (LDL)**. Some of the circulating cholesterol is used by body tissues to build cells, and some of the cholesterol is returned to the liver. A problem arises if the bloodstream is carrying excess cholesterol. The excess is deposited on the lining of the arteries and contributes to plaque formation and atherosclerosis (discussed later in the chapter). For this reason LDL cholesterol is called the "bad" cholesterol. People with high levels of LDL cholesterol have a greater risk for cardiovascular disease.

Another type of lipoprotein is called **high density lipoprotein (HDL)**. HDL cholesterol picks up other cholesterol circulating in the bloodstream and returns it to the liver for reprocessing or excretion. Because HDL cholesterol clears cholesterol out of the system, it is known as the "good" cholesterol. Individuals with a higher ratio of HDL cholesterol to LDL cholesterol have a lower risk for CVDs. African American men and women have lower HDL levels than Anglo American men and women. This may be related to cultural dietary factors, as the African American diet tends to be higher in saturated fat than the average Anglo diet.

Table 8.1
Medications for Hypertension

Category	Action
Diurectics	Rid the body of excess water and salt
Beta blockers	Reduce heart rate and heart's output of blood
Sympathetic nerve inhibitors	Discourage nerves from constricting blood vessels
Vasodialators	Cause muscles in artery walls to relax and allow artery to widen
ACE inhibitors	Interfere with body's production of angiotensin, which causes arteries to constrict
Calcium channel blockers	Reduce heart rate and relax blood vessels

Facts About Stroke

Stroke killed 144,070 people in the United States in 1991 and is the third largest cause of death, ranking behind diseases of the heart and cancer.

✳ Stroke is the leading cause of serious disability in the United States.

✳ 28% of the people who suffer a stroke in a given year are under age 65.

✳ The incidence of stroke more than doubles in each successive decade over age 55.

✳ The incidence of stroke is about 19% higher for males than for females; for males under age 65, the difference is even greater.

✳ The 1990 death rates for stroke were 27.7% for Anglo American males and 56.1% for African American males; and 23.8% for Anglo American females and 42.8% for African American females.

✳ From 1981 to 1991 the death rate from stroke declined 30.5% overall.

Source: *Heart and Stroke Facts: 1994 Statistical Supplement,* American Heart Association.

4. Ruptured **aneurysm:** A sac formed by distention or dilation of the artery wall breaks open.

A stroke resulting from cerebral embolism or thrombosis usually is related to atherosclerosis and hypertension. A stroke also can occur if an aneurysm bursts as a result of a blow or injury to the head. Ultrasound can be used to help assess the risk for a stroke. Scientists from the Framingham Heart Study discovered that the larger the heart's lower left ventricle is in relation to the person's height, the greater the danger of stroke.

Warning signs and symptoms of a stroke are:

✳ sudden loss of feeling in the face, arm, or leg

☎ Call for information

> National Stroke Association
> 800-787-6537
> 303-771-1887 TTY/TTD

✳ sudden severe headache with no known cause

✳ dizziness, unsteadiness, or sudden falls, especially with any of the other signs

✳ twisting of the mouth to one side or dropping of the bottom lip

✳ temporary blurred, double, or loss of vision (especially in one eye)

✳ temporary loss of speech; difficulty speaking or understanding speech.

Sometimes warning signs last only a few moments and then disappear. These brief episodes, known as **transient ischemic attacks** or **TIAs,** are sometimes called "mini-strokes." They identify an underlying serious condition that is progressive; half of them predate a major stroke by a year or less. Unfortunately, because TIAs do go away temporarily, many people ignore them.

The most common form of TIA is called **transient monocular blindness,** in which a person experiences blurred vision in one eye. A second form is **transient hemispheral attack,** in which the person may have difficulty thinking and communicating and, in addition, numbness or weakness in one arm, one leg, or the face, because of diminished blood flow to one side of the brain.

Preventing stroke requires reducing the risk factors. One of these not discussed thus far is alcohol consumption. More than two drinks a day can raise blood pressure, according to the National Institutes of Health. Many studies have shown that, conversely, cutting back on drinking lowers blood pressure, often within days after becoming a

KEY TERMS

Stroke (cerebrovascular accident) (CVA) disruption of blood flow to the brain, causing destruction of brain cells

Cerebral embolism moving blood clot that partially blocks a blood vessel in the brain

Cerebral thrombus blood clot that gets caught on plaque in a blood vessel in the brain, causing complete blockage of the blood vessel

Cerebral hemorrhage bleeding from a ruptured blood vessel in the brain

Aneurysm sac formed by distention or dilation of an artery wall

Transient ischemic attack (TIA) brief occurrence of stroke symptoms

Transient monocular blindness form of TIA characterized by blurred vision in one eye

Transient hemispheral attack form of TIA in which difficulty thinking and communicating occur along with numbness in one arm, leg, or the face because of less blood flow to one side of the brain

"teetotaler."

Women can cut their risk of stroke in half by increasing their consumption of three common vitamins — betacarotene, vitamin E, and vitamin C — according to a major Harvard study of 87,000 female nurses. Most powerful of these was beta carotene, found in yellow vegetables such as carrots and squash (see Chapter 9).

In addition, some relatively new treatment methods show promise. In one study, funded by the National Institute of Neurological Disorders and Stroke, two drugs that reduce the tendency of the blood to clot — aspirin and warfarin — lowered the risk of stroke 50% to 80% in patients with atrial fibrillation, a type of irregular heartbeat. People with this condition have five times the normal risk for stroke. It is associated with some 70,000 strokes each year in the United States, and about 15% of all patients who have had a stroke have atrial fibrillation.

For people who have already had one stroke or its warning signs and have severe stenosis (narrowed arteries), a surgical procedure called **carotid endarterectomy** has proved beneficial in preventing future strokes. In this procedure fatty deposits are removed from one of the two main arteries in the neck that supply blood to the brain. About 91,000 carotid endarterectomies were performed in the United States in 1992.

KEY TERMS

Carotid endarterectomy removal of fatty deposits from one of the two main arteries in the neck that supply blood to the brain

Summary

1 The cardiovascular system consists of the heart and blood vessels, responsible for pumping oxygen throughout the body.

2 The major risk factors for cardiovascular disease are the predisposing factors of heredity, age, and sex, and more important, variables that can be changed including high blood pressure, physical inactivity, poor blood lipid profile, high triglyceride level, cigarette smoking, diabetes, obesity, and stress and hostility.

3 Coronary heart disease (heart attack and angina) results from an insufficient supply of blood to the arteries of the heart and subsequent lack of oxygen to the heart muscle.

4 Arrhythmias, which result from atherosclerosis, hypertension, or a mineral imbalance in the body, range from imperceptible to life-threatening.

5 Congenital heart defects, the most frequent congenital condition in newborns, are classified as stenoses, septal defects, and cyanotic defects.

6 The four conditions leading to stroke are cerebral embolism, cerebral thrombus, cerebral hemorrhage, and cerebral aneurysm.

Select Bibliography

American Heart Association. *1992 Heart and Stroke Facts*. Dallas: AHA, 1994.

Byron, Peg. "The Most Common Misdiagnoses." *Lear's*, March, 1994.

Dixon, Barbara M. *Good Health for African Americans*. New York: Crown Publishing, 1994.

Good Housekeeping *Family Health and & Medical Guide*. New York: Hearst Books, 1980.

"Good News About Heart Disease." *American Health*, Dec. 1994.

Hoeger, Werner W. K. and Sharon A. Hoeger. *Lifetime Physical Fitness and Wellness*. Englewood, CO: Morton Publishing, 1994.

Huddleston, James. In The *Wellness Book*, edited by Herbert Benson and Eiken Stuart. New York: Birch Lane Press, 1992.

Joint National Committee on Detection, Evaluation, and Treatment of High Blood Pressure. "The 1988 Report of the Joint National Committee on Detection, Evaluation, and Treatment of High Blood Pressure." *Archives of Internal Medicine*, 148: (1988), 1023-1038.

Saunders, Elijah, editor. "Cardiovascular Diseases in Blacks." *Cardiovascular Clinics*, 21:3 (1981).

Wilson, Thomas W., and Clarence E. Grimes. "Biohistory of Slavery and Blood Pressure Differences in Blacks Today: A Hypothesis." *Hypertension*, 17:1, January, 1991. [Supplement]

University of California at Berkley. *Wellness Letter*, Sept. 1994, p. 8.

American Heart Association℠
Fighting Heart Disease and Stroke

RISKO
A Heart Health Appraisal

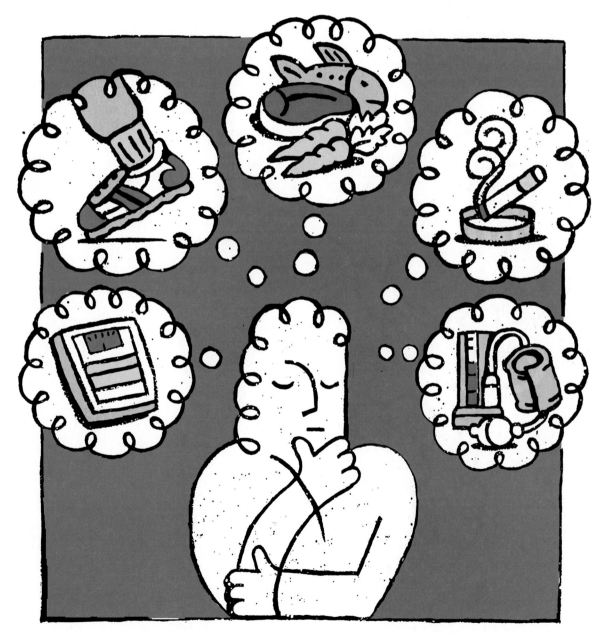

Understanding Heart Disease

Estimates are that almost 500,000 Americans die of coronary heart disease every year. It's the single leading cause of death in the United States – as well as in many other countries.

Scientists have identified certain factors linked with an increased risk of developing coronary heart disease. Some of these factors are unavoidable, like increasing age, being male or having a family history of heart disease. However, many other risk factors can be changed to lower the risk of heart disease. High blood pressure, high blood cholesterol, cigarette smoking and physical inactivity are the four major modifiable risk factors; obesity is a contributing risk factor. Diabetes also strongly influences the risk of heart disease.

This RISKO brochure is a way for you to evaluate your risk of coronary heart disease based upon your risk factors. RISKO scores are based on blood pressure, cholesterol, smoking and weight. Physical inactivity is also an important risk factor but was not part of the statistical base from which RISKO was derived.

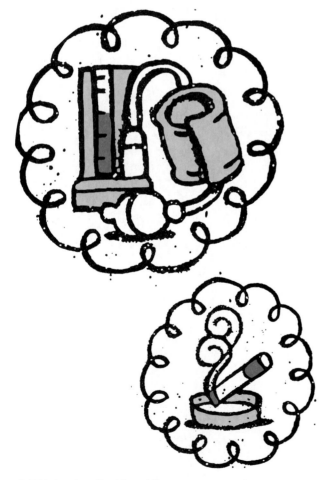

© 1994, American Heart Association

MEN

1. Systolic Blood Pressure

If you **are not** taking anti-hypertensive medications and your blood pressure is...

124 or less	0 points
between 125 and 134	2 points
between 135 and 144	4 points
between 145 and 154	6 points
between 155 and 164	8 points
between 165 and 174	10 points
between 175 and 184	12 points
between 185 and 194	14 points
between 195 and 204	16 points
between 205 and 214	18 points
between 215 and 224	20 points

SCORE

If you **are** taking anti-hypertensive medications and your blood pressure is...

120 or less	0 points
between 121 and 127	2 points
between 128 and 135	4 points
between 136 and 143	6 points
between 144 and 153	8 points
between 154 and 163	10 points
between 164 and 175	12 points
between 176 and 190	14 points
between 191 and 204	16 points
between 205 and 214	18 points
between 215 and 224	20 points

2. Blood Cholesterol

Locate the number of points for your total and HDL cholesterol in the table below.

SCORE

		HDL							
		25	30	35	40	50	60	70	80
TOTAL	140	4	2	0	0	0	0	0	0
	160	5	3	2	0	0	0	0	0
	180	6	4	3	1	0	0	0	0
	200	7	5	4	3	0	0	0	0
	220	7	6	5	4	1	0	0	0
	240	8	7	5	4	2	0	0	0
	260	8	7	6	5	3	1	0	0
	280	9	8	7	6	4	2	0	0
	300	9	8	7	6	4	3	1	0
	340	9	9	8	7	6	4	2	1
	400	10	9	9	8	7	5	4	3

3. Cigarette Smoking

If you...

SCORE

do not smoke	0 points
smoke less than a pack a day	2 points
smoke a pack a day	5 points
smoke two or more packs a day	9 points

4. Weight

Locate your weight category in the table below. If you are in...

weight category A	0 points
weight category B	1 point
weight category C	2 points

SCORE

FT	IN	A	B	C
5	1	up to 162	163-250	251+
5	2	up to 167	168-257	258+
5	3	up to 172	173-264	265+
5	4	up to 176	177-272	273+
5	5	up to 181	182-279	280+
5	6	up to 185	186-286	287+
5	7	up to 190	191-293	294+
5	8	up to 195	196-300	301+
5	9	up to 199	200-307	308+
5	10	up to 204	205-315	316+
5	11	up to 209	210-322	323+
6	0	up to 213	214-329	330+
6	1	up to 218	219-336	337+
6	2	up to 223	224-343	344+
6	3	up to 227	228-350	351+
6	4	up to 232	233-368	359+
6	5	up to 238	239-365	366+
6	6	up to 241	242-372	373+

TOTAL SCORE

WOMEN

1. Systolic Blood Pressure

If you **are not** taking anti-hypertensive medications and your blood pressure is...

125 or less	0 points
between 126 and 136	2 points
between 137 and 148	4 points
between 149 and 160	6 points
between 161 and 171	8 points
between 172 and 183	10 points
between 184 and 194	12 points
between 195 and 206	14 points
between 207 and 218	16 points

If you **are** taking anti-hypertensive medications and your blood pressure is...

117 or less	0 points
between 118 and 123	2 points
between 124 and 129	4 points
between 130 and 136	6 points
between 137 and 144	8 points
between 145 and 154	10 points
between 155 and 168	12 points
between 169 and 206	14 points
between 207 and 218	16 points

SCORE

2. Blood Cholesterol

Locate the number of points for your total and HDL cholesterol in the table below.

TOTAL	HDL							
	25	30	35	40	50	60	70	80
140	2	1	0	0	0	0	0	0
160	3	2	1	0	0	0	0	0
180	4	3	2	1	0	0	0	0
200	4	3	2	2	0	0	0	0
220	5	4	3	2	1	0	0	0
240	5	4	3	3	1	0	0	0
260	5	4	4	3	2	1	0	0
280	5	5	4	4	2	1	0	0
300	6	5	4	4	3	2	1	0
340	6	5	5	4	3	2	1	0
400	6	6	5	5	4	3	2	2

SCORE

3. Cigarette Smoking

If you...

do not smoke	0 points
smoke less than a pack a day	2 points
smoke a pack a day	5 points
smoke two or more packs a day	9 points

SCORE

4. Weight

Locate your weight category in the table below. If you are in...

weight category A	0 points
weight category B	1 point
weight category C	2 points
weight category D	3 points

SCORE

FT	IN	A	B	C	D
4	8	up to 139	140-161	162-184	185+
4	9	up to 140	141-162	163-185	186+
4	10	up to 141	142-163	164-187	188+
4	11	up to 143	144-166	167-190	191+
5	0	up to 145	146-168	169-193	194+
5	1	up to 147	148-171	172-196	197+
5	2	up to 149	150-173	174-198	199+
5	3	up to 152	153-176	177-201	202+
5	4	up to 154	155-178	179-204	205+
5	5	up to 157	158-182	183-209	210+
5	6	up to 160	161-186	187-213	214+
5	7	up to 165	166-191	192-219	220+
5	8	up to 169	170-196	197-225	226+
5	9	up to 173	174-201	202-231	232+
5	10	up to 178	179-206	207-238	239+
5	11	up to 182	183-212	213-242	243+
6	0	up to 187	188-217	218-248	249+
6	1	up to 191	192-222	223-254	255+

TOTAL SCORE

What Your Score Means

Note: If you're diabetic, you have a greater risk of heart disease. Add 7 points to your total score.

0-2 You have a low risk of heart disease for a person of your age and sex.

3-4 You have a low-to-moderate risk of heart disease for a person of your age and sex. That's good, but there's room for improvement.

5-7 You have a moderate-to-high risk of heart disease for a person of your age and sex. There's considerable room for improvement in some areas.

8-15 You have a high risk of developing heart disease for a person of your age and sex. There's lots of room for improvement in all areas.

16 & Over You have a very high risk of developing heart disease for a person of your age and sex. You should act now to reduce all your risk factors.

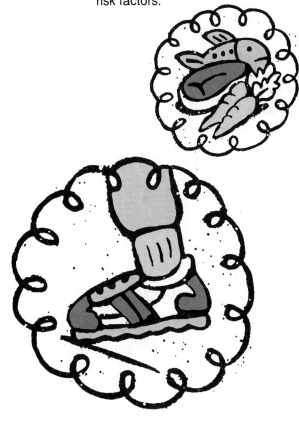

Some Words of Caution

- RISKO is a way for adults who don't have signs of heart disease now to measure their risk. If you already have heart disease, it's very important to work with your doctor to reduce your risk.

- RISKO is not a substitute for a thorough physical examination and assessment by your doctor. It's intended to help you learn more about the factors that influence the risk of heart disease, and thus to reduce your risk.

- If you have a family history of heart disease, your risk of heart disease will be higher than your RISKO score shows. If you have a high RISKO score and a family history of heart disease, taking action now to reduce your risk is even more important.

- If you're a woman under 45 years old or a man under 35 years old, your real risk of heart disease is probably lower than your RISKO score.

- If you're overweight, have high blood pressure or high blood cholesterol, or smoke cigarettes, your long-term risk of heart disease is higher even if your risk of heart disease in the next several years is low. To reduce your risk, you should eliminate or control these risk factors.

How To Reduce Your Risk

- **Quit smoking for good.** Many programs are available to help.

- **Have your blood pressure checked regularly.** If your blood pressure is less than 130/85 mmHg, have it rechecked in two years. If it's between 130-139/85-89, have it rechecked in a year. If your blood pressure is 140/90 or higher, you have high blood pressure and should follow your doctor's advice. If blood pressure medication is prescribed for you, remember to take it.

- **Stay physically active.** Physical inactivity, besides being a risk factor for heart disease, contributes to other risk factors including obesity, high blood pressure and a low level of HDL cholesterol. To condition your heart, try to get 30-60 minutes of exercise 3-4 times a week.
  Activities that are especially beneficial when performed regularly include:
  - brisk walking, hiking, stair-climbing, aerobic exercise and calisthenics;
  - jogging, running, bicycling, rowing and swimming;
  - tennis, racquetball, soccer, basketball and touch football.

  Even low-intensity activities, when performed daily, can have some long-term health benefits. Such activities include:
  - walking for pleasure, gardening and yard work;
  - housework, dancing and prescribed home exercise.

- **Lose weight if necessary.** For many people, losing weight is one of the most effective ways to improve their blood pressure and cholesterol levels.

- **Reduce high blood cholesterol through your diet.** If you're overweight or eat lots of foods high in saturated fats and cholesterol (whole milk, cheese, eggs, butter, fatty foods, fried foods), then make changes in your diet. Look for *The American Heart Association Cookbook* at your local bookstore; it can help you.

- **Visit or write your local American Heart Association for more information and copies of free pamphlets.**
  Some subjects covered include:
  Reducing your risk of heart attack and stroke.
  Controlling high blood pressure.
  Eating to keep your heart healthy.
  How to stop smoking.
  Exercising for good health.

Your contributions to the American Heart Association will support research that helps make publications like this possible.

For more information, contact your local American Heart Association or call 1-800-AHA-USA1 (1-800-242-8721).

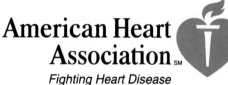

American Heart Association℠
Fighting Heart Disease and Stroke

National Center
7272 Greenville Avenue
Dallas, Texas 75231

Reproduced by permission.
© American Heart Association, 1994.

The Basics of Nutrition

9

*A*mericans are living on the fast-track. Our bodies are examples not only of what we eat but also of what we do not eat. During our lifetime we will spend approximately 6 years eating about 60 tons of food prepared in 70,000 meals, with only 100 foods accounting for 75% of the total amount of food we consume. About a fourth of all Americans eat dinner at fast-food restaurants each day. Fast-food restaurants serve approximately 200 hamburgers every second.

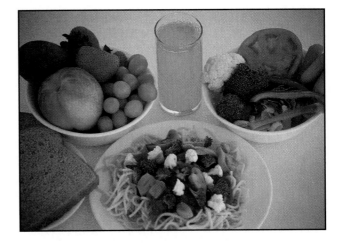

While millions of people are dying each year of starvation throughout the world, many Americans are dying as an indirect result of an overabundance of food. In addition to overeating, the diet of most Americans is not balanced. The American diet is too high in calories, sugar, sodium, fats, cholesterol, and alcohol. The *Healthy People 2000* report highlights some of the most important dietary changes that Americans can make to safeguard their health and well-being, including reducing the consumption of fat and sodium, increasing the consumption of complex carbohydrates (starch) and dietary fiber, and consuming adequate amounts of iron and calcium, among others.

Among the many diseases related to poor nutritional habits are coronary heart disease, stroke, cancers, atherosclerosis, and adult-onset diabetes. Consuming the proper nutrients over time is essential to prevent disease and improve health and well-being.

NUTRITION AND NUTRIENTS

Nutrition is the sum of all the interactions between an organism and the food it consumes. **Nutrients** are chemical substances or nourishing elements found in food. Foods contain approximately 50 nutrients that the body is unable to make. These are used for three essential purposes:

1. To provide energy.

2. To form body structures (growth and repair of body tissues).

3. To help regulate the body's biochemical reactions, collectively called metabolism.

The nutrients are grouped into six main categories: carbohydrates, fats, proteins, vitamins, minerals, and water. The first three are sources the body uses to supply energy, and the latter three regulate body processes; they have no caloric value. Energy is measured in **kilocalories** (kcal), commonly referred to simply as calories. A **calorie** is the amount of energy required to raise the temperature of 1 gram of water 1°C.

The **energy value** of a food is computed by multiplying the number of grams of each energy nutrient in a serving of food by the caloric values per gram of carbohydrate, protein, and fat, as follows: For example, if a food has 10 grams of carbohydrates, 5 grams of protein, and 4 grams of fat, the caloric value is calculated as follows:

	Total grams	× kcal		
Carbohydrate	10	× 4	=	40
Protein	5	× 4	=	20
Fat	4	× 9	=	36
		Total	=	96 calories

Figure 9.1 graphically depicts the caloric value of major energy foods. Alcohol is not a nutrient because the body cannot use it to promote growth, for maintenance, or for repair. Even though serves as an energy source, it is high in calories. Therefore, alcohol often is said to contain "empty calories." Chapter 12 presents additional information on alcohol.

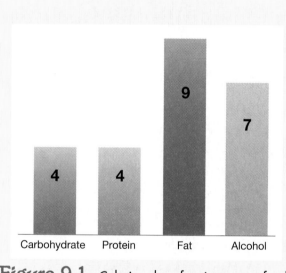

Figure 9.1 Caloric value of major energy foods

The process of converting nutrients into body tissue and functions is known as **metabolism,** The number of calories needed per day depends on the body's **metabolic rate** (MR), the total amount of energy the body expends in a given time. Metabolic rate depends upon the person's age, sex, size, muscle mass, climate, emotional state, glandular function, and exercise level. The **basal metabolic rate** (BMR) is the number of calories used while resting. MR is a combination of BMR and calories expended in normal daily activities. These concepts are expanded in Chapter 10.

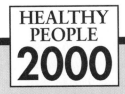

HEALTHY PEOPLE 2000

OBJECTIVES FOR NUTRITIONAL IMPROVEMENTS

❋ Reduce dietary fat intake to an average of 30% of calories or less and average saturated fat intake to less than 10% of calories among people aged 2 and older.

❋ Increase complex carbohydrate and fiber-containing foods in adult diet to five or more daily servings for vegetables (including legumes) and fruits, and to six or more daily servings for grain products.

❋ Decrease salt and sodium intake.

THE PROCESS OF DIGESTION

What happens to the food and nutrients the food contains when you eat? **Digestion** is the process of breaking down food and drink into substances the body can easily absorb. Food not broken down is passed as waste out of the body. Several body organs contribute to the digestive process by breaking down food substances chemically or mechanically into small molecules that can be absorbed into body cells.

The digestive system is illustrated in Chapter 7. Assimilation and breakdown of food take place within the **digestive tract**, a winding channel totaling more than 30 feet in length. Muscles along this tract propel the food forward, and the mucous lining of the tract lubricates it and prevents irritation.

Food first enters the digestive tract through the mouth, where the tongue, teeth, and saliva work together to break down the food initially so it can enter the throat and **esophagus**, the tube that carries the food to the **stomach**. There, acids and enzymes further break down the food into a thick liquid, which enters the small intestine.

In the first 10" of the small intestine, the **duodenum**, digestive juices from the liver and pancreas continue to break down the food into nutrients that comprise it. The multifaceted **liver** (a) produces bile, which is necessary for absorption of fat, (b) removes some of the wastes from the blood, (c) produces and stores glucose (a form of sugar), and (d) produces many substances needed by the body. The **gallbladder** performs an indirect digestive function by storing the bile manufactured by the liver and releasing it into the small intestine as needed. The gallbladder is not an essential organ; if it is removed surgically, the liver can take over its role.

Other digestive juices needed to digest and absorb food come from the **pancreas**. The pancreas

KEY TERMS

Nutrition the sum of all the interactions between an organism and the food it consumes

Nutrients chemical substances or nourishing elements found in food

Kilocalorie the amount of energy required to raise the temperature of 1 gram of water 1°C

Calorie a term meaning the same as kilocalorie

Energy value the result of multiplying the number of grams of each energy nutrient in a serving of food by the caloric values per gram of carbohydrate, protein, and fat

Metabolism process of converting nutrients into body tissue and functions

Metabolic rate (MR) total amount of energy the body expends in a given amount of time

Basal metabolic rate (BMR) amount of energy (calories) a person uses when totally inactive

Digestion process of breaking down food and drink into substances the body can absorb

Digestive tract 30-foot long channel where breakdown and assimilation of food and drink take place in the body

Esophagus the tube that carries the food to the stomach

Stomach the organ containing acids and enzymes that break down food

Duodenum the first 10 inches of the small intestine

Liver digestive organ that produces bile, removes some waste from the body, produces and stores glucose

Gallbladder stores bile and releases it into the small intestine as needed

Pancreas digestive organ that secretes insulin and other digestive juices

also secretes hormones. Among these is insulin, responsible for the body's utilization of glucose. In the remaining portions of the small intestine (the jejunum and the ileum), the digested food is absorbed into the bloodstream.

Solid substances that are not assimilated into bloodstream through the small intestine move on to the large intestine, or **colon**. There wastes are processed into feces. The feces leave the body through the rectum and out of the anus.

THE ENERGY NUTRIENTS

Carbohydrates

The basic body fuel is **carbohydrates**. The body receives approximately 90% of its energy from metabolism of carbohydrates. Carbohydrates are compounds composed of carbon, hydrogen, and oxygen. They can be categorized as either simple carbohydrates (simple sugars) or complex carbohydrates (starches).

Simple carbohydrates are sugars found naturally in foods such as fruit, vegetables (peas and beets), and milk. Words that end in "ose" (glucose, fructose, galactose, sucrose, maltose, dextrose) designate simple carbohydrates. Refined and processed sugars, including corn syrup and sorghum, are also simple carbohydrates. Foods containing simple sugars include cakes, candy, jellies, rolls, and colas. Simple sugars have little or no nutritional value and often are called "empty calories." A diet in which too many simple carbohydrates are consumed can contribute to dental cavities, obesity, and health conditions such as diabetes, hyperglycemia, hypoglycemia, and heart disease.

Foods containing **complex carbohydrates**, or **starches**, are rich in protein and nonenergy nutrients (vitamins, minerals), and lower in calories and fat and higher in dietary fiber. The best sources of complex carbohydrates are fruits, vegetables, peanuts, potatoes, and legumes such as beans, black-eyed peas, and kidney beans.

Dietary fiber or "roughage" is found in the walls of plant cells and in the tough structural part of plants. It is a non-nutrient complex carbohydrate. High-fiber foods (indigestible leaves, stems, seeds, hulls, and skins of grains and plants) are high in B vitamins, iron, and protein. These foods include whole-grain and enriched breads and cereals, needed to keep the digestive system in order.

Fiber may be soluble or insoluble. **Soluble** fibers dissolve in water and are digested in the large intestine. These fibers (pectin, some hemicellulose, and gums) help lower blood cholesterol level. They stay in the stomach longer (give a sense of fullness), slow the absorption of sugars from the small intestine, and may assist in controlling blood sugar levels. Soluble fiber is present in wheat bran, dried beans, barley, oats, oat bran, corn bran, fruits such as citrus, apples, prunes, pears, oranges, and many vegetables. Whole-grain breads are excellent sources of fiber, opposed to breads made with white or refined wheat flour in which the fiber-rich bran may have been removed mechanically. Food

Boosting the Fiber Content of Your Diet

If your diet is low in fiber:

* Substitute brown rice for white rice.

* Substitute whole wheat products for white-wheat products.

* Add brown rice, millet, bulgur, or barley to soups, stews, and casseroles.

* Cook with recipes that include bran and other good sources of fiber.

* Don't overcook vegetables. Steaming and stir-frying are two methods that prevent the breakdown of fiber.

* Sprinkle wheat germ or bran on applesauce, pudding, yogurt, cottage cheese, custard, ice cream.

* Whenever you can, eat unpeeled fresh fruits and vegetables (scrubbed well).

* Choose high-fiber snacks (popcorn, fruits, raw vegetables).

* Read labels. Look for whole-grain breads, macaroni, egg noodles, and cereals.

* When buying bread, look for "stone-ground wheat" or "whole wheat" as the first ingredient. Other breads usually are made from refined flour (with the bran removed) that has been colored brown.

From *Wellness: Guidelines for a Healthy Lifestyle* by Werner W. K. Hoeger and Brent Q. Hafen (Englewood, CO: Morton, 1994), p. 183.

labels list the fiber content in breads.

Insoluble fibers, those that cannot be dissolved in water, speed the passage of food through the digestive tract. This may inhibit the action of cancer-causing agents in the colon and thus reduce the risk of colon cancer. Insoluble fiber increases bulk in the feces, preventing constipation, hemorrhoids, obesity, and diverticulosis (formation of pouches in the intestine). Excellent sources of insoluble fibers are leafy greens, wheat, rice, corn bran (outer layer), seeds of fruits (such as strawberries), skins of fruits, and root vegetables.

The National Cancer Institute recommends about 20 to 35 grams of fiber per day, the equivalent of five or six servings of high-fiber foods such as whole-grain cereals and fruits. Fiber intake should be distributed throughout the day to avoid intestinal gas, cramps, diarrhea, and bloating (from fermentation of fiber and sugars in the colon).

Dietary Fat

The average American eats a greater amount of fat than is considered healthy. The diet of African Americans is even higher in fat than the average American diet. Diets that are high in fat can lead to diabetes, heart disease, high blood pressure, stroke,

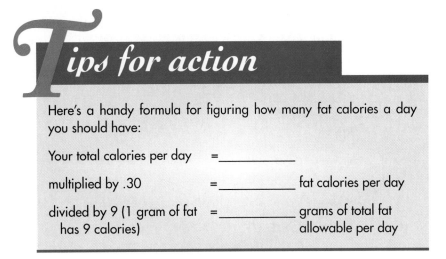

Tips for action

Here's a handy formula for figuring how many fat calories a day you should have:

Your total calories per day = _____

multiplied by .30 = _____ fat calories per day

divided by 9 (1 gram of fat = _____ grams of total fat
has 9 calories) allowable per day

and cancers of the colon, uterus, breast, and prostate. Fats, or **lipids**, however, do serve significant purposes in the body.

1. They provide insulation against the cold.
2. They suppress hunger pangs.
3. They protect vital organs against injury.
4. They transport four fat-soluble vitamins (A, D, E, K) in the body.
5. They contribute to growth.
6. They regulate hormones.
7. They are essential for healthy skin.

In addition, fat supplies 9 calories of energy per gram, and it is a concentrated source of energy when carbohydrate supplies are insufficient, such as during prolonged exercise.

Too Much Fat in Children's Lives

Two-thirds of U.S. children fail the Children's Health Index, a measure of good health and safety, according to *Prevention* magazine data released in September, 1994. About 31% of children ages 3 to 17 are overweight, an increase of 29% since 1984. The Health Index is based on a telephone survey of 424 parents by Princeton Survey Associates.

Only 50% of the parents surveyed try to limit fat in their children's menus, down from 64% in 1991. Competing information on what's best to eat might be overwhelming parents. *Prevention's* Tom Dybdahl wrote, "Lot's of people are feeling, 'I might as well eat what I want.'"

KEY TERMS

Colon large intestine where wastes are processed
Carbohydrates compounds composed of carbon, hydrogen, and oxygen used by the body to create 90% of its energy
Simple carbohydrates sugars found naturally in foods; contribute no nutritional value
Complex carbohydrates (starches) important source of energy for the body found in fruits, vegetables, and legumes
Dietary fiber (roughage) non-nutrient complex carbohydrate needed to keep the digestive system in order
Soluble dissolvable in water
Insoluble not dissolvable in water
Lipids blood fats

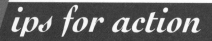

Tips for action

To cut fat from your diet:

❋ Eat less fried food.

❋ Go easy on adding fats, such as butter or margarine on toast and mayonnaise on sandwiches.

❋ Drink fortified skim milk, and choose dairy products (such as cheeses) made from skim or low-fat milk.

❋ Eat meatless main dishes at least several times a week.

❋ Eat more fish; bake, broil, or stew it.

❋ Eat no more than 4 to 6 ounces of lean meat, poultry, and fish a day and no more than 1 to 3 teaspoons of oils/fats daily.

❋ Avoid fatty meats, such as corned beef, sausage, hotdogs, luncheon meats, spareribs, regular ground beef, and heavily marbled meat.

❋ Eat red meat only a few times a week. Choose lean cuts, such as round, rump, or flank. Trim all visible fat before you cook, and cook the meat so the fat can drain away from it.

❋ Use meat for flavoring, as in chili, rather than as a main dish.

❋ Remove skin from chicken and turkey before you cook it.

❋ Cook stews, soups, and gravies a day ahead; refrigerate and lift off congealed fat.

❋ Bake, broil, roast, steam, stir-fry, or stew foods instead of frying them.

❋ Eat no more than four egg yolks a week, including the ones you use in cooking.

❋ Eat in moderation. Know when to stop.

❋ Learn to read food labels. Fat grams are listed on most food labels.

Dietary fats are either saturated (solid at room temperature) or unsaturated (liquid at room temperature). **Saturated fats** usually are found in animal products including lard, butter, cheese, milk, pork, beef, bacon, veal, lamb, poultry skin, hotdogs, luncheon meats, non-dairy cream substitutes, chocolate, and cocoa. Exceptions to the "solid" rule are coconut oil, palm oil, and palm kernel oil (tropical oils), which are liquid at room temperature. Saturated fats increase the levels of blood cholesterol.

Unsaturated fats include monounsaturated fats and polyunsaturated fats. **Monounsaturated fats** are found in foods such as olives, peanuts, and cashews, as well as canola oil, peanut oil, and olive oil. **Polyunsaturated fats** are found in mayonnaise, margarine, pecans, almonds, walnuts, sunflower oil, soybean oil, sesame oil, safflower oil, and corn oil, among others. Table 9.1 lists examples of each of the types of fat.

Cholesterol (Sterols)

To understand the role of fats in the body, we have to understand their relationship to cholesterol. **Cholesterol** is a yellow, waxy, fatlike substance (steroid alcohol) produced by the liver and found in the cells of humans and animals. The human body produces 800 to 1500 milligrams of cholesterol each day. It has several functions.

1. It is required for metabolism and production of certain hormones, including sex hormones (estrogen, progesterone, and androgen).

2. It aids in digestion.

3. It helps produce vitamin D, a major component of cell membranes.

4. It protects the nerve fibers.

Cholesterol is present only in animal products such as egg yolks, cheese, milk, dairy products, and meat. It is found primarily in the liver, kidneys,

Table 9.1
Types of Fats and Examples

Saturated Fats		Monounsaturated Fats	Polyunsaturated Fats
Bacon	Meat	Canola oil	Corn oil
Butter	Milk, whole	Cashews	Cottonseed oil
Cheese	Palm kernel oil	Olive oil	Fish
Chocolate	Palm oil	Peanut oil	Nuts (most varieties)
Coconut oil	Poultry		Safflower oil
Cream cheese	Shortening		Soybean oil
Egg yolk	Sour cream		Sunflower oil
Hydrogenated (hard) Fats			Margarine, tub
Lard			Mayonnaise
			Unhydrogenated peanut butter

Tips for action

To raise HDL ("good" cholesterol) levels:

❋ Exercise, especially aerobic exercise (5 times per week; 45–60 minute sessions).

❋ Maintain proper body weight or lose weight.

❋ If you smoke, quit smoking.

❋ Do not take anabolic steroids.

❋ Substitute monounsaturated oils for saturated fat in your diet, and do not exceed 30% of all calories from fat.

❋ Eat foods rich in betacarotene ("yellow" foods).

❋ Take cholesterol medications if prescribed by your physician.

spinal cord, adrenal glands, and brain. The liver manufactures about 80% of total cholesterol found in the blood and tissues; dietary sources furnish the other 20%.

Figure 9.2 depicts the movement of cholesterol throughout the body. Fats first must be combined with protein. In this form cholesterol is a **lipoprotein**. The three types of lipoprotein involved in transporting protein in the body are low density lipoprotein (LDL), very low density lipoprotein (VLDL), and high density lipoprotein cholesterol (HDL). The **LDL** or "bad cholesterol" molecule contains large amounts of

KEY TERMS

Saturated fats fats found in animal product; increase levels of blood fat cholesterol

Monounsaturated fats fats with only one double bond of unsaturated carbons in carbon atom chain

Polyunsaturated fats fats that contain two or more double bonds between unsaturated fats along the carbon atom chain

Cholesterol yellow, waxy substance produced by the liver and found in animal products; used by the body for metabolism and production of certain hormones

Lipoprotein form of cholesterol combined with protein when transported through the body

LDL "Bad cholesterol" molecule containing large amounts of cholesterol

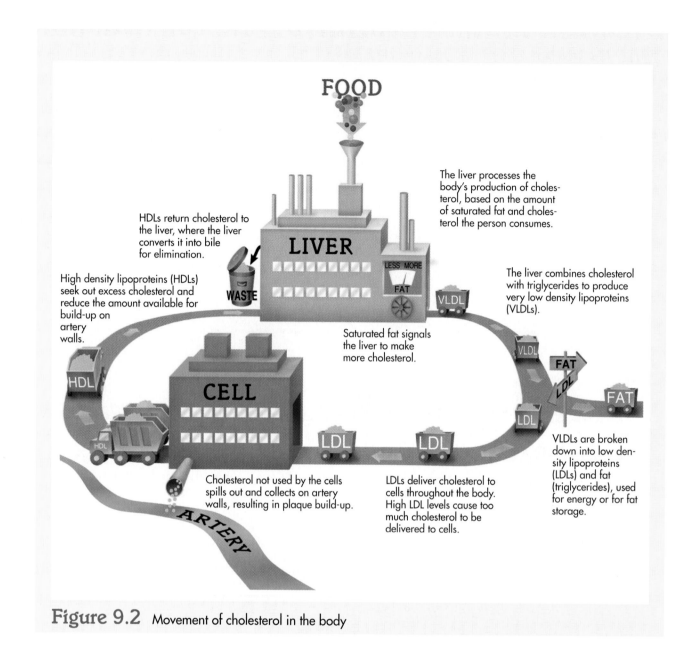

Figure 9.2 Movement of cholesterol in the body

The following labels appear within the figure:

FOOD

LIVER

The liver processes the body's production of cholesterol, based on the amount of saturated fat and cholesterol the person consumes.

HDLs return cholesterol to the liver, where the liver converts it into bile for elimination.

WASTE

LESS MORE

FAT

The liver combines cholesterol with triglycerides to produce very low density lipoproteins (VLDLs).

High density lipoproteins (HDLs) seek out excess cholesterol and reduce the amount available for build-up on artery walls.

VLDL

VLDL

FAT

LDL

FAT

HDL

CELL

Saturated fat signals the liver to make more cholesterol.

HDL

LDL

LDL

LDL

VLDLs are broken down into low density lipoproteins (LDLs) and fat (triglycerides), used for energy or for fat storage.

Cholesterol not used by the cells spills out and collects on artery walls, resulting in plaque build-up.

LDLs deliver cholesterol to cells throughout the body. High LDL levels cause too much cholesterol to be delivered to cells.

ARTERY

cholesterol and transports two-thirds of the cholesterol in the blood. The **HDL** or "good cholesterol" molecule has a high concentration of protein. These molecules remove other cholesterol from the walls of the arteries and transport it to the liver, where it is processed and excreted. In addition, **VLDL**, largest of the lipoproteins, allows cholesterol to circulate in the bloodstream.

Most research indicates that HDL-cholesterol is determined by heredity and decreases with age. Women tend to have higher levels than men, and most African Americans have higher levels than Anglo-Americans. Low levels of HDL cholesterol may be the best predictor of coronary heart disease, more significant than the total cholesterol values. Because HDL cholesterol rids the body of cholesterol, a high HDL cholesterol level is desirable.

LDL cholesterol contains about 45% cholesterol and carries the cholesterol in the blood for use by the cells. Some of it becomes deposited on the arterial walls. Limiting the saturated fat content of foods helps reduce the production of cholesterol in the body. To see a significant effect in lowering LDL cholesterol, total fat consumption should be lower than 30% of total daily caloric intake guidelines (see discussion on cholesterol testing later in the chapter).

Butter Versus Margarine

The process of hydrogenation produces transfatty acids (TFAs) in margarine. Butter, on the other hand, contains saturated fats. Both are bad, but which is worse? The controversy of butter versus margarine arose in the summer of 1994 with a statement by Dr. Walter Willett and Dr. Alberto Ascherio of the Harvard School of Public Health that TFAs (in margarine) could be responsible for 30,000 deaths from heart disease each year in the United States. Here's the response:

✳ Dr. Margo Denhe, American Heart Association Nutrition Committee:

"[TFAs] are not worse than saturates [such as butter]. And they're still better than coconut oil..."

✳ Dr. Neil Stone, Northwestern University School of Medicine:

"Thanks to Dr. Willett's group, there is concern about transfatty acids. But it won't be clear what the public messages should be until more studies are done."

✳ Dr. Ed Blonz, author, *The Really Simple No Nonsense Nutrition Guide* (Coneri Press, 1993):

"With the small amount of butter I use, I don't worry about it. Let's face it — butter has flavor."

✳ Jeanne Jones, nationally syndicated columnist on low-fat cooking:

"I usually avoid butter and use margarine only in tub form because of the TFAs."

✳ Mindy Herman, American Dietetic Association:

"If Americans follow the Food Guide Pyramid and use fats sparingly, transfatty acids will fall into line."

Triglycerides

Phospholipids and sterols make up 5% of the fats in the diet. **Triglycerides**, the most common fatty substance in the blood, comprise 95% of our dietary fat intake. These fatty acids are carried in the bloodstream primarily by VLDLs and chylomicrons and cannot travel in the bloodstream without the phospholipids. Combined with cholesterol, triglycerides speed formation of plaque in the arteries (Figure 9.3). Triglycerides should be less than 125 milligrams per deciliter (mg/dl) of blood, and less than 100 mg/dl is ideal. As triglyceride levels increase, HDL cholesterol levels decrease.

Triglycerides are found in foods including luncheon meats, shellfish, and poultry skin, and are manufactured mainly in the liver, from refined sugars, starches, and alcohol. Diets high in sugars and alcohol raise triglyceride levels. Aerobic exercise, weight loss, and reducing consumption of foods can lower the triglyceride level.

Research has shown that **omega-3 oils** reduce triglycerides but do not alter cholesterol. Eskimos have traditional diet consisting of 40% fat, but they have a low rate of heart disease. This may be attributable to a diet replete with fish.

Omega-3 oils are found in foods such as sardines, salmon, tuna, herring, and mackerel. Studies indicate that fish-oil capsules are not as effective as eating fish once a week and can be dangerous if too many capsules are consumed.

Monounsaturated fats tend to lower LDL cholesterol levels and may lower blood pressure and the blood sugar level as well. Polyunsaturated fats lower HDL cholesterol in the bloodstream. Some mono- and polyunsaturated fats are **hydrogenated**. Hydrogen is added to increase shelf life and make the product more spreadable. This process also increases the saturation, and the resulting **transfatty acids (TFAs)** may increase the risk of heart disease and cancer. Therefore hydrogenated fat may be as dangerous as saturated fat. Stick margarine is more hydrogenated and contains more transfatty acids than tub margarine.

KEY TERMS

HDL "Good cholesterol" molecule containing high concentration of protein

VLDL largest of the lipoproteins; allows cholesterol to circulate in blood stream

Hydrogenated hydrogen added to fats to increase shelf life and make the product more spreadable; increases saturation of the fat

Transfatty acids (TFAs) product of hydrogenation; may increase risk of heart disease and cancer

Triglycerides the most common fatty substance in the blood

Omega-3 oils oils found in fish

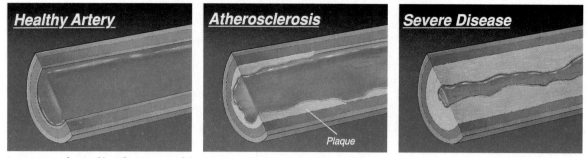

THE ATHEROSCLEROTIC PROCESS

Healthy Artery   **Atherosclerosis**   **Severe Disease**

Plaque

From *Heart of a Healthy Life*. Courtesy of the American Heart Association, © 1992.

Figure 9.3 The atherosclerotic process

Four Great Reasons to Eat Fish

✳ *Heart Attack*: Eating only 7 ounces of fish a week (a regular-sized can of tuna) can cut your risk of heart attack in half.

✳ *Stroke*: Blood clots cause 80% of strokes. Eating oily fish may act as a mild anticoagulant to thwart the formation of dangerous clots.

✳ *Arthritis*: Fish oil, an anti-inflammatory, can help relieve the pain, swelling, and stiffness of rheumatoid arthritis. It will not cure arthritis, though.

✳ *Cancer*: Fish eaters are less likely than non-fish eaters to die of cancer. The Japanese eat three times more fish than Americans eat, and their rate of breast cancer is five times lower. By the way — life expectancy in Japan is the world's highest: 83 years for women and 76 for men — compared with the USA's 79 years for women and 72 years for men.

All of this assumes, of course, that the fish is not fried, smothered in cheese or cream, or covered with tarter sauce. The best ways to eat seafood are baked, broiled, blackened, grilled, or steamed. Flounder, cod, haddock, sole, shrimp, scallops, crabs, and clams are the best choices because of their low fat and high vitamin and mineral content.

Source: "Eat Smart" column by Jean Carper, *USA Weekend*, August 19-21, 1994; Center for Science in the Public Interest.

Cholesterol Testing

After a person has an initial normal baseline test, a blood lipid analysis should be done every 3–4 years prior to age 35 and every year after age 35 in conjunction with a regular medical physical examination. Your cholesterol level is not affected as much by the cholesterol you eat as by the overall percentage of fat in your diet. Of the 30%, less than one-third should come from saturated fats, the rest from monounsaturated fats.

The American Heart Association advises that the intake of cholesterol be limited to 300 mg/dl per day. The National Cholesterol Education Program (NCEP) recommends keeping serum (blood) cholesterol levels below 200 mg/dl per day. Other researchers recommend that for individuals age 30 and younger, total cholesterol should not be higher than 180 mg/dl per day, and for preteens the level should be below 170 mg/dl per day.

The ratio of total cholesterol to HDL cholesterol can be determined by dividing the total cholesterol level by the value for HDL cholesterol. For example:

Total Cholesterol	200 mg/dl
HDL	÷ 45 mg/dl = 4.4

The recommended ratio of HDL cholesterol to total cholesterol should be less than 4.5 for men and less than 4.0 for women. Before menopause, women tend to have higher levels of HDL cholesterol.

Snacking Facts

Pretzels, which are almost fat-free, are the fastest growing snack food in the United States. Per-capita consumption is up 100% since 1988. The mid-Atlantic states have been dubbed the "Pretzel Belt," as pretzel consumption there is twice the national average. Americans still prefer high-fat snacks, though. We eat three times as many pounds of potato chips and twice as many pounds of tortilla chips as pretzels.

Proteins

Proteins are chains of **amino acids,** chemical compounds that contain carbon, oxygen, hydrogen and nitrogen. They comprise about 16% of body weight and supply 4 calories of energy per gram. The "building blocks" of body tissues, proteins are essential to build and repair tissues such as blood, bones, muscles, skin, hair, nails, and internal organs. They regulate the body's chemical processes, carry nutrients to body cells, form enzymes, formulate hormones, and protect against disease because they are the major ingredient in antibodies. Nutrients, oxygen, and iron are transported to the cells of the body through protein.

There are 20 amino acids. The nine *essential amino acids* can be obtained from foods we consume, and the body can manufacture the other 11 amino acids. *Complete proteins* contain all nine essential amino acids. They tend to be from animal sources. *Incomplete proteins,* which contain only some of the essential amino acids, come from vegetable sources (beans, brown rice). An incomplete protein source must be combined with another food or more to make it a complete protein. Table 9.2 shows how to combine incomplete proteins to make a complete protein.

Excess protein is broken down for energy or is stored as fat. Therefore, red meat should be limited to no more than 3 to 6 ounces a day. More protein is needed for females who are pregnant and those who are breast-feeding.

Approximately 12% of our daily caloric intake should come from proteins. Females require approximately 48 grams daily; males require about 60 grams. To determine your protein needs, use the following equation:

body weight (in pounds) $\times$ 0.36 grams

For example:

160 lb. male $\times$ 0.36 grams = 57.6 grams protein

The Leanest Red Meats

	Percent of Calories From Fat
Buffalo top sirloin	15
Venison	18
Veal cutlets	24
Pork tenderloin	27
Beef top round	29
Beef eye of round	32
Lamb, leg of	34
Beef round tip	35
Rabbit, domestic	37
Beef sirloin	38

Cuts are raw, trimmed of visible fat

Source: U.S. Department of Agriculture, Handbook 8.

Table 9.2
Combinations for Complete Protein

To make a complete protein, select foods from two or more items in column 1.

Food Group	Examples
Grains	oats, rice, whole-grain breads, pasta
Legumes	peanuts, soy products, black-eyed peas, lima beans, kidney beans, red beans
Vegetables	all other vegetables
Seeds and nuts	cashews, nut butters
Eggs and milk products	eggs, milk, yogurt, cheese, cottage cheese

Examples	red beans and rice
	peanut butter and wheat bread
	eggplant parmesan

KEY TERMS

Proteins chains of amino acids
Amino acids chemical compounds that contain carbon, oxygen, hydrogen, and nitrogen

THE REGULATORY NUTRIENTS

Water

Water is the most important nutrient. Approximately 60% of the body's weight is made up of water apportioned differently among body tissues. Bones, for example, consist of about 20% water, and brain tissue is 75% water.

The body's need for water depends upon the individual person and factors such as sweat loss, activity patterns, body weight, loss through expired air and urine, and the amount of liquid consumed in foods and drinks. The adult body contains approximately 10 gallons of water. The percentage of water may be as low as 40% in obese individuals and as high as 70% in muscular individuals, because fat tissue is low in water content and muscle tissue is high in water content.

Water is essential to digest and absorb nutrients, regulate body temperature (particularly during exercise in the heat), lubricate the joints, remove waste products, transport oxygen and nutrients, and build and rebuild cells. A loss of 5% body water causes **dehydration**, dizziness, fatigue, and weakness. A 10%-15% loss can be harmful or even fatal. A person can survive only 3 days without drinking water. Water loss occurs from drinking coffee or alcohol (because this increases urination), skipping a meal, exercising, flying in a plane, and living in a hot, dry climate.

Although most foods provide water to the body, fruits and vegetables are the best sources because of

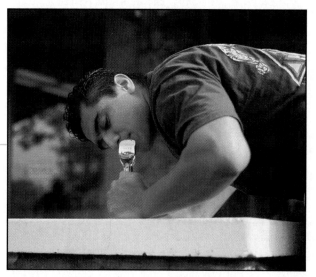

Water is the most important nutrient.

their high water content — lettuce (96%), tomatoes (94%;), apples (84%), oranges (86%). Foods such as bread and meat can contain from 33% to 50% water. As a general guideline, individuals should consume at least six to eight 8-ounce glasses of water each day (soft drinks, tea, coffee, and alcoholic beverages don't count). This amount is needed to maintain adequate water balance in the body. Consuming sugar and protein (waste from proteins builds up in the kidneys) also increases the need for water.

A person should drink before becoming thirsty — approximately a half cup every 30–45 minutes. Before and during exercise, participants should drink water to prevent dehydration. Liquids containing dissolved sugars or sodium stay in the stomach longer, delaying the usefulness of the fluids. Plain water is absorbed faster in the stomach and gets into the bloodstream more quickly. Cool water is best because it cools the body and leaves the digestive tract rapidly to enter tissues where it is needed.

A pale yellow urine output at least four times a day is a good indicator of hydration, that water is being added to tissue. Dark yellow urine indicates that the kidneys had to concentrate waste material into a smaller volume of water.

Vitamins

Vitamins are organic substances essential for normal growth and are needed in small amounts to carry out a variety of metabolic and nutrition functions. Vitamins produce the chemical reactions involved in manufacturing hormones and blood cells, enable good vision, promote strong bones and teeth, and ensure proper functioning of the nervous system and the heart. The 13 vitamins are divided into two types: fat-soluble (A, D, E, and K) and water-soluble (B-complex and C). Table 9.3 summarizes the functions of the vitamins and gives good sources for each, as well as deficiency symptoms.

Fat-soluble vitamins are found in foods associated with fats (lipids). They are stored in the body and normally are not excreted in the urine but, instead, tend to remain stored in the body in the

KEY TERMS

Dehydration abnormal depletion of body fluids
Vitamins organic substances essential for normal growth

✳ Table 9.3
Sources and Functions of Vitamins

Vitamin	Good Sources	Major Functions	Deficiency Symptoms
A	Milk, cheese, eggs, liver, and yellow/dark green fruits and vegetables	Required for healthy bones, teeth, skin, gums, and hair. Maintenance of inner mucous membranes, thus increasing resistance to infection. Adequate vision in dim light.	Night blindness, decreased growth, decreased resistance to infection, rough-dry skin.
D	Fortified milk, salmon, tuna, egg yolk	Necessary for bones and teeth. Needed for calcium and phosphorus absorption	Rickets (bone softening), fractures, and muscle spasms
E	Vegetable oils, yellow and green leafy vegetables, margarine, wheat germ, whole-grain breads, cereals	Related to oxidation and normal muscle and red blood cell chemistry	Leg cramps, red blood cell breakdown
K	Green leafy vegetables, cauliflower, cabbage, eggs, peas, potatoes	Essential for normal blood clotting	Hemorrhaging
B_1 (Thiamine)	Whole-grain or enriched bread, lean meats and poultry, organ fish, liver, pork, poultry, organ meats, legumes, nuts, dried yeast	Assists in proper use of carbohydrates. Normal functioning of nervous system. Maintenance of good appetite.	Loss of appetite, nausea, confusion, cardiac abnormalities, muscle spasms
B_2 (Riboflavin)	Eggs, milk, green leafy vegetables, whole grains, lean meats, dried beans and peas	Contributes to energy release from carbohydrates, fats, and proteins. Needed for normal growth and development, good vision, and healthy skin	Cracking of the corners of the mouth, inflammation of the skin, impaired vision.
Vitamin B_6 (Pyridoxine)	Vegetables, meats, whole-grain cereals, soybeans, peanuts, potatoes	Necessary for protein and fatty acids metabolism of, and formation of normal red blood cell	Depression, irritability, muscle spasms, nausea
Vitamin B_{12}	Meat, poultry, fish, liver, organ meats, eggs, shellfish, milk, cheese	Required for normal growth, red blood cell formation, nervous system and digestive tract functioning	Impaired balance, weakness, drop in red blood cell count
Niacin	Liver and other organ meats, fish, poultry, whole grains, enriched breads, nuts, green leafy vegetables, dried beans and peas	Contributes to energy release from carbohydrates, fats, and proteins. Normal growth and development, and formation of hormones and nerve-regulating substances	Confusion, depression, weakness, weight loss
Biotin	Liver, kidney, eggs, yeast, legumes, milk, nuts, dark green vegetables	Essential for carbohydrate metabolism and fatty acid synthesis	Inflamed skin, muscle pain, depression, weight loss
Folic Acid	Green leafy vegetables, organ meats, whole grains and cereals, dried beans	Needed for cell growth and reproduction and red blood cell formation	Decreased resistance to infection
Pantothenic Acid	All natural foods, especially liver, kidney, eggs, nuts, yeast, milk, dried peas and beans, green leafy vegetables	Related to carbohydrate and fat metabolism	Depression, low blood sugar, leg cramps, nausea, headaches
Vitamin C (Ascorbic Acid)	Fruits and vegetables	Helps protect against infection. Formation of collagenous tissue. Normal blood vessels, teeth, and bones	Slow-healing wounds, loose teeth, hemorrhaging, rough-scaly skin, irritability

Adapted from *Principles & Labs for Physical Fitness & Wellness*, 2d edition, by Werner W. K. Hoeger, and Sharon Hoeger (Englewood CO: Morton Publishing, 1994), p. 185.

liver and fatty tissues until they are needed. The body does not require an everyday supply, and overdoses can interfere with or disrupt the action of other nutrients.

Water-soluble vitamins (B and C complex) are transported in the fluids of cells and tissues and can be lost from the body through sweat and urine. These vitamins are not stored in the body in large quantities. In addition, they can be lost in varying amounts through cooking methods when the water in which the food is cooked or soaked is discarded. Water-soluble vitamins must be replaced daily.

Antioxidants are intrepid disease-fighters that can protect your body from the harmful effects of free radicals. **Free radicals** are chemicals produced when the body burns fuel for energy. When the body produces too many free radicals, it can lead to a chain reaction in which the the free radicals attack and damage the body's cells. The damage has been implicated in the cause of more than fifty diseases including various forms of cancer, heart disease, cataracts, premature aging, and AIDS.

Antioxidants occur naturally in our bodies, but a person can increase the intake of certain nutrients to help guard against free radicals. The vitamins C and E and the plant source of Vitamin A, **beta-carotene,** are the most common food sources. Studies of antioxidants as related to heart disease and cancer show a reduction in the risk even with short-term intake. Recent studies have suggested that these nutrients, especially vitamin E, may lower the

About Niacin

The B vitamin niacin, also known as nicotinic acid, is an effective treatment for high blood cholesterol, dramatically lowering total and LDL ("bad") cholesterol and triglycerides, and at the same time boosting HDL ("good") cholesterol. It's the least expensive treatment, costing as little as one-tenth as much as the standard cholesterol-lowering drugs, and is available alongside other OTC vitamin supplements and by prescription . A recent study in the *Journal of the American Medical Association* confirmed the strengths of high-dose niacin as a cholesterol fighter, but it also showed that at the high doses needed to be effective, niacin is no longer a vitamin but a drug with a drug's potential side effects.

Source: *UC Berkeley Wellness Letter*, Sept, 1994, p. 2

risk of heart disease by preventing oxidation of the LDL ("bad") cholesterol, thereby reducing the build-up of plaque in coronary arteries. Additional studies have found that antioxidants may reduce the risk of infectious disease and may boost the immune system in elderly people. Author Dr. Kenneth Cooper believes antioxidants delay the onset of premature aging and decrease the risk for early Parkinson's disease. Foods rich in antioxidants are listed in Table 9.4.

Table 9.4
Foods Rich in Antioxidants

Antioxidant Nutrient	Primary Food Sources
Vitamin C (ascorbic acid)	Papaya, cantaloupe, cauliflower, melons, citrus fruits, tomatoes, dark green vegetables, grapefruit, green and red pepper, strawberries, raspberries, asparagus, broccoli, cabbage, collard greens, orange juice, tomato juice, brussels sprouts, kiwi fruit
Vitamin E	Vegetable oils (safflower, corn, cottonseed, sunflower), nuts, egg yolk, liver, dried beans, yellow and green leafy vegetables, sunflower seeds, almonds, wheat germ, 100% whole-wheat bread, 100% whole-grain cereals, oatmeal, hazelnuts, mayonnaise
Beta-carotene	Yellow, orange, and dark green leafy vegetables and fruits (sweet potatoes, carrots, squash, tomatoes, mango, cantaloupe, pumpkin, asparagus, broccoli, apricots, peaches, spinach, romaine lettuce, papaya
Vitamin A	milk, eggs, cheese, liver, butter, fish oil
Selenium (mineral)	Lean meat, nonfat milk, seafood, 100% whole-grain cereal, 100% whole-wheat bread, skinless chicken

Minerals

Minerals are inorganic substances that make up 4% of our body weight. The other 96% of our body weight is composed of carbon, oxygen, hydrogen, and nitrogen in some combination. The body contains 25 known minerals that have several important functions:

1. They build bones and teeth.
2. They maintain the acid-base balance of the blood.
3. They promote normal blood clotting.
4. They promote normal heart rhythm.
5. They transmit messages of the nervous system.
6. They maintain water balance.
7. They regulate muscular contraction and metabolic process. Table 9.5 outlines the salient features of the most important minerals.

KEY TERMS

Antioxidants disease-fighters that protect the body from the harmful effects of free radicals

Free Radicals chemicals produced when the body burns fuel for energy

Beta-carotene plant source of vitamin A; helps guard against free radicals

Minerals inorganic substances that make up 4% of our body weight

Table 9.5
Major Sources and Functions of Minerals

Nutrient	Good Sources	Major Functions	Deficiency Symptoms
Calcium	Milk, yogurt, cheese, green leafy vegetables, dried beans, sardines, salmon	Required for strong teeth and bone formation. Maintenance of good muscle tone, heartbeat, and nerve function	Bone pain and fractures, periodontal disease, muscle cramps
Iron	Organ meats, lean meats, seafoods, eggs, dried peas and beans, nuts, whole and enriched grains, green leafy vegetables	Major component of hemoglobin. Aids in energy utilization	Nutritional anemia; overall weakness, chronic fatigue, sleeplessness, susceptibility to infection
Phosphorus	Meats, fish, milk, eggs, dried beans and peas, whole grains, processed foods	Required for formation of bones and teeth. Energy release regulation.	Bone pain and fracture, weight loss, weakness
Zinc	Milk, meat, seafood, whole grains, nuts, eggs, dried beans	Essential component of hormones, insulin, and enzymes. Used in normal growth and development	Loss of appetite, slow-healing wounds, skin problems
Magnesium	Green leafy vegetables, whole grains, nuts, soybeans, seafood, legumes	Needed for bone growth and maintenance. Carbohydrate and protein utilization. Nerve function. Temperature regulation	Irregular heartbeat, weakness, muscle spasms, sleeplessness
Sodium	Table salt, processed foods, and meat	Body fluid regulation. Transmission of nerve impulse. Heart action	Rarely seen
Potassium	Legumes, whole grains, bananas, orange juice, dried fruits, potatoes	Heart action. Bone formation and maintenance. Regulation of energy release. Acid-base regulation	Irregular heartbeat, nausea, weakness
Selenium	Seafood, meat, whole grains	Component of enzyme; functions in close association with vitamin E	Muscle pain, possible heart muscle deterioration; possible hair and nail loss

Adapted from *Principles & Labs For Physical Fitness & Wellness*, 2d edition, by Werner W. K. and Sharon Hoeger (Englewood, CO: Morton Publishing, 1994), p. 186.

5. *Milk, yogurt, cheese* (2–3 servings daily). Dairy products such as milk, buttermilk, yogurt, cottage cheese, and ice cream are high in calcium, riboflavin, protein and vitamins A and B$_{12}$. Most adults should consume two servings daily, but teenagers, young adults up to age 24, and women who are pregnant or breast-feeding should consume three servings of milk, yogurt, or cheese products per day. Nonfat plain yogurt could be substituted for sour cream, and part-skim or low-fat cheeses for the traditional cheeses. To ease the transition from whole milk, a person might first switch to 2%-fat (low-fat), then to 1% (extra light), and finally to nonfat (skim) milk. Table 9.9 lists the calories and percentage of calories from fat for the different milk products.

6. *Fats, oils,* and *sweets.* The final component of the Food Guide Pyramid consists of fats, oils, and sugars. The reasons for avoiding fats (and oils) have been dis-

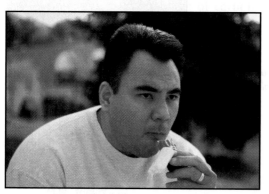

Sweets should be eaten sparingly.

Caution in Reading Labels

❋ Don't be misled by what the manufacturer says on other parts of the product. "Reduced Fat" doesn't mean no fat or low fat.

❋ Just because a product label says "No Preservatives" doesn't mean other chemicals have not been used in processing.

❋ When comparing products, make sure to check serving size. A 7-ounce serving will be higher in nutrients simply because it's larger than a 3-ounce serving used by another brand.

❋ Pull or sell date is the last date on which the product should be sold, assuming that it has been stored and handled properly. The pull date allows for some storage time in the home refrigerator. Cold cuts, milk, ice cream, and refrigerated baked products are examples of foods with pull dates.

❋ Expiration date is the last date on which the food should be eaten or used. Baby formula and yeast are examples of products that carry an expiration date.

❋ Freshness date may allow for normal home storage. Some bakery products that have a freshness date are sold at a reduced price for a short time after the date.

Adapted from "No More Label Fables," *Tufts University Diet and Nutrition Letter 10* (February 1993); and Safeway Stores, 430 Jackson Street, Oakland, CA 94660.

cussed. In addition, sugars are hidden in cola drinks (10 teaspoons of sugar per can), low-fat fruit yogurt (7 teaspoons per cup), fruit pie (6 teaspoons per serving) and ketchup (1 teaspoon in every tablespoon). Also sweeteners — jams, jellies, syrups, corn sweeteners, molasses, fruit juice, concentrate, and sugar in candy, cake, and cookies — should be used sparingly.

Figure 9.7 gives two sample meal plans based on the Food Guide Pyramid.

❋ Table 9.9
Calories in Variations of Milk

Milk (1 cup)	Calories	Grams of fat	% of Calories from fat	% of calories from fat
Whole milk (3.3%)	150	8.5	51	51 ÷ 150 = 34%
2% milk ("low-fat")	120	4.7	35	35 ÷ 120 = 29%
1% milk ("low-fat")	100	0.5	22	22 ÷ 100 = 22%
Skim (nonfat) milk	85	0.4	trace	trace
Buttermilk	80	trace	trace	trace
Chocolate 2%	170	4	36	36 ÷ 170 = 21%

1400-Calorie Diet

Serving	Breakfast	Serving	Dinner
1	1/2 cup blueberries	1	1/2 cup tomato sauce
1	8 oz nonfat yogurt (plain or fruit)	1	1/2 cup steamed vegetables
2	whole small bagel, 1 tablespoon jam	1	2 oz steamed shrimp
		1	1 oz Parmesan cheese
	Lunch	2	1 cup pasta
1	banana		
1	1 cup raw vegetables		**Snack**
1	1/4 cup cottage cheese	1	1 peach
2	large baked potato	1	1 cup skim milk
		1	2 graham crackers

Comparison to Food Pyramid

	Suggested	Actual
Fats, Oils, & Sweets	use sparingly	
Milk, Yogurt, & Cheese	2–3 servings	3 servings
Vegetables	3–5 servings	3 servings
Fruits	2–4 servings	3 servings
Meat, Poultry, Fish, Dry Beans, Eggs, & Nuts	2–3 servings	2 servings
Bread, Cereal, Rice, & Pasta	6–11 servings	7 servings

2000-Calorie Diet

Serving	Breakfast	Serving	Dinner
1	banana	1	1/2 cup fruit salad
1	1 cup skim milk	2	1 cup steamed vegetables
1	1 tsp. margarine	1	3 oz fish broiled
1.5	1½ cups cold cereal	1	1 T. butter on fish
2	2 slices toast	2	1 cup rice
		1	1 small roll
	Lunch		
1	apple		**Snack**
2	salad with 2 cups raw vegetables	1	orange
1	3 oz roast turkey	1	8 oz. nonfat yogurt (plain or fruit)
1	2 T. low-calorie salad dressing	1	1/2 small bagel
2	2 slices bread for sandwich	1	3 cups air-popped popcorn

Comparison to Food Pyramid

	Suggested	Actual
Fats, Oils, & Sweets	use sparingly	
Milk, Yogurt, & Cheese	2–3 servings	2 servings
Vegetables	3–5 servings	4 servings
Fruits	2–4 servings	4 servings
Meat, Poultry, Fish, Dry Beans, Eggs, & Nuts	2–3 servings	2 servings
Bread, Cereal, Rice, & Pasta	6–11 servings	10.5 servings

Figure 9.7 Sample meal plans

This Spud's For You

We all know by now that it's the topping, not the potato, that piles on the calories. Here's how some favorite choices add up.

Food	Measure	Calories	Fat (grams)	Sodium (milligrams)
Baked potato with skin	1 medium	220	0.2	16
Butter	1 tablespoon	102	11.5	117
Margarine, diet, corn oil	1 tablespoon	50	5.6	139
Sour cream	2 tablespoons	62	6	15
Low-fat sour cream	2 tablespoons	41	3.6	12
Low-fat yogurt	2 tablespoons	18	0.4	20
Cheddar cheese	1 ounce	114	9.4	176
Part-skim mozzarella cheese	1 ounce	72	4.5	132
Salsa	¼ cup	24	0	600
Bacon, fried crisp	1 slice	43	3.7	120

Source: Reprinted by permission from *Cooking Light*.

What is a Serving?

The Food Guide Pyramid does not state the difference between skim milk and whole milk or between meat and poultry. One ounce of boneless beef contains 70–100 calories, whereas an ounce of boneless chicken has 50–55 calories. And although the pyramid tells how many servings of each food to eat each day, it does not specify how much a "serving" is.

The number of servings that will be right for you depends on how many calories you need, which in turn depends on your age, sex, size, and activity level. Almost everyone should have at least the lowest number of servings in each range.

How many servings do you need each day? Do you need to measure servings? Absolutely not! Servings should be used only as a general guide. For mixed foods you should do the best you can to estimate the food group servings of the main ingredients. For example, a generous serving of pizza counts in the bread group (crust), milk group (cheese), and vegetable group (tomato); a helping of beef stew counts in the meat group and the vegetable group. Both examples have some fat (in the cheese on the pizza and in the beef in the stew). A serving adds up quicker than you think!

Mediterranean Diet Pyramid

Another pyramid has been developed recently, this one by the World Health Organization in association with experts from Harvard School of Public Health and Oldways Preservation & Exchange Trust. The Mediterranean Diet, depicted in Figure 9.8, is modeled after the typical eating pattern of men in the Mediterranean region around 1960. This population had notably low rates of diet-linked diseases and a longer life expectancy.

Like the Food Guide Pyramid, this one recommends high consumption of complex carbohydrates and fruits and vegetables. It differs, however, in its recommendation of olive oil, which is high in monounsaturated fat and is suggested for use "sparingly" in the Food Guide Pyramid.

Is Eating Nuts a Good Idea?

Contrary to popular opinion, nuts may be healthy for you. They do have a lot of calories and fat, but 50% to 80% of the fat is monounsaturated fat, the kind in olive oil, recommended in the Mediterranean Diet Pyramid. These fats help lower bad LDL cholesterol and blood pressure. Nuts also provide protein, fiber, magnesium, potassium, folic acid, calcium, and vitamin E. Like other nonanimal foods, they have no cholesterol. An ounce a day shouldn't add any pounds.

Seven good nuts are almonds, pecans, hazelnuts, walnuts, macadamia nuts, Brazil nuts, and pistachios. By the way, peanuts are not nuts at all; they are legumes. They, too, are rich in micronutrients tied to less cancer, heart disease, and diabetes.

Source: Jean Carper, author of *Food — Your Miracle Medicine*, in a column appearing in *USA Weekend*, December 2–4, 1994.

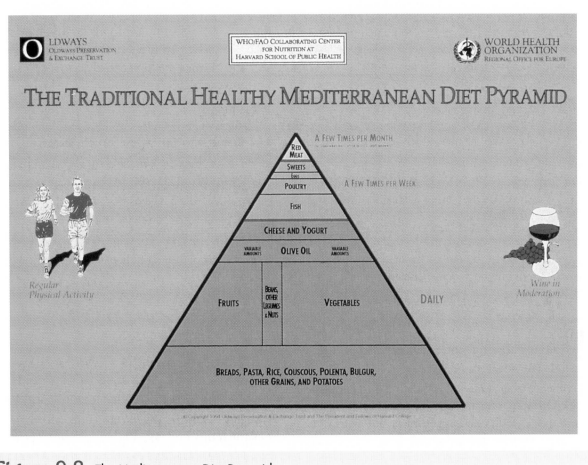

Figure 9.8 The Mediterranean Diet Pyramid

Another major difference is the recommendation: "Exercise daily, wine in moderation." The recognition of exercise is not debatable. Critics of the Mediterranean diet, however, believe that wine drinking could lead to alcohol abuse and liver damage and should not be encouraged. Proponents counter them in citing studies that show a glass or two of wine a day may prevent certain cardiovascular diseases. While the verdict is still out, the Greeks may have the best advice: moderation in all things.

☎ Call for information

For more information on Mediterranean Diet:
Oldways Preservation & Exchange Trust
617-695-0600
617-426-7696 Fax

VEGETARIANS

Several million Americans follow a **vegetarian** diet because of religious, health, ethical, or philosophical reasons, or they think foods of plant origin provide more natural nourishment for the body. Vegetarians must obtain sufficient amounts of protein, iron, vitamin B_{12}, vitamin D, and calcium from fewer food sources.

Research studies show that vegetarians' cholesterol levels tend to be lower. They have a lower incidence of breast, colon, and prostate cancers, lower blood pressure, and less osteoporosis.

KEY TERMS

Vegetarian person who eats foods of plant origin and not meat

Meat Eaters Versus Vegetable Eaters

Mammals can be separated into three categories based on their natural diet: meat eaters (carnivores such as lions, tigers, dogs, and cats), leaf and grass eaters (herbivores or grazers such as horses and cows), and fruit and vegetable eaters (monkeys, apes, chimpanzees). Humans obviously do not survive on grass and leaves, but are we by nature meat eaters or fruit and vegetable eaters? Follow the digestive tract when the food enters the mouth.

	Meat Eaters	Vegetable Eaters
Teeth and mouth	Sharp, pointed fangs	No fangs
	No molars or grinding teeth; no carbohydrate-digestive enzymes in saliva	Well-developed molars to grind food and mix it with enzymes that digest carbohydrates
Stomach	Produce 20 times the hydrochloric acid as human stomach; needed to digest animal flesh	Have less hydrochloric acid, as digesting fruits and vegetables requires less acid
Intestines	Short digestive tract because meat spoils quickly	Digestive tract 12 times body length to allow complete digestion of carbohydrates

Are you convinced that people are fruit and vegetable eaters? If not, also consider that humans are one of the slowest mammals on earth, outrun by all others except a species of sloth. "Man as mighty hunter" is a myth; evidence clearly shows that early humans subsisted primarily on fruits and vegetables.

Source: Adapted from *Reversing Heart Disease* by Julian M. Whitaker (New York: Warner Books, 1985).

Vegetarians usually are not overweight. The four styles of vegetarians are:

※ **Lactovegetarian** One who eats dairy products (milk, milk products, and cheese) as well as plant foods (fruits and vegetables) but does not eat meat, poultry, fish or eggs.

What Is Pica?

One of the more unusual practices that survived the journey from Africa is *pica*, the practice of eating clay and other nonfood items. Clay eating was common in West Africa because it alleviated hunger and soothed the irritation caused by intestinal parasites. Clay eating also may have been part of religious rituals. Eating clay also may have added calcium, iron, and phosphorus to mineral-deficient diets.

In America clay eating was present during slavery and is still fairly common in some parts of the South and even in northern cities, especially by pregnant women. In rural areas clay is the substance of choice. In urban areas, laundry starch is often preferred, though some people eat coffee grounds, plaster, paraffin, and milk of magnesia.

Pica eating seems to be passed on from mother to daughter. Whether it is harmful is not known. It may lead to weight gain and hypertension (from the sodium in clay), and it may interfere with nutrition, blocking the absorption of vitamins and minerals and substituting for real food.

Source: *Good Health for African Americans* by Barbara Dixon (New York: Crown Publishers, 1994), p. 25.

※ **Ovolactovegetarian** One who eats eggs, dairy products, and plant foods (fruits and vegetables) but does not eat meat, poultry, or fish.

※ **Vegan** A pure vegetarian, one who eats only plant foods and often takes vitamin B_{12} supplements because this vitamin normally is found only in animal products.

※ Partial or **semivegetarian** One who eats plant food, dairy products, eggs, and usually a small selection of poultry, fish, and other seafood, but not beef or pork.

Eating a wide variety of foods is necessary to ensure that all nutritional needs are met. Careful planning and time should be devoted to selecting a proper vegetarian diet.

VITAMIN AND MINERAL SUPPLEMENTS

Do you need to take vitamin/ mineral supplements? The answer lies with your diet. Men more often than women are meeting their nutrient needs. Some

Tips for action

If You Are a Vegetarian:

1. Eat proteins from a variety of sources, and include several protein sources at each meal.

2. Apportion protein so that 60% is from grains; 35% from legumes (black-eyed peas, peanuts, split peas, garbanzos, tofu [soybean curd], lentils, and various beans and peas; and 5% from dark green leafy vegetables.

3. To obtain *riboflavin* and boost iron intake, eat dark green leafy vegetables (at least a cup a day), whole grains, yeast, and legumes.

4. To obtain *iron*, eat whole grain, dried fruit, nuts, legumes.

5. To obtain *zinc*, eat whole grains and legumes.

6. To obtain *calcium*, eat tofu, nuts, and green leafy vegetables, and consume fortified orange juice and soy milk. Supplements may be necessary.

7. To obtain *vitamin B_{12}*, found only in animal foods, eat foods fortified with vitamin B_{12} such as soy milk, breakfast cereals, and special yeast products. Supplements may be necessary.

8. To obtain *vitamin D*, spend at least 30 minutes a day in the sun, or take a supplement of 200 I. U. or 5 micrograms.

9. Eat fruits with meals, because *vitamin* C will improve iron absorption. The iron in plants is more difficult to absorb than that in animal sources.

10. Because vegetarian diets are low in fat, make sure you get at least 1 gram of fat a day so your body will absorb fat-soluble vitamins.

women may need more nutrients to compensate for their loss in heavy menstrual flows.

Vitamins may have significant health benefits for some people. In 1992 the U. S. Public Health Service recommended a vitamin supplement — **folic acid**, a B vitamin — for all women of child-bearing age. This vitamin may play a protective role in preventing neural tube defects (abnormalities of the brain and spinal cord) such as spina bifida, in which a segment of the spinal cord protrudes through the spinal column. Folic acid (folate) also may play a role in preventing cervical and other cancers by strengthening the chromosomes.

Vitamins A, C, and E may safeguard cells from damage by oxygen molecules, thus preventing heart disease and cancer. According to a 1992 study by the National Cancer Institute, individuals taking vitamin E supplements have a 50% lower risk of cancer of the mouth and pharynx than those who do not take it as a supplement.

Beta-carotene, the compound that turns into Vitamin A in the body, can reduce the risk for heart attack and stroke. Most researchers recommend 6 mg per day (equivalent of a quarter pound of carrots or sweet potatoes). Larger amounts of beta-carotene may lower the vitamin E level. In addition, antioxidants (substances that protect cells from the damaging effects of oxidation), including vitamins C, E, and beta-carotene, may reduce dangerous blood fats, thus lowering the risk for heart disease and cancer.

According to the National Research Council's report *Diet and Health*, "The desirable way for the

KEY TERMS

Lactovegetarian one who eats dairy products and plants but not meat, poultry, fish, or eggs

Ovolactovegetarian one who eats eggs, dairy products and plants but not meat, poultry, or fish

Vegan one who eats only plant foods

Semivegetarian one who eats plant food, dairy products, eggs, small amounts of poultry and fish, but no beef or pork

Folic acid a B vitamin important in preventing neural tube defects of the fetus

Food Allergy Versus Intolerance

Many people who believe they are allergic to certain foods do not have a true food allergy. In an allergic reaction the body erroneously reacts to a harmless substance and produces histamines, which evoke the symptoms of an allergy. The most common symptoms are rash or hives, swelling body parts, and nausea and vomiting. In the most severe cases, if untreated, disruption of normal breathing and heartbeat can lead to death. The foods that most commonly provoke an allergic reaction are soybeans, shellfish, peanuts, legumes (beans), wheat, and milk.

Food intolerance, in contrast, is the result of a deficiency in digestive enzymes. The most common perhaps is **lactose intolerance**, in which the person cannot digest milk sugar because of a lack of the enzyme lactase. As many as three-fourths of all African Americans, American Indians, Mexican-Americans, and Jewish people are born with lactose deficiency or develop the intolerance to milk and dairy products after infancy. After ingesting dairy products, they develop abdominal cramps, gas pains, and diarrhea. The cause is a lack of the enzyme lactase, which aids in digesting the lactose in dairy products. Control of the symptoms is the only treatment for lactose intolerance, as lactose production in the digestive system cannot be stimulated.

general public to obtain recommended levels of nutrients is by eating a variety of foods." The report also suggests several instances in which supplements may be appropriate. Those who might benefit from nutrient supplements include:

✳ Pregnant and breast-feeding women, who have hard-to-meet needs for nutrients such as folate, iron, and calcium.

✳ Women who have excessive menstrual bleeding, who may need iron to help replenish iron stores lost in blood.

✳ Individuals on very low-calorie diets or strict vegetarian regimens, which often lack sufficient zinc, calcium, iron, and vitamin B_{12}.

✳ Individuals who have chronic illnesses or diseases or take medications that interfere with appetite or the way the body handles certain nutrients.

✳ People who smoke, drink a considerable amount of alcohol, and take drugs such as aspirin and oral contraceptives.

Perhaps people at risk of heart attack, elderly people, and high-performance athletes may need to take a supplement. African Americans may not get enough vitamin D because their darker skin screens out the vitamin-D-activating property of sunlight. People who are taking supplements because of an illness or drug therapy should be under professional guidance because some vitamins and minerals counteract the actions of certain medications.

The Council on Scientific Affairs of the American Medical Association recommends a supplement containing between 50% and 150% of the adult RDA for vitamins.

Balance between vitamin and mineral supplements is necessary. This lessens the chances of

Tips for action

Dietary factors contribute substantially to illness and premature death. What you eat is a significant controllable risk factor affecting long-term health. Leading causes of death associated with dietary factors include artery disease, coronary heart disease, some types of cancer, stroke, and diabetes.

1. Reduce dietary fat intake. Be aware that most fast-food and junk foods contain more than 50% saturated fat.

2. Examine food labels when purchasing food. Be aware of the amount of sodium, fat, and sugar in foods you are consuming. Know the amounts recommended for daily consumption for your sex, age, and size. Do not exceed the recommended daily values.

3. Do not add table salt to food. Adding a small amount of salt when the food is being cooked or prepared is healthier. Substitute selected herbs and spices that can enhance the taste and add flavor.

Do You Need Supplements?

If you are in any of the following categories, you may need supplements:

* **Women on birth control pills:** B vitamins (thiamine, riboflavin, B_6, B_{12}, folic acid, vitamin C)

* **Pregnant and breast-feeding women:** all vitamins, especially vitamin D, vitamin E, calcium, iron, and folic acid

* **Heavy smokers:** vitamin C and E

* **Heavy drinkers:** thiamine, niacin, B_6, folic acid

* **Taking antibiotics:** can destroy healthy bacteria in the intestinal tract and interfere with absorption of vitamin K and several B vitamins

* **People with chronic health conditions:** may be unable to absorb enough vitamins from food (people with bile duct blockage; chronic diarrhea; chronic disorders of stomach and intestine)

* **Those who have had a heart attack:** vitamin E, under physician's supervision

* **People undergoing surgery:** vitamin C for healing

* **Elderly:** B vitamins, thiamine, vitamin C

* **People on low-calorie diets for weight loss:** all vitamins and minerals

* **Vegetarians:** calcium, iron, zinc, vitamin B_{12}

From *Good Health for African Americans*, by Barbara Dixon (New York: Crown, 1994), pp. 190-191.

If you do take supplements:

* Look at the expiration date and buy ones that will last you awhile.

* Keep them in a cool, dark, dry place, such as the refrigerator.

* Choose a supplement high in beta-carotene rather than one high in vitamin A. Large quantities of vitamin A can be toxic.

* Buy vitamin C separately. Multivitamins containing a lot of vitamin C usually are expensive.

* Make sure multivitamins contain folic acid.

* Be sure the supplement does not contain additives.

* Dr. Kenneth Cooper recommends a daily "antioxidant cocktail" consisting of 1000 mg of vitamin C, 400 I.U. of natural vitamin E, and 25,000 I.U. (15 mg of beta-carotene — all of which costs less than $5 a month)

competition between the two, causing an imbalance. As examples, a high amount of folate can hide the symptoms of a vitamin B_{12} deficiency, and a high amount of copper can inhibit zinc absorption.

Synthesized vitamins and "natural" vitamins have the same chemical composition and are not different from vitamins found in generic vitamin tablets. The only exception is vitamin E; the body absorbs natural forms faster. The main consideration is to keep vitamin supplementation reasonable. Megadoses can be unhealthy.

☎ *Call for information*

Consumer Nutrition Hot Line
800-366-1655
Weekends 8 a.m.–8 p.m.
Weekdays 9 a.m.–4 p.m. central time

FAST FOODS

When selecting fast foods, we need to be wise consumers. Most fast foods are high in calories, fat, sugar, and salt, and low in nutrients and fiber. Not all fast foods are unhealthy, though, especially when combined with additional foods in your daily diet.

Most fast-food chains have switched from beef tallow or fat (lard) to unsaturated vegetable oils for frying, but the total fat content is still high. Because of consumer pressure, they offer lighter menu items such as salads, grilled chicken sandwiches on oat-bran buns, and nonfat yogurt. Other measures include lowering sodium levels, removing additives from fish breading products, and taking MSG out of sausages. Many states require fast-food restaurants to post nutritional information about their

KEY TERMS

Lactose intolerance adverse reaction to dairy products because of lack of digestive enzyme

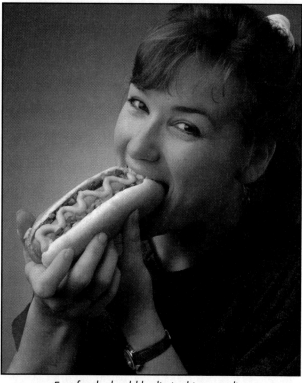
Fast foods should be limited in your diet.

foods. You can get the best nutritional value at a cafeteria or restaurant by requesting salad dressing (low-calorie) on the side, selecting or ordering an appetizer with a salad and vegetable, and asking that the entree be baked or broiled without fat.

SUBSTITUTES AND ADDITIVES

Artificial Sweeteners

An artificial sweetener is often 220 times sweeter than sucrose, or table sugar. Current evidence suggests that artificial sweeteners ingested in moderate amounts pose no health problems to the consumer. Other studies indicate that artificial sweeteners do nothing to ease hunger pains and actually may increase the desire for sweets. Individuals who use these sweeteners tend also to increase the amount of fats in their diet. Examples of artificial sweeteners are aspartame (Nutra-Sweet and Equal), acesulfame-K (Sunette), saccharin, sucralose, sweetener 2000, and thaumatin.

Tips for action

When eating out:

✳ Select plain scrambled eggs, pancakes without butter or syrup, English muffins.

✳ Select plain hamburgers (no cheese) or roast beef (leaner than hamburger, lower in fat and calories). Skip the mayonnaise (and save 100–150 calories), bacon, and cheese (save 200 calories from saturated fat and cholesterol).

✳ Avoid fried foods, foods prepared with sauces, gravies, or sauteed in butter. Avoid fried chicken, processed chicken (contains fatty, ground-up skin). Be cautious of fish sandwiches (trapped oil in breading) and creamy tartar sauce (high in fat and calories).

✳ Request unsalted items.

✳ Include dairy products for additional calcium.

✳ Include fresh fruits and vegetables for vitamins A, C, and fiber.

✳ Eat a baked potato instead of french fries, and skip toppings made with sour cream, melted cheese, or butter.

✳ At the salad bar be cautious of mayonnaise, oily vegetable salads, and rich dressings. Get salad dressing on the side. Use low-calorie dressing in moderation (two small ladles can contain nearly as much fat as a large burger, even though the fat is largely unsaturated).(At home, make your own salad dressing using lemon juice or vinegar as basic ingredients.)

✳ Avoid frosted desserts and cakes. Choose fruit, or sherbet.

What About Aspartame?

The artificial sweetener aspartame is used in 99% of all diet soft drinks. It was introduced in 1983 as Nutra Sweet and Equal and became popular because it was just as sweet as saccharin but did not leave a metallic aftertaste.

Diet doctor Robert Atkins, in his monthly newsletter *Heart Revelations*, says aspartame can cause insomnia, heart palpitations, joint pain, vomiting, headache, dizziness, anxiety, memory loss, confusion, and even weight gain. Recent evidence points to aspartame as a cause of depression. Diana Korte, author of *Every Woman's Body* (Bantam) suggests avoiding as many food additives as possible, including aspartame.

In rebuttal, Martha Stone, nutrition advisor to *Prevention* magazine, says that aspartame was the most studied additive ever approved by the FDA. "Aspartame wouldn't have gotten to the market if it caused problems in humans," she said. "The bottom line is that the complaints have never checked out scientifically." In 1993 the American Dietetic Association reviewed the research on aspartame and endorsed it as "safe to consume." Michelle Hoeting, a chemical dietitian at the Barbara Davis Center for Childhood Diabetes in Denver, views aspartame as a safe alternative for people with diabetes.

The bottom line seems to be moderation. Jean Olivia-Rasbach, director of nutrition for Healthmark Centers, suggests no more than two servings a day with aspartame. In addition to soda, it appears most commonly in desserts, yogurt, Jell-O, and chewing gum.

The Food and Drug Administration has set 22.7 milligrams per pound of body weight as the acceptable daily intake of aspartame. A 12-ounce can of aspartame-sweetened soda contains about 180 milligrams of aspartame.

Saccharin is relatively safe in low to moderate doses. Some evidence, however, links it to a higher incidence of bladder cancer. The risk increases with the amount of saccharin used. In sum, artificial sweeteners should be used in moderation, in keeping with FDA guidelines.

Fake Fat

Simplesse (low-calorie substitute for fat) is made from protein that has been heated and blended to form tiny round particles, to create a sense of creaminess. **Fake fat** mimics the taste of fat and contains a small percentage of calories, fat, and cholesterol. It can be found in yogurt, ice cream, sour cream, and salad dressing, among other foods. Simplesse contains 130 calories in one-half cup of ice cream but only 1 gram of fat, compared to regular ice cream, which contains about 150 calories and 8 grams of fat.

Olestra is another artificial fat, derived from sucrose and fatty acids. It is found in ice cream, snacks, margarine, and desserts. Additional artificial fat substitutes include polydextrose (Litesse); corn protein (Lita), used in mayonnaise, ice cream, salad dressing, sour cream, and yogurt; and modified corn starch (Stellar). Many "light" desserts do not have much nutritional value. It's best to eat more fruits and vegetables.

Salt Substitutes

The best idea is to go easy on foods that are high in salt and forego the salt shaker. Salt substitutes aren't for everyone, particularly people with diabetes. Some substitutes to avoid or use sparingly are onion, celery, or garlic salt, seasoned salt, meat tenderizer, bullion, monosodium glutamate (MSG), soy sauce, worcester sauce, dill pickles, sauerkraut, and tomato juice.

Food Additives

Today, more than 2,800 substances are added to foods to improve their nutritional quality, to maintain freshness, to aid in processing or preparation, or to alter the taste or appearance. The most widely used additives are sugar, salt, and corn syrup. Others include citric acid, baking soda, vegetable colors, mustard, and pepper.

If the additive is known to cause cancer in animals, the FDA will not approve it in foods for humans. Negative health consequences from food additives is minimal for people who eat sensibly.

KEY TERMS

Fake fat a substance that mimics the taste of fat

Food Safety

✳ Cook foods thoroughly, especially beef, poultry, fish, pork, and eggs. Cooking kills most microbes. Don't eat raw animal products.

✳ Trim fat from meat, poultry, and fish and remove skin (which also contains most of the fat) from poultry and fish. Discard fats and oils found in broths and pan dripping. (Pesticide residues concentrate in the animals' fat).

✳ Cook stuffing separately from poultry; or wash poultry thoroughly, stuff immediately before cooking, and then transfer the stuffing to a clean bowl immediately after cooking.

✳ Avoid coughing or sneezing over foods, even when you are healthy, and cover any cuts on your hands.

✳ Thoroughly wash hands with hot soapy water before and after handling food, especially raw meat, fish, poultry, or eggs, which may contain *Salmonella* bacteria.

✳ Don't buy food in containers that leak, bulge, or are severely dented. The deadly botulism toxin may be present.

✳ Don't let groceries sit in warm car; bacteria will grow in warm temperatures. Get them home to the refrigerator or freezer promptly.

✳ Store foods below 40°F. Do not leave cooked or refrigerated foods, such as meats or salads, at room temperature for more than 2 hours.

✳ Make sure counters, cutting boards, dishes, and other equipment are thoroughly cleaned before and after use, especially if they have come in contact with raw meat, fish, poultry, or eggs.

✳ Thoroughly rinse and scrub fruits and vegetables. Remove outer leaves of leafy vegetables, such as lettuce and cabbage.

✳ If possible, use separate cutting boards for meat and for foods that will be eaten raw, such as fruits or vegetables.

Adapted from "Safety First: Protecting America's Food Supply." *FDA Consumer*, November, 1988 p 26.

ETHNIC FOODS

Ethnic foods may be part of your culture or that of friends. As people migrate to other countries, they bring with them their eating practices, food choices, and manner of preparing foods. The predominant minority ethnic groups in America are African American and Hispanic. African Americans brought some of their food traditions from West Africa — foods such as peanuts, black-eyed peas, and okra — and these foods were combined with American Indian foods such as sweet potatoes, wild game, fish, and greens. Table 9.9 lists some foods to choose often and less often when dining at various ethnic restaurants.

✳ Table 9.9
Multicultural Eating Guide

	Choose Often	Choose Less Often
Chinese	Beef with broccoli Chinese greens Rice, brown or white Steamed beef with pea pods Steamed rice Stir-fry dishes Teriyaki beef or chicken Wonton soup	Crispy duck Egg rolls Fried Rice Kung pao (fried chicken) Peking duck Pork spare ribs
East Indian	Chapati (tortilla-like bread) Chicken tandoor Dal (lentils) Kami (chick-pea soup) Khur (milk/rice dessert) Tandoori, chicken or fish	Bhatura (fried bread) Coconut milk or soup Fried shrimp with poori Ghee (clarified butter) Korma (rich meat dish) Samosa (fried meat and vegetables in dough)
Japanese	Chiri nabe (fish stew) Grilled scallops Sushi, sashimi (raw fish) Teriyaki Yakitori (grilled chicken)	Tempura (fried chicken, shrimp, or vegetables) Tonkatsu (fried pork)
Thai	Forest salad Larb (minty chicken salad) Po tak (seafood soup) Yum neua (broiled beef with onions)	Fried fish, duck, or chicken Curries with coconut milk Yum koon chaing (sausage with peppers)
Italian	Cioppino (seafood stew) Minestrone soup (vegetarian) Pasta with marinara sauce Pasta primavera (pasta with vegetables) Steamed clams	Antipasto Cannelloni, ravioli Fettucini alfredo Garlic bread White clam sauce
Mexican	Beans and rice Black bean/vegetable soup Burritos, bean Chili Enchiladas, bean Fajitas Gazpacho Taco salad Tamales Tortillas, steamed	Chilies rellenos Chimichangas Enchiladas, beef or cheese Flautas Guacamole Nachos Quesadillas Tostadas
Middle Eastern	Gyros Lentil soup Pita bread Rice pilaf Shish kebab	Baklava Falafel Mousaka
French	Poached salmon Spinach salad	Beef Wellington Escargot French onion soup Sauces in general
Soul Food	Baked chicken Baked fish Roasted pork (not smothered) Sauteed okra Baked sweet potato	Southern fried chicken Fried fish Smothered pork tenderloin Okra in gumbo Sweet potato casserole

Summary

1 The two major types of nutrients are energy nutrients (carbohydrates, fats, and proteins) and the regulatory nutrients (water, vitamins, and minerals).

2 The process of digestion begins when the food enters the mouth, moves through the esophagus to the stomach, small and large intestines, and exits through the rectum and anus.

3 Dietary fats are either saturated (animal) fats or unsaturated fats (which are further separated into monounsaturated and polyunsaturated fats).

4 Lipoproteins (fats combined with protein) are of three types: low density lipoprotein (LDL, or "bad" cholesterol), high density lipoprotein (HDL, or "good" cholesterol), and VLDL (very low density lipoprotein, which allows cholesterol to circulate in the bloodstream).

5 Complete proteins (usually from animal sources) contain the nine essential amino acids; incomplete proteins (from vegetable sources) contain only some of the essential amino acids.

6 Water is the most important nutrient, as it is needed in all bodily functions. Without it, the individual will die in less than a week.

7 Vitamins are of two major types: fat-soluble (associated with lipids) and water-soluble (cannot be stored long in the body).

8 The three essential minerals that the body needs daily are calcium, iron, and sodium (salt).

9 The U.S. government has established the Dietary Guidelines for Americans and the U.S. Recommended Dietary Allowances (RDAs), more recently replaced by the Daily Values (DVs).

10 The Food Guide Pyramid is the standard that replaced the Basic Four Food Groups with six categories: grain products; vegetables; fruits; meat, poultry, fish, dry beans, eggs, and nuts; milk, yogurt, cheese; and fats, oils, and sweets.

11 The Mediterranean Diet Pyramid recommends high consumption of complex carbohydrates, fruits, and vegetables but differs from the Food Guide Pyramid in the recommendation for use of olive oil (high in monounsaturated fat) and "wine in moderation."

12 The styles of vegetarians (plant food eaters) are lactovegetarian, ovolactovegetarian, vegan, and semivegetarian, based on whether dairy products and eggs are included.

13 Some people need vitamin and mineral supplements for specific purposes, but a balanced nutritional diet should preclude a blanket recommendation for supplementation.

14 Food substitutes and additives should be used advisedly.

15 Like the American menu, all ethnic foods include good and poor choices, usually based on the fat and salt content and method of preparation.

Select Bibliography

"Antioxidants: Never Too Late." *University of California Berkeley Wellness Letter*, 10:8 (1994), 2.

Applegate, L. "Ethnic Food Options." *Runner's World*, 10 (1993), 26-29. 26–27.

"American Cancer Society Guidelines on Diet, Nutrition, and Cancer." *Cancer Journal for Clinicians*, 41:6 (1991), 334–338.

"Are We Eating Right?" *Consumer Reports*, October, 1992.

Bean, A. "Iron Stores." *Runner's World*. 29:5 (1994), 34.

"Better Eating for Better Aging." *Food Insight Reports*, 1990, pp. 1-3.

Brody, J. *Jane Brody's Nutrition Book*. New York: Bantam, 1987.

Bruess, C. E. and Richardson, G. E. *Healthy Decisions*. Dubuque, IA: Wm C. Brown & Benchmark, 1994.

Cooper, Kenneth, *Antioxidant Revolution*. Nashville: Thomas Nelson, 1994.

"Dairy Does a Body Good." *Focus*, 1992, pp 1, 7.

"Diet May Shield Against Two Leading Cancer Killers." *Environmental Nutrition*, 15:2 (1992), 1, 3.

Dixon, Barbara. *Good Health for African Americans*. New York: Crown, 1994.

Dunne, Lavon J. *Nutrition Almanac*. New York: McGraw-Hill, 1990.

Floyd, P. A., et al. *Wellness: A Lifetime of Commitment*. Winston-Salem, NC: Hunter Publishing, 1993.

"Food Irradiation: The Controversy Heats Up." *Tufts University Diet & Nutrition Letter*, 10:1 (1992), A–6.

Garrison, R. H., and Somer, E. *The Nutrition Desk Reference*. New Canaan, CT: Keats, 1990.

"Growing Old Healthfully: Are Antioxidants the Answer?" *Environmental Nutrition*, 15:1 (1992), 1, 3.

Hafen, B. Q. and W. W. K. Hoeger. *Wellness: Guidelines for a Healthy Lifestyle*. Englewood, CO: Morton, 1994.

Hales, D. *An Invitation to Health*, 6th edition. Redwood City, CA: Benjamin/Cummings Publishing, 1994.

"The HDL Triglyceride Trap." *Nutrition Action Newsletter*, 17:7 (1990), 1–7.

Hoeger, W.W. K. *Principles and Labs*, 3d edition. Englewood, CO: Morton, 1994.

Human Nutrition Information Service. *Food Guide Pyramid*. Hyattsville, MD: U. S. Department of Agriculture, 1992.

Hunter, B. T. "Strategies to Reduce Dietary Fat." *Consumers' Research*, 72:4 (1989), 29–31.

"The Importance of Fiber." *University of California Berkeley Wellness Letter*, 8:4 (1992), 2–3.

"Lactose Intolerance." In *Newsletter of Glaxo Institute For Digestive Health*, December, 1993.

"Lactose: Truth or Intolerance?" *Nutrition Action Newsletter*, 18:3, (1991), 8–9.

"The Latest on Caffeine and Pregnancy," *University of California Berkeley Wellness Letter*, 10:6 (1994), 2.

Miller, L. "Antioxidants to the Rescue." *Runner's World*, 28:10 (1993), 30–32.

Nutrition and Your Health: Dietary Guidelines For Americans, 3d edition. Washington DC: Government Printing Office, 1990.

"Nutrition Counselors: Whom Can You Trust?" *Environmental Nutrition*, 15:2 (1992), 1, 3.

Stamford, B. "What Cholesterol Means to You." *Physician and Sportsmedicine*, 18:1 (1990), 150.

"Taking Supplements Seriously." *Nutrition Action Newsletter*, 18:8 (1991), 1–8.

"What Cholesterol Means to You." *Physician and Sportsmedicine*, 18:1 (1990), 149–150.

"Udder Confusion." *University of California Berkeley Wellness Letter*, 10:8 (1994), 1-2.

Fruits and Vegetables In Your Diet

NAME _____ DATE _____

COURSE _____ SECTION _____

Food Guide Pyramid
A Guide to Daily Food Choices

_____, _____, & _____

USE _____

_____

_____ & _____
Group
_____ SERVINGS

_____

Group
_____ SERVINGS

KEY
● Fat (naturally occurring and added)   ▼ Sugars (added)

These symbols show fats, oils, and added sugars in foods.

_____

_____, _____, _____,
_____ & _____
_____ **Group**
_____ SERVINGS

_____

_____ **Group**
_____ SERVINGS

_____, _____,
_____, & _____
Group
_____ SERVINGS

Does Your Diet Measure Up?

NAME _____ DATE _____

COURSE _____ SECTION _____

The 40 questions below will help you focus on the key features of your diet. The (+) or (−) numbers under each set of answers instantly pat you on the back for good habits or alert you to problems you may not even realize you have.

The Grand Total rates your overall diet, on a scale from "Great" to "Arghh!"

The quiz focuses on fat, cholesterol, sodium, sugar, fiber, and vitamins A and C. It doesn't attempt to cover everything in your diet. Also, it doesn't try to measure precisely how much of these key nutrients you eat. What the quiz will do is give you a rough sketch of your current eating habits and, implicitly, suggest what you can do to improve them.

Don't despair over a less-than-perfect score. A healthy diet isn't built overnight.

INSTRUCTIONS

Under each answer is a number with a + or − sign in front of it. Circle the number that is directly beneath the answer you choose. That's your score for the question. (If you use a pencil, you can erase your answers and give the quiz to someone else.)

Circle only one number for each question, unless the instructions tell you to "average two or more scores if necessary."

How to average: In answering question 18, for example, if you drink club soda (+3) and coffee (−1) on a typical day, add the two scores (which gives you +2) and then divide by 2. That gives you a score of +1 for the question. If averaging gives you a fraction, round it to the nearest whole number.

If a question doesn't apply to you, skip it.

Pay attention to serving sizes. For example, a serving of vegetables is 1/2 cup. If you usually eat one cup of vegetables at a time, count it as two servings.

Add up all your + scores and your − scores.

Subtract your − scores from your + scores. That's your GRAND TOTAL.

QUIZ

1. How many times per week do you eat unprocessed red meat (steak, roast beef, lamb or pork chops, burgers, etc.)?

   (a) never   (b) 1 or less   (c) 2–3   (d) 4–5   (e) 6 or more
      +3   +2   0   −1   −3

2. After cooking, how large is the serving of red meat you usually eat? (To convert from raw to cooked, reduce by 25%. For example, 4 oz. of raw meat shrinks to 3 oz. after cooking. There are 16 oz. in a pound.)

   (a) 8 oz. or more   (b) 6–7 oz.   (c) 4–5 oz.   (d) 3 oz. or less
        −3   −2   −1   0

   (e) don't eat red meat
        +3

3. Do you trim the visible fat when you cook or eat red meat?

   (a) yes   (b) no   (c) don't eat red meat
     +1   −3   0

4. How many times per week do you eat processed meats (hot dogs, bacon, sausage, bologna, luncheon meats, etc.)? *(OMIT products that contain 1 gram of fat or less per serving.)*

   (a) none   (b) less than 1   (c) 1-2   (d) 3–4   (e) 5 or more
     +3   +2   0   −1   −3

5. What kind of ground meat or poultry do you usually eat?

   (a) regular ground beef   (b) lean ground beef
          −3   −2

   (c) ground round   (d) ground turkey
         0   +1

   (e) Healthy Choice™   (f) don't eat ground meat
         +2   +3

6. What type of bread do you usually eat?

   (a) whole wheat or other whole grain   (b) rye
              +3   +2

   (c) pumpernickel   (d) white, "wheat," French, or Italian
         +2   −2

7. How many times per week do you eat deep-fried foods (fish, chicken, vegetables, potatoes, etc.)?

   (a) none   (b) 1–2   (c) 3–4   (d) 5 or more
      +3   0   −1   −3

8. How many servings of non-fried vegetables do you usually eat per day? *(One serving = 1/2 cup. INCLUDE potatoes.)*

   (a) none   (b) 1   (c) 2   (d) 3   (e) 4 or more
      −3   0   +1   +2   +3

9. How many servings of cruciferous vegetables do you usually eat per week? *(ONLY count kale, broccoli, cauliflower, cabbage, Brussels sprouts, greens, bok choy, kohlrabi, turnip, and rutabaga. One serving = 1/2 cup.)*

   (a) none   (b) 1–3   (c) 4–6   (d) 7 or more
      −3   +1   +2   +3

10. How many servings of vitamin-A-rich fruits or vegetables do you usually eat per week? *(ONLY count carrots, pumpkin, sweet potatoes, cantaloupe, spinach, winter squash, greens, and apricots. One serving = 1/2 cup.)*

    (a) none   (b) 1-3   (c) 4–6   (d) 7 or more
       −3   +1   +2   +3

11. How many times per week do you eat at a fast-food restaurant? *(INCLUDE burgers, fried fish or chicken, croissant or biscuit sandwiches, topped potatoes, and other main dishes. OMIT meals of just plain baked potato, broiled chicken, or salad.)*

    (a) never   (b) less than 1   (c) 1   (d) 2   (e) 3
       +3   +1   0   −1   −2

    (f) 4 or more
       −3

12. How many servings of grains rich in complex carbohydrates do you eat per day? *(One serving = 1 slice of bread, 1 large pancake, 1 cup whole grain cold cereal, or 1/2 cup cooked cereal, rice, pasta, bulgur, wheat berries, kasha, or millet. OMIT heavily-sweetened cold cereals.)*

    (a) none   (b) 1–3   (c) 4–5   (d) 6–8   (e) 9 or more
       −3   0   +1   +2   +3

13. How many times per week do you eat fish or shellfish? *(OMIT deep-fried items, tuna packed in oil, shrimp, squid, and mayonnaise-laden tuna salad — a little mayo is okay.)*

    (a) never   (b) 1–2   (c) 3–4   (d) 5 or more
       −2   +1   +2   +3

14. How many times per week do you eat cheese? *(INCLUDE pizza, cheeseburgers, veal or eggplant parmigiana, cream cheese, etc. OMIT low-fat or fat-free cheeses.)*

    (a) 1 or less   (b) 2–3   (c) 4–5   (d) 6 or more
       +3   +2   −1   −3

15. How many servings of fresh fruit do you eat per day?

    (a) none   (b) 1   (c) 2   (d) 3   (e) 4 or more
       −3   0   +1   +2   +3

16. Do you remove the skin before eating poultry?

    (a) yes   (b) no   (c) don't eat poultry
       +3   −3   0

17. What do you usually put on your bread or toast? *(AVERAGE two or more scores if necessary.)*

    (a) butter/cream cheese   (b) margarine/peanut butter
           −3   −2

    (c) diet margarine   (d) jam or honey
         −1   0

    (e) fruit butter   (f) nothing
         +1   +3

18. Which of these beverages do you drink on a typical day? *(AVERAGE two or more scores if necessary.)*

    (a) water or club soda   (b) fruit juice   (c) diet soda
          +3   +1   −1

    (d) coffee or tea   (e) soda, fruit "drink," or fruit "ade"
         −1   −3

19. Which flavorings do you add to your foods most frequently? *(AVERAGE two or more scores if necessary.)*

    (a) garlic or lemon juice   (b) herbs or spices
          +3   +3

    (c) salt or soy sauce   (d) margarine   (e) butter   (f) nothing
          −2   −2   −3   +3

20. What do you eat most frequently as a snack? *(AVERAGE two or more scores if necessary.)*

    (a) fruits or vegetables   (b) sweetened yogurt   (c) nuts
          +3   +2   −1

    (d) cookies or fried chips   (e) granola bar
          −2   −2

    (f) candy bar or pastry   (g) nothing
          −3   0

21. What is your most typical breakfast? *(SUBTRACT an extra 3 points if you also eat bacon or sausage.)*

    (a) croissant, danish, or doughnut   (b) eggs
                 −3   −3

    (c) pancakes or waffles   (d) cereal or toast
           −2   +3

    (e) low-fat yogurt or cottage cheese (f) don't eat breakfast
             +3   0

22. What do you usually eat for dessert?

    (a) pie, pastry, or cake   (b) ice cream
           −3   −3

    (c) fat-free cookies or cakes   (d) frozen yogurt or ice milk
              −1   +1

    (e) nonfat ice cream or sorbet   (f) fruit
             +1   +3

    (g) don't eat dessert
         +3

23. How many times per week do you eat beans, split peas, or lentils?

(a) none   (b) 1   (c) 2   (d) 3 or more
   −2   +1   +2   +3

24. What kind of milk do you drink?

(a) whole   (b) 2% low-fat   (c) 1% low-fat
   −3   −1   +2

(d) 1/2% or skim   (e) none
      +3   0

25. What dressings or toppings do you usually add to your salads? *(ADD two or more scores if necessary.)*

(a) nothing, lemon, or vinegar   (b) fat-free dressing
         +3   +2

(c) low- or reduced-calorie dressing   (d) regular dressing
            +1   −1

(e) croutons or bacon bits
         −1

(f) cole slaw, pasta salad, or potato salad
         −1

26. What sandwich fillings do you eat most frequently? *(AVERAGE two or more scores if necessary.)*

(a) luncheon meat   (b) cheese or roast beef
      −3   −1

(c) peanut butter   (d) low-fat luncheon meat
      0   +1

(e) tuna, salmon, chicken, or turkey
         +3

(f) don't eat sandwiches
         0

27. What do you usually spread on your sandwiches? *(AVERAGE two or more scores if necessary.)*

(a) mayonnaise   (b) light mayonnaise
     −2   −1

(c) ketchup, mustard, or fat-free mayonnaise   (d) nothing
               0   +2

28. How many egg yolks do you eat per week? *(ADD 1 yolk for every slice of quiche you eat.)*

(a) 2 or less   (b) 3–4   (c) 5–6   (d) 7 or more
     +3   0   −1   −3

29. How many times per week do you eat canned or dried soups? *(OMIT low-sodium, low-fat soups.)*

(a) none   (b) 1–2   (c) 3–4   (d) 5 or more
   +3   0   −2   −3

30. How many servings of a rich source of calcium do you eat per day? *(One serving = 2/3 cup milk or yogurt, 1 oz. cheese, 1½ oz. sardines, 3½ oz. salmon, 5 oz. tofu made with calcium sulfate, 1 cup greens or broccoli, or 200 mg of a calcium supplement.)*

(a) none   (b) 1   (c) 2   (d) 3 or more
   −3   +1   +2   +3

31. What do you usually order on your pizza? *(Vegetable toppings include green pepper, mushrooms, onions, and other vegetables. SUBTRACT 1 point from your score if you order extra cheese.)*

(a) no cheese with vegetables   (b) cheese with vegetables
            +3   +1

(c) cheese   (d) cheese with meat toppings
     0   −3

(e) don't eat pizza
      +2

32. What kind of cookies do you usually eat?

(a) graham crackers or ginger snaps   (b) oatmeal
            +1   −1

(c) sandwich cookies (like Oreos)
         −2

(d) chocolate coated, chocolate chip, or peanut butter
                  −3

(e) don't eat cookies
      +3

33. What kind of frozen dessert do you usually eat? *(SUBTRACT 1 point from your score for each topping you use — whipped cream, hot fudge, nuts, etc.)*

(a) gourmet ice cream   (b) regular ice cream
        −3   −1

(c) sorbet, sherbet, or ices
         +1

(d) frozen yogurt, fat-free ice cream, or ice milk
                  +1

(e) don't eat frozen desserts
         +3

34. What kind of cake or pastry do you usually eat?

(a) cheesecake, pie, or any microwave cake
                  −3

(b) cake with frosting or filling   (c) cake without frosting
         −2   −1

(d) unfrosted muffin, banana bread, or carrot cake
                  0

(e) angelfood or fat-free cake
         +1

(f) don't eat cakes or pastries
         +3

35. How many times per week does your dinner contain grains, vegetables, or beans, but little or no animal protein (meat, poultry, fish, eggs, milk, or cheese)?

(a) none   (b) 1–2   (c) 3–4   (d) 5 or more
   −1   +1   +2   +3

36. Which of the following salty snacks do you typically eat? *(AVERAGE two or more scores if necessary.)*

(a) potato chips, corn chips, or packaged popcorn
−3

(b) reduced-fat potato or tortilla chips   (c) salted pretzels
−2   −1

(d) unsalted pretzels or baked corn or tortilla chips
+1

(e) homemade air-popped popcorn
+3

(f) don't eat salty snacks
+3

37. What do you usually use to saute vegetables or other foods? *(Vegetable oil includes safflower, corn, canola, olive, sunflower, and soybean.)*

(a) butter or lard
−3

(b) more than one tablespoon of margarine or vegetable oil
−1

(c) no more than one tablespoon or margarine or vegetable oil
0

(d) no more than one tablespoon of olive oil
+1

(e) water or broth
+2

38. What kind of cereal do you usually eat?

(a) whole grain (like oatmeal or shredded wheat)
+3

(b) low-fiber (like cream of wheat or corn flakes)
0

(c) sugary low-fiber (like frosted flakes)   (d) granola
−1   −2

39. With what do you make tuna salad, pasta salad, chicken salad, etc.?

(a) mayonnaise   (b) light mayonnaise
−2   −1

(c) nonfat mayonnaise   (d) low-fat yogurt
0   +2

(e) nonfat yogurt
+3

40. What do you typically put on your pasta? *(ADD one point if you also add sauteed vegetables. AVERAGE two or more scores if necessary.)*

(a) tomato sauce   (b) tomato sauce with a little parmesan
+3   +3

(c) white clam sauce   (d) meat sauce or meat balls
+1   −2

(e) Alfredo, pesto, or other creamy sauce
−3

YOUR GRAND TOTAL

+59 to +116	GREAT!	You're a nutrition superstar. Give yourself a big (non-butter) pat on the back.
0 to +58	GOOD	Pin your quiz on the nearest wall.
−58 to −1	FAIR	Hang in there
−117 to −59	ARGHH!	Empty your refrigerator and cupboard. It's time to start over.

Copyright © 1994, Center for Science in the Public Interest. Reprinted by permission.

Weight Management

10

OBJECTIVES

* Explain body composition and the metabolic rate.

* Differentiate *overweight* and *obesity* and describe their relationship to major health problems.

* Explain three theories of obesity.

* Discuss three unhealthy eating disorders and the differences between them.

* Identify three aids to determine if you are overweight or underweight.

* Describe three methods for assessing body composition.

* Discuss gimmicks and diet aids.

* Design a personal weight management program.

The American culture is obsessed with thinness, manifested in weight-loss programs, exercise equipment, health clubs, appetite-reducing pills, cellulite creams, gels, liquid diets, and books to assist us in our ultimate dream of having that perfect, thin body. Chubby Americans have tried at least one diet or "miracle" weight product — diet drinks, low-protein formulas, "miracle" creams — that promises to melt fat away. Americans are getting fatter as the diet industry is booming. The annual cost of diet products and services is estimated to exceed $40 billion. This

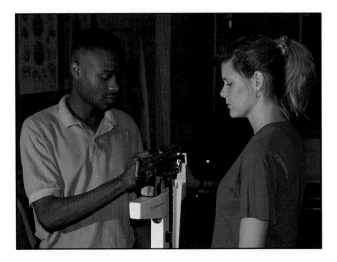

represents about 15% of the total health-care costs in the United States. Even though Americans spend enormous amounts of time and money to adjust their weight, few keep the weight off. They lose 10 pounds or so only to find that these pounds return — and more.

Another population consists of individuals with eating disorders — anorexia nervosa, bulimia nervosa, and binge eating. The physical and psychological forces at work in eating disorders are complex, and the cultural focus on thinness is a contributor.

Weight *management* is stressed in this chapter. If a person is too heavy or too light, changes are necessary for a healthier future. Despite the emphasis on thinness in our society, obesity and overweight remain a major health problem. What are the reasons people eat? The usual answers are: "I'm frustrated . . . bored . . . sad . . . for social reasons." Almost never is *hunger* given as an answer.

At the core of weight change are theories based on body composition and metabolism including genetic predisposition, setpoint, and fat cell hypertrophy and hyperplasia. People can apply this knowledge to weight loss or gain by first assessing their body composition and taking steps to produce the desired results. Aids to measure thinness or fatness are height/weight tables, body mass index (BMI), and waist-to-hip ratio. Tools used to measure body composition include hydrostatic weighing, skinfold measurements, and bioelectrical impedance analysis. The remaining variables — attitude, commitment, determination, and motivation — are psychological.

BODY COMPOSITION AND METABOLIC RATE

Body composition refers to the proportion of body tissue that consists of fat (adipose tissue), referred to as **% body fat,** and nonfat tissue (muscles, bone, and organs such as the heart, brain, liver, and kidneys), called **lean body mass.** The ratio of body fat to lean body mass, rather than total body weight, is what is important. Excessive fat is unhealthy because it increases the risk for chronic diseases.

Total body fat is further broken down into two types: (a) **essential fat,** needed for normal physiological functioning, and (b) **storage fat,** stored mainly beneath the skin and around major organs. Its basic functions are as an insulator to retain body heat, as a source of energy for metabolism, and as padding against physical trauma. Storage fat is lost through exercise and lean diet, but if a person loses too much storage fat, the body will resort to using up essential fat for producing energy. This may be detrimental to health.

Body composition is one of the four components of health-related fitness. The others are cardiovascular endurance, muscular flexibility, and muscular strength and endurance (discussed in Chapter 11). Because diet is a major determinant of body composition, and of health-related fitness, its regulation is essential to a healthy life.

One pound of fat equals 3500 calories.

A balance between caloric intake and caloric expenditure is necessary to maintain proper body fat content. The **energy-balancing equation** basically states that when caloric input equals caloric output, the individual does not gain or lose weight. If caloric intake exceeds output, the person gains weight. When caloric output exceeds input, the person loses weight. One pound of fat equals 3500 calories. If a person's daily caloric expenditure is 2500 calories, this person should be able to lose about 1 pound of fat in 1 week by decreasing the daily intake of calories by 500 calories per day (500 × 7 = 3500). Or the calories could be expended by doing various exercises. Table 10.1 lists the caloric expenditure of selected activities.

By consulting calorie charts for various foods and exercises, a person theoretically should be able to achieve an optimum weight by following a precisely determined formula of diet and physical activity. Unfortunately, translating the energy-balancing equation to one's life is not that simple. It relates to differences in human metabolism and other lifestyle factors such as physical activity and composition of one's diet.

Metabolism refers to how the body utilizes its fuel from nutrients (food) to carry on vital processes. The metabolic rate is the total amount of energy the body expends in a given time and, hence, the number of calories it uses, either at rest or while active. Most of the energy (55% to 75%) is required to maintain vital bodily functions including respiration, temperature regulation, and blood pressure while the body is at rest (called

Table 10.1
Expenditure of Calories for Selected Activities

Activity	Approximate Calories Expended per Hour
Ballroom dancing	330
Bicycling 5½ miles	210
Bowling	264
Desk work	132
Driving a car	168
Gardening	220
Golf	300
Horseback riding (trot)	480
Ironing (standing up)	252
Lawn mowing (hand mower)	462
Painting at an easel	120
Piano playing	150
Preparing a meal	198
Roller skating	350
Running 10 mph	900
Sitting and eating	84
Sitting in a chair reading	72
Skiing	594
Sleeping (basal metabolism)	60
Standing up	138
Swimming (leisurely)	300
Tennis	420
Volleyball	350
Walking (2.5 miles per hour)	216
Walking downstairs	312

Source: *Nutrition Almanac*, 3d edition, by Lavon J. Dunne (New York: McGraw-Hill, 1990).

basal metabolic rate (BMR) or resting metabolic rate). The energy required to digest food accounts for 5% to 15% of the daily energy expenditure, and 10% to 40% of energy is expended during physical activity.

The metabolic rate depends on a variety of factors including:

❋ *Body size and composition.* The more muscle and less fat you have, the more energy your body will use even when at rest. If an obese person and a person who is not obese weigh exactly the same, the obese person has a lower metabolic rate.

❋ *Sex.* In general, males develop more muscle tissue than females. Therefore, men tend to have a higher metabolic rate than women.

❋ *Diet.* Diet has little effect on the resting metabolic rate, but when, what, how much, and how often you eat all have a temporary effect on metabolic rate. Constant dieting may lower the metabolic rate. After repeatedly losing and gaining weight, the body may increase its metabolic efficiency by reducing the number of calories required to maintain body functions (the set-point theory, discussed next). Each time a person diets, he or she loses weight more slowly and gains it back more quickly.

❋ *Age.* Lean body mass decreases after age 30, at an average rate of 3% per decade for active people and 5% per decade for sedentary people. Therefore, as we age, we lose muscle mass, and our metabolic rate slows down.

❋ *Genetic factors.* Inherited factors have a relatively minor effect on resting metabolism.

❋ *Hormones.* Thyroid hormone helps to regulate metabolic rate. Therefore, certain thyroid disorders affect metabolic rate. Thyroid pills will not increase metabolic rate in healthy people except when taken in dangerously high amounts.

❋ *Activity level.* By exercising regularly and watching your weight, you can increase your overall metabolic rate. Exercise is important to long-term weight control. Exercise increases the resting metabolic rate and lean body mass (associated with higher metabolic rate). Exercise expends calories, thus raising total energy expenditure. The more energy is expended, the more calories a person can consume without gaining weight.

KEY TERMS

Body composition proportionate amounts of fat tissue and nonfat tissue in the body

Total body fat (% body fat) adipose tissue as a percent of total body tissue

Lean body mass nonfat body tissue made up of muscle, bone, and organs

Essential fat body fat needed for normal physiological functioning

Storage fat fat found beneath the skin and around major organs that acts as an insulator, as padding, and as a source of energy for metabolism

Energy-balancing equation formula stating that when caloric input equals caloric output, an individual does not gain or lose weight

THEORIES OF WEIGHT DETERMINATION

Several theories have emerged concerning weight determination. Inherited factors undoubtedly play a role, but the true extent has not been determined. Other factors probably have a more significant influence. Two contemporary theories that have some credibility are the setpoint theory and a theory of fat cell hypertrophy and hyperplasia.

Genetic Predisposition

You have your parents' eyes, body build, and even their smile. If you have a weight problem, did you inherit that from your parents as well? Yes, your natural weight has a genetic component. An estimated 80% of identical twins reared apart weigh almost the same as each other throughout their lives. These studies suggest that you have a genetically given weight that your body wants to maintain.

A diet high in complex carbohydrates, low in fat and sugar, plus regular aerobic exercise will lower the fat thermostat.

Genetic predisposition theory holds that inherited genes influence weight. Children inherit their general body type (height, bone structure) from their parents. Body fat can be altered, but body type cannot be changed. If both parents are overweight or obese, the child has an 80% chance of being overweight; if one parent is overweight or obese, 40%; and with neither parent overweight or obese, a 7% chance of being overweight or obese. Therefore, if obesity runs in the family, the chances of the children being overweight are higher.

Genes influence body weight, size, type, and the propensity toward obesity. Also, the pattern of fat distribution in the body (hips, waist, abdomen) is a function of heredity. Your food preferences are not inherited, however. They are set during childhood for the most part. If you were brought up on sweets and junk foods, they probably remain an important part of your diet. On the other hand, if you were brought up on healthy foods, you probably include them regularly in your diet.

In sum, heredity forms a strong foundation for obesity. Even so, family environment, parents' food consumption patterns, and your exercise habits strongly influence what is built on that foundation.

Setpoint Theory

Satiety is defined as a feeling of fullness. You stop eating when you feel satisfied. A common habit acquired during childhood is to eat long after we have eaten enough. As kids, we were told, "Children are starving in Africa; finish what's on your plate." Therefore, we learned to clean our plates out of guilt, not hunger. This is especially true when dining out because people feel compelled to eat food they pay for.

The **setpoint** theory holds that each individual has a weight-regulating mechanism in the hypothalamus of the brain, which controls how much we weigh. When the body's fat falls too low, this internal thermostat triggers an increase in food intake by increasing our appetite, so we eat more.

A low-calorie diet will not lower the setpoint. Even though a person will lose fat and weight, the weight will return when the person returns to regular eating patterns. Under no circumstances should a woman eat fewer than 1200 calories a day (small women, 1000 calories a day), and men should not eat fewer than 1800 calories a day (small men, 1500 calories a day). Very low-calorie diets deprive the body of basic nutrients needed for normal functioning and lower the resting metabolic rate.

A combination of a diet high in complex carbohydrates and low in fat and sugar plus regular aerobic exercise is the most practical way to lower the fat thermostat. Amphetamines and nicotine have been shown to lower the fat thermostat, but the drawbacks outweigh the benefits.

Fat Cell Hypertrophy and Hyperplasia Theory

According to the **fat cell hypertrophy** and **hyperplasia** theory, the quantity of fat in the body is the result of the size (hypertrophy) and the number (hyperplasia) of fat cells a person has. Hyperplasia occurs after birth, again at age 5–6, and during puberty. Most researchers believe that at these times increasing body fat increases the number of fat cells in the body. On the other hand, losing body fat does not change that number. Therefore, when weight is gained, the number of fat cells increases, but when weight is lost, the fat cells are still there.

Childhood-onset obesity is thought to be the result of developing too many fat cells. Adult-onset obesity is thought to be the result of developing larger, rather than more, fat cells. Some obese people have the combined problem of large fat cells *and* too many fat cells. The more fat cells, the greater is the capacity to store more energy in the form of fat.

OVERWEIGHT AND OBESITY

The terms *overweight* and *obese* often are used interchangeably. This is incorrect because the two have different meanings. **Overweight** designates the body weight that exceeds the normal or standard weight for an individual based on population averages for frame size and height. Using these height/weight tables (discussed later) a professional athlete or weight lifter could be considered overweight, yet have a body fat content that is average or below average. According to these standards, individuals often are overweight but few are overfat. On the other end of the spectrum are individuals who are within the normal range of body weight for their frame size and height but still might have too much body fat.

Obesity is a condition in which the person has an excessive amount of body fat. Obesity is a major contributor to coronary heart disease (hypertension, atherosclerosis, congestive heart failure). The more a person weighs, the more blood vessels the body needs to circulate blood throughout the body. It often is said that every pound of extra fat requires a mile of blood vessels. The heart takes on a heavy burden as it has to pump harder to force the blood flow through so many vessels. As a result, the heart grows in size and blood pressure tends to rise. Overweight also is a factor in osteoarthritis (because of the extra weight placed on the joints), gout, bone and joint diseases (including ruptured intervertebral discs), varicose veins, respiratory ailments, gallbladder disease, complications during pregnancy and delivery, and higher accidental death rate.

Obesity can alter hormone levels, which may cause impotence in men and reproductive problems in women. Women who are 30% overweight are twice as likely to die of endometrial cancer, and those who are 40% overweight have four times the risk. Obese women are also more likely to incur cancers of the breast, cervix, ovaries, and gallbladder. Obese men are more likely to develop cancers of the rectum, colon, esophagus, bladder, pancreas, stomach, and prostate.

According to Dr. Richard J. Flanigan, Denver cardiologist, people who are obese are "digging their own grave with their teeth." They eat too much, and they eat the wrong kind of food in the wrong amounts. Suffice it to say, individuals who want to be healthy cannot ignore their weight. And minority groups, particularly women, are at even greater risk because of their higher prevalence of overweight and obesity.

An obese person has 20% or more body weight above the recommended weight for a person of that height and sex. That is about 25 pounds for an average 5'4" woman and 30 pounds for a 5'10" man. According to the National Institutes of Health Technology Assessment Conference Panel's 1992 report, one-quarter to one-third of all Americans are 20% or more overweight. The categories for obesity are:

Mild obesity:
    20%–40% above recommended weight

Moderate obesity:
    41%–99% above recommended weight

Severe obesity:
    100% or more above recommended weight

Prevalence

In the past 10 years the average weight of American adults has increased by approximately 15 pounds. At any given time an estimated 20% of men and 40% of women are trying to lose weight.

KEY TERMS

Genetic predisposition theory stating that inherited genes influence weight

Satiety feeling of fullness

Setpoint theory stating that individuals have a weight-regulating mechanism in the hypothalamus of the brain that controls how much we weigh

Fat cell hypertrophy and hyperplasia theory stating that the quantity of fat in the body is the result of the size and number of fat cells a person has

Overweight body weight that exceeds the normal or standard weight for an individual

Obesity a condition in which a person has an excessive amount of body fat

---

Telltale Signs of a Fatter America

"As a whole, we are probably the fattest people ever." So proclaimed Dr. Boyd Eaton, an Atlanta-based radiologist and anthropology professor at Emory University who has studied the course of health across the history of human beings.

Consider the following:

❋ In the past 7 years young adults age 25–30 have gained an average of 10 pounds.

❋ The sale of queen-size mattresses has passed that of double-size mattresses in the 1990s.

❋ The average man now wears a size 42 regular suit, up from a size 40 a decade ago.

❋ A third of American women now wear a size 16 or larger, and some manufacturers are cutting their clothes fuller but still applying the same size, so a size 10 is not the same as a size 10 was 5 years ago.

❋ The average woman wears a size 36B or C bra, up from the former 34B.

❋ Automakers like Ford have lengthened their seat tracks from about 5½" a decade ago to about 9" now, which allows drivers to push back from the steering wheel.

❋ Steelcase, leading manufacturer of office furniture, is introducing the Criterion Plus, an office chair that can handle up to 500 pounds (up from the current capacity of 225 pounds).

❋ A popular new toilet model has a seat about 2" longer and 1/2" wider than the standard model.

❋ Liposuction procedures in hospitals numbered about 300,000 in 1994.

❋ Yankee Stadium lost 7,465 seats when it was renovated in 1976, mainly because of the wider replacement seats needed.

❋ 60% of the U. S. population did not pursue any leisure-time physical activity in 1990, according to the U. S. Centers for Disease Control and Prevention.

Source: David Jacobson, *Detroit News*, reprinted in the *Denver Post*, September 28, 1994, p. F1.

Dr. F. Xauler Pi-Sunyer wrote in the *Journal of the American Medical Association*, "The proportion of the population that is obese is incredible. If this was about tuberculosis, it would be called an epidemic." Dr. Robert Suskind, co-director of the Weight Reduction Clinic at the Children's Hospital of New Orleans, stated that at least one-fourth of U. S. children are overweight, and 70% of children who are overweight at ages 10–13 will become overweight adults. The Centers for Disease Control and Prevention reported in the winter of 1994 that 21% of America's teenagers are overweight, up from 15% in the 1970s. Experts are blaming too much junk food, and TV watching instead of exercising. Figure 10.1 shows the trends in weight gain for adults by age group and gender.

A study by the National Center for Health Statistics (NCHS), and the Centers for Disease Control and Prevention (CDC), reported in the summer of 1994 that African American and Mexican-American women had the highest proportion of overweight (defined as 20% or more above recommended weight) individuals — approaching half!

The percentage of overweight Anglo-American women was 33%. Weight gain was most likely among African American women ages 25–34. By way of comparison, about 31% of African American men were overweight. In the age ranges of 20–44, only 10% of African American men were overweight, compared to 16% of Anglo American men. Further, African American women and men and Anglo-American men tend to carry their weight above the waist, which is associated with higher risk for heart disease. Anglo-American women tend to accumulate pounds below the waist, which is less risky but also more difficult to lose.

A limited study by NCHS for the Hispanic Health and Nutrition Examination Survey (HHANES) in 1992–94 found that 39% of the Mexican-American women and 30% of the Mexican-American men were overweight. The rates varied by ethnic origin (e. g., Puerto Rico, Cuba). We can assume that these groups, too, have not escaped the burgeoning increase in the number of overweight and obese people during the last decade.

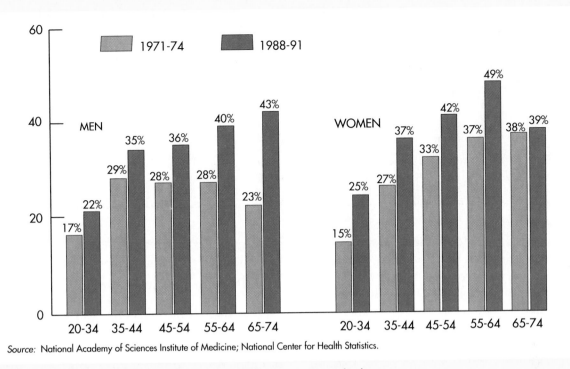

Source: National Academy of Sciences Institute of Medicine; National Center for Health Statistics.

Figure 10.1 Percentage of Americans who are overweight, by age group

People of lower education and income levels, regardless of race, tend to weigh more than people who are better educated and earn more. Rural and southern populations are more overweight than city dwellers and northern and western populations of the United States.

The most obvious culprit is diet. The heavier populations consume a diet high in fatty and fried foods, exemplified by the typical "soul food." Another factor is a cultural group's overall attitude toward weight. Many African American women, for example, do not consider overweight to be a problem, and they tend to think they should weigh much more than is healthy for them. Cultural differences in the standard for beauty (a "fine brown frame") give the message to many African American women that being a little larger is okay. Although this flies in the face of the prevailing societal overemphasis on being slim, ignoring or underestimating the consequences of being overweight is destructive, too.

Diets and Dieting

U. S. government studies recommend that losing even a moderate amount of weight can improve the

health of millions of people. But diets are not the answer. Diets do not teach people how to eat properly even though some people may lose weight by dieting.

Almost no strict, low-calorie diet works over the long term. Diets merely restrict one's food intake temporarily, so when the diet ends, weight gain resumes. Results of dozens of scientific studies in clinical settings show that 90% to 95% of obese persons gain back the weight lost in 5 years; only approximately 10% remain thin. Robert E. T. Stark, chairman of the board of the American Society of Bariatric Physicians (specializing in the treatment of obesity), said, "Of course they gain it back. They've used unrealistic diet methods." He added that food deprivation has a way of backfiring.

Many experiments have been done with rats that were overfed until they were obese, then put on a restricted diet. After reaching a lean weight, they were overfed again. The cycle was repeated. The second time the rats took more than twice as long to lose the same amount of weight. Even though experiments have not used humans, humans may follow the same pattern. After a strict

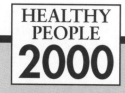

HEALTHY PEOPLE 2000

OBJECTIVES FOR WEIGHT LOSS

❋ Reduce overweight among low-income women age 20 and older.

❋ Reduce overweight among black women age 20 and older, Hispanic women age 20 and older, and American Indians and Alaska Natives.

❋ Reduce overweight among men and women with high blood pressure.

❋ Increase the proportion of overweight people age 12 and older who adopt sound dietary practices combined with regular physical activity to attain appropriate body weight.

diet, the human body's metabolism seems to change. In one experiment researchers divided women of the same weight into two groups: those who had slimmed down to that weight and those who had never dieted. The first group used fewer calories doing normal activities then the second, even burning 10% fewer calories during sleep. The formerly obese people in the study who dieted and stayed thin ate an average of 1298 calories a day to maintain their new weight, whereas people of the same weight who had not restricted their diet could eat nearly 50% more and stay at that level. These results indicate that dieters always may have to eat less food if they want to stay thin.

EATING DISORDERS

While as many as a third of Americans are struggling with real concerns of overweight, more and more Americans are enmeshed in the relatively recent phenomenon of eating disorders. An eating disorder is a severe disturbance in eating behavior. As a result of the cultural emphasis on thinness, in combination with psychological and physiological factors that are not fully understood, people with eating disorders have a perception of being "too fat," which may not be the case at all. They engage in destructive eating behaviors under the veneer of weight control. These disorders are obsessive and in most cases require intensive intervention. In addition to the psychological component, possible physical components are hypothesized to be:

❋ a predisposition to eating disorders caused by a biological factor linked to clinical depression

❋ insufficient serotonin (a neurotransmitter that sends nerve messages to and from the brain)

❋ malfunctioning of the hypothalamus.

The three forms of eating disorders — anorexia nervosa, bulimia nervosa, and binge eating — are taking a toll on the health of a growing number of people. Eating disorders are more prevalent in adolescent girls and young women than in males, more common in Anglo-Americans than in African Americans, and more frequent in people under age 30 than in older people. The U. S. Department of Agriculture has estimated that 5% to 20% of college-age women are bulimic and that 1 in 100 females between ages 12 and 18 is anorexic. Males account for 5% to 10% of all cases of eating disorders.

More precise figures are not available because these are secretive diseases. Eating disorders, however, seem to be more common in middle and upper-middle socioeconomic groups, those to whom the cultural message of slimness may have the greatest appeal. Perhaps because African Americans have not subscribed as fully to the preoccupation with slimness, eating disorders are not as prevalent in that population. Even so, tennis star and Wimbledon finalist Zina Garrison-Jackson has acknowledged her battle with bulimia that began in 1983 following the death of her mother. Athletes as a whole, both male and female, have a greater prevalence of eating disorders, probably because they perceive (or have been coached to believe, in some cases) that they must sacrifice the nutritional principles that govern the general population if they are to win competitive events. Gymnasts and figure skaters are two examples. Occupations such as ballet and modeling also carry higher risks for eating disorders. A study out of Cornell University and Ithaca College (New York) reveals that 40% of 131 lightweight football players had dysfunctional eating patterns including binging and purging.

Eating disorders typically begin with a weight-loss diet. Food, of course, is not the real problem. Individuals with eating disorders usually have a poor self-image and low self-esteem.

Anorexia Nervosa

Anorexia nervosa is an eating disorder in which the person does not eat enough food to maintain normal body weight. This leads to severe weight loss, malnutrition, and possibly death. Of all anorexics, 90%–95% are female, and most are in the upper teen and college-age group, although the condition has been documented in middle-aged women and in children as young as 9. These individuals are more afraid of gaining weight or becoming fat than death from starvation. The typical anorexic starves herself on 50 to 100 calories a day. Often the pre-occupation with weight begins with a distressing situation, such as the loss of a boyfriend or parents' divorcing. Anorexia nervosa is characterized by:

✳ intense fear of becoming fat, even though the person is underweight

✳ a distorted body image that allows the person to "see" herself as overweight when she actually is underweight

✳ refusal to maintain body weight

✳ cessation of menstrual cycle

✳ failure to mature sexually or, if mature, loss of interest in sex.

Figure 10.2 points out the physical characteristics of anorexia nervosa. Physiologically, the anorexic's body tries to protect itself by lowering

KEY TERMS

Anorexia Nervosa an eating disorder in which a person does not eat enough food to maintain normal body weight

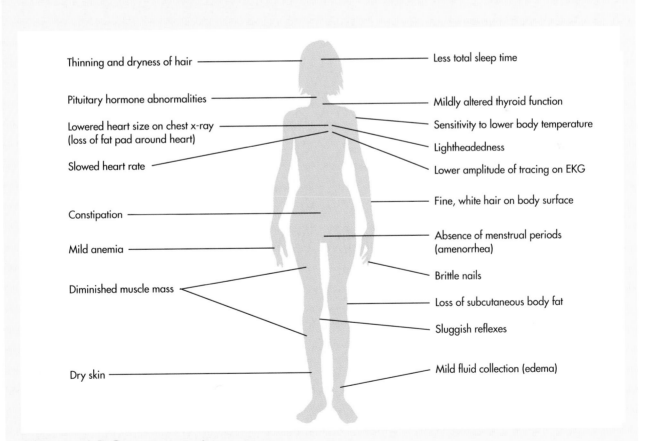

Thinning and dryness of hair

Pituitary hormone abnormalities

Lowered heart size on chest x-ray (loss of fat pad around heart)

Slowed heart rate

Constipation

Mild anemia

Diminished muscle mass

Dry skin

Less total sleep time

Mildly altered thyroid function

Sensitivity to lower body temperature

Lightheadedness

Lower amplitude of tracing on EKG

Fine, white hair on body surface

Absence of menstrual periods (amenorrhea)

Brittle nails

Loss of subcutaneous body fat

Sluggish reflexes

Mild fluid collection (edema)

Figure 10.2 Symptoms of anorexia nervosa

the metabolism. As thyroid activity decreases, the hair and nails become brittle, and the skin becomes dry. Depletion of body fat causes the person to be intolerant to cold. The electrolyte imbalance can result in less bone density and heart failure.

Bulimia Nervosa

Bulimia nervosa is characterized by a pattern of **binging** (consuming a lot of food in a short time), followed by **purging** (self-induced vomiting) or taking laxatives or diuretics. For bulimics overeating is an attempt to gain comfort and compensate for anxiety, depression, anger, or loneliness. To offset the ensuing guilt and fear of getting fat, the bulimic's "solution" is to purge the food consumed during the binge. A binge can last as long as 8 hours with the consumption of 20,000 calories (approximately 210 brownies), although the average binge involves about 3,400 calories (the equivalent to an entire pecan pie).

The pattern of gorging and purging eventually becomes ingrained. Bulimia is characterized by:

✳ a feeling of lack of control during binges

✳ any or some combination of: self-induced vomiting, taking laxatives and/or diuretics, fasting, exercising excessively and strenuously

✳ excessive concern with body shape and weight.

Bulimics may retain close to normal weight and may not present obvious signs of their eating disorder because they binge and purge in private. In college they are most often "discovered" by friends and roommates who share bathrooms and eat with them in cafeterias. An estimated one in five women on college campuses is bulimic.

Eventually, bulimia can lead to serious physical problems including trauma to the lining of the mouth, esophagus, and stomach; erosion of tooth enamel and receding gums; electrolyte imbalance in

☎ *Call for information*

National Association of Anorexia Nervosa and Associated Disorders
708-831-3438

the bloodstream; fatigue and muscle cramps; endocrine and metabolic changes affecting the menstrual cycle, and it can contribute to osteoporosis and heart failure. Repeated use of laxatives causes constipation. Bulimia has been recognized as an eating disorder only since 1980, so research is sparse.

Binge Eating

Binge eating is the most recently recognized eating disorder. The binge eater often is overweight, and dieters may be more susceptible to the disorder. The condition is similar to bulimia nervosa except that the person does not purge or use other compensatory behaviors such as misuse of laxatives or excessive exercise. Characteristics of binge eating include:

✳ rapidly consuming large amounts of food in a short time

✳ feeling unable to stop eating

✳ feeling disgusted with oneself, depressed, or guilty after eating

✳ eating more rapidly than other people

✳ eating large amounts of food when not hungry

✳ eating until an uncomfortable feeling sets in

✳ eating a lot of food when alone

✳ eating throughout the day with no planned mealtimes

Some binge eaters develop bulimia nervosa, induce vomiting at times, or use laxatives to avoid weight gain. Others continue to binge or overeat. Treatment almost always requires professional assistance by psychologists and physicians who use therapeutic methods such as individual and group therapy. In some cases an antidepressant drug has been helpful.

What Is "Too Thin"

Over a 10-year period (1979–88), 60% of Miss America contestants and 69% of *Playboy* centerfolds were 15% or more below the average weight for their age and height. That degree of thinness is a major indicator of anorexia nervosa, according to the American Psychiatric Association.

Differences Between Eating Disorders

Although all eating disorders are based on food intake, the dynamics and manifestations of each are quite different. Dr. Jennifer Hagman, a psychiatrist and co-director of the Eating Disorders Program at Children's Hospital, Denver, has identified essential differences between anorexia and bulimia. Anorexics like the way they look and find thinness attractive. They never look too thin to themselves, and they actually may perceive themselves as being "too fat" even when they are extremely thin. To anorexics, the mirror is not an accurate reflection, because their thinking is distorted. By contrast, bulimics despise themselves and what they are doing. Because they are more realistic, and they are not as nutritionally deprived, bulimia does not have as potentially severe consequences as anorexia, and anorexia is harder to treat.

Although the groundwork most often is laid in high school, eating disorders often emerge as a problem during college. According to Dr. Hagman, leaving home at that stage in life involves **individuation**, separating from family and developing a self-identity. Part of that identity is one's body. Anorexia has a total or partial recovery rate of about 85% overall. Dr. Hagman stresses that the longer people wait to get help, the longer they take to recover.

In African Americans bulimia is more common than anorexia, again because they do not tend to subscribe to the culture of thinness. Many African Americans who do have eating disorders are involved in sports and the performing arts.

ASSESSING THINNESS AND FATNESS

Height/Weight Tables

In the past the most common assessment tool to determine recommended body weight was the **height/weight table**. The numbers in these tables originally were derived by measuring the height

Some Clues to an Eating Disorder

❋ Excessive weight loss (15%–25% below recommended weight)

❋ Frequent weight fluctuations (rollercoaster dieting may show up in erratic weight gains or losses)

❋ Unusual eating habits (taking tiny bites, moving food around on the plate)

❋ No longer eating meals with the family or group ("too busy," etc.)

❋ Secretive behavior, especially in eating and bathroom use

❋ Taking laxatives or diet pills

❋ Food disappearing regularly

❋ Overdoing exercise

❋ Menstrual periods stopping

❋ More dental cavities and gum disease (induced by malnutrition and vomiting)

❋ Extreme sensitivity to cold

❋ Distorted body image (continually saying "I'm too fat")

Source: *Facts About Eating Disorders* (Denver: Children's Hospital, 1994).

and weight of 4.2 million people insured by major life insurance companies. The companies determined the average weight of the longest-lived people of a given height, and that weight was called "ideal."

These tables have drawbacks. First, they rarely take age into account. Age is important because the weights associated with minimum mortality rise with age. Thus, overweight in a younger person is riskier than overweight in an older person. Further, the skeletal structure or frame size is inaccurate. Some people naturally weigh more than their

KEY TERMS

Bulimia nervosa an eating disorder in which a person consumes a lot of food in a short time, followed by self-induced vomiting or taking laxatives or diuretics

Binging Consuming a large amount of food in a short time; gorging

Purging self-induced vomiting

Binge eating an eating disorder characterized by consuming a lot of food in a short time

Individuation separating from family and developing a self-identity

Height/weight table assessment tool used to determine recommended body weight

"ideal weight" because they have a heavy bone structure. The ranges of weights recommended in height/ weight tables as "healthy" are too narrow. Minorities and women are underrepresented in the database. The U. S. Food and Drug Administration (FDA) and the Department of Health and Human Services (DHHS) published a new height/weight table in 1990 (Table 10.2) giving a range of suggested weights based on height and age.

Table 10.2
Height/Weight Table

Height (ft-in.)	19 to 34 years	35 Years and Over
5–0	97–128	108–138
5–1	101–132	111–143
5–2	104–137	115–148
5–3	107–141	119–152
5–4	111–146	122–157
5–5	114–150	126–162
5–6	118–155	130–167
5–7	121–160	134–172
5–8	125–164	138–178
5–9	129–169	142–183
5–10	132–174	146–188
5–11	136–179	151–194
6–0	140–184	155–199
6–1	144–189	159–205
6–2	148–195	164–210
6–3	152–200	168–216
6–4	156–205	173–222

Note: Both sexes are combined in one table; the higher weights generally apply to men, the lower to women.

Source: U. S. Department of Health and Human Services, *Nutrition and Your Health: Dietary Guidelines for Americans* (Washington, DC: U. S. Government Printing Office, 1990).

Waist-to-Hip Ratio

The **waist-to-hip ratio** technique focuses on the distribution of body fat. Fat in the waist and abdomen (the "apple shape") is more active metabolically and is associated with higher risk for disease and premature death than is fat in the thighs, hips and buttocks (the "pear shape"). The higher the ratio of waist-to-hip measurement, the greater is the risk. More men are apples, and more women are pears.

To determine the waist-to-hip ratio, the waist circumference measurement is divided by the measurement of the widest circumference around the hips. For men this ratio should be less than .95,

and for women the ratio should be less than .8. Higher ratios suggest a higher risk. Table 10.3 shows the risk for disease according to the waist-to-hip ratio.

Table 10.3
Risk for Disease According to Waist-to-Hip Ratio

Waist-to-Hip Ratio		
Men	Women	Disease Risk
≤0.95	≤0.80	Very Low
0.96–0.99	0.81–0.84	Low
≥1.00	≥0.85	High

Body Mass Index (BMI)

Another technique used to determine thinness and excessive fatness is the **body mass index (BMI)**. This index incorporates height and weight to estimate critical fat values at which the risk for disease increases. BMI is calculated by multiplying your weight in pounds by 705, dividing this figure by your height in inches, and then dividing by the same height gain (or weight in kilograms divided by the same height in meters). For example, the BMI for an individual who weighs 172 pounds and is 67 inches tall would be 27 (172 × 705 ÷ 67 ÷ 67). According to BMI, the lowest risk for chronic disease is in the 20 to 30 range (see Table 10.4). Individuals are classified as overweight between 25 and 30. BMIs above 30 are defined as obese and below 20 as underweight. BMI is a useful tool to

Table 10.4
Disease Risk According to Body Mass Index (BMI)

BMI	Disease Risk
<20.00	Moderate to Very High
20.00 to 21.99	Low
22.00 to 24.99	Very Low
25.00 to 29.99	Low
30.00 to 34.99	Moderate
35.00 to 39.99	High
>40.00	Very High

screen the general population, but, similar to height/weight charts, it fails to differentiate fat from lean body mass or where most of the fat is located.

Figuring Recommended Body Weight

Figure 10.3 provides a general guideline to determine your recommended body weight using basal metabolic rate. Because African Americans tend to have denser bones than Anglo-Americans, they are allotted an extra 4-6 pounds on the average. The recommended weight determined in Figure 10.3 is the basis used in Figure 10.4 to calculate your caloric needs using the BMR plus sex and activity factors. The BMR factor for men is higher than for women because muscle tissue is more active than fat tissue, and men generally have more muscle tissue than women do.

Although age is not factored into the figure, the younger you are, the higher your BMR will be, generally speaking. The BMR is highest during infancy, puberty, and pregnancy, when the body is undergoing rapid changes and thus requires the most energy. After age 30, the BMR decreases by 1% or more each year, so people find that they have to work harder to take off extra pounds as they get older.

Men

106 pounds for the first 5 feet of height
+ 6 pounds for each additional inch

For example:

For a 6-foot-tall man:

106 + (12 x 6)
= 106 + 72 =
178 pounds
recommended weight

5 ft.
106 lbs.

12 in. x 6 lbs.
72 lbs.

Women

100 pounds for first 5 feet of height
+ 5 pounds for each additional inch

For example:

For a 5'4" woman

100 + (4 x 5)
= 100 + 20 =
120 pounds
recommended weight

5 ft.
100 lbs.

4 in. x 5 lbs.
20 lbs.

± 10% to account for individual differences (small or large frame)

Modifications for African Americans*
Men: 110 lbs. for the first 5 feet of ht.
Women: 104 lbs. for the first 5 feet of ht.

* According to Barbara Dixon, *Good Health for African Americans* (New York: Crown, 1994), p. 89.

Figure 10.3 Guidelines to determine recommended body weight

Daily caloric needs =
Weight (pounds) × BMR factor
× 24 (hours/day) × activity factor
= _____ BMR caloric needs

BMR Factor
Men = .45   Women = .41

Activity Factors	Range
Sedentary	1.40 – 1.50
Light Activity	1.55 – 1.65
Moderate Activity	1.65 – 1.70
Heavy Work	1.75 – 2.00

For example: How many calories a day does a male 180-pound construction worker need?

Daily caloric needs =
180 (pounds) × .45 × 24 hours × 1.75
(activity factor) = 3402 daily calorie needs

BMR = Basal metabolic rate

Figure 10.4 Calculation of caloric needs

KEY TERMS

Waist-to-hip ratio waist circumference measurement divided by measurement of the widest circumference around the hips

Body mass index (BMI) technique incorporating height and weight to estimate critical fat values

ASSESSING BODY COMPOSITION

Body composition can be assessed in a number of ways. Some techniques are highly accurate but inaccessible, and others almost anyone can do but they may not be as accurate. These methods include hydrostatic or underwater weighing, skinfold measurements, and bioelectrical impedance analysis.

Hydrostatic Weighing

One of the most accurate methods for assessing body composition is underwater or **hydrostatic weighing**. While under water the person sits in a chair, exhales air, and bends over, feet not touching the floor. Because the density of fat is different from that of lean tissue, these masses can be estimated by measuring the amount of water displaced or by comparing the difference between the underwater and dry weighing.

This method can be intimidating, especially for those who have a fear of water. On the plus side, it covers both essential and storage fat and is rather inexpensive compared to utilizing specialized labs and hospitals. It is inconvenient, though, and not widely available. Measurements can be affected by eating foods that create internal gas or engaging in

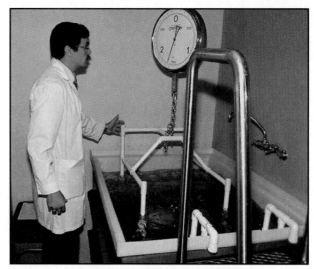

Hydrostatic weighing is one technique used to assess body composition.

activities that affect fluid retention or cause dehydration. Reliability depends on the individual doing the weighing, the person taking the test, and the respiration effort. The standards used for assessment were developed by testing middle-aged sedentary males, so they may be inaccurate for most people.

Table 10.5 gives suggested guidelines for body composition. It also should be mentioned that too little body fat (less than 8% for women and 5% for men) can cause health problems, including muscle

Table 10.5
Suggested Guidelines for Body Composition

MEN					
Age	Excellent	Good	Moderate	Overweight	Obese
≤19	12.0	12.1-17.0	17.1-22.0	22.1-27.0	≥27.1
20-29	13.0	13.1-18.0	18.1-23.0	23.1-28.0	≥28.1
30-39	14.0	14.1-19.0	19.1-24.0	24.1-29.0	≥29.1
40-49	15.0	15.1-20.0	20.1-25.0	25.1-30.0	≥30.1
≥50	16.0	16.1-21.5	21.6-26.0	26.1-31.0	≥31.1
WOMEN					
Age	Excellent	Good	Moderate	Overweight	Obese
≤19	17.0	17.1-22.0	22.1-27.0	27.1-32.0	≥32.1
20-29	18.0	18.1-23.0	23.1-28.0	28.1-33.0	≥33.1
30-39	19.0	19.1-24.0	24.1-29.0	29.1-34.0	≥34.1
40-49	20.0	20.1-25.0	25.1-30.0	30.1-35.0	≥35.1
≥50	21.0	21.1-26.0	26.1-31.0	31.1-36.0	≥36.1

Source: Principles & Labs for Physical Fitness and Wellness, 3d edition, by Werner W. K. Hoeger and Sharon A. Hoeger (Englewood, CO: Morton, 1994).

wasting and fatigue. In women a low percentage of body fat is associated with amenorrhea (lack of menstruation) and loss of bone mass.

Skinfold Measurements

The **skinfold measurement** is a more convenient method to measure body composition. It measures the thickness of fat under the skin. A technician grasps a fold of skin at a predetermined location and measures it using an instrument called a **caliper.** The skinfold measurement assessment usually is available at colleges, universities, and health clubs. Repeated measurements are taken from several areas of the body (see Figure 10.5), and the results are computed from formulas that predict body fatness from skinfold thickness (Tables 10.6

and 10.7). The more sites measured, the more valid is the measure of percentage of body fat.

The distribution of body fat is not uniform, so taking the measurements can be difficult. Differences in age, sex, and ethnic group can cause measurement errors, as can pinching muscles in conjunction with the skin. Because criteria have not

KEY TERMS

Hydrostatic weighing method of determining body composition by measuring the amount of water displaced when a person exhales and sits under water

Skinfold measurement method of determining body composition by measuring the thickness of fat under the skin

Caliper instrument used to measure the thickness of fat under the skin

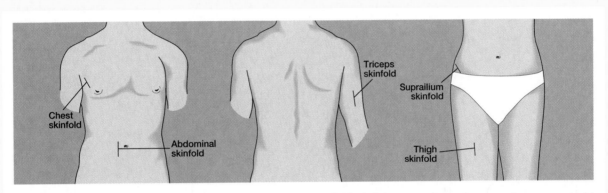

1. Select the proper anatomical sites. For men, use chest, abdomen, and thigh skinfolds. For women, use triceps, suprailium, and thigh skinfolds. Take all measurements on the right side of the body with the person standing. The correct anatomical landmarks for skinfolds are:

   Chest: a diagonal fold halfway between the shoulder crease and the nipple.

   Abdomen: a vertical fold taken about 1" to the right of the umbilicus.

   Triceps: a vertical fold on the back of the upper arm, halfway between the shoulder and the elbow.

   Thigh: a vertical fold on the front of the thigh, midway between the knee and hip.

   Suprailium: a diagonal fold above the crest of the ilium (on the side of the hip).

2. Measure each site by grasping a double thickness of skin firmly with the thumb and forefinger, pulling the

fold slightly away from the muscular tissue. Hold caliper perpendicular to the fold, and take the measurement 1/2" below the finger hold. Measure each site three times and read the values to the nearest .1 to .5 mm. Record the average of the two closest readings as the final value. Take the readings without delay to avoid excessive compression of the skinfold. Release and refold the skinfold between readings.

3. When doing pre- and post-assessments, conduct the measurement at the same time of day. The best time is early in the morning to avoid water hydration changes resulting from activity or exercise.

4. Obtain percent fat by adding the three skinfold measurements and looking up the respective values.

For example, if the skinfold measurements for an 18-year-old female are: (a) triceps = 16, (b) suprailium = 4, and (c) thigh = 30 (total = 50), the percent body fat is 20.6%

Source: *Principles & Labs for Physical Fitness and Wellness*, 3d edition, by Werner W. K. Hoeger and Sharon A. Hoeger (Englewood, CO: Morton, 1994).

Figure 10.5 Anatomical landmarks and technique for skinfold measurements

Table 10.6
Percent Fat Estimates for Women

Sum of 3 Skinfolds	Under 22	23 to 27	28 to 32	33 to 37	38 to 42	43 to 47	48 to 52	53 to 57	Over 58
				Age to the Last Year					
23– 25	9.7	9.9	10.2	10.4	10.7	10.9	11.2	11.4	11.7
26– 28	11.0	11.2	11.5	11.7	12.0	12.3	12.5	12.7	13.0
29– 31	12.3	12.5	12.8	13.0	13.3	13.5	13.8	14.0	14.3
32– 34	13.6	13.8	14.0	14.3	14.5	14.8	15.0	15.3	15.5
35– 37	14.8	15.0	15.3	15.5	15.8	16.0	16.3	16.5	16.8
38– 40	16.0	16.3	16.5	16.7	17.0	17.2	17.5	17.7	18.0
41– 43	17.2	17.4	17.7	17.9	18.2	18.4	18.7	18.9	19.2
44– 46	18.3	18.6	18.8	19.1	19.3	19.6	19.8	20.1	20.3
47– 49	19.5	19.7	20.0	20.2	20.5	20.7	21.0	21.2	21.5
50– 52	20.6	20.8	21.1	21.3	21.6	21.8	22.1	22.3	22.6
53– 55	21.7	21.9	22.1	22.4	22.6	22.9	23.1	23.4	23.6
56– 58	22.7	23.0	23.2	23.4	23.7	23.9	24.2	24.4	24.7
59– 61	23.7	24.0	24.2	24.5	24.7	25.0	25.2	25.5	25.7
62– 64	24.7	25.0	25.2	25.5	25.7	26.0	26.2	26.4	26.7
65– 67	25.7	25.9	26.2	26.4	26.7	26.9	27.2	27.4	27.7
68– 70	26.6	26.9	27.1	27.4	27.6	27.9	28.1	28.4	28.6
71– 73	27.5	27.8	28.0	28.3	28.5	28.8	29.0	29.3	29.5
74– 76	28.4	28.7	28.9	29.2	29.4	29.7	29.9	30.2	30.4
77– 79	29.3	29.5	29.8	30.0	30.3	30.5	30.8	31.0	31.3
80– 82	30.1	30.4	30.6	30.9	31.1	31.4	31.6	31.9	32.1
83– 85	30.9	31.2	31.4	31.7	31.9	32.2	32.4	32.7	32.9
86– 88	31.7	32.0	32.2	32.5	32.7	32.9	33.2	33.4	33.7
89– 91	32.5	32.7	33.0	33.2	33.5	33.7	33.9	34.2	34.4
92– 94	33.2	33.4	33.7	33.9	34.2	34.4	34.7	34.9	35.2
95– 97	33.9	34.1	34.4	34.6	34.9	35.1	35.4	35.6	35.9
98–100	34.6	34.8	35.1	35.3	35.5	35.8	36.0	36.3	36.5
101–103	35.2	35.4	35.7	35.9	36.2	36.4	36.7	36.9	37.2
104–106	35.8	36.1	36.3	36.6	36.8	37.1	37.3	37.5	37.8
107–109	36.4	36.7	36.9	37.1	37.4	37.6	37.9	38.1	38.4
110–112	37.0	37.2	37.5	37.7	38.0	38.2	38.5	38.7	38.9
113–115	37.5	37.8	38.0	38.2	38.5	38.7	39.0	39.2	39.5
116–118	38.0	38.3	38.5	38.8	39.0	39.3	39.5	39.7	40.0
119–121	38.5	38.7	39.0	39.2	39.5	39.7	40.0	40.2	40.5
122–124	39.0	39.2	39.4	39.7	39.9	40.2	40.4	40.7	40.9
125–127	39.4	39.6	39.9	40.1	40.4	40.6	40.9	41.1	41.4
128–130	39.8	40.0	40.3	40.5	40.8	41.0	41.3	41.5	41.8

Note: Calculated from triceps, suprailium, and thigh skinfold thickness. Body density is calculated based on the generalized equation for predicting body density of women developed by A. S. Jackson, M. L. Pollock, and A. Ward. *Medicine and Science in Sports and Exercise* 12, (1980), 175–182. Percent body fat is determined from the calculated body density using the Siri formula.

Source: *Lifetime Physical Fitness and Wellness,* 4th edition, by Werner W. K. Hoeger and Sharon A. Hoeger (Englewood, CO: Morton, 1994).

Table 10.7

Percent Fat Estimates for Men

	Age to the Last Year							
Sum of 3 Skinfolds	**Under 19**	**20 to 22**	**23 to 25**	**26 to 28**	**29 to 31**	**32 to 34**	**35 to 37**	**38 to 40**
8– 10	.9	1.3	1.6	2.0	2.3	2.7	3.0	3.3
11– 13	1.9	2.3	2.6	3.0	3.3	3.7	4.0	4.3
14– 16	2.9	3.3	3.6	3.9	4.3	4.6	5.0	5.3
17– 19	3.9	4.2	4.6	4.9	5.3	5.6	6.0	6.3
20– 22	4.8	5.2	5.5	5.9	6.2	6.6	6.9	7.3
23– 25	5.8	6.2	6.5	6.8	7.2	7.5	7.9	8.2
26– 28	6.8	7.1	7.5	7.8	8.1	8.5	8.8	9.2
29– 31	7.7	8.0	8.4	8.7	9.1	9.4	9.8	10.1
32– 34	8.6	9.0	9.3	9.7	10.0	10.4	10.7	11.1
35– 37	9.5	9.9	10.2	10.6	10.9	11.3	11.6	12.0
38– 40	10.5	10.8	11.2	11.5	11.8	12.2	12.5	12.9
41– 43	11.4	11.7	12.1	12.4	12.7	13.1	13.4	13.8
44– 46	12.2	12.6	12.9	13.3	13.6	14.0	14.3	14.7
47– 49	13.1	13.5	13.8	14.2	14.5	14.9	15.2	15.5
50– 52	14.0	14.3	14.7	15.0	15.4	15.7	16.1	16.4
53– 55	14.8	15.2	15.5	15.9	16.2	16.6	16.9	17.3
56– 58	15.7	16.0	16.4	16.7	17.1	17.4	17.8	18.1
59– 61	16.5	16.9	17.2	17.6	17.9	18.3	18.6	19.0
62– 64	17.4	17.7	18.1	18.4	18.8	19.1	19.4	19.8
65– 67	18.2	18.5	18.9	19.2	19.6	19.9	20.3	20.6
68– 70	19.0	19.3	19.7	20.0	20.4	20.7	21.1	21.4
71– 73	19.8	20.1	20.5	20.8	21.2	21.5	21.9	22.2
74– 76	20.6	20.9	21.3	21.6	22.0	22.2	22.7	23.0
77– 79	21.4	21.7	22.1	22.4	22.8	23.1	23.4	23.8
80– 82	22.1	22.5	22.8	23.2	23.5	23.9	24.2	24.6
83– 85	22.9	23.2	23.6	23.9	24.3	24.6	25.0	25.3
86– 88	23.6	24.0	24.3	24.7	25.0	25.4	25.7	26.1
89– 91	24.4	24.7	25.1	25.4	25.8	26.1	26.5	26.8
92– 94	25.1	25.5	25.8	26.2	26.5	26.9	27.2	27.5
95– 97	25.8	26.2	26.5	26.9	27.2	27.6	27.9	28.3
98–100	26.6	26.9	27.3	27.6	27.9	28.3	28.6	29.0
101–103	27.3	27.6	28.0	28.3	28.6	29.0	29.3	29.7
104–106	27.9	28.3	28.6	29.0	29.3	29.7	30.0	30.4
107–109	28.6	29.0	29.3	29.7	30.0	30.4	30.7	31.1
110–112	29.3	29.6	30.0	30.3	30.7	31.0	31.4	31.7
113–115	30.0	30.3	30.7	31.0	31.3	31.7	32.0	32.4
116–118	30.6	31.0	31.3	31.6	32.0	32.3	32.7	33.0
119–121	31.3	31.6	32.0	32.3	32.6	33.0	33.3	33.7
122–124	31.9	32.2	32.6	32.9	33.3	33.6	34.0	34.3
125–127	32.5	32.9	33.2	33.5	33.9	34.2	34.6	34.9
128–130	33.1	33.5	33.8	34.2	34.5	34.9	35.2	35.5

Note: Calculated from chest, abdomen, and thigh skinfold thickness. Body density is calculated based on the generalized equation for predicting body density of men developed by A. S. Jackson and M. L. Pollock, *British Journal of Nutrition* 40, (1978) 497–504. Percent body fat is determined from the calculated body density using the Siri formula.

Source: *Lifetime Physical Fitness and Wellness,* 4th edition, by Werner W. K. Hoeger and Sharon A. Hoeger (Englewood, CO: Morton, 1994).

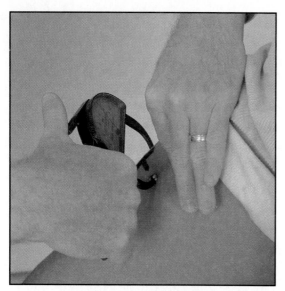

Skinfold thickness technique for body composition assessment.

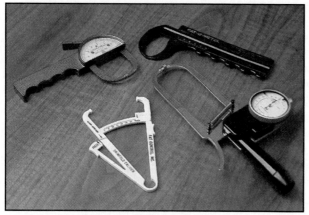

Various type of skinfold calipers used to assess skinfold thickness.

been defined to take these differences into account, measurements always should be taken by trained personnel.

Bioelectrical Impedance Analysis

To measure **bioelectrical impedance**, electrodes are attached to the body in several areas, usually on the right hand and right foot. A weak, harmless electrical current is transmitted from electrode to electrode. Electrical conduction through the body favors the path of the lean tissues over the fat tissues. The easier the conductance, the leaner the person. A computer is used to calculate fat percentage from these measurements.

For accurate measurements, prior to the test the person being measured has to avoid consuming

alcohol for 24–48 hours, avoid eating and drinking at least 4 hours, and urinate within 30 minutes before the test. The test results may be inaccurate if a person has used diuretic medications within the previous 7 days or has exercised 12 hours before testing. This may cause water retention or affect the body's electrolyte balance. Excessive fluid during the menstrual cycle and dehydration both skew the results by showing a higher body fat.

The accuracy of equations used to estimate percent body fat with this technique is debatable. An advantage, though, is that the results are readily reproducible and, unlike the tests that require experienced technicians, almost anyone can administer this test. Even though the results may not be completely accurate, they are useful in assessing changes in body composition over time.

WEIGHT-LOSS GIMMICKS

Gimmicks are everywhere around us. A gimmick is a tricky device or deceptive thing. Americans are beginning to realize that gimmicks do not produce lasting results. Research studies recommend losing weight slowly and consistently — no more than 1/2 to 1 pound weekly. The American Heart Association advises that no more than 30% of daily calories should come from fat. Of the remaining 70%, at least 55%–60% should come from complex carbohydrates (rice, potatoes, pasta, vegetables, cereal, fruits) and 10%–12% from protein (lean meats, fish, beans, poultry).

To lose 1 pound of fat per week, the caloric deficit should be no more than 500 calories a day (7 × 500 = 3500 calories a week) below the normal diet and should be a minimum of 1200 calories per day for overweight females and 1500 calories per day for overweight males. Furthermore, weight loss must be accompanied by a proper exercise program. Oprah Winfrey is a prime example of a person who went for the quick fix and found it did not work. Not until she stepped up her exercise program and went on a sensible diet did she *keep* the weight off.

Fad Diets

Diets can deceive people with weight problems. Any diet that promises to "take off weight fast" is misleading and dangerous. Commercially advertised

How Safe is a Diet

When selecting a diet, ask yourself:

❋ Does the diet contain foods found primarily in supermarkets?

❋ Does it include a variety of foods from which to select?

❋ Can you follow the diet at home, work, parties, restaurants?

❋ Is the cost of the foods reasonable?

If you answered *no* to any of these questions, do not try the diet. Seek another solution.

---

diets usually are low in nutrients and calories and can cause a metabolic imbalance, which can even result in death. On a very-low-calorie diet, as much as half of the weight lost may be lean protein tissue, and because the heart is a muscle, it can become weak and unable to pump enough blood through the body. When the body uses protein instead of carbohydrates and fat as a source of energy, the weight lost is in the form of water, causing a faster loss of weight. Water loss, however, results in the loss of essential vitamins and minerals. Blood pressure may drop, causing dizziness, fatigue, and lightheadedness. A person may lose hair, become nauseous, and have abdominal pain. The menstrual cycle may become irregular.

Cutting calories slows down the metabolism, too. A person may eat as few as 800 calories a day and still not lose weight. Once the person goes off the diet, the metabolism remains slow. The body continues to use fewer calories and the pounds come back.

Liquid Diets

Liquid diets consist of protein formula and water and generally are earmarked for people who are at least 20% overweight. Only 10%–20% of the people who have followed a liquid diet manage to stay within 10 pounds of their target weight a year and a half after embarking on the diet. Today's liquid diets, however, contain more carbohydrates, vitamins, minerals, and protein than the 1970s liquid diets did.

Liquid diet programs should be administered by medical professionals who provide weekly screening of heart function, blood pressure, electrolyte levels, urine content, and potassium — all indicators of how the body is coping without real food.

Side effects of liquid diets can include hair loss, dry skin, gum disease, constipation, sensitivity to cold, and mood swings. Examples of liquid diets are Medifast and Optifast, which supply 420–800 calories a day and include sufficient protein to preserve muscle tissue.

Over-the-Counter Diet Pills and Diet Aids

The "magic pill" — that's the American way. Among the numerous over-the-counter gimmicks are amino acids (L-glutamine, L-arginine) and grapefruit juice extract. The two most common diet aids sold in drugstores are phenyl propanolamine hydrochloride (PPA) and fiber. PPA is similar to amphetamines (available legally only by prescription). It acts as a mild stimulant and suppresses the appetite or desire to eat. PPA may cause dizziness, headaches, insomnia, hypertension, heart palpitations, and rapid pulse in some people. It is not approved by the FDA for use longer than 12 weeks.

Fiber diets containing oat bran, hemicellulose, corn bran, pectin, cellulose, guar gum, pectin, psyllium seed, lignin, and apple fiber are marketed as weight-loss aids. Manufacturers say these fibers swell in the stomach and absorb liquids, thereby providing a feeling of fullness. Dietary fiber in reality acts as a bulking agent in the large intestine, not in the stomach. Most of these products provide 1 to 3 grams of fiber per day, which is not close to the recommended daily intake of 20 to 35 grams. The FDA has found no data to warrant classifying any type of fiber as an aid in weight control or as an appetite suppressant. The slogan "buyer beware" was coined in ancient Rome to warn people to investigate before buying. It's still a good idea.

Passive Exercise

Gimmicks such as vibrators, steam baths, rubber suits, body wraps, motor-driven cycles, and motor-driven rowing machines are not necessary in a

---

KEY TERMS

Bioelectrical impedance method of determining body composition by analyzing electrical conduction through the body successful weight management plan. They basically are a waste of time and money.

* *Vibrators* (tables, belts, pillows) result in negligible caloric expenditure and do not generate weight loss. They may aggravate the back and can be dangerous to pregnant women.

* Attempted weight loss by using *rubber suits* causes the person to sweat. Weight loss comes from the loss of body fluid, which causes unhealthy changes in water metabolism and in kidney and circulatory functions.

* *Massage.* It is relaxing and may improve circulation, but it will not reduce weight.

* *Body wraps* (wrapping the body in bandages soaked in a "special formula") may alter the body circumference temporarily, but the body will regain its shape within hours after unwrapping. Body wraps also are potentially dangerous.

* *Steam baths* and *saunas* remove fluids from the body. Rapid fluid loss can cause severe dehydration and chemical imbalance. Consuming water immediately after a sweat session will return the body to normal weight.

* *Motor-driven cycles* and *motor-driven rowing machines* are devices that do the work for the person. They may help maintain flexibility and increase circulation, but the most effective means of weight reduction is for the body, not a machine, to do the work.

Commercial and Medical Programs

Many commercial and medical programs are available for both weight loss and weight gain. Perhaps some of these programs work for some individuals. Commercial weight-loss programs include sessions on nutrition, exercise, counseling, and behavior modification. Often these programs are expensive and may require purchasing special supplements and foods. Information on diet centers is generally lacking because they don't follow up with statistics or don't divulge them freely. No long-term data exist on these programs except before-and-after photos and testimonials. In lieu of commercial programs, the local university or college, hospital, or

physician can help a person select a reputable weight management program. Also, registered dietitians can be found in hospitals, and some conduct weight management programs in private practice.

ROLE OF EXERCISE

Moderate exercise — expending 2000 calories per week — has been linked to a longer life. It also is a necessary component of any weight-management program. A combination of strength-training exercises and aerobics expends the greatest amount of calories. During the first few minutes of exercise, the body uses readily available carbohydrates for energy. During sustained exercise the body switches to fat for fuel.

For various reasons, African American women have much lower rates of physical activity than Anglo-American women (and higher rates of overweight and obesity). Exercise *must* be a part of any weight management program. Physical fitness is the topic of the next chapter. The discussion here is limited to the role of exercise in weight management. In brief, strength-training increases lean body mass, and aerobic exercise lowers the setpoint. Losing body fat through exercise takes time, patience, and persistence. Some individuals do not see results for a long time. The underlying principle is that body fat requires fewer calories to maintain itself than lean muscle tissue does. By adhering to an exercise and proper nutritional program, the desirable weight change will follow.

The safest and best way to increase metabolism is to increase physical activity. Increasing the metabolism increases the delivery of oxygen to the exercising muscles. The more capable the body is of utilizing oxygen, the more fat is expended.

People who diet without some type of exercise lose not only fat tissue but lean tissue as well. If they regain weight without exercising, the gain is mostly in the form of fat. Fat tissue expends fewer calories to maintain itself, so if the person eats the same amount of food as before, he or she will gain weight. Obesity is risky, but repeated "yo-yo" dieting (losing and regaining weight again and again) can be also. Large-scale studies reveal that weight

The safest and best way to increase metabolism is to increase physical activity.

fluctuation (primarily caused by dieting) may shorten the lifespan. Losing weight too quickly may result in illness or injury, and most often the person will discontinue the program. The safest and most effective way to lose unwanted pounds is *gradually*.

Time and intensity are important in total energy expenditure. More exercise results in a greater total weekly caloric expenditure and, therefore, more weight change. Briskly walking a mile three to six times per week, for example, is sufficient for most people.

A person cannot lose **cellulite** (lumpy fat) in specific body locations by doing localized, isolated exercises. Fat cells release fat into the blood (not the muscle), and all the muscles share the fat. Fat cells are reduced throughout the body as a result of lower caloric intake, not by **spot-reducing** exercises such as curl-ups for the abdominal area or side bends in an attempt to have a smaller waist. A program of exercise will tone muscles in those areas by strengthening muscle tissue under the stored body fat. Spot reduction does not work. Endurance exercise and proper caloric intake do.

ATTITUDE AND BEHAVIOR MODIFICATION

Eating healthier often requires a person to make fundamental changes. In contrast to dieting, which promotes the myth that we can produce long-lasting changes from the outside-in, weight change should be considered from the inside-out. First, people must correct their attitudes and habits, according to Jennifer Carney, Denver nutritional consultant. She says people should find ways other than eating to nurture themselves.

Many people have to unlearn habits ingrained since childhood, such as being rewarded with sweets, being urged to "hurry up and eat," and "clean up your plate." In conflicting messages, the media promote slimness to the point of emaciation, which makes overweight people feel guilty and leads to the loss of self-esteem and to depression.

There are no miracles in controlling weight. No one gadget can do it for a person. Conscious effort and determination are rewarded.

Weight management is promoted most successfully as a key to *health*. Individuals in weight

Choices in Eating

Which of the following would you choose?

Breakfast

Good Choices	Poor Choices
English muffin	Biscuits and gravy
Boiled egg	Cheese omelet
Cereal with low-fat milk	Sugared cereal with cream
Wheat toast, plain	Bagel and cream cheese
Whole-grain muffin	Chocolate muffin
Low-fat yogurt	Bacon or sausage

Lunch/Dinner

Good Choices	Poor Choices
Steamed perch	Deep-fried shrimp
Baked chicken breast	Southern-fried chicken
Baked potato, plain	French fries
Vegetable soup	Cream soup
Tossed salad	Cole slaw
Chili	BBQ ribs
Black-eyed peas	Ham hocks and beans
Bean burrito	Cheese nachos
Spaghetti	Hush puppies
Stir-fried vegetables	Egg roll

The hidden ingredient in the "poor choices" is fat — in the form of butter and other dairy products, oil, mayonnaise. Or the key may lie in the method of cooking. Methods that require fat or oil are poor choices. Better methods are roasting, baking, broiling, braising, poaching, stir-frying, steaming, microwaving.

Some ethnic fast-food restaurants have been chastised recently for the high calorie counts of their items. The foods themselves usually are not the problem. The problem is in the cooking methods and "add-ons."

management programs first must recognize their bad habits and be motivated to lose the weight. The behaviors of the person who is overeating must be modified. When the behaviors of eating fewer calories and expending more energy through exercise are attained, the outcome is a healthier person.

KEY TERMS

Cellulite fat cells
Spot-reducing exercising to reduce fat in a specific location of the body

LIFETIME WEIGHT MANAGEMENT PLAN

Half the battle of breaking bad habits lies in recognizing them. Jotting down what you eat and what your feelings are at the time you eat is important. You may realize that you reach for snacks when you are bored or worried. The weight gain has developed over several years. Likewise, weight loss should be a slow and gradual process. It takes time. To make specific lifestyle changes:

✳ Set realistic expectations, tackling one bad habit at a time. Consider each step in the right direction a success. As you change your habits, remember that what you are doing is good for *you*. You are doing this for yourself, not to please anyone else.

✳ Make sure your weight management plan is medically safe.

✳ Include both short- and long-term goals. Break long-term goals into small, reasonable steps to get you where you want to go.

✳ Keep a record (chart or journal) of your weight and daily eating behaviors so you can measure your progress. Write down the quantity and the caloric content of the foods you eat.

✳ Make a mental note of what makes you want to eat (examples: It's lunchtime. I'm bored. Someone offered me food). Anticipate problems, and plan ways to avoid them.

✳ Don't buy and store ice cream, cookies, soft drinks, candy.

✳ Keep nutritious foods on hand, and encourage the people around you to eat these foods with you.

✳ Eat small meals frequently. Include more complex carbohydrates.

✳ Do not skip meals, and avoid snacking after the evening meal.

✳ Measure and weigh the foods if this helps you. Keep up-to-date records of food intake, exercise, and weight change.

✳ Make specific changes. For instance, substitute low-fat frozen yogurt for ice cream.

✳ Eat breakfast. It increases metabolism. To lose weight, consume approximately 75% of your daily calories before 1:00 p.m.

✳ Eat meals slowly (20–30 minutes), pausing often. Put down utensils between bites. Swallow before reloading the fork. It takes the appetite control center about 20 minutes to receive the message that you have eaten enough.

✳ Feeling bored or down? Reach for the phone instead of food. Take a break by walking. Post a list of substitute activities you enjoy.

✳ Do not eat while watching television or talking on the telephone. Eat at regular mealtimes and in designated areas (kitchen or dining room).

✳ Avoid stimulants, diuretics, laxatives, diet pills, and dehydration techniques (steam baths, saunas).

✳ Limit your alcohol intake. Alcohol may slow the body's ability to burn fat, and it favors fat storage. Alcohol is also high in calories (7 calories per gram) and may increase your appetite.

✳ Drink a minimum of eight 6–8 ounce glasses of water daily. Limit beverages such as colas and other caffeinated drinks.

✳ Maintain a regular aerobic exercise program. Walking after a meal will expend fat while it is still in the bloodstream and before it reaches the fat storage stage. Choose activities you enjoy.

Tips for action

A few suggestions when eating out are:

Appetizer: shrimp cocktail, fruit cup, steamed mussels

Soup: bean or lentil, minestrone, won ton, clear soups

Bread: whole grain, plain rolls without butter

Salad: greens with dressing on the side

Entree: baked fish, vegetable plate or extra vegetables, pasta with red sauce

Dessert: fruit cup, sorbet, fruit ice

Source: *High-Fiber Fitness Plan*, by James W. Anderson with Nancy J. Gustafson (Lexington, KY: University Press of Kentucky, 1994), p. 111.

* Ask for help from others. Eat and exercise with friends and family members who offer support and encouragement. Avoid negative environments and people.

* Praise yourself, think positive, and avoid self-criticism even when you fail. Reward yourself with nonfood treats when you are successful even in a small step. Buy a new outfit or go to the movies.

* Learn from failure. Everyone backslides. You are only human. Do not demand too much from yourself. Instead decide how you can avoid failure so you can be successful in the future.

* Wean yourself from fat. Some experts say it is best to go cold turkey. After 8–12 weeks you should lose your taste for fatty foods. Also avoid foods made with fat substitutes.

* Prepare foods wisely. Use less fat and refined foods. Bake, broil, and boil instead of frying. Eat plenty of fruits and vegetables. Remove all visible fat from meats. Do not use coconut oil, cocoa butter, or palm oil.

Remember this rule: If caloric intake is more than caloric output, weight increases. If caloric intake is less than caloric output, weight decreases. If caloric intake equals caloric output, weight is maintained. People must realize that fat can not be starved off, slept off, or melted off. Weight management is a lifetime adventure of setting and achieving one goal at a time. No quick, easy methods or devices can help you change body weight. Weight management takes time, patience, and persistence. Selecting foods wisely, modifying unhealthy eating behaviors, and doing aerobic exercise are the safest and best ways to achieve a healthy body.

Summary

1 The metabolic rate depends on body size and composition, gender, diet, age, genetic factors, hormones, and activity level.

2 The three theories of weight determination are genetic predisposition, fat cell hypertrophy and hyperplasia theory, and setpoint theory, the latter of which is receiving the most attention currently.

3 Americans in general are becoming fatter, weighing an average of 15 pounds more than they did a decade ago.

4 Health hazards of overweight and obesity include higher incidences of cardiovascular diseases, respiratory problems, diabetes, arthritis, some cancers, and other conditions.

5 The three classifications of eating disorders are anorexia nervosa, bulimia, and binge eating, all of which are most prevalent in young Anglo-American women.

6 To determine recommended body weight, a person can consult height/weight tables or figure basal metabolic rate and caloric needs.

7 Determining body composition — the proportion of fat tissue (% body fat) to lean body mass — is the basis for making a weight change.

8 Three means to assess body composition include hydrostatic weighing, skinfold measurements, and bioelectrical impedance analysis.

9 Weight-loss gimmicks include fad diets, unsupervised liquid diets, over-the-counter diet pills and aids, passive exercise devices, and some commercial and medical programs.

10 Weight change requires not only changes in eating habits but also a regular exercise program and attitude and behavior modification including a commitment to a lifetime of weight management program.

Select Bibliography

American Journal of Public Health, 80 (Dec, 1990). (special supplement)

Applegate, L. "Spring Clean Your Diet." *Runner's World*, 29:5 (1994), 30.

"Ask the Experts." *University of California Berkeley Wellness Letter*, 10:6 (1994), 8.

Brody, J. *Jane Brody's Nutrition Book*. New York: Bantam, 1994.

Brownell, K. D. "The Ups and Downs of Yo-Yo Dieting." *Reebock Instructor News*, 3:1 (1989), 3.

Cahil, D. M. "The Fat Eating Experiment." *Walking Magazine*, 5:1 (1990), 29–35.

Chinnici, M. "Picking the Perfect Diet." *Walking Magazine*, 1989, 41–43.

Dixon, Barbara. *Good Health for African Americans*. New York: Crown, 1994.

Floyd, P. A., et al. *Wellness: A Lifetime Commitment*. Winston-Salem, NC: Hunter, 1993.

Garrison, R. H., and E. Somer. *The Nutrition Desk Reference*. New Canaan, CT: Keats, 1990.

Hafen, B. Q., and W. W. K. Hoeger. *Wellness: Guidelines for a Healthy Lifestyle*, Englewood, CO: Morton, 1994.

Hales, D. *An Invitation to Health*, 6th edition. Redwood City, CA: Benjamin/Cummings, 1994.

"Healthfront." *Prevention*, 46:5 (1994), 11–24.

Hoeger, W. W. K., and S. A. Hoeger. *Lifetime Physical Fitness & Wellness*. Englewood, CO: Morton Publishing, 1994.

Hoeger, W. W. K., and S. A. Hoeger. *Principles & Labs for Physical Fitness and Wellness*. Englewood, CO: Morton Publishing, 1994.

"How to Lose Those 10 Stubborn Pounds. " *Prevention*, 46:6 (1994), 58–60.

Insel, P. M., and W. T. Roth, *Core Concepts in Health*, 7th edition. Mountain View, CA: Mayfield, 1994.

"Join the Prevention Program." *Prevention*, 45:2 (1993), 37–38.

Journal of the American Medical Association, 265:2 (Jan. 9, 1991). (entire issue)

Kitay, L. "Are You Too Good?" *Weight Watchers Magazine*, 27:7 (1994), 23–26.

Lohman, Timothy G. *Advances in Body Composition Assessment*. Champaign, IL: Human Kinetics Publishers, 1992.

"Nutrition Counselors: Whom Can You Trust?" *Environmental Nutrition*,15:2 (1992), 1,3.

Seligman, M. E. "Dump That Diet." *Reader's Digest*, May, 1994, pp. 123–125.

Tannen, N. "My Mother, My Weight." *Weight Watchers*, 27:5 (1994), 38–42.

"Train Your Body to Trim Your Tummy." *Prevention*, 46:5 (1994), 51–53.

Westcott, W. I. "You Can Sell Exercise for Weight Loss." *Fitness Management*, 7:12 (1991), 33–34.

Calculating Recommended Body Weight

NAME _____ DATE _____

COURSE _____ SECTION _____

Women:

100 pounds for the first 5 feet	=	_____
104 pounds for the first 5 feet (African American)	=	_____
+ 5 pounds for each additional inch	=	_____
± 10% to account for individual differences (small or large frame)	=	_____

Men:

106 pounds for the first 5 feet	=	_____
110 pounds for the first 5 feet (African American)	=	_____
+ 6 pounds for each additional inch	=	_____
± 10% to account for individual differences (small or large frame)	=	_____

Note: To lose 1 pound of fat, subtract 500 calories per day (exercising = 250 calories and proper nutrition = 250 calories, a total of 500 calories) 7 days per week $\times$ 500 calories = 3500 calories per week.

Determining Caloric Assessment

NAME _____ DATE _____

COURSE _____ SECTION _____

Weight in pounds: _____ × _____ (BMR Factor)

= _____ × 24 (hrs/day) _____ = _____ × (activity factor) = _____

Daily caloric needs = _____

BMR Factor

Men   = .45

Women = .41

Activity Factor	Range
Sedentary (sitting)	1.40 – 1.50
Light Activity (washing dishes)	1.55 – 1.65
Moderate activity (postman delivery person)	1.65 – 1.70
Heavy work (manual laborer)	1.75 – 2.00

Note: To maintain your present weight, consume the number of calories calculated above. To lose weight, consume fewer calories and increase your activity.

Calculating Waist-to-Hip Ratio

NAME _____ DATE _____

COURSE _____ SECTION _____

Waist (inches):   =   _____

Hip (inches):   =   _____

Ratio: $\dfrac{\text{Waist}}{\text{Hip}}$ =   _____

Men   Women
0.95 or less   0.80 or less

Daily Diet Recording Form

NAME _____ DATE _____

COURSE _____ SECTION _____

See Food Pyramid, Chapter 9

No.	Food	Amount	Bread, Cereal, Rice & Pasta	Vegetable	Fruit	Milk, Yogurt & Cheese	Meat, Poultry, Fish, Dry Beans, Eggs, & Nuts
			Food Groups (servings)				
1							
2							
3							
4							
5							
6							
7							
8							
9							
10							
11							
12							
13							
14							
15							
16							
17							
18							
19							
20							
21							
22							
23							
24							
25							
26							
27							
28							
29							
30							
Totals							
Recommended Amount			6–11	3–5	2–4	2–3	2–3
Deficiencies							

Health-Related Components of Fitness

11

OBJECTIVES

* Define *physical fitness*.
* Cite several physical and psychological benefits of fitness.
* Explain the FITT formula.
* List and define the components of health-related fitness.
* Explain the differences between aerobic and anaerobic exercise.
* Calculate resting, target, and recovery heart rates, and explain their relationship to cardiovascular fitness.
* Name the three phases of an exercise session.
* Explain the principles of overload, progression, specificity, and retrogression.
* Define and explain static, ballistic, and PNF stretching.
* Name the muscle groups exercised during strength/endurance training.
* Be able to wisely select attire, shoes, fitness products, facilities, and health and fitness spas/clubs.
* Name and explain three heat-related injuries and two cold-related injuries.
* Explain the RICES injury treatment concept.

When speaking of physical fitness, the term has different meanings for different people. Some narrow their focus to top athletes. For them Michael Jordan may be the personification of physical fitness. In the past, physical fitness was identified with strength, à la Charles Atlas. With the emphasis on aerobics recently, many equate physical fitness to cardiorespiratory fitness — to the exclusion of the other components of fitness. And how does overall health fit into the physical fitness picture? The answer is that physical fitness is

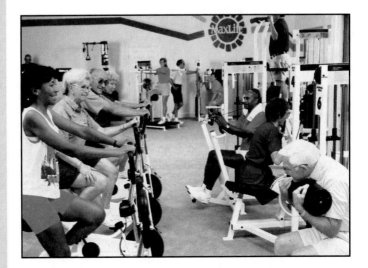

all of these things. The American Medical Association has defined **physical fitness** as the general capacity to adapt and respond favorably to physical effort. Physically fit people are able to meet the ordinary and the extraordinary demands of daily life effectively without being exhausted and with energy to spare for recreational activities.

The opposite of physical fitness is a sedentary life, ironically misnamed the "good life" on occasion. Contemporary society has cars, golf carts, elevators, remote controls, and other labor-saving devices to make life easier. Unfortunately, that is not what we need. These conveniences hasten the rate of deterioration of the body, threaten health, and shorten life. Sedentary people have twice as many health problems as active people. Exercise is essential to fitness and adds years to our life and life to our years. An active person has more energy, a leaner physique, and a stronger and more flexible body.

Physical fitness can be classified into two categories: skill-related fitness and health-related fitness. Skill-related fitness, primarily the domain of athletes, is composed of agility, balance, coordination, power, reaction time, and speed. Because the emphasis of this book is on health, we are concerned here with the basic components of **health-related fitness**: cardiorespiratory endurance, body composition, muscular flexibility, muscular strength and endurance. These components are shown in Figure 11.1. Body composition was discussed in

Chapter 10, so that information will not be repeated here.

BENEFITS OF EXERCISE

When asked why they exercise, most people indicate that it makes them "feel better." These two words cover a multitude of benefits, the greatest of which is an improved quality of life. More specific health benefits of physical activity are summarized below:

* Lowers the blood pressure
* Increases energy
* Improves muscle strength, flexibility, and tone
* Improves posture; tightens and firms abdomen
* Alleviates back problems
* Allows greater mobility of joints
* Increases muscle strength and tone
* Strengthens bones, thereby reducing risk of osteoporosis
* Reduces risk for cardiovascular disease
* Improves cardiorespiratory system
* Prevents blood pooling and varicose veins in legs
* Improves blood circulation
* Improves digestion and fat metabolism
* Boosts the immune system
* Promotes faster recovery following injury and disease
* Alleviates premenstrual syndrome (PMS)
* Lowers the risk for chronic illness and cancer
* Lowers LDL ("bad") cholesterol and increases HDL ("good") cholesterol
* Promotes better sleep habits
* Aids in weight control
* Lowers stress and anxiety levels
* Relieves chronic pain
* Improves self-image and helps fight depression
* Boosts sexual vitality
* Improves quality of life
* Delays aging and extends longevity

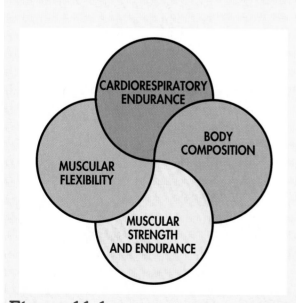

Figure 11.1 Health-related fitness components

OBJECTIVES FOR PHYSICAL FITNESS

✳ Increase the proportion of people age 6 and older who engage regularly, preferably daily, in light to moderate physical activity at least 30 minutes per day.

✳ Increase the proportion of people who engage in vigorous physical activity that promotes the development and maintenance of cardiorespiratory fitness 3 or more days per week for 20 or more minutes per occasion.

✳ Reduce the proportion of people age 6 and older who engage in no leisure-time physical activity.

✳ Increase the proportion of people age 6 and older who regularly perform physical activities that enhance and maintain muscular strength, muscular endurance, and flexibility.

✳ Increase the proportion of overweight people age 12 and older who have adopted sound dietary practices combined with regular physical activity to attain an appropriate body weight.

✳ Increase the proportion of worksites offering employer-sponsored physical activity and fitness programs.

In contrast, a sedentary lifestyle promotes high blood pressure, coronary heart disease, ulcers, insomnia, low back pain, blood vessel disorders, atherosclerosis, strokes, obesity, cancer, and diabetes, among other conditions. In general, diseases associated with a sedentary lifestyle are called **hypokinetic** (hypo = under, kinetic = activity) disorders.

According to Susan Johnson, Director of Continuing Education, Cooper Institute for Aerobics Research, Dallas, the psychological benefits of exercise include:

✳ Less stress — because a physically fit person is better able to cope with minor stresses and because exercise is a way to get rid of excess energy and stress-related emotions.

✳ Less anxiety — for the same reasons regular exercise decreases stress.

✳ Less depression. Some mental health specialists are recommending that people with depression start a regular exercise program as part of their treatment.

✳ Increased alertness.

✳ Greater productivity.

✳ Enhanced self-image. People who exercise regularly look good — and they know it. Therefore, they feel good.

✳ Higher self-esteem. All of the above factors combine to raise self-esteem.

✳ Improved sense of general well-being.

To achieve the benefits of exercise, the **FITT formula** — frequency, intensity, time, and type of activity — can be applied to each of the physical fitness components discussed in this chapter. Generally, the formula works this way:

✳ **Frequency (F)**

Ideally, a person should exercise 3 to 5 days per week. Beginning exercisers should start with three times and may progress to five times per week. With more than 5 days of physical activity per week, extra improvements are minimal. One or two days of rest per week will enable the body to recuperate and prevent injury. Individuals on a weight-loss program should

KEY TERMS

Physical fitness the general capacity to adapt and respond favorably to physical effort

Health-related fitness has four components: body composition, cardiovascular endurance, muscular flexibility, muscular strength/endurance

Hypokinetic underactive

FITT formula frequency, intensity, time, and type of workout applied to each of the physical fitness components exercise 45 to 60 minutes at low to moderate intensity, 5 to 6 days per week. Exercising longer increases caloric expenditure for quicker weight loss.

✳ **Intensity (I)**

Intensity refers to how hard a person must work to improve physical fitness. This is discussed specifically under each of the health-related fitness components.

✳ **Time (T)**

The American College of Sports Medicine recommends a workout session of 20–60 minutes. Beginners and older people should start at 20 minutes and gradually build up to 30–60 minutes.

✳ **Type of Activity (T)**

The type of activity a person selects is a function of cardiorespiratory endurance, flexibility, and muscular strength and endurance. Exercises in each of these areas are suggested throughout this chapter.

PHASES OF EXERCISE

Each exercise session has three basic phases: the warm-up, the workout, and the cool-down. These phases apply to whichever health-related component (cardiorespiratory, flexibility, muscular strength/endurance) is to be developed, though the specific exercises are unique to each.

Warm-up

The **warm-up**, the beginning phase of each session, helps the body progress gradually from rest to exercise as blood moves more freely in the joints and increases the speed of nerve impulses to the active muscles. The warm-up has the following features:

1. Slowly stretching while concentrating on movements and flexibility exercises raises the temperature of heart and skeletal muscles.

2. The heart rate should reach about 120 beats per minute.

3. Warm-up activities help prevent injury and muscle soreness.

4. Preparation for cardiorespiratory training should include approximately 2 minutes of walking, jogging, or mild exercises in place.

5. Static stretching of the major muscle groups (discussed later) is emphasized.

6. The entire warm-up should be 5 to 10 minutes.

Workout Session

After the warm-up comes the time to work out. The heart and lungs obtain their best benefits when the workout is continuous, using the large muscle groups for about 30 minutes. When people first start exercising, they may not be able to exercise continuously for 30 minutes without resting. As they exercise each day, they will find that they will be exercising longer without tiring. If a person is not sweating or breathing hard or the heart rate has not increased, he or she is not exercising hard enough. People who are getting a good workout, will be sweating, their heart will be beating faster, and they will be breathing harder, but they should be able to converse at the same time.

Cool-Down

During a vigorous workout the heart pumps blood to all of the body's muscles. These muscles contract and return the blood to the heart for reoxygenation, preventing blood from pooling in the arm and leg muscles. Ceasing activity abruptly can cause the

---

Warm-Ups

The best warm-ups are those that mirror your real workout to come.

✳ *Runners:* Start with a brisk walk or jog a slow mile.

✳ *Golfers:* Take some practice swings.

✳ *Swimmers:* Do some slow laps.

✳ *Aerobics:* Before class, do a couple of easy dance routines.

✳ *Tennis players:* Practice footwork and do some easy serves and groundstrokes.

Exercise-equipment workouts require a warm-up, too. Involve arms and legs by combining work on a stationary bike, rowing machine, or treadmill to loosen major muscles. Then have a go at the stair-climbing machine.

All warm-ups start gently and gradually gear up to 10 minutes of light exercise.

Adapted from *Well-Body Almanac,* edited by Tracy Minkin; research assistance by Editorial Advisory Committee, Medical Center, University of Alabama, Birmingham.

Why Do We Sweat?

Many people think of sweat as an annoyance, but without it we might literally cook to death. Sweat cools the body as it evaporates. When the humidity climbs close to 100%, however, sweat cannot evaporate into the air. That's when it turns the body sticky and runs off the face and body in rivulets.

Sweating indicates that the body is working fine. A fit person sweats at a lower temperature than a person who is not fit — about twice as much as a sedentary person. During a 2-hour workout on a hot day, an athlete can lose as much as a gallon of water from the body.

Men sweat more than women. A woman's body temperature has to climb a degree higher than a man's before she begins to perspire. Hairy people sweat more because their more numerous hair follicles provide homes to more apocrine glands. The apocrine glands, found in the armpits, genitals, and any place we have hair, produce a substance that becomes rank smelling when mixed with bacteria. Asians have fewer apocrines than Anglos or African Americans, so they sweat less. The odor is so rare in Japanese men that it would have disqualified a man from military service at one time.

Indeed, body odor is what gives sweat a bad name. The negative reaction to sweating hasn't always been the case, however. Sweat once was considered an aphrodisiac. Elizabethan lovers exchanged peeled apples they had worn under their arms. In a letter to Josephine, Napoleon wrote, "I will be arriving in Paris tomorrow. Don't wash."

Source: "Be Grateful for Sweat," by Ken Scales, *Ebony Magazine*, November 1994.

FITNESS TRAINING PRINCIPLES

Training principles that are incorporated in any exercise program are:

1. *Overload.* According to the **overload principle**, to improve physical fitness, the body must be subjected gradually to more stress than it is accustomed to. The body is an adaptive mechanism. When the level of stress increases, the body will adjust and must work harder to see improvement. Overload is specific to each body part, as well as each component of fitness (cardiorespiratory, flexibility, strength/endurance).

2. *Progression.* The **progression principle** combines overload and adaptation. If fitness is to be achieved, additional stress (overload) must be placed on the body once it has adapted to stress. If the overload is increased too soon before the body has had time to adapt to that stress, exhaustion or regression may result.

3. *Specificity.* The principle of **specificity of training** states that overload must be aimed specifically at the desired outcome of the fitness component. Physical exercise programs should be designed or closely resemble the activity with specific results in mind. For example, if you are training for *strength*, you must lift weights (a resistance) to get the desired results.

4. *Retrogression.* During the exercise process, the exerciser will reach plateaus when improvement stops temporarily. Performance may level off for a time before it improves again. This is the **retrogression principle**. Once the body has adjusted to the overload, performance levels will improve.

exerciser to become faint, dizzy, or even pass out.

Stretching plus an aerobic activity (walking or light jogging) are recommended **cool-down** activities to immediately follow each exercise session. The person continues to exercise at a lower level so the body can return safely to its resting state. The cool-down phase should last about 5 to 10 minutes or until the heart rate generally is below 120 beats per minute. The cool-down should be longer for more intense and longer workouts.

KEY TERMS

Warm-up the beginning phase of each workout session that helps the body progress gradually from rest to exercise

Cool-down the ending phase of a workout that helps the body begin to return to its resting state

Overload principle gradually subjecting the body to more stress than it is accustomed to

Progression principle placing additional stress on the body once it has adapted to its current stress factor

Specificity of training aiming overload specifically at the desired outcome of the fitness component

Retrogression principle leveling of performance for a period of time before performance improves again

5. *Slow and gradual exercise.* The key to success in an exercise program is to begin slowly and be consistent. Increasing the frequency, intensity, time, and type of exercise too rapidly may invite injury. The body requires time to adjust to a sudden change in lifestyle. Training must be sensible.

CARDIORESPIRATORY ENDURANCE

The single most important component of health-related physical fitness is cardiorespiratory endurance or aerobic exercise. **Cardiorespiratory endurance** is the ability of the heart, lungs, and blood vessels to deliver blood and nutrients to the cells efficiently to meet the demands of prolonged, aerobic physical activity. The term *cardiovascular* often is used instead. The American College of Sports Medicine prefers to use *cardiorespiratory* because it may describe the total function, including that of the lungs, more accurately.

Cardiorespiratory fitness is achieved by **aerobic exercises,** which improve the heart and lung functioning by boosting the body's consumption of oxygen. Aerobic means "with oxygen." Any activity that requires oxygen to produce energy is called aerobic. Some common examples are brisk walking, running, swimming, and cycling. These generally are continuous and rhythmic, and they require the heart to beat faster to produce the oxygen necessary to perform the activity.

In contrast to aerobic exercise is **anaerobic exercise,** which does not require oxygen to produce the necessary energy. Anaerobic exercises are high-intensity and can be preformed for only short periods. They do not develop the cardiorespiratory system. Examples of anaerobic exercise are sprinting and weight lifting.

Exercises that have frequent rest intervals between outlays of energy are called **nonaerobic exercises.** They, too, do not give the heart and lungs a good workout. Examples are bowling, softball, golf, and doubles tennis.

Benefits of Aerobic Exercise

The primary benefits of aerobic exercise are that it:

❋ Improves the ability of the heart, lungs, and circulatory system to carry oxygen to the body's cells

❋ Requires the heart to pump more blood per beat, which increases its efficiency

❋ Slows the resting heart rate

❋ Improves the supply of blood to the tissues

FITT Formula for Cardiovascular Endurance

F = Frequency   3–5 days per week

I = Intensity   60%–85% heart rate reserve

T = Time   30–60 minutes of continuous aerobic activity

T = Type of activity   Aerobic (walking, race walking, jogging, water jogging, skipping rope, stair climbing, bench stepping, cycling, aerobic dance, soccer)

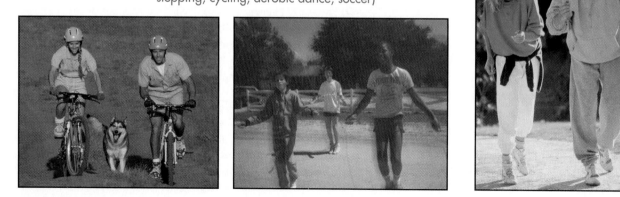

What time of day should you exercise?

The best time for exercise is the time that is right for you. If you're a "morning person," set your alarm 30 minutes earlier. Others like to exercise in late afternoon or after work to relax. Some say that if they exercise too late in the day, they have trouble falling asleep. Most important is to find the time of day that feels best so you will stick to your exercise program.

❋ Decreases the resting blood pressure

❋ Improves cardiorespiratory system so it works less at rest and during lower levels of exercise

❋ Has positive effects on blood lipids (fats)

❋ Helps protect a person from the effects of stress

❋ Improves the body's metabolism, thus providing better control of body fat

❋ Improves psychological and emotional well-being

Aerobic exercise also is classified in two ways. **High-impact aerobics** have a running or jumping component. These exercises are not recommended for individuals with a low level of fitness. **Low-impact aerobics** place minimal stress on the joints and are recommended for people with low fitness levels. Examples of these nonweight-bearing activities are walking, cycling, rowing, water jogging, and swimming. Computerized and noncomputerized machines have been manufactured to simulate many of these activities — rowing machines, treadmills, stationary bicycles, and cross country-skiing machines, to name a few.

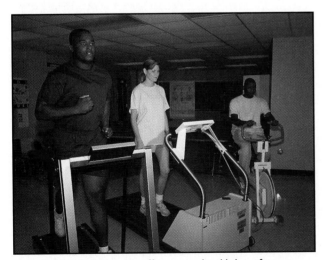

Aerobic exercise offers many health benefits.

Principles and Concepts of Aerobic Exercise

Some basic principles apply to cardiorespiratory or aerobic endurance for health-related purposes.

1. Frequency, intensity, and time should be considered in relation to the person's fitness level.

2. Low-impact activities are safer, especially for older people and for those who need to minimize strain to the joints.

3. The rate of progression usually is slower for individuals who are not fit.

4. Self-concept and motivation are important when continuing a health-fitness program for a lifetime.

The selected activity must be continuous and sufficiently strenuous to elevate the heart rate to the **proper training intensity** — the intensity that gives the best cardiorespiratory development results. "Continuous" is defined as an activity that takes 3 minutes or longer and marks the approximate point at which the contracting skeletal muscle shifts to aerobic metabolism to produce energy.

Before undertaking an aerobic program, a person should understand the applicable concepts, including resting and maximal heart rates, recovery heart rate, and rate of perceived exertion. A physician's approval is necessary if you have any concerns regarding your state of health to safely start an exercise program.

KEY TERMS

Cardiorespiratory endurance the ability of the heart, lungs, and blood vessels to deliver blood and nutrients to the cells efficiently during aerobic activity

Aerobic exercises any activity that requires oxygen to produce energy

Anaerobic exercise high-intensity activity that does not require oxygen to produce the desired energy

Nonaerobic exercises activities that have frequent rest intervals between outlays of energy

High-impact aerobics aerobic exercise that has a running or jumping component

Low-impact aerobics activities that place minimal stress on the joints and are recommended for people with low fitness levels

Proper training intensity the intensity that gives the best cardiorespiratory development results determined by heart rate

Risk Factors for Exercising

Precede an exercise program with a medical exam if you have any of the following risk factors:

❋ elevated blood pressure

❋ cigarette smoking

❋ family history of coronary heart disease in parents or siblings before age 55

❋ any heart, lung, or metabolic disease, such as diabetes

Resting Heart Rate

To calculate target heart rate, you first must learn how to measure resting heart rate. Resting heart rate can be a good indicator of your fitness level. Slow resting heart rates tend to indicate an active lifestyle, and fast rates are associated with sedentary habits.

Resting heart rate can be determined by counting the heart rate for 1 minute upon waking naturally early in the morning (without an alarm). Perhaps to get the best results, you should take your resting heart rate several days in a row and get an average. Table 11.1 gives resting heart rate ratings.

You can take your pulse in two different ways. The **carotid pulse** is taken by locating the carotid artery in the neck and gently tilting the head back slightly to one side. You should use the middle finger or forefinger (or both) to feel the pulse. You should not use the thumb, because it has a beat of

its own. Pressure to the carotid artery should be applied lightly; a firm pressure will result in a reflex response, causing a temporary drop in heart rate. The **radial pulse** may be taken by placing your fingers on the thumb side of your upturned wrist below the heel of the hand. Some people have trouble counting the pulse at this site while resting but find it easy to count when exercising.

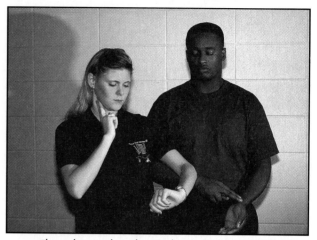

The pulse can be taken at the carotid artery (left) or the radial artery (right)

Target Heart Rate

To determine your target heart rate, you must first learn to estimate your **maximal heart rate (MHR)**, the highest rate obtained during all-out exercise. This is done by subtracting your age from 220. Cardiorespiratory development takes place when working between 50% and 85% of **heart rate reserve**. For health purposes the 60% level allows conversation during exercise and is considered safe. "Moderate" is about 70%. Starting too low is better than starting too high. The goal is to increase the intensity gradually until you can tolerate the 85% intensity.

Factors including emotional stress, high humidity, and hot temperatures must be taken into account, as they may affect the heart rate response. (These factors are discussed later in the chapter.) Infections and fever elevate the body temperature, increasing the heart rate response. Medications such as **beta blockers**, prescribed to control high blood pressure and heart conditions, decrease the heart activity and may constrict air passages in the lungs. Any person taking prescription medications should exercise with the physician's knowledge and recommendations.

Table 11.1
Resting Heart Rate Ratings

Heart Rate (beats/minute)	Rating
<59	Excellent
60–69	Good
70–79	Average
80–89	Fair
> 90	Poor

Source: *Principles & Labs for Physical Fitness and Wellness*, by Werner W. K. Hoeger and Sharon A. Hoeger (Englewood, CO: Morton Publishing, 1994). Reprinted by permission of the authors.

The best way to determine if the exercise is intense enough to condition the heart and lungs, but not too intense, is to take the pulse often during an exercise session. A heart responding normally to exercise shows a rapid increase during the first 3–5 minutes, followed by a steady state or plateau. Beginning exercisers should aim for the lower end of the target zone (60%) and gradually increase to 85% of the maximum heart rate. To determine target zone, according to the **Karvonen formula:**

1. Determine your resting heart rate (RHR)

2. Find your maximal heart rate (MHR) by subtracting your age from 220 (for example: 220 − 20 (age) = 200.)

3. Check your pulse immediately after completing the exercise session.

To find the upper limits of your target zone, compute as follows:

upper limit = (MHR − RHR) × .85 + RHR = ____

To find the lower limits of the target zone:

lower limit = (MHR − RHR) × .60 + RHR = ____

Figure 11.2 shows the target zone for a 20-year-old male in average physical shape.

KEY TERMS

Carotid pulse pulse taken by locating the carotid artery in the neck

Radial pulse pulse taken by locating the radial artery in the wrist

Maximal heart rate (MHR) the fastest heart rate obtained during all-out exercise

Heart rate reserve (HRR) the difference between resting heart rate and maximal heart rate

Beta blockers medications prescribed to control high blood pressure and heart conditions

Karvonen formula a method for determining if exercise is demanding enough to condition the heart and lungs by ascertaining the optimal target zone

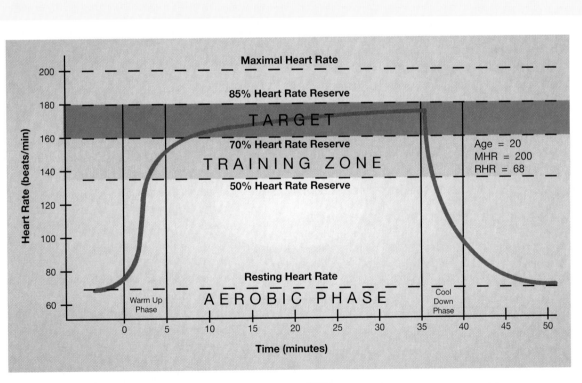

Reprinted with permission. *Lifetime Physical Fitness & Wellness: A Personalized Approach* by Werner W. K. Hoeger and Sharon A. Hoeger. Copyright © 1994, 4th Edition, Morton Publishing Co.

Figure 11.2 Typical cardiovascular or aerobic training pattern

Recovery Heart Rate

Recovery time after exercising helps determine whether the exercise demands are appropriate or excessive. As part of the cool-down, the pulse should be checked at 5 minutes and 10 minutes after exercising. After 5 minutes the pulse rate should be below 120 beats per minute, and after 10 minutes the pulse rate should be below 100 beats per minute. The closer the pulse is to your resting heart rate, the better is your condition. If it takes a long time for your pulse to recover and return to its resting level, you are unfit. Fast recovery indicates a good fitness level.

The pulse rate of most individuals decreases to under 100 beats per minute during the first minute of rest and decreases during the first 2 to 3 minutes after exercise at about the same rate it increased during exercise. For healthy young people, cool-down should last until the heart rate is about 120 or below. For middle-aged and older adults, the rates should be 100 and below.

Rate of Perceived Exertion (RPE)

An alternative method of determining the intensity of exercise is the **rate of perceived exertion (RPE)** scale developed by Gunnar Borg. Individuals may perceive less or do more than they think they do while exercising. Therefore, associating your own inner perception of the exercise with the phrases given on the scale in Figure 11.3 is important. This

From "Perceived Exertion: A Note on History and Methods," by Gunnar Borg, *Medicine and Science in Sports and Exercise*, 5 (1983), 90–93.

Figure 11.3 Rate of perceived exertion scale

scale from 6 to 20 is preferred because adding a 0 to each number provides a rough estimate of heartbeats per minute. For example, *hard* corresponds to a heart rate of 150. *Very hard* is comparable to a heart rate of 170. Generally, warm-ups and cool-downs range between 7 and 11. The typical intensity for training is 11 to 16 (110–160).

RPEs eliminate the problem of counting pulse rate during aerobic activities. Perhaps for safety, exercisers should check the target zone against the rate of perceived exertion during the first weeks of an exercise program to ensure that they are within the proper heart rate intensity guidelines.

Frequency and Time

Frequency of exercise is an important variable in increasing the body's ability to use oxygen (aerobic capacity). Beyond a certain

---

Teenage Girls and Exercise

When asked what they thought about physical education class, fifteen teenage girls from Edison High School, New Jersey, wrinkled their noses in disgust. The reasons for this disdain of exercise? Not wanting to mess up their hair and simply not wanting to be bothered.

Their reactions were not unusual. The national increase in inactivity across the board seems especially pronounced in teenage girls. Reasons for the laziness in this particular group are elusive, but the aversion to exercise does extend to sports. This puts boys at an advantage, because they still tend to place a much higher priority on sport activity than girls do.

Unfortunately, lack of activity is leading girls down a path toward obesity and serious health problems throughout life.

frequency and duration, exercise does not benefit the exerciser and can be risky. According to Dr. Kenneth Cooper, a pioneer in the field of aerobics, unless you are preparing for a race, running more than 15 miles a week is not necessary for fitness. Cooper's research indicates that exercising more than five times a week triples the injury rate in amateur athletes. Further, increasing the duration of each exercise session from 30 to 45 minutes doubles the risk, unless it is done gradually over several months.

Fast heart rate recovery indicates a good fitness level.

Cross-Training

Cross-training means combining more than one activity to attain cardiorespiratory fitness. It also can be used to allow certain muscles to rest. Most of all, it can provide relief from monotony and renewed motivation. For example, swimming and running might be alternated, or a person could try a new activity such as canoeing to substitute for the usual tennis.

Assessment of Cardiorespiratory Fitness

Laboratory measurements (treadmill, bicycle ergometer) or field tests (distance/speed measures and step tests) can be used to determine aerobic function. The most commonly used tests for health-related purposes are the field tests used to estimate aerobic fitness level, such as step tests, distance runs, and walking tests. Distance runs (12-minute or 1.0 to 1.5 miles) maintaining a constant speed or pace, are popular. Fast walking is recommended for unfit persons and older adults. The Rockport Fitness Walking Test provides a good measure of aerobic fitness. The goal of this test is to walk 1 mile as fast as possible. To make valid comparisons, the same test should be used for both pre- and post-assessments. Field test results should be considered only estimates of the person's ability. (See Self-Assessment at the end of this chapter.)

FLEXIBILITY

Flexibility is defined as the ability of a joint to move freely through its full range of motion. The full range of motion in a joint or group of joints is necessary to perform most active sports and daily activities without straining the muscles and developing back problems, as well as to maintain good posture. The degree of flexibility depends on hereditary factors, age, sex, occupation, posture, body composition, and musculoskeletal differences. Generally, flexibility improves from childhood through adolescence. Afterward a gradual loss of joint mobility continues throughout adult life.

At all ages females tend to be more flexible than males. Stretching exercises can increase flexibility. Because range of motion is specific to body parts (trunk, shoulder, ankle), a complete stretching program should include all body parts and follow basic guidelines for improving flexibility. Figure 11.4 shows the major muscle groups exercised, and representative exercises are presented on the next few pages.

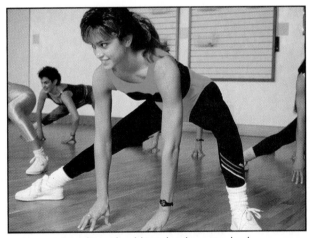

Stretching should involve the entire body.

KEY TERMS

Rate of perceived exertion (RPE) an alternative method of determining the intensity of exercise

Cross-training combining more than one activity to attain cardiorespiratory fitness

Flexibility the ability of a joint to move freely through its full range of motion

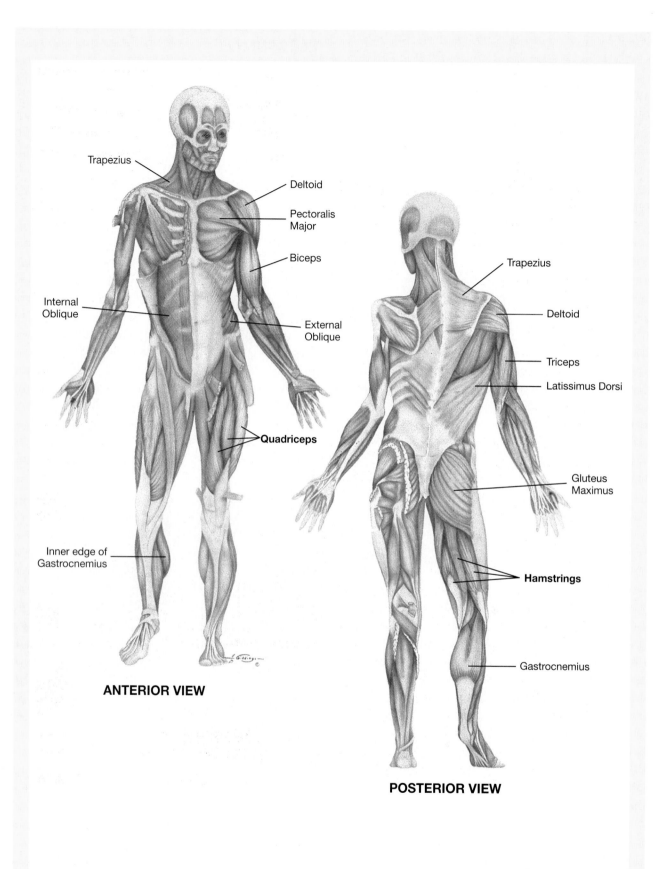

Trapezius

Deltoid

Pectoralis Major

Biceps

Internal Oblique

External Oblique

Quadriceps

Inner edge of Gastrocnemius

ANTERIOR VIEW

Trapezius

Deltoid

Triceps

Latissimus Dorsi

Gluteus Maximus

Hamstrings

Gastrocnemius

POSTERIOR VIEW

Figure 11.4 Major muscle groups of the body

FITT Formula for Flexibility

F = **Frequency** After initial daily stretching, 8 weeks, 2–3 days per week to maintain
I = **Intensity** Stretch to the point of mild discomfort
T = **Time** Five times per exercise, final stretch position 10–60 seconds
T = **Type of activity** Static (slow-sustained)

Types of Stretching

Stretching exercises are of three types:

1. Static or slow-sustained

2. Ballistic or dynamic

3. Proprioceptive neuromuscular facilitation (PNF)

Static or **slow-sustained stretching** is the most frequently used and recommended of the stretching exercises. In this technique the muscles are relaxed and lengthened gradually through a joint's complete range of motion and are held for a short time (10–60 seconds). This type of stretch should not be painful. It also has a low injury rate. Therefore, it should be used especially by beginners and older adults.

The **ballistic** or **dynamic stretching** technique uses rapid, bouncy, or bobbing movements to stretch muscle fibers. It can be dangerous and counterproductive. The bounces can overstretch muscle fibers, causing the muscle to contract rather than stretch. This may produce muscle soreness and injury from small tears to the soft tissue. This type of stretching is not recommended for health-related purposes.

Proprioceptive neuromuscular facilitation (PNF) is based on the contraction and relaxation of muscles. It requires the assistance of another person. The procedure is as follows:

1. The person assisting with the exercise provides initial force by slowly pushing in the direction of the desired stretch. The first stretch does not cover the entire range of motion.

2. The person being stretched then applies force in the opposite direction of the stretch, against the assistant who tries to hold the initial degree of stretch as close as possible. An isometric contraction is being performed at that angle.

3. After four or five seconds of isometric contraction, the muscle being stretched is completely relaxed. The assistant then slowly increases the degree of stretch to a greater angle.

4. The isometric contraction then is repeated for another 4 or 5 seconds, following which the muscle is relaxed again. The assistant then can slowly increase the degree of stretch one more time. Steps one to four are repeated two to five more times, until the exerciser feels mild discomfort. On the last trial the final stretched position should be held for several seconds.

Some researchers believe the PNF technique results in greater muscle length and therefore is more effective than the static stretch. The disadvantages of this type of stretch are that two people are needed, more time is required, and the probability of injury is greater.

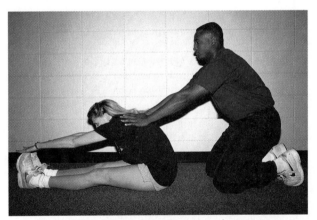

The PNF stretching technique requires the assistance of another person.

KEY TERMS

Static (slow-sustained) stretching technique in which muscles are relaxed and lengthened gradually through a joint's complete range of motion
Dynamic (ballistic) stretching technique using rapid, bouncy, or bobbing movements to stretch muscle fibers
Proprioceptive neuromuscular facilitation (PNF) technique based on the contraction and relaxation of muscles

Quad Stretch

Action: Grasp the foot and lift the foot to buttocks level and pull backward with opposite hand.

Areas Stretched: Quadriceps muscle.

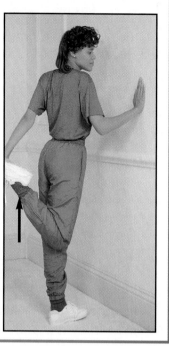

Trunk Rotation and Lower Back Stretch

Action: Sit on the floor and bend the left leg, placing the left foot on the outside of the right knee. Place the right elbow on the left knee and push against it. At the same time, try to rotate the trunk to the left (counterclockwise). Hold the final position for a few seconds. Repeat the exercise with the other side.

Areas Stretched: Lateral side of the hip and thigh; trunk, and lower back.

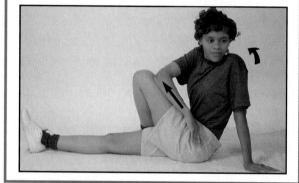

Single-Knee to Chest Stretch

Action: Lie down flat on the floor. Bend one leg at approximately 100° and gradually pull the opposite leg toward your chest. Hold the final stretch for a few seconds. Switch legs and repeat the exercise. Lower back should remain in contact with floor.

Areas Stretched: Lower back and hamstring muscles, and lumbar spine ligaments.

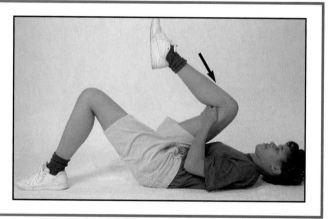

Double-Knee to Chest Stretch

Action: Lie flat on the floor and then slowly curl up into a fetal position. Hold for a few seconds. Lower back should remain in contact with floor.

Areas Stretched: Upper and lower back and hamstring muscles; spinal ligaments.

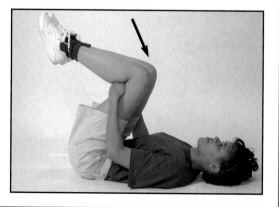

Triceps Stretch

Action: Place the right hand behind your neck. Grasp the right arm above the elbow with the left hand. Gently pull the elbow backward. Repeat the exercise with the opposite arm.

Areas Stretched: Back of upper arm (triceps muscle) and shoulder joint.

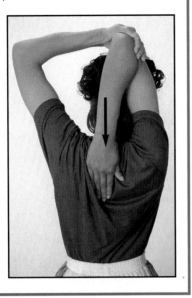

Heel Cord Stretch

Action: Stand against the wall or at the edge of a step and stretch the heel downward, alternating legs. Hold the stretched position for a few seconds.

Areas Stretched: Heel cord (Achilles tendon), gastrocnemius, and soleus muscles.

Hamstring Stretch

Action: Extend right leg. Position the left leg with knee bent with the bottom of the foot touching the extended leg. Reach with both hands toward the ankle or foot and pull head to knee while keeping the leg straight. Hold for a few seconds. Repeat other side.

Areas Stretched: Hamstrings.

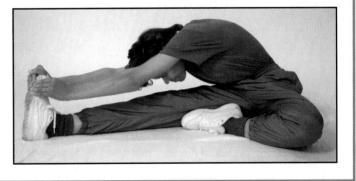

Sit-and-Reach Stretch

Action: Sit on the floor with legs together and gradually reach forward as far as possible. Hold the final position for a few seconds. This exercise may also be performed with the legs separated, reaching to each side as well as to the middle.

Areas Stretched: Hamstrings and lower back muscles, and lumbar spine ligaments.

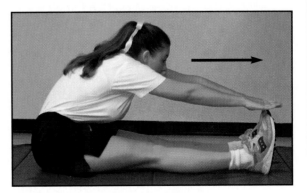

Lateral Head Tilt

Action: Slowly and gently tilt the head laterally. Repeat several times to each side.

Areas Stretched: Neck muscles and ligaments of the cervical spine.

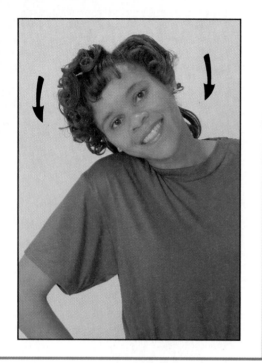

Side Stretch

Action: Stand straight up, feet separated to shoulder width, and place your hands on your waist. Now move the upper body to one side and hold the final stretch for a few seconds. Repeat on the other side.

Areas Stretched: Muscles and ligaments in the pelvic region.

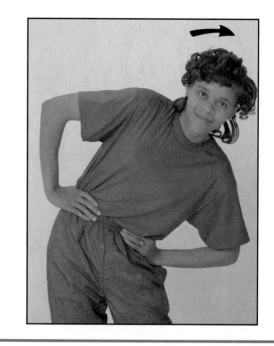

Shoulder Hyperextension Stretch

Action: Have a partner grasp your arms from behind by the wrists and slowly push them upward. Hold the final position for a few seconds.

Areas Stretched: Deltoid and pectoral muscles, and ligaments of the shoulder joint.

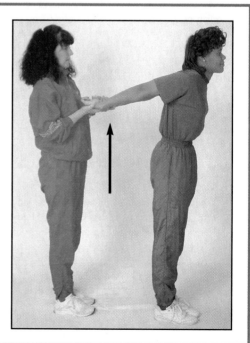

Assessment of Flexibility

Flexibility is specific to each muscle group. Therefore, different tests determine the range of motion in various groups of muscles. Two tests commonly used for an indication of flexibility levels are the Sit-and-Reach and the Total Body Rotation tests. The most widely known test, the Modified Sit-and-Reach, estimates hip, hamstring, and spine flexibility. An improvement over the traditional Sit-and-Reach test, arm and leg lengths are taken into consideration. When these muscle groups are tight, chronic lower back problems and injury may result. Tightness of these muscles is associated with too much sitting, an indicator of a sedentary lifestyle. Stretching prior to testing is necessary before performing any flexibility testing. The Backsaver Sit-and-Reach test is commonly substituted for the modified Sit-and-Reach. The Modified Sit-and-Reach is presented as a self-assessment at the end of the chapter.

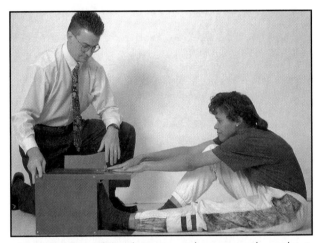

Backsaver Sit-and-Reach Test is another commonly used test in place of the Modified Sit-and-Reach Test.

MUSCULAR STRENGTH AND ENDURANCE

Muscular strength is the ability or capacity of a muscle or muscle group to exert maximum force against resistance. This means the absolute maximum weight that can be lifted, pushed, pulled, or pressed in one effort. Examples of muscular strength are pull-ups and rope climbing. Strong muscles provide greater endurance, resistance to fatigue, and power, and they help to maintain correct posture. In addition, strong muscles protect the body joints, resulting in fewer strains, sprains, and muscular difficulties such as back pain.

Age and sex differences parallel changes in muscle mass. Strength in females tends to decline after age 30, and this decline usually is the result of decreasing physical activity. Males gain strength rapidly at puberty (13–14 years) because of their sex hormone, testosterone, which stimulates muscle growth. The continuing production of testosterone contributes to strength. Women's strength may increase from strength training, but women do not develop muscle bulk as males do because they produce much smaller amounts of testosterone. Thus, the average male is stronger than the average female.

Closely related to muscular strength is **muscular endurance**, the ability of muscles to exert force or sustain a muscle contraction repeatedly for an extended period. A person who is strong is more resistant to fatigue because less effort is required to produce repeated muscular contractions. Muscular endurance usually implies specific groups of muscles — for example, abdominals, thighs, chest. Examples of exercises to increase endurance are abdominal curl-ups, push-ups, and sit-ups when these can be repeated more than ten times.

If muscles are not used, they will degenerate and **atrophy** (decrease in strength and size). Muscles begin to atrophy after 3 to 4 days if they are not exercised. If muscles are used regularly and vigorously, they will increase in size and improve in strength, termed **hypertrophy**.

Muscular training is highly specific, and specific muscles must be exercised to achieve certain results. A workout with weights should exercise major muscle groups: the deltoids (shoulders), pectorals (chest), triceps and biceps (back and front of upper arm), quadriceps (front thigh), gluteus maximums (buttocks), and abdomen (refer to Figure 11.4). Numerous machines and freeweight routines

KEY TERMS

Muscular strength the ability or capacity of a muscle or muscle group to exert maximum force against resistance

Muscular endurance the ability of muscles to exert force or sustain a muscle contraction repeatedly for an extended period

Atrophy to decrease in strength or size of tissue from disuse

Hypertrophy an increase in size and strength of muscles that are used regularly and vigorously

FITT Formula for Muscular Strength and Endurance

F = **Frequency**   2–3 times per week

I = **Intensity**   8–12 repetitions of each exercise to near maximum fatigue

T = **Time**   30 minutes

T = **Type of Activity**   Isotonic — major muscle groups

focus on each muscle group. When the weight is raised and lowered, muscle fibers lengthen (eccentric) and shorten (concentric) during muscle contraction. The exercise routine is repeated until the muscle group is fatigued.

Types of Muscular Contractions

Strength and endurance can be developed by doing three types of exercise: isotonic, isometric, and isokinetic. In **isotonic (dynamic) muscle contraction** the muscle changes length, either shortening (concentrically) or lengthening (eccentrically). Isotonic exercises are those in which a resistance is raised and then lowered, such as in weight lifting (bench press), or the resistance comes from the body's own weight (push-ups, sit-ups).

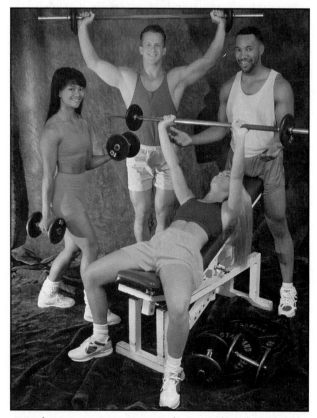

Weight training increases muscular strength and endurance.

Isotonic exercise develops the most muscular strength when the resistance is high with few repetitions. Isotonic exercise equipment includes free weights, barbells (dumbbells), floor, wall, or ceiling pulleys, bars for pull-ups, and Nautilus and Universal (variable resistance) machines. Nautilus and Universal weight-training machines follow the

Abdominal Crunch and Abdominal Curl-Up

Action: Start with your head and shoulders off the floor, hands in center of your chest, elbows to the side and knees slightly bent (the greater the flexion of the knee, the more difficult the curl-up). Now curl up to about 30° (abdominal crunch). Return to the starting position without letting the head or shoulders touch the floor, or allowing the hips to come off the floor. If you allow the hips to raise off the floor and the head and shoulders to touch the floor, you will most likely "swing up" on the next repetition, which minimizes the work of the abdominal muscles. If you cannot curl up with the arms on the chest, place the hands by the side of the hips or even help yourself up by holding on to your thighs. Do not perform the crunch exercise with legs completely extended, as this will cause strain on the lower back.

Muscles Developed: Abdominal muscles.

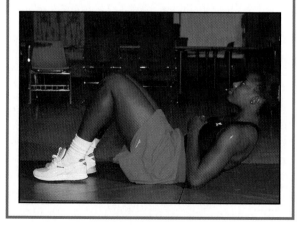

Heel Raise

Action: From a standing position with feet flat on the floor, raise and lower your body weight by moving at the ankle joint only (for added resistance, have someone else hold your shoulders down as you perform the exercise).

Muscles Developed: Gastrocnemius.

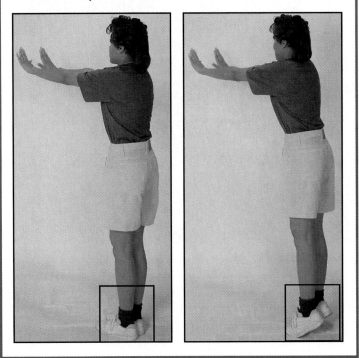

principle of variable resistance. These machines are equipped with mechanical devices that provide different amounts of resistance, with the intent of overloading the muscle group maximally through the entire range of motion.

In **isometric (static) muscle contraction** the muscle remains the same length and no movement occurs while a force is exerted against an immovable object. Squeezing a tennis ball to develop hand grip strength, pressing against doorways or walls, and pulling against ropes or towels with the arms or legs are examples of isometric exercise. Isometrics are most useful for individuals who are recovering from an injury, are bedridden, or are limited in movements for reasons other than cardiorespiratory disease.

Isokinetic exercises are isotonic concentric activities utilizing constant resistance machines that regulate movement velocity and resistance to overload muscles throughout the entire range of motion. Isokinetic exercises are most effective in

strengthening specific muscle groups. The machines are more expensive than traditional weight training equipment and are found principally in hospitals and commercial fitness clubs. Machines illustrative of this type are Exer-Genie, Cybex II, and Hydra-Fitness.

Assessment of Muscular Endurance/Strength

Strength and endurance are specific to the angle of the joint at which movement occurs. Therefore, when assessing muscular endurance and strength, the principle of specificity is important. The exercise must target the muscles identified for development.

The most widely accepted tests include the abdominal crunches and exercises involving the upper arm and shoulder (modified pull-up, pull-up, push-up, flexed arm hang), and hip and thigh (distance jump or sprint). Abdominal crunches are done with heels 12" to 18" from the buttocks. Pull-ups use different muscle groups when the palms are facing inward (easier to do) than when palms are facing outward.

Valsalva Effect

The **valsalva effect** is defined as an increase in pressure in the abdomen and chest that results from holding your breath during exercise (for example, straining to lift a heavy object or exerting maximal force). This increased pressure decreases the return

KEY TERMS

Isotonic (dynamic) muscle contraction muscle changes in length, either shortening or lengthening

Isometric (static) muscle contraction muscle remains the same length and no movement occurs while a force is exerted against an immovable object

Isokinetic exercises isotonic concentric activities utilizing constant resistance machines that regulate movement and resistance to overload muscles

Valsalva effect an increase in pressure in the abdomen and chest that results from holding one's breath during exercise

Leg Extension

Action: Sit in an upright position with the feet under the padded bar and grasp the handles at the sides. Extend the legs until they are completely straight, then return to the starting position.

Muscles Developed Quadriceps.

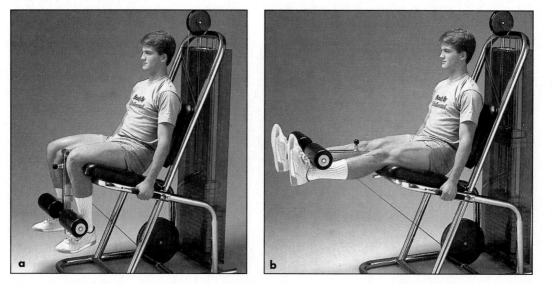

Photos courtesy of Universal Gym® Equipment Inc., 930 27th Ave., S.W., Cedar Rapids, IA 52406.

Rowing Torso

Action: Sit in the machine with your arms in front of you, elbows bent and resting against the padded bars. Press back as far as possible, drawing the shoulder blades together. Return to the original position.

Muscles developed Posterior deltoid, rhomboids, and trapezius.

Photos courtesy of Nautilus®, a registered trademark of Nautilus® Sports/Medical Industries, Inc., 709 Powerhouse Road, Independence, VA.

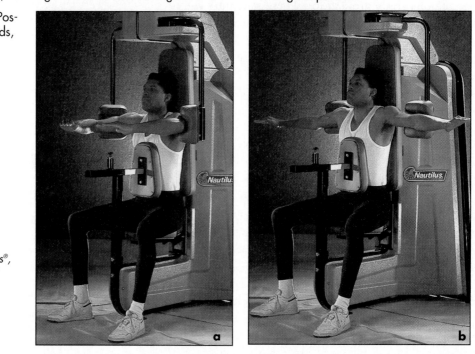

Tips for action

To prevent injury during strength/endurance training:

❋ Avoid training without medical supervision if you have high blood pressure, hernia, recent surgery, heart disease, infection, or fever.

❋ Train for muscular endurance before you train for muscular strength.

❋ Warm up 10 minutes, and stretch before and after training.

❋ Wear proper shoes with good traction.

❋ Use proper form, and progress slowly.

❋ Avoid training alone for reasons of safety as well as motivation.

❋ Do not hold your breath while lifting, as this can cause hernia or blackout (the Valsalva effect).

❋ Train the entire body, beginning with larger muscle groups.

❋ Keep weights close to the body.

❋ Avoid lifting from a stooped position.

❋ When lifting from the floor, do not allow hips to come up before the upper body.

❋ Avoid full squats, and stay in squat position as little as possible.

❋ Avoid too much overload or intensity. Allow the body to adapt to new stress without soreness.

❋ Control weights. Do not let them drop or bang.

❋ Allow 48 to 72 hours between training sessions for your body to recover from a workout and to avoid overtraining.

of blood to the heart, which in turn raises the blood pressure and slows the heart rate. In addition, tissues may be ruptured, especially in the abdominal region (hernias) and in the eyes when pathology is already present (such as glaucoma). Torn or detached retina of the eye may result when holding the breath. Obviously, this tendency is not good, and exercisers have to guard against it. The rule of breathing during resistance exercise is: Exhale while exerting force; inhale when relaxed.

Anabolic Steroids

Anabolic steroids are synthetic derivatives of the male hormone testosterone. They are approved for prescription and have been used by physicians in treating severe burns and injuries. These steroids stimulate the development of bone, muscle, skin, and hair growth, as well as emotional responses. Competitive athletes looking for an extra edge and young men and women attempting to transform their bodies sometimes use black-market and quack steroid products. Many steroids come from underground laboratories or foreign countries and often are not even steroids. Anabolic steroids are dangerous, with serious side effects as presented in Figure 11.5. Olympian Ben Johnson was stripped of his medal when tests showed he had been taking anabolic steroids.

CONDITIONS AND CLOTHING FOR EXERCISE

People exercise in all kinds of conditions and settings, from tropical islands and ski resorts to the outdoor basketball court at the community center.

KEY TERMS

Anabolic steroids synthetic derivatives of the male hormone testosterone

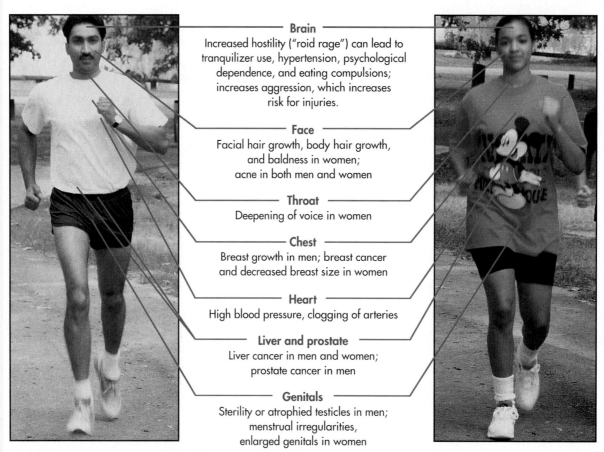

Brain
Increased hostility ("roid rage") can lead to tranquilizer use, hypertension, psychological dependence, and eating compulsions; increases aggression, which increases risk for injuries.

Face
Facial hair growth, body hair growth, and baldness in women; acne in both men and women

Throat
Deepening of voice in women

Chest
Breast growth in men; breast cancer and decreased breast size in women

Heart
High blood pressure, clogging of arteries

Liver and prostate
Liver cancer in men and women; prostate cancer in men

Genitals
Sterility or atrophied testicles in men; menstrual irregularities, enlarged genitals in women

Source: *Weight Training For Life* 3d Edition by James Hesson, Englewood, CO: Morton Publishing, 1994).

Figure 11.5 Adverse effects of steroids on the body

Life-sustaining processes require a fairly constant internal temperature, and deviations to either extreme can cause problems. Exercise is most difficult in hot and humid weather because the excess heat generated in the body is more difficult to dispel. The optimum temperature range for exercising is below 70° F when the humidity is below 45%.

Figure 11.6 presents guidelines for exercise in heat and humidity. The higher the percent humidity, the lower the temperature must be for safe exercise. Conversely, the lower the humidity, the higher the temperature can be.

The type of clothing worn during exercise is critical to optimum performance and benefit. Exercisers should dress appropriately for the environment and the specific workout. In general, the clothes worn should enable free movement and be comfortable and safe.

Exercise during a moderate workout raises the body temperature, which can make the body feel that the surrounding temperature is 20° F warmer than the actual temperature. When exercising on a 40° F day, the person should dress for a 60° F day. Dressing in several layers of loose-fitting, thin clothing is best, as the layers insulate and trap heat generated by the workout. This also allows the person to remove a layer of clothing at a time as body heat increases. Fabrics made from Capilene, Thermax, polypropylene, and synthetics are best.

In warm weather minimum clothing should be worn. It should be loose, airy, light in color, and lightweight, and should not restrict movement when exercising. Example products include Coolmax, Nike's Dri-F.I.T., Asic's Perma-Plus, and Aquator. These garments are made to wick (draw) moisture away from the skin to the surface,

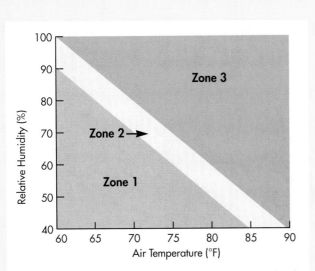

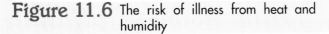

From *The Physiological Basis for Exercise and Sport,* 5th ed. Edward Fox, Richard Bowers, and Merle Foss, Copyright © 1993 Wm. C. Brown Communications, Inc., Dubuque, Iowa. All rights reserved. Reprinted by permission.

Figure 11.6 The risk of illness from heat and humidity

providing more efficient evaporation and cooling of the body.

During wet, icy, cool, and snowy weather the materials worn (such as Gortex) should allow moisture to escape from the body. A visor or cap may be necessary to keep water out of the face.

Acrylic socks are most absorbent and prevent blisters and foot irritation. They dry more quickly than cotton and draw moisture away from the skin, preventing blistering and chafing. Socks with extra cushioning at the toes, balls of the feet, and heel areas may be more expensive, but these features reduce friction better than regular socks do.

During warm weather a light-colored straw-type hat or visor will allow air to circulate around the head and protect the eyes and forehead from sun rays. During cold weather 40% of the body's heat can be lost if the head is left

uncovered. A wool or synthetic cap or hood will help to hold in body heat.

Mittens keep the fingers close together, so the surface area from which to lose heat is smaller — an advantage over gloves. Inner liners made of polypropylene or other materials are recommended to draw moisture from the skin.

Shoes are perhaps the most important piece of equipment for any exercise. Properly fitting shoes are essential to avoid injuries (Achilles tendon strain, blisters, heel bruises). In selecting the correct shoe, body type, degree of pronation or supination, if any, the activity itself, and surfaces should be considered. Walking shoes, court shoes (tennis or basketball), and shoes for aerobics have different characteristics and should be purchased for that specific exercise program. Figure 11.7 shows the characteristics of an ideal running shoe.

Additional attire to consider when exercising may be athletic bra, athletic supporter, workout watches, reflective materials (night), heart rate monitors, sunglasses, and sunscreens. Wearing rubberized suits during hot weather is dangerous. They do not allow body moisture to evaporate and may cause heat-related injuries.

When Selecting Shoes:

✳ Choose shoes according to your *specific activity*.

✳ Be sure the shoes have good stability, motion control, durability, and fit.

✳ Get fitted for shoes in the middle of the day when your feet have expanded and may be one-half size larger. (Also, each foot may be a different size.)

✳ To allow the feet to breathe, choose shoes with nylon or mesh uppers (cooler).

✳ Buy shoes at a reputable shoe store where the salespersons are knowledgeable. Expect to pay more for a good shoe.

✳ Break in new shoes slowly. Examine your shoes closely after 6 months or so, as that is the point at which many shoes begin to lose their cushioning. Discard your shoes when they wear out.

✳ For special conditions (unusual foot width; rigid, high arch; flat feet; obesity; pronation; toe shape), ask an expert to assist you. An evaluation from a podiatrist may be necessary.

✳ Ask to "test-drive" the shoes on a noncarpeted surface to help you determine the amount of comfort and cushion of the shoes.

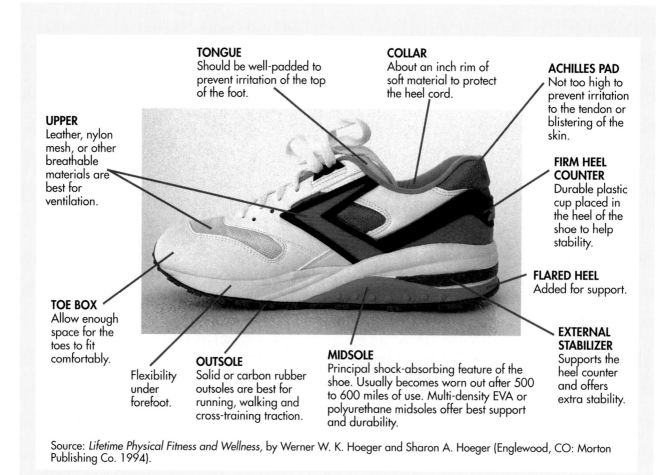

TONGUE
Should be well-padded to prevent irritation of the top of the foot.

COLLAR
About an inch rim of soft material to protect the heel cord.

ACHILLES PAD
Not too high to prevent irritation to the tendon or blistering of the skin.

UPPER
Leather, nylon mesh, or other breathable materials are best for ventilation.

FIRM HEEL COUNTER
Durable plastic cup placed in the heel of the shoe to help stability.

TOE BOX
Allow enough space for the toes to fit comfortably.

FLARED HEEL
Added for support.

Flexibility under forefoot.

OUTSOLE
Solid or carbon rubber outsoles are best for running, walking and cross-training traction.

MIDSOLE
Principal shock-absorbing feature of the shoe. Usually becomes worn out after 500 to 600 miles of use. Multi-density EVA or polyurethane midsoles offer best support and durability.

EXTERNAL STABILIZER
Supports the heel counter and offers extra stability.

Source: *Lifetime Physical Fitness and Wellness,* by Werner W. K. Hoeger and Sharon A. Hoeger (Englewood, CO: Morton Publishing Co. 1994).

Figure 11.7 Characteristics of ideal running shoe

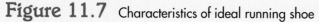

EXERCISE-RELATED INJURIES

Studies show that the benefits of exercise outweigh the risks of injury. Even when activities are planned carefully, however, injury does occur. Usually injuries are not serious or permanent. Most injuries occur simply because people take unnecessary risks when exercising. If an injury does not receive the proper attention, it can escalate into a serious problem, sometimes to the point of permanent damage. If you experience pain during a workout, stop. Your body is telling you something is amiss.

The best treatment for injuries, of course, is prevention. Prevention is more important than any physician or self-treatment. Half or more of all new exercisers suffer exercise-related injuries during the first 6 months of their program. The injuries often result from anatomical problems. Few individuals have perfect body alignment. Other injuries result from training errors, improper shoes, and environmental conditions. Surfaces such as asphalt, concrete, and Astroturf can pose problems, as they absorb and hold heat. Grass softens the impact and reduces stress on the body. Holes, cracks in pavement, gravel, and slippery spots are potentially dangerous. Being alert and placing the feet securely on surfaces deters injuries.

Heat-Related Concerns

Hot, humid weather raises caution signs. Prolonged exposure to or hot temperatures coupled with high relative humidity can result in heat cramps, heat exhaustion, or heat stroke.

Heat cramps are the least severe of the heat-related health concerns, but they are extremely painful. Muscle spasms occur in the arms, legs (calf), and abdominal muscles as a result of heavy exertion. Heat cramps result from tightness of the

Tips for action

When exercising in hot, humid weather:

✳ Drink 12 to 20 ounces of fluid such as gatorade 15 to 30 minutes before exercising. Water stimulates the production of urine, leaving less liquid for sweating.

✳ Drink 6 to 8 ounces every 15 minutes during exercise.

✳ Avoid alcoholic and caffeinated beverages; these, too, stimulate the production of urine.

✳ If need be, modify your exercise program by
   — working out during cooler times of day
   — choosing a cooler place to exercise
   — slowing your pace and shortening the duration of exercise
   — wearing light, porous clothing.

In cold weather:

✳ Dress in layers to trap air warmed by the body, which provides an insulating effect.

✳ Adequately protect exposed areas — fingers, nose, ears, facial skin, toes.
   — wear mittens rather than gloves, and thick socks.
   — wear a stocking cap that also covers the ears.

In very cold weather:

   — wear a ski mask or scarf that covers the mouth so you will be breathing moist air.
   — consider polypropylene underwear plus wool outer garments.

---

muscles, fatigue, or imbalance between water and electrolytes (sodium, calcium, potassium), which are essential to muscle contraction.

Heat cramps may be prevented by proper stretching before exercising, drinking plenty of water, and consuming sufficient electrolytes, sodium (salting food), calcium (milk/cheese), and potassium (bananas). People should avoid exercising during the hottest part of the day (11 a.m.– 4 p.m.). The temperature usually is highest at about 4 p.m. Massaging the affected area sometimes helps.

Heat exhaustion results from depletion and inadequate replacement of fluids as a result of heavy sweating during vigorous exercise in a warm, humid place. It is not a serious threat to life. Symptoms include cold/clammy skin, dilated pupils, profuse sweating, mildly elevated temperature, headache, dizziness, rapid, weak pulse, nausea/vomiting, and hyperventilation. Immediate treatment of heat exhaustion requires relocating the person to a cooler place, loosening clothing, having the person drink large quantities of cool water, and applying cold packs to the skin.

Heat stroke is the most severe of the heat-related disorders. It is a life-threatening emergency. The temperature control system that produces sweat to cool the body stops working. Symptoms include relatively dry skin, serious disorientation, constricted pupils, very high body temperatures (105°F or higher), sudden collapse, and loss of consciousness.

If the body temperature is lowered to normal within 45 minutes, the possibility of death from heat stroke can be reduced significantly. Treatment includes cooling the person rapidly by immersing the person in cool water or wrapping wet sheets and ice packs around the body, especially the head, torso, and joints. Fanning the person and giving plenty of cold liquids is helpful. The affected person should be taken immediately to the hospital or an emergency treatment facility.

Cold-Related Concerns

When exercising in cold weather, conserving heat is a major concern. Wind chill is a contributing factor. The wind chill index is given in Figure 11.8. Cold-related injury concerns include frostbite, hypothermia, and hyperthermia.

Frostbite is a common injury caused by overexposure to cold temperatures. When blood flow is restricted, ice crystals form in body tissues on the feet, hands, ears, nose, cheeks, and chin. The frozen body parts should be immersed in warm, not hot water, then loosely covered or bandaged. The affected area should not be rubbed or massaged. Medical attention should be sought immediately. Amputation is the most extreme treatment when tissue has been destroyed irretrievably.

Hypothermia usually occurs in damp, windy conditions and temperatures in the 50°F to 60°F range. The body's temperature drops below 95°F, and heat is lost faster than it can be produced. Symptoms include shivering, followed by loss of coordination and difficulty speaking. When the shivering stops, the muscles stiffen and the person becomes unconscious. Treatment includes warming the body slowly, placing dry clothing on the person immediately, and not giving anything to eat or drink unless the person is fully conscious. Medical attention should be sought immediately.

Abnormally high body temperature, **hyperthermia,** can occur when a person is wearing too much clothing. To prevent hyperthermia, the exerciser should dress in several layers of light clothing and remove clothing as the body temperature increases.

RICES Concept for Treatment of Injury

The standard recommended treatment for acute injuries is:

R = Rest
I = Ice application
C = Compression
E = Elevation
S = Support and Stabilization

Wind Speed (mph)	What the Thermometer Reads (°F)											
	50	40	30	20	10	0	−10	−20	−30	−40	−50	−60
	What It Equals in its Effect on Exposed Flesh											
Calm	50	40	30	20	10	0	−10	−20	−30	−40	−50	−60
5	48	37	27	16	6	−5	−15	−26	−36	−47	−57	−68
10	40	28	16	4	−9	−21	−33	−46	−58	−70	−83	−95
15	36	22	9	−5	−18	−36	−45	−58	−72	−85	−99	−112
20	32	18	4	−10	−25	−39	−53	−67	−82	−96	−110	−124
25	30	16	0	−15	−29	−44	−59	−74	−88	−104	−118	−133
30	28	13	−2	−18	−33	−48	−63	−79	−94	−109	−125	−140
35	27	11	−4	−20	−35	−49	−67	−82	−98	−113	−129	−145
40*	26	10	−6	−21	−37	−53	−69	−85	−100	−116	−132	−148
	Little danger if properly clothed					Danger of freezing exposed flesh			Great danger of freezing exposed flesh			

* Wind speeds greater than 40 mph have little additional effect.

Source: *Physiology of Fitness,* by B. J. Sharkey (Champaign, IL: Human Kinetics Books, 1990). Reprinted by permission.

Figure 11.8 Wind chill index

The purpose of **RICES** is to minimize injury and its risks. An injury may require one or more of these treatments:

1. *R = Rest.* If you experience pain, stop immediately. Listen to your body. Resting a few days will help stop excess bleeding and pain and promote healing of damaged tissues without complications. "Train, don't strain; if stressed, get rest." Unless indicated by a physician, absolute rest should not exceed 48 hours because muscles may become weak, joints may stiffen, and scar tissue may form around the injured part.

2. *I = Ice.* Icing is the most effective, safest, and cheapest form of treatment. Ice (icebag, cold whirlpool) acts as a local anesthetic by reducing the impulses of pain receptors, blood flow, muscle spasm, and inflammation (though inflammation is a part of the healing process, too much of it can impede healing). Ice helps to limit tissue damage and hastens the healing process.

   Apply ice compresses for 10 to 20 minutes, then reapply every 2 waking hours for the next 48 to 72 hours. Once the skin is numb, stop icing. Be sure not to exceed the 20-minute limit; longer than that may damage skin and nerves. Packs that remain flexible when frozen, such as a gel pack, two plastic bags of ice, or even a bag of frozen peas, can provide more cooling because they conform to the body. Self-freezing chemical packs or refreezable packs may be colder than regular ice. Chemicals in the packs can burn if allowed to be in direct contact with the skin.

   Do not use ice if you are hypersensitive to cold or have a circulatory problem. Never place an unwrapped ice pack over the elbow or the outside of the knee, because it may cause nerve damage (nerves are near the surface).

3. *C = Compression.* Pressure reduces swelling and blood flow to the injured part. Use an Ace-type elastic bandage or wet wrap for compression (not so tight that you cut off circulation).

4. *E = Elevation.* Combine elevation of the affected part with icing and compression. Elevation reduces internal bleeding and pooling of blood in the injured part. Elevate the injury above heart level to reduce swelling and

KEY TERMS

Frostbite a condition caused by overexposure to cold temperatures

Hyperthermia abnormally high body temperature

Hypothermia a condition in which body temperature drops below 95° and loses its ability to produce heat because heat is lost faster than it can be produced

RICES standard recommended treatment for acute injuries: rest, ice application, compression, elevation, support, and stabilization

Tips for action

To prevent injury from low-impact aerobics:

* Wear recommended shoes.
* Work out on resilient wood floors.
* Keep arm movements smooth and controlled.
* Use good form
  — abdomen tight
  — pelvis tucked in
  — rib cage up
  — knees bent slightly.
* Warm up beforehand and cool down afterward.

Exercise and Nutrition

During heavy exercise glycogen is broken down into glucose, which then becomes available to the muscles for energy production. Glucose provides about 6% more energy per unit of oxygen consumed than fat does. Heavy and prolonged exercise over several days depletes glycogen faster than the body can replace it through nutritive intake.

Therefore, athletes and people with similar physical demands are advised to switch to a carbohydrate-rich diet to restore glycogen levels. People who exercise less than an hour a day need not worry, as the regular recommended diet is sufficient to restore glycogen stores.

Following an exhaustive workout, eating a combination of carbohydrates and protein (tuna sandwich) within 30 minutes of exercise seems to speed up glycogen storage at an even faster rate. Protein intake increases insulin activity, thus enhancing glycogen replenishment. A 70% carbohydrate intake then should be maintained throughout the rest of the day.

dry heat (heating pad or heating lamp) or moist heat (hot bath, hot water bottle, heat pack, whirlpool). Those who have heart conditions or a fever should avoid hot baths and whirlpools. If infection or loss of sensation is present, heat should not be applied.

Warm (not hot) heat should be applied for 20 to 30 minutes, two to three times a day. Using warm heat 5 to 10 minutes before exercising reduces stiffness. A hot water bottle, heating pad, or hot pack that does not have a cover can be wrapped in a towel. If in doubt about the nature of the injury, medical evaluation should be sought immediately. If the area becomes inflamed or painful after heating an injury, self-treatment should be stopped immediately.

eliminate pain caused by blood rushing to the injured part.

5. S = *Stabilization and support*. Support or surround the injured part as much as possible to prevent further injury. Keep this support on the injured part until all indications of the injury are gone. By bracing, taping or strapping an injury, the person can still be active. Supports/splints are available from medical supply companies and pharmaceutical agencies.

RICES is not a substitute for seeing a doctor in case of a serious injury and or an injury that does not respond to self-treatment in 24 hours. RICES does not include heat treatment, which is indicated for some injuries.

Heat Treatment

Heat stimulates blood flow and may increase inflammation. Therefore, it should be applied with caution. Only after the swelling has subsided (in approximately 2–3 days) should a person apply heat. At that point the increased blood flow caused by heating promotes healing. Heat also helps to relax muscles, prevent spasms, reduce joint stiffness, and relieve pain.

Before using heat on an injury, a physician should be consulted to determine whether to use

BACKACHE

Backache is one of the most prevalent physical health problems in America today. It is the second-leading reason people go to doctors (after the common cold). Only rarely does a back problem have a serious cause or prognosis, but it still debilitates huge numbers of people. About 75% consists of chronic low back pain. Much of the backache problem is caused by (a) physical inactivity, (b) poor postural habits and body mechanics, and (c) overweight.

Near the end of 1994 a special task force of the Agency for Heath Care Policy and Research (AHCPR) presented guidelines for low back pain sufferers. In essence, the report recommended surgical intervention only as a last resort. It suggested that about nine of 10 people who have lower back problems will recover on their own within a month. The task force did not find a scientific basis for spinal traction or acupuncture, and it said that some formerly recommended treatments, such as bed rest, actually can weaken muscles or bones.

Instead, the experts advised that people with lower back pain do low-stress exercises such as walking, swimming, and biking, and take aspirin (or other acetaminophen or NSAID) for pain. Spinal manipulation (chiropracty) also was found to be helpful. Back pain can be prevented. Some recommendations include:

— regular exercise

— comfortable, low-heeled shoes

— work surfaces placed at comfortable heights

— chair with good back support

— lifting objects close to the body

— resting feet on a low stool when sitting a long time

— placing a pillow or rolled-up towel behind the small of the back when driving long distances

Figure 11.9 gives some basic guidelines on how to care for the back.

FITNESS PRODUCTS AND FACILITIES

Being an informed consumer will help a person distinguish between valid information and health fraud. Books, magazine articles, and other non-advertised printed materials are available to help people select products and facilities.

Fitness Equipment

Good equipment enhances the enjoyment and decreases the risk of injury from exercise. Active equipment improves fitness because the exerciser has to provide the muscle and aerobic power to perform the activity. Active exercise devices include stair climbers, stationary cycles, treadmills, weight machines, and ski machines. In contrast, passive equipment does not work for you and, therefore, is a waste of time and money. Passive equipment includes steam and sauna baths, rubberized suits (also dangerous because they do not permit sweating), hot tubs, vibrators (tables, pillows, belts), and motor-driven cycles.

Guidelines for selecting fitness equipment include the following:

1. Investigate the equipment before purchasing. Seek advice from knowledgeable personnel in local colleges or universities, community wellness centers, and YMCAs, as well as sports instructors and coaches. Ask questions and shop around for the best buys.

2. Make sure the equipment is safe, is in good working order, and fits properly.

3. "Test-drive" equipment before you buy it. Does it provide a good workout? Select equipment according to your physical and lifestyle needs.

4. Don't be in a hurry. Give yourself a cooling-off period so you will not buy on impulse.

5. Buy quality equipment, or wait until you can afford it. Check the length of warranty. Look for warranties of 1 or 2 years or more.

Tips for action

To prevent future injuries:

❋ Keep fit. Yo-yo exercising invites injury.

❋ Warm up before exercising.

❋ Use proper techniques when lifting objects and executing sports skills.

❋ Rest when you are ill or have been overexercising

❋ Use safe equipment, and use it properly.

❋ Wait for injuries to heal before returning to your normal fitness program.

HOW TO STAY ON YOUR FEET WITHOUT TIRING YOUR BACK

To prevent strain and pain in everyday activities, it is restful to change from one task to another before fatigue sets in. Housewives can lie down between chores; others should check body position frequently, drawing in the abdomen, flattening the back, bending the knees slightly.

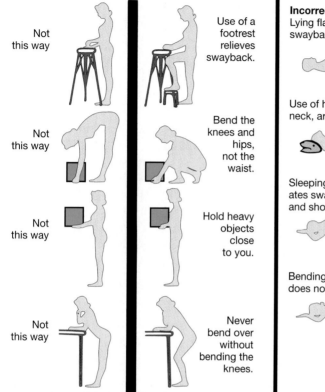

Not this way — Use of a footrest relieves swayback.

Not this way — Bend the knees and hips, not the waist.

Not this way — Hold heavy objects close to you.

Not this way — Never bend over without bending the knees.

HOW TO PUT YOUR BACK TO BED

For proper bed posture, a firm mattress is essential. Bedboards, sold commercially, or devised at home, may be used with soft mattresses. Bedboards, preferably, should be made of 3/4 inch plywood. Faulty sleeping positions intensify swayback and result not only in backache but in numbness, tingling, and pain in arms and legs.

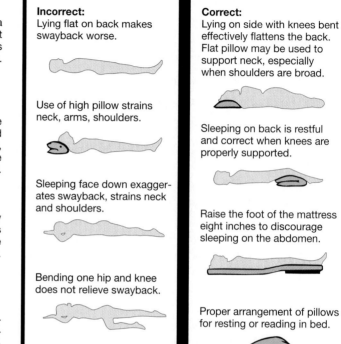

Incorrect:
Lying flat on back makes swayback worse.

Use of high pillow strains neck, arms, shoulders.

Sleeping face down exaggerates swayback, strains neck and shoulders.

Bending one hip and knee does not relieve swayback.

Correct:
Lying on side with knees bent effectively flattens the back. Flat pillow may be used to support neck, especially when shoulders are broad.

Sleeping on back is restful and correct when knees are properly supported.

Raise the foot of the mattress eight inches to discourage sleeping on the abdomen.

Proper arrangement of pillows for resting or reading in bed.

HOW TO SIT CORRECTLY

A back's best friend is a straight, hard chair. If you can't get the chair you prefer, learn to sit properly on whatever chair you get. To correct sitting position from forward slump: Throw head well back, then bend it forward to pull in the chin. This will straighten the back. Now tighten abdominal muscles to raise the chest. Check position frequently.

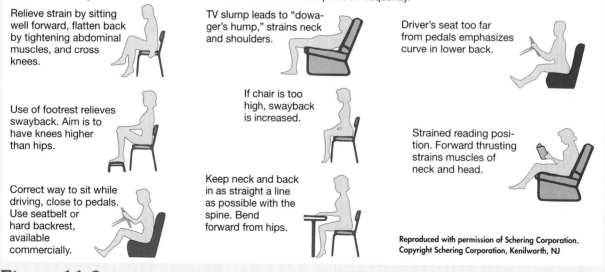

Relieve strain by sitting well forward, flatten back by tightening abdominal muscles, and cross knees.

Use of footrest relieves swayback. Aim is to have knees higher than hips.

Correct way to sit while driving, close to pedals. Use seatbelt or hard backrest, available commercially.

TV slump leads to "dowager's hump," strains neck and shoulders.

If chair is too high, swayback is increased.

Keep neck and back in as straight a line as possible with the spine. Bend forward from hips.

Driver's seat too far from pedals emphasizes curve in lower back.

Strained reading position. Forward thrusting strains muscles of neck and head.

Reproduced with permission of Schering Corporation. Copyright Schering Corporation, Kenilworth, NJ

Figure 11.9 Your Back and How to Care For It.

6. Buy according to your needs, and buy equipment you will continue to use. Will the equipment fit into your lifestyle and exercise space? Can it be stored easily?

Health and Fitness Clubs

Most people who join a health or fitness club do not go regularly or quit within 6 months. Still, clubs may provide motivation and expert advice on better ways to exercise. Before joining one of these facilities, a person should consider:

1. *Location/hours.* The facility should be within 15 minutes of you and open at convenient hours.

2. *Individual concerns.* Are you allowed, before signing the contract, to discuss your physical limitations, risk factors, individual problems? Does the facility recommend that you consult with your doctor before beginning an exercise program?

Exercise improves the body from the outside in; nutrition improves the body from the inside out.

3. *Stress test.* If you have any doubts regarding your present state of health, consult your physician, who may recommend an exercise stress test.

4. *Facility/equipment.* Is the facility in good order, clean, well-ventilated? Is it overcrowded (waiting line)? Does the club have programs such as aerobics classes and enough cardiorespiratory fitness equipment, such as treadmills, stair-climbing machines, stationary bicycles, running track, swimming pool, rowing machines? Does it include devices for strength and flexibility development? Is the equipment maintained properly and in good condition? What type of floor is used for aerobic workouts — suspended wood floor, high-density matting, carpet over cushioning? Beware of aerobic floors made of tile, linoleum, or cement.

5. *Qualified/certified personnel.* What type of in-house training does the club require of its instructors? Certification is not mandated by law, but it should be considered. Exercisers may find that working with a trained professional makes exercise enjoyable, prevents injury, and provides motivation. Are warm-up and cool-down periods included? Ask to observe instructors and classes, and talk with club members.

Do the instructors address the participants' various ability levels? Do they give personalized attention and move around? Is safety stressed? Are they CPR- and first aid-certified? If not, look elsewhere!

6. *Membership.* Does membership include lockers, showers, towels, classes, or will you have to pay extra for these amenities? Select a no-contract if possible. If not, choose a short-term contract before you commit to join for a year or more. Read the contract carefully. Many clubs go out of business, and some change ownership often. Get all agreements in writing. "Pay as you go" is the best plan.

7. *People.* Are the participants older or younger than you? Are they in better or worse shape? Perhaps you will enjoy the exercise program more if you feel compatible with the people who exercise with you.

8. *Visit.* Visit the club at the time of day you plan to use it. How many people are using the facility when you plan to exercise?

9. *Check it out.* Call the Better Business Bureau to see if complaints have been filed.

HEALTH/WELLNESS PRESCRIPTION

Personal health is unique to the individual. No single exercise program is suitable for all people. Your wellness prescription should consist of your own interests, objectives, time, and schedule. The following guidelines will help you in planning your health/wellness prescription:

1. *Goals/Objectives.* What is my purpose for this program? My short-term (days, weeks) and long-term (months, years) goals? Objectives? Are these attainable and realistic?

☎ Call for information

National Wellness Institute
715-342-2969

Tips for action

At the fitness starting line:

❋ Select one or more activities you enjoy. Books, videos, and magazines are available to help you learn about various activities.

❋ Set a time and schedule. Among your day's activities, make exercise a top priority.

❋ Make a personal contract stating a realistic goal and your commitment to reach it. Include the beginning date, clear description of what your want to accomplish, ways to measure your progress, and the date you expect to accomplish your goal. Start by listing your major goal, then list smaller objectives to accomplish it.

❋ Don't overdo it. Overexertion can cause soreness and fatigue, which might discourage you.

❋ Seek support. Network with family, friends, a partner, a group, and ask them to join you. Make exercise a social event. Talk with people and discover the strategies that worked for them. Borrow from their experience.

❋ Listen to music. Music enhances your training and helps the time pass quickly.

❋ Do not feel guilty or blame yourself when you slip in your exercise program. Deal with your reasons and move on.

❋ Seek assistance when you need it. Controlling counterproductive behaviors such as alcohol and drug abuse, overeating, and cigarette smoking may require outside help. Programs such as Weight Watchers, Alcoholics Anonymous, Smoke Enders, and services provided by health departments and counseling centers are just a few of the community resources available.

❋ Get plenty of rest and sleep.

❋ Make exercise a daily choice. Once you have started, don't stop. See yourself as a capable person in charge of your health and well-being. Notice how much better you look and feel.

❋ Participate in team sports — volleyball, softball, basketball, bowling.

❋ Park the car a few blocks away from where you're going, and then walk the rest of the way.

❋ Always take stairs instead of elevators.

❋ Walk the dog at a brisk pace.

❋ Mow the lawn and work in the yard.

❋ Vary your routine to prevent monotony and boredom.

❋ Keep a record of your progress, and reward *yourself* when you show improvement.

❋ Be patient.

❋ Have fun and enjoy your new lifestyle!

2. *Medical readiness.* Am I ready for this exercise program? Do I have any health risk factors? Have I consulted with my physician if indicated?

3. *Attire.* Am I ready to exercise in hot or cold weather? Do I have comfortable clothing and shoes?

4. *Present level of health/fitness.* What is my health/fitness status? Have I had a pre-evaluation as to my current status on health-related components of physical fitness?

5. *Activity.* Do I have a method for maintaining a written record of my daily and weekly exercise plan?

6. *Time and convenience.* Do I have a set daily and weekly time to devote to my exercise program? How far do I have to go to exercise? Are the equipment and facilities convenient?

7. *Does my exercise prescription include*:
   Warm-up, activity session, cool-down?
   Overload principle?
   Principle of progression?
   Principle of specificity?
   Active exercise?
   Safe exercise?
   Target zone (FITT) for:
      cardiovascular
      flexibility
      muscular strength/endurance

8. *Nutrition.* How am I doing with basic nutrients? Do I need more vitamins, minerals, water? Does my diet provide sufficient complex carbohydrates (grains, fruits, and vegetables). Have I cut down fat intake to less than 30% of total dietary calories?

9. *Drugs.* Am I drug-free? If not, do I plan to become drug-free?

10. *Stress management activities.* Do I take time for myself? What relaxation techniques do I use?

11. *Do I need to add, modify, or adjust* my current exercise program?

12. *Enjoyment and motivation.* Am I enjoying and happy with the results of my exercise program? Do I look forward to exercising?

13. *Cost.* Can I afford to purchase the necessary equipment? Fees for a fitness/health club? Can I find other means to exercise with little or no cost involved?

14. *Rewards.* How am I going to reward myself after achieving short-term goals? Long term-goals?

Summary

1 Exercise has both physical and psychological benefits including reduced risk for many diseases, plus more energy and vitality.

2 The FITT formula is an acronym for frequency, intensity, time, and type of activity. It applies to each of the physical fitness components.

3 The health-related physical fitness components are cardiorespiratory endurance, muscular flexibility, and muscular strength and endurance.

4 Phases of exercise include the warm-up, the actual workout, and the cool-down.

5 Principles of fitness training include the overload principle, the progression principle, and specificity of training.

6 The purpose of aerobic exercise is to increase your heart rate to higher levels and thus increase cardiorespiratory fitness.

7 The three types of stretching are static, or slow-sustained; dynamic or ballistic; and proprioceptive neuromuscular facilitation (PNF).

8 Types of muscular contractions are isotonic (dynamic) and isometric (static).

9 Clothing should be comfortable and allow the person to move freely. Proper shoes are particularly important.

10 Heat-related concerns include muscle cramps, heat exhaustion, and heat stroke.

11 The most common cold-weather concerns are frostbite and hypothermia.

12 The RICES treatment for injury consists of: rest, ice, compression, elevation, and stabilization and support. In addition, heat treatment sometimes is indicated.

Select Bibliography

American Alliance for Health, Physical Education, and Recreation. *Health-related Physical Test Manual.* Reston VA: AAHPER, 1980.

American Alliance for Health, Physical Education, Recreation and Dance. *Physical Best.* Reston, VA: AAHPERD, 1988.

American College of Sports Medicine. *Resource Manual for Guidelines for Exercise Testing and Prescription.* Philadelphia: Lea & Febiger, 1988.

American College of Sports Medicine. "The Recommended Quantity and Quality of Exercise for Developing and Maintaining Cardiorespiratory and Muscular Fitness in Healthy Adults." *Medicine and Science in Sports and Exercise,* 22 (1990), 265–274.

American College of Sports Medicine. *Guidelines for Exercise Testing and Prescription,* 4th edition. Philadelphia: Lea & Febiger, 1991.

Benson, Herbert., and Eileen M. Stuart. *The Wellness Book.* New York: Birch Lane Press, 1992.

Bloom, M. "Pooling Your Efforts." *Runner's World,* 26:8 (1991), 40–45.

Borg, G. "Psychophysical Bases of Perceived Exertion." *Medicine and Science in Sports and Exercise,* 14 (1982), 377–381.

Boskin, W., and G. Graf. *Health Dynamics: Attitudes and Behaviors.* St. Paul: West Publishing, 1990.

Bowers, R. W., and E. L. Fox. *Sports Physiology.* Dubuque, IA: Wm. C. Brown, 1992.

Buroker, K. C., and J. A. Schwane. "Does Postexercise Static Stretching Alleviate Delayed Muscles Soreness?" *Physician and Sports-medicine,* 17 (June 1989), 65–83.

"Common Overuse Injuries." *Reebok Instructor News,* 4:4 (1991), 6–7.

Cooper, K. H. *The Aerobics Program for Total Well-Being.* New York: Mount Evans and Co., 1982.

"Does Lactic Acid Cause Muscle Soreness?" *Reebok Instructor News,* 3:6 (1990), 8.

Durkin, J. F. "If the Shoe Fits." *Runner's World,* 25:4 (1991), 46–48.

Ellis, J. "Between a Sock and a Hard Place." *Runner's World,* 24:8 (1989), 28.

Ellis, J. "Run Injury-Free." *Runner's World,* 29:3 (1994), 40–48.

"Equipment and Props for Exercise." *Reebok Instructor News,* 3:4 (1990), 7.

"Exercise Without Injury." *University of California Berkeley Wellness Letter,* 6:6 (1990), 4–5.

Floyd, P. A., and J. E. Parke, *Walk, Jog, Run for Wellness Everyone,* 2d edition. Winston-Salem: Hunter Publishing, 1992.

Floyd, P. A., et al. *Wellness: A Lifetime Commitment,* 2d edition. Winston-Salem: Hunter Publishing, 1993.

Fox, E. L., R. W. Bowers, and M. L. Fossand, *The Physiological Basis for Exercise and Sport.* Philadelphia: Saunders College Publishing, 1992.

Gautier, M. M. "Continuous Passive Motion: The No-Exercise Exercise." *Physician and Sportsmedicine,* 15:142 (1987).

Hafen, B. Q., and Karren, K. J. *First Aid,* 5th edition. Englewood Cliffs NJ: Prentice Hall, 1993.

Hesson, J. L. *Weight Training for Life.* Englewood, CO: Morton, 1994.

Hoeger, W. W. K., and S. A. Hoeger. *Principles and Labs for Physical Fitness and Wellness,* 3d edition. Englewood, CO: Morton, 1994.

"How Fit Is Your Health Club?" *University of California Berkeley Wellness Letter,* 7:2 (1990), 6.

"Meditation in Motion." *University of California Berkeley Wellness Letter,* 10:5 (1994), 7.

Miller, L. "The Best Medicine." *Runner's World,* 28:2 (1993), 40–47.

"Muscle Cramps: S-T-R-E-T-C-H Spells Relief." *University of California Berkeley Wellness Letter,* 6:4 (1990), 6.

"New Year's Resolution." *Runner's World,* 29:1 (1994), 40–43.

Nieman, D. C. *Fitness & Your Health.* Palo Alto, CA: Bull Publishing, 1993.

"Relief: Exercise Injuries." *University of California Berkeley Wellness Letter,* 6:8 (1990), 4–5.

"The R.I.C.E. Principles." *Reebok Instructor News,* 4:4 (1991), 4.

Rippe, J. M., and A. Ward. *The Rockport Walking Program.* New York: Prentice Hall, 1989.

Robertson, J. W. "An Ounce of Prevention." *Runner's World,* 26:2 (1991), 40–46.

Rosato, Frank. *Jogging and Walking for Health and Fitness,* 3d edition. Englewood, CO: Morton Publishing, 1994.

Runner's World Shoe Guide. Emmaus, PA: Rodale Press, 1990.

Scales, Ken. "Be Grateful for Sweat." *Ebony,* November, 1994.

Schnatter, M. J. "Care Package for the Sport Minded." *McCall's,* April, 1991, pp. 140–145.

Sheehan, G. "Heat Success." *Runner's World,* 24:7 (1989), 16.

Shephard, R. J. "Risks of Exercise." *President's Council on Physical Fitness and Sports,* 1:5 (1994), 1.

Silvester, L. J. *Weight Training for Strength and Fitness.* Boston: Jones and Bartlett Publishers, 1992.

Voelker, R. "A Little Exercise Goes a Long Way in Cardiovascular Health." *American Medical News,* July, 20, 1992.

Waldron, M. "Fitness Equipment: Are These Your Symptoms?" *Runner's World,* 29:1 (1994), 30.

"Wellness Tips." *University of California Berkeley Wellness Letter,* 10:1 (1993), 7.

"When to Ice/When to Heat." *University of California Berkeley Wellness Letter,* 10:8 (1994), 6.

Wilmore, J. H., and D. L. Costill. *Training for Sport and Activity.* Dubuque, IA: Wm. C. Brown, 1988.

Counting The Heart Rate

NAME _____ DATE _____

COURSE _____ SECTION _____

Count your heart rate (pulse) at two locations: the carotid artery (side of neck) and the radial artery (wrist).

1. Practice locating both your carotid and radial artery heartbeats, or pulses. Count your pulses as soon as possible after exercising.

2. Count your pulse at both the carotid (neck) and radial (wrist) locations. Use a watch or clock to count for 10, 15, or 30 seconds. To establish your heart rate in beats per minute, multiply the 10-second count by 6, the 15-second count by 4, or the 30-second count by 2.

3. Count the pulse of a partner using both the carotid and radial locations.

4. Record the results in the spaces below.

Carotid pulse count:

	Self Heart rate/min.	Partner Heart rate/min.
_____ 10 seconds × 6 =	_____	_____
_____ 15 seconds × 4 =	_____	_____
_____ 30 seconds × 2 =	_____	_____

Radial pulse count:

	Self Heart rate/min.	Partner Heart rate/min.
_____ 10 seconds × 6 =	_____	_____
_____ 15 seconds × 4 =	_____	_____
_____ 30 seconds × 2 =	_____	_____

Which method do you prefer when counting your heart rate? Why ?

Total Fitness: How Do You Rate?

NAME _____ DATE _____

COURSE _____ SECTION _____

Before you begin

Precede an exercise program with a medical exam if you have any of the following risk factors:

* ❋ Elevated blood pressure or cholesterol
* ❋ Cigarette smoking
* ❋ Family history of coronary disease in parents or siblings before age 55, any heart, lung, or metabolic disease, such as diabetes
* ❋ Man over 40 years of age
* ❋ Woman over 50 years of age

Flexibility
MODIFIED SIT-AND-REACH

The Test

To perform this test, you need a yardstick on a 12" box or the Acuflex I Sit-and-Reach Flexibility Tester.

Warm up and remove your shoes prior to the test. Sit on the floor with legs straight out and hips, back, and head against the wall. An assistant now places the box against the bottom of your feet. Put one hand on top of the other and reach forward as far as possible leaving the head and back touching the wall. At this point, the assistant places the yardstick on top of the box and slides the stick along the top of the box until it touches the person's fingers. The yardstick now is held firmly in place. Gradually reach forward, releasing head and back from the wall stretching as far as possible on the yardstick and holding the final position 2 seconds. Repeat and average the two scores.

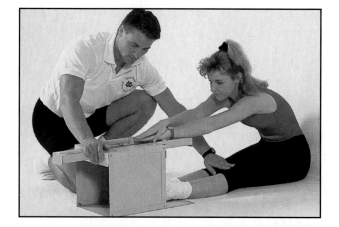

The Results

Men in their 20s with good flexibility should be able to reach 15 inches. In their 30s, 14 inches, in their 40s 13.5 inches and in their 50s, 11.5 inches. Women in their 20s should be able to reach 16 inches. In their 30s 15.5 inches, in their 40s 14.5 inches and in their 50s 12.5 inches.

The Future

Add some stretching to your daily routine. Stretch your muscles only after they are warm.

Aerobic Exercise

THE ROCKPORT WALKING TEST

One way to measure your aerobic fitness is by taking the Rockport Walking Test, which measures your heart rate after brisk exercise. The more fit you are, the lower your heart rate.

The Test

❋ Warm up, then walk one mile as fast as you can. Record your time to the nearest second.

❋ Count your heart rate for 15 seconds immediately after the walk, then multiply by 4 to get a one-minute heart rate. Record your heart rate.

❋ Use your walking time and your post-exercise heart rate to determine your rating using Chart 1 for males or Chart 2 for females.

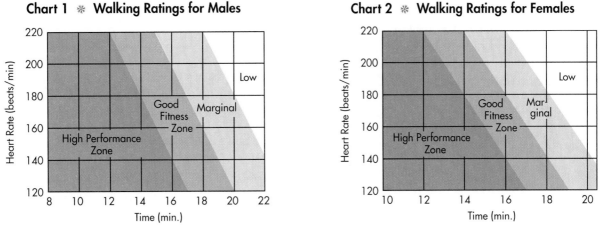

Chart 1 ❋ **Walking Ratings for Males**

Chart 2 ❋ **Walking Ratings for Females**

The ratings in these charts are for ages 20–29. They provide reasonable ratings for people of all ages.

The Results

Men in good condition should have a pulse rate of 79 to 97 beats per minute (BPM), with younger men (ages 18 to 25) closer to 79 and older men (ages 56 to 65) closer to 97. If your pulse does not fall within this range, you need more aerobic exercise.

Women who are in good condition should measure 85 to 104 BPM, with younger women closer to 85 and older women closer to 104. Try to get more regular aerobic exercise if your pulse rate does not fall within this range.

The Future

Over a period of 2 months, gradually work up to 30- to 60-minute sessions of aerobic activity — anything from brisk walking to swimming — at least three times a week. Then take the walk test again and see how far you have come.

Reprinted by permission of the Rockport Company Inc. © 1993

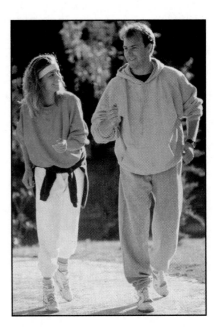

Strength Training

PUSH-UPS

Push-ups involve the muscles of your chest, shoulders, and arms. They are a good measure of upper-body strength.

The Test

Men should use the standard push-up position, with their hands and toes on the floor. Women may modify the standard push-up by putting their knees on the floor. Do as many push-ups in a row as you can. Be sure to keep count as you go. Also make sure that your chest comes within 3 inches of the floor with each push-up.

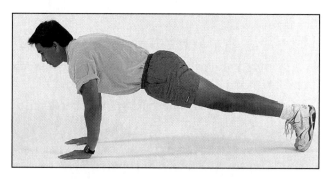

The Results

Men in their 20s with good upper-body strength should be able to do at least 30 push-ups. Men in their 30s should be able to do 25 to 36. Men in their 40s should be able to do 21 to 30 push-ups, and men in their 50s, 18 to 27.

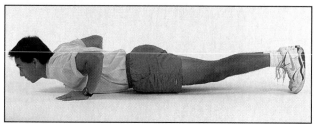

Women in their 20s with good upper body strength should be able to do at least 23 push-ups. Women in their 30s should be able to do 22 to 33. Women in their 40s should be able to 18 to 27 push-ups, and women in their 50s, 15 to 22 push-ups.

The Future

Working out with weights is the best way to improve your strength. To reduce your risk of injury, always warm up before doing any lifting, and remember to start slow. You might start out with body-weight exercises, relying on push-ups, sit-ups, and pull-ups. Then try machines or free weights.

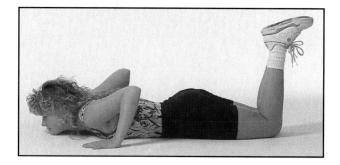

Put It All Together

Use your results to see which areas you're strong in and which areas need improvement. Be sure to include some strength training, aerobic activity, and stretching in all your workouts, and you'll be closer to achieving total fitness.

	Scores	Rating
Flexibility		
Aerobic		
Strength		

Adapted with permission. Madison Publishing Company.

Tobacco and Alcohol

12

*O*f all the drugs used by the American public, from aspirin to heroin, the two that have the largest negative impact and result in the most deaths — tobacco and alcohol — are both legal. Tobacco, either smoked or smokeless, has no redeeming value. Its hold on people stems from its addictive properties. Alcohol, on the other hand, can provide some beneficial effects when consumed in moderation. Its misuse, however, can have adverse psychological, social, and relational impacts.

The rate of tobacco smoking, on the decline in American society at large, is

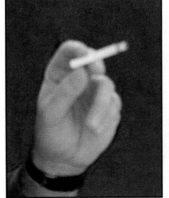
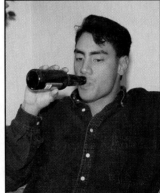

climbing in young Anglo women. Binge drinking has reached epidemic proportions on college campuses throughout the country. In this chapter we discuss tobacco and alcohol and their psychological, and social effects. Chapter 13 covers the other psychoactive drugs.

TOBACCO USE

Tobacco is a plant, *Nicotiana tobacum* or *Nicotiana rustica*, grown in the United States and other countries. Although the American Indians harvested and used tobacco years before introducing it to European explorers, Jean Nicot of France is credited with popularizing tobacco uses in 1559. Nicot tested tobacco on people and reported that it cured migraine headaches, other persistent headaches, and colds. His reports and the number of people of the aristocracy praising and using the drug in France caused its use to spread rapidly. By 1565 the plant had been named *nicotiana*, with the active ingredient isolated and called nicotine in 1828.

The leaves of the tobacco plant are dried and processed into cigarettes, cigars, and pipe tobacco for smoking. Strips of leaves are processed to make chewing tobacco, and the leaf is pulverized into a fine powder to make snuff. Cigarette smoking is the most popular use of tobacco.

In the early 1980s, **clove cigarettes** from India began entering the United States, and imports now have surpassed 150 million clove cigarettes. Although some people assume that these cigarettes are made entirely of cloves, they actually contain about 40% cloves and about 60% tobacco. Their levels of tar, nicotine, and carbon monoxide are even higher than regular cigarettes. The active ingredient in cloves, eugenol, has a numbing effect in the back of the throat that enables users to inhale the smoke more deeply. Most smokers of clove cigarettes are teenagers and young adults.

Strong pressure is placed on individuals, especially through the media, to smoke and to use tobacco products. The tobacco industry advertises products and continues to target specific groups, especially younger users, females, and minority groups. The Joe Camel ads are illustrative of the strategy to reach young audiences. Many of the tobacco companies produce ads displaying beautiful, handsome, well-dressed, athletic models in fancy cars and impressive environments. In truth, physical attractiveness and sunny beaches with romantic overtones are far removed from the realities of smoking and its effects.

Prevalence of Smoking

Health concerns and fears have caused a considerable overall drop in tobacco smoking. It has reached its lowest level since 1942. Teenagers, however, are smoking just as much. A breakdown of smokers by ethnic group and sex is given in Figure 12.1 for the year 1992. Presently, young Anglo women (ages 18–44) are smoking even more. In contrast, young African American women have virtually given up smoking, according to Michael Eriksen, director of the Office on Smoking and

Smoking Worldwide

Worldwide deaths from cigarettes may reach 10 million people a year — triple the rates now — if current smoking patterns continue. That means one death every 3 seconds, or 20 deaths every minute by the year 2020, say scientists at Britain's Imperial Cancer Research Fund, the World Health Organization, and the American Cancer Society. The report, considered the most comprehensive to date, covers 45 countries.

Scientists compared U.S. lung-cancer death rates to those in other nations to estimate numbers of smokers worldwide. They also figured in deaths from related maladies — heart attacks, strokes, and other cancers — to find:

* 10% of British men will die from smoking by the time they are 35 to 59 years old.

* In Poland, 20% of men will die from smoking.

* In Spain, smoking will kill millions of women within decades, even though their lung cancer rates are low now because they traditionally have not been smokers.

Dr. Clark Heath, American Cancer Society, says the warnings aren't new "but people ignore them at their peril."

From "Deaths From Smoking May Triple by 2020," by Dennis Kelly, in *USA Today*, September 20, 1994, p.1.

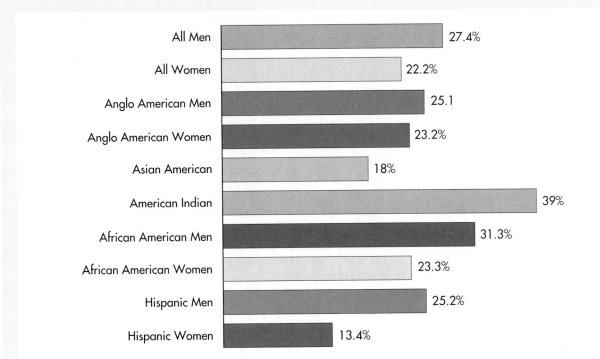

All Men	27.4%
All Women	22.2%
Anglo American Men	25.1
Anglo American Women	23.2%
Asian American	18%
American Indian	39%
African American Men	31.3%
African American Women	23.3%
Hispanic Men	25.2%
Hispanic Women	13.4%

Sources: AMC Cancer Research Center, Denver, July 1994; for Asian-Americans and American Indians, Centers for Disease Control.

Figure 12.1 Breakdown of smokers by ethnic group and sex, 1992

Health of the Centers for Disease Control and Prevention. Of the groups surveyed, Hispanic women continue to have the lowest rates of smoking.

Components of Tobacco

Nicotine

Nicotine is a powerful and addictive chemical component in tobacco that initially acts as a stimulant. It gives the person a brief "kick." The first cigarette of the day can raise the heart rate by 10 to 20 beats per minute and blood pressure by 5 to 10 points as the blood vessels constrict. In addition, nicotine decreases HDL ("good") cholesterol levels, steps up the release of glycogen by the liver, slightly deadens the taste buds and the sense of smell, causes halitosis (bad breath), weakens tooth enamel, and causes dry throat and hoarseness.

The 1988 Surgeon General's report concluded that all forms of tobacco are addicting. Nicotine is the chemical that causes the addiction, and the tobacco addiction is similar to addictions of drugs such as cocaine and heroin.

Gases

Among the more than 4,000 elements, compounds, and toxic chemicals in cigarette smoke are the gases nitrogen, carbon monoxide, carbon dioxide, acetone, vinyl chloride, hydrogen cyanide, formaldehyde, and ammonia. **Carbon monoxide** is an extremely poisonous gas in tobacco smoke. When the smoker inhales carbon monoxide, it combines with the hemoglobin of red blood cells. When this happens, carbon monoxide reduces the red blood cells' capacity to carry oxygen to major organs such as the brain and heart.

KEY TERMS

Tobacco a plant, *Nicotiana tobacum* or *Nicotiana rustica*, in which the leaves are dried and processed for smoking

Clove cigarettes cigarettes containing about 40% cloves, with a numbing ingredient, eugenol

Nicotine an addictive chemical component in tobacco

Carbon monoxide extremely poisonous gas in tobacco smoke

Facts about Smoking

Did You Know . . .

❋ Smokers' blood has from two to five times more carbon monoxide than nonsmokers' blood.

❋ Smoking is a cause of low-birthweight babies.

❋ Smoking reduces lung capacity 50% faster than normal aging alone.

❋ Smokers have more facial wrinkles than nonsmokers.

❋ 85% of adult smokers today started when they were teenagers.

❋ Smoking increases the risk for strokes, cancer, heart attacks, impotence, and osteoporosis — not just to the smoker but to the whole family.

❋ Smoking is more powerful than heroin or cocaine.

❋ Smoking is not a habit. It's an addiction.

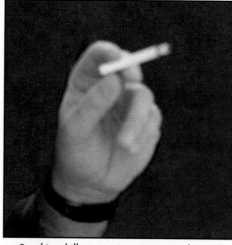

Smoking kills more Americans each year than died in World War II.

Tobacco Tar

Tobacco **tar** is composed of particles that form a yellowish-brown, sticky residue on hands, ashtrays, and lungs. When smokers inhale, these particles remain in the lungs. Among the carcinogenic (cancer-causing) substances in tar are nitrosamines, pyrenes, chrysenes, phenols, and cresols. Tar is the agent that causes cancers of the lung, oral cavity, and others.

Smokers inhale dangerous tars into the lungs, where carcinogenic components are dispersed into the bloodstream. In smokeless tobacco carcinogens in the tar and nicotine are absorbed through the mucous membrane lining of the mouth or digestive system and passed to the bloodstream.

Adverse Effects of Tobacco

Despite the decline in cigarette smoking and the fact that choosing not to smoke is the most preventable cause of death, at least one in six deaths per day (more than 1,000 a day) are still attributed to tobacco use (see Figure 12.2). Dr. Louis Sullivan, former Secretary of the U. S. Department of Health and Human Services, reported that smoking cigarettes kills approximately 400,000 people each year. This is more than the number of Americans who died in

World War II, and more than those who die from AIDS, multiple sclerosis, diabetes, accidents, gunshot wounds, and breast and prostate cancers combined. Smoking accounts for 87% of all deaths from lung cancer and 30% of all cancer deaths. It is the cause of 40% of preventable deaths and 30% of all adult early deaths. As shown in Figure 12.3, female deaths are rising along with the increased smoking by women since 1965.

Tobacco destroys the lungs, weakens the heart, deadens the esophagus, and damages the kidneys, eyes, bladder, and uterus, according to Dr. Robert

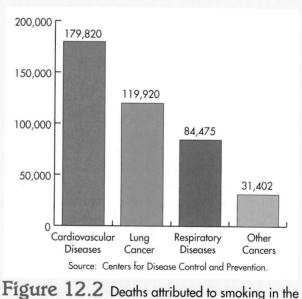

Source: Centers for Disease Control and Prevention.

Figure 12.2 Deaths attributed to smoking in the United States in 1990

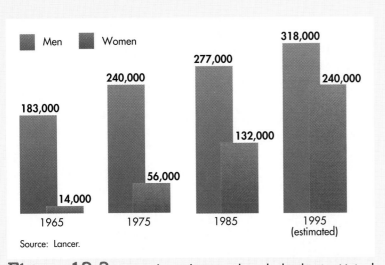

Figure 12.3 Annual smoking-attributed deaths in United States comparing men and women.

gases, tar, and other chemicals that have been inhaled.

The results of a study by the American Health Foundation revealed that African Americans may be more likely biologically than Anglos to develop lung cancer from smoking. African Americans have long been shown to have a 50% higher incidence of lung cancer and death from the disease. Initial data seem to indicate that African Americans have less capacity to detoxify NNk, one of the most important tobacco-related carcinogens linked to lung cancer. Though African American men smoke fewer cigarettes a day, the cigarettes they smoke tend to contain more tar and nicotine.

Cancer ravages the lungs with a vast number of wildly multiplying cells. Most often it begins with constant irritation of the bronchial lining. Because of this irritation, the hairlike cilia, which filter the

Schrier, chairman of medicine at the University of Colorado Health Sciences Center. The National Center for Environmental Health reports that smoking may inhibit sexual function. Federal researchers found that smokers were more likely to be impotent than nonsmokers. Smoking may clog the blood vessels in the penis just as it clogs vessels in the rest of the body. The good news is that the impotence may cease after the smoker quits smoking. It may be responsible for 14% of all leukemias and 80% of all laryngeal cancers.

Figure 12.4 illustrates some of the wide-range effects of smoking on the body. Here we will discuss the two most common of these — cancers and cardiorespiratory diseases — as well as effects on pregnant women and children.

Cancers

Smoking is the major cause of lung cancer in women and men in the United States. The incidence of lung cancer is closely associated with the length of time one has smoked, the number of cigarettes smoked each day, the accumulation of tar in the lungs, and the amount of

KEY TERMS

Tar yellowish-brown, sticky residue in tobacco that causes cancer

Cigarette Smoking ⟶ Cancer

The facts are clear.

❋ Cigarette smoking is a major cause of cancers of the lung, larynx, oral cavity, and esophagus and a contributing cause in cancers of the bladder, pancreas, and kidney.

❋ Lung cancer risk increases steadily with the number of cigarettes smoked per day. In those who smoke 40 or more cigarettes a day (2 or more packs), the rate of lung cancer is 12–25 times the rate for nonsmokers.

❋ The 5-year survival rate for people diagnosed with lung cancer is 13%.

❋ The risk of lung cancer is less in people who quit smoking, and the risk decreases as the number of years since quitting increases.

❋ Smoking increases the risk of lung cancer more than ten-fold.

❋ Smoking has made lung cancer the No. 1 cancer killer of American women.

❋ More than 80% of the current smokers started before age 21.

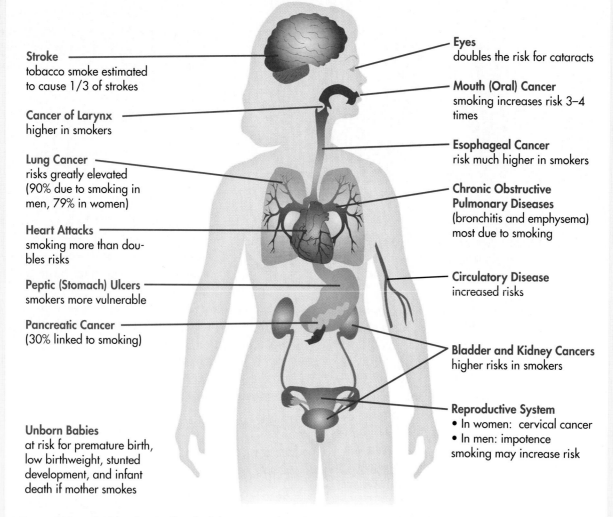

Stroke
tobacco smoke estimated to cause 1/3 of strokes

Cancer of Larynx
higher in smokers

Lung Cancer
risks greatly elevated (90% due to smoking in men, 79% in women)

Heart Attacks
smoking more than doubles risks

Peptic (Stomach) Ulcers
smokers more vulnerable

Pancreatic Cancer
(30% linked to smoking)

Unborn Babies
at risk for premature birth, low birthweight, stunted development, and infant death if mother smokes

Eyes
doubles the risk for cataracts

Mouth (Oral) Cancer
smoking increases risk 3–4 times

Esophageal Cancer
risk much higher in smokers

Chronic Obstructive Pulmonary Diseases
(bronchitis and emphysema) most due to smoking

Circulatory Disease
increased risks

Bladder and Kidney Cancers
higher risks in smokers

Reproductive System
• In women: cervical cancer
• In men: impotence smoking may increase risk

Source: *Wellness: Guidelines for a Healthy Lifestyle*, by Brent Q. Hafen and Werner W. K. Hoeger (Englewood, CO: Morton Publishing, 1994), p. 286.

Figure 12.4 Health effects of smoking

air we breathe, disappear from the lining of the bronchi. Although extra mucus is secreted to substitute for the cilia and trap pollutants, this mucus itself becomes a problem. It remains trapped until finally forced out of the lung by a "smoker's cough."

If the smoker quits before cancerous lesions are present, the bronchial lining will return to normal. If the smoker does not quit and cancerous lesions are present, the abnormal cell growth will spread, blocking the bronchi and invading the lung tissue. In the latter stages of lung cancer, abnormal cells break away from the lungs and are carried by the lymphatic system to other vital organs, where new cancers begin (metastasis).

Smokeless tobacco (chewing tobacco and snuff) and cigar smoking are linked to high rates of cancer of the oral cavity (mouth, lips, gums, cheeks, throat), esophagus, and pharynx. A pinch of snuff or a larger wad of chewing tobacco is placed between the gum and cheek, where the nicotine is absorbed into the bloodstream via capillaries. Within approximately 5 minutes the effects — such as elevated blood pressure and heart rate — are similar to the effects of smoking.

A major hazard of smokeless tobacco is the presence of carcinogens, specifically **nitrosamines**. Various changes may occur in the mouth after only a few weeks of use. The user may feel a burning

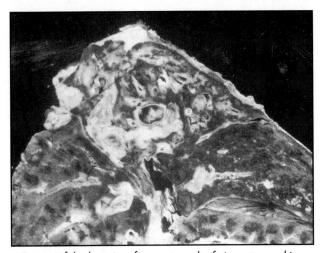

Cancer of the lung is a frequent result of cigarette smoking.

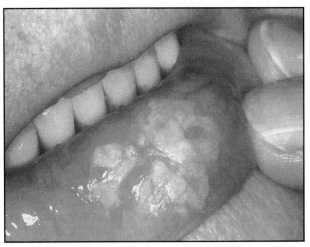

Smokeless tobacco was the cause of this squamous cell carcinoma on the lower lip.

sensation of the gums and lips, have cracked and bleeding lips, and develop precancerous lesions in oral cavity tissue. In a condition known as **leukoplakia**, the oral cavity tissue turns white, thickens, and hardens. If the use of smokeless tobacco continues, these precancerous lesions can develop into cancer. In addition, smokeless tobacco irritates the gums causing gingivitis and, eventually tooth loss.

Cardiorespiratory Diseases

Tobacco smokers have high rates of coronary heart disease, pulmonary emphysema, and chronic bronchitis. When pulmonary emphysema and chronic bronchitis are diagnosed together, this condition is called chronic obstructive lung disease, discussed in Chapter 8.

Emphysema destroys the elasticity of the alveoli (air sacs) of the lung. It greatly reduces the smoker's ability to inhale and exhale properly, and the smoker is chronically short of breath. The tissue affected by emphysema can never be repaired or replaced. The disease progresses slowly but steadily and turns its victims into respiratory cripples. People with emphysema spend years literally gasping for breath. Many die because of an overworked heart. Emphysema changes the lung's normal appearance. Some of the air sacs burst and collapse, creating tiny craters in the lung. Others balloon in the body's desperate struggle to obtain oxygen and expel carbon dioxide. Emphysema, once a relatively rare disease, now is common in smokers. It has been associated strongly with the

cigarette smoke that causes intense "air pollution" in the lungs.

Chronic bronchitis is an inflammation of the bronchial tubes. When the lining of the bronchial tubes becomes irritated, it secretes excessive mucus, causing bronchial congestion. This congestion produces chronic coughing and makes breathing extremely difficult. Chronic bronchitis and emphysema are included in the discussion of respiratory disorders in Chapter 8.

Effects on Pregnant Women and Children

Smoking during pregnancy can jeopardize the fetus' long-term physical growth and intellectual development. Women who smoke during pregnancy have high rates of low-birthweight infants, premature deliveries, spontaneous abortions (miscarriages), bleeding during pregnancy, death of the fetus (stillbirth), and children who die during infancy. Women who use oral contraceptives (the pill) and smoke are at higher risk for stroke, heart attack, and problems associated with the circulatory system. Smoking can affect a woman's reproductive health. In addition, smoking women have higher rates of cervical cancer.

KEY TERMS

Smokeless tobacco chewing tobacco and snuff

Nitrosamines cancer-causing substance found in tobacco

Leukoplakia a condition in which tissue in the oral cavity turns white, thickens, and hardens; a common effect of smokeless tobacco

Secondhand Smoke

Passive smoking or involuntary smoking can do serious harm to nonsmokers. The smoke emitted from these tobacco products (sidestream smoke) contains dangerous substances including carbon monoxide, nicotine and other carcinogens. The amount of exposure depends upon the concentration of tobacco smoke in the nonsmoker's environment. Annual deaths induced by secondhand smoke are 3,000 to 50,000, mostly from heart attacks. One study, reported by the American Cancer Society, found that women exposed to husbands who smoked 20 or more cigarettes a day at home had double the risk of lung cancer as women who were married to nonsmokers.

Environmental tobacco smoke can cause eye irritation, elevated heart rate and blood pressure, dry scratchy throat, and breathing difficulty. Children of parents who smoke have higher rates of respiratory illnesses and infection (pneumonia and bronchitis), colds, chronic coughs, allergies, ear infections, as well as reduced lung functioning. Parents' cigarette smoke also lowers HDL ("good") cholesterol in children with high cholesterol levels (about 2.9 million U. S. children). These children subsequently have a greater risk for heart disease.

Help on the Way for Nonsmokers

A major tobacco company has developed a low-smoke cigarette. The cigarette still has as much of the addictive nicotine and the toxic carbon monoxide, but it reduces 90% of the tars along with secondhand smoke. Only a carbon tip is lit, then warm air is pulled through the tobacco, where glycerine is vaporized and carries the nicotine and tobacco flavor to the smoker — but not the smoke to the nonsmoker.

Infants are three times more likely to die from sudden infant death syndrome (SIDS) if their mothers smoke during and after pregnancy.

In light of the Surgeon General's warning and additional health and medical findings, restrictions on smoking in the workplace and public places are being legislated rapidly. As more research about the harmful effects of passive smoking is being reported, the public's interest concerning nonsmokers' health and safety is increasing.

How To Quit

At any given time, about 70% of the 46 million smokers say they would gladly quit — if they

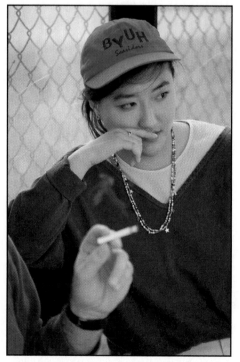

Legislation to protect nonsmokers' rights is being stepped up.

Warnings From the Surgeon General Required for Tobacco Products

SURGEON GENERAL'S WARNING: Cigarette Smoke Contains Carbon Monoxide.

SURGEON GENERAL'S WARNING: Smoking Causes Lung Cancer, Heart Disease, Emphysema and May Complicate Pregnancy.

SURGEON GENERAL'S WARNING: Quitting Smoking Now Greatly Reduces Serious Risks to Your Health.

SURGEON GENERAL'S WARNING: Smoking by Pregnant women may result in Fetal Injury, Premature Birth, and Low Birth Weight.

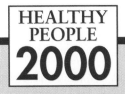
* Reduce cigarette smoking in adults (special target groups are blue-collar workers, adults who have not graduated from high school, military personnel, pregnant women and women of reproductive age, African Americans, Hispanics, American Indians, Alaska natives, and southeast Asian men)

* Reduce cigarette smoking by children so fewer go on to smoke as adults.

* Have at least one-half the adult smokers stop for at least 1 day a year.

* Have women who smoke cigarettes stop while they are pregnant.

* Expose fewer children age 6 and under to cigarette smoke at home.

* Decrease use of smokeless tobacco by males ages 12–24.

* Establish all elementary, middle, and secondary schools as tobacco-free environments, and include tobacco prevention in all curricula.

* Establish smoke-free environments in the majority of the nation's workplaces and enclosed public places (including health-care facilities, schools, public transportation).

* Enact comprehensive clean indoor air acts that prohibit smoking in all 50 states.

* Eliminate or severely restrict all forms of tobacco product advertising and promotion to which youth younger than age 18 are likely to be exposed.

could. The dependence — physical, psychological, or both — has a strong hold on tobacco users. Of those who try to quit, only about 8% succeed the first time. Many have been smoking since their teen years, to the point where it is a totally ingrained pattern. Some fear quitting because they believe they will inevitably gain weight. Although the metabolism does slow somewhat, ex-smokers in a 117,000-woman study conducted by the Nurses' Health Study from 1977 to 1983 weighed an average of only 3 to 6 pounds more after 2 nonsmoking years than those who continued to smoke.

Consider the following benefits:

* Among former smokers, the decline in risk of death, compared with continuing smokers, begins shortly after quitting and continues at least 10 to 15 years.

* Stopping smoking reduces the risks for cancers of the oral cavity and the esophagus by 50% as

> "To cease smoking is the easiest thing I ever did; I ought to know because I've done it a thousand times."
> — Mark Twain

soon as 5 years after cessation. Further reduction of risk occurs over time.

* The risk for cervical cancer is substantially lower among former smokers than continuing smokers, even in the first few years after cessation.

* The excess risk of heart disease caused by smoking is reduced by about half after 1 year of quitting smoking and then declines gradually.

* After quitting smoking, the risk of stroke eventually returns to the level of the "never smoker." In some studies this has occurred within 5 years, and in others as long as 15 years.

* For those without overt chronic obstructive lung disease, smoking cessation improves

KEY TERMS

Passive smoking inhaling smoke in the environment by the nonsmokers; involuntary smoking

Tips for action

To help curb the craving:

The following are different ways smokers can retrain themselves to live without cigarettes. Any one of several of these methods in combination might be helpful to you.

❋ Don't smoke after you get a craving for a cigarette until 3 minutes have passed. During those 3 minutes, change your thinking or activity.

❋ Don't store up cigarettes. Never buy a carton. Wait until one pack is finished before you buy another.

❋ Never carry cigarettes around with you at home or at work. Keep your cigarettes as far from you as possible. Leave them with someone or lock them up.

❋ Never carry matches or a lighter with you.

❋ Put away your ashtrays or fill them with objects so they cannot be used for ashes.

❋ Change your brand of cigarettes weekly so you are always smoking a brand of lower tar and nicotine content than the week before.

❋ Always ask yourself, "Do I need this cigarette, or is it just a reflex?"

❋ Each day try to put off lighting your first cigarette.

❋ Decide arbitrarily that you will smoke only on even- or odd-numbered hours of the clock.

❋ Keep your hands occupied. Try playing a musical instrument, knitting, or fiddling with hand puzzles.

❋ Take a shower. You can't smoke in the shower.

❋ Brush your teeth frequently to get rid of the tobacco taste and stains.

❋ If you have a sudden craving for a cigarette, take ten deep breaths, holding the last breath while you strike a match. Exhale slowly, blowing out the match. Pretend the match was a cigarette by crushing it out in a ashtray. Now immediately get busy on some work or activity.

❋ Smoke only half a cigarette.

❋ Get out of your old habits. Seek new activities or perform old activities in a new way. Don't rely on the old ways of solving problems. Do things differently.

❋ If you are a stay-home "kitchen smoker" in the morning, volunteer your services to schools or nonprofit organizations to get you out of the house.

❋ Stock up on light reading materials, crossword puzzles, and vacation brochures that you can read during your coffee breaks.

❋ Frequent places where you can't smoke, such as libraries, buses, theatres, swimming pools, department stores, or just go to bed.

❋ Give yourself time to think and get fit by walking a half hour each day. If you have a dog, take it for a walk with you.

Source: American Cancer Society, Texas Division. Used by permission.

Who Quits Smoking?

❋ Women are more likely than men to try to quit smoking.

❋ An equal proportion of men and women have been off cigarettes 1 to 4 years, though men are more likely than women to have been off cigarettes 5 or more years.

❋ African Americans are more likely than Anglos to try to quit smoking, Anglos, however, are more likely than African Americans to have been off cigarettes 1 or more years.

❋ Younger smokers (ages 20–44) are more likely than older smokers to try to quit smoking.

❋ People with any college education are more likely than those without to both try to quit and to stay off cigarettes 1 or more years.

Source: American Cancer Society; a report of the U. S. Surgeon General, 1990.

pulmonary function about 5% within a few months after quitting.

❋ Pregnant smokers who stop smoking at any time up to the 30th week of gestation have infants with higher birthweights than do women who smoke throughout pregnancy. Quitting in the first 3 to 4 months of pregnancy and abstaining throughout the remainder of pregnancy protects the fetus from the adverse effects of smoking on birthweight.

❋ Smokers with gastric or duodenal ulcers who stop smoking heal more rapidly.

Nicotine is thought to be among the most addictive of substances, an addiction with both physical and psychological aspects. Physical symptoms of withdrawal may include headaches, muscle aches, cramps, nausea, and visual disturbances. Physical withdrawal takes about a week while nicotine is being flushed from the body via the kidneys. The first 3 or 4 days are the most difficult due to withdrawal symptoms.

The psychological component is more difficult to pin down but is equally problematic. Psychological withdrawal can last years, although the first 2 to 3 months are most critical. Although nicotine is classified as a stimulant because of its physical properties, the primary psychological symptom of withdrawal is intense anxiety. Tobacco seems to have dual stimulating and antianxiety or tranquilizing properties. For example, intense anxiety is the most prevalent symptom of withdrawal, but sleepiness is also a

Tips for action

After you've quit smoking:

❋ Don't skip meals (smokers often skip meals because they get an adrenaline rush from cigarettes that takes the place of eating).

❋ Eat less more often. Snack on low-calorie vegetables and fruits.

❋ Drink six to eight glasses of water a day.

❋ Cut back on caffeine and alcohol, both are often associated with smoking.

❋ Plan exercise into your daily routine. Run up stairs. Do some yardwork.

❋ Soak in the bathtub at the end of the day. This is a great relaxer.

❋ Don't use weight gain as an excuse to resume smoking. You must be 90 pounds overweight to rival the cardiovascular risk of smoking a pack of cigarettes a day.

❋ Chew gum.

❋ Visit your dentist and get your teeth cleaned to get rid of the tobacco stains.

common symptom. These seemingly contradictory properties of nicotine make psychological withdrawal difficult.

Many products and programs have been offered as aids to quit smoking (see Table 12.1), ranging from tablets to nicotine gum to hospital-based clinics. Studies generally have shown that none of these aids is as effective as unaided individual effort, though some people are helped by these products and services.

The newest product on the market is the **nicotine patch**, available by medical prescription only. This is a rectangular pad, usually affixed to the arm, that delivers a steady amount of nicotine through the skin over a 24-hour period. Each day a new patch containing increasingly less nicotine is

❋ Table 12.1
Methods To Quit Smoking

Method	What it is	How it works	Average Cost	Success rate	How to get it
Cold turkey	Abrupt and total smoking cessation	Willpower. Initial nicotine withdrawal takes about 3 to 4 days, but symptoms can persist for weeks	$0	Less than 10%	Steel your resolve
Nicotine gum	Marketed by SmithKline Beecham under the name Nicorette, this Chiclet-sized nicotine-laced chewing gum currently is sold only by prescription	Aids in cold-turkey quitting by replacing some of the nicotine smoking provides	$35 to $75 a box, depending on dosage (Manufacturer recommends 9 to 12 boxes over a 6-month period, but some people use less)	About 33% with counseling	Ask your physician
Nicotine patch	Sold under the names Habitrol, Nicoderm, Prostep, Nicotrol. All are prescription adhesive pads about 2″ square	Applied to a quitter's upper arm or torso for 18 to 24 hours daily over a number of weeks. A continuous supply of nicotine is absorbed into the bloodstream	$25 to $30 weekly, for 6 to 12 weeks	About 33% with counseling	Ask your physician
Smokenders®	Weekly 2-hour sessions for 6 weeks. Sometimes used in conjunction with patches	Gradual withdrawal until quit date; relapse support	About $325; often corporate sponsored	55% to 65%*	Call 800-828-HELP
Smokeless®	Seven or eight 1-hour or 1½-hour group sessions over 4 weeks	Uses behavioral techniques to teach stop-smoking, stress and weight management	About $120; often corporate sponsored	45% to 62%*	Call 800-345-2476
Freedom From Smoking®	American Lung Assn's not-for-profit program: eight 1-hour to 2-hour group classes over 7 to 8 weeks	Motivational lectures, tips on quitting, group support	$50 to $150	28%	Contact local chapter of ALA by calling 800-LUNG USA
Freshstart®	American Cancer Society's not-for-profit program: four 1-hour group sessions over a 2-week period	By third session smokers quit. Lectures cover stopping strategies, stress and weight control, relapse prevention	$0 to $25	27%	Contact local chapter of ACS or call 800-227-2345
How to Quit™	Sponsored by American Medical Association, this new self-help kit contains instructional video and booklets as well as relaxation and support tapes	Over a 4-week period helps smoker prepare, quit, develop stress-management techniques, work on relapse prevention	$70	New; success studies in progress	Call 800-214-2299

*Success claims based only on "graduates," not dropouts

Source: *Remedy*, Nov./Dec. 1994. Reprinted by permission of the author Kathleen Madden.

self-applied. The rationale is that the patch gradually reduces the addictive craving for nicotine through lower doses. Meanwhile, the person is not taking in all of the carcinogenic substances contained in tobacco smoke. After 3 months — the maximum allowed prescription — the craving for nicotine presumably will be reduced to the point where the person can be tobacco-free. The nicotine patch is recommended for use within a comprehensive program that addresses the psychological aspects of smoking as well.

About a third of the people who quit smoking resume smoking later. Most people who have stopped for good, however, have made more than one previous attempt to stop. This should motivate smokers to keep trying even though they may not be successful until several attempts.

ALCOHOL USE

For centuries beer, wine, and distilled spirits have been used in economic, social, political and religious ceremonies and various other celebrations. Except for the brief period of Prohibition in the United States (1917-1932), alcohol has been socially acceptable and legal.

Americans have desired the effects produced from consuming the beverage **ethyl alcohol**, also known as ethanol or grain alcohol. The major types of alcoholic beverages are:

1. *Distilled spirits* or hard liquor: made by distilling brewed or fermented grains. Contains 40%–50% alcohol by volume. Distilled liquor includes gin, scotch, whiskey, rum, vodka, and various liqueurs. The alcohol content of distilled beverages is expressed in terms of **proof**, which is equal to twice the percent of alcohol. One degree of proof, then, equals one-half of 1% of alcohol. For example if a beverage is 86 proof, the product contains 43% alcohol by volume, and a 90-proof beverage contains 45% alcohol by volume.

2. *Wine*: made by fermenting grapes and other fruits. Table wine contains 9% to 14% alcohol by volume and often is served with food. Dessert wine or fortified wine has distilled alcohol added and contains 18% to 21% alcohol by

---

Facts About Beer

※ A 12-ounce can of domestic beer contains 3.4% alcohol.

※ A 12-ounce Ice beer and specialty beers contain 4%+ alcohol. (The process extracts water, leaving a higher alcohol content.)

※ A 12-ounce can of "lite" beer must contain at least 3.2% alcohol by law.

※ A 12-ounce can of beer sold in supermarkets must be under 3.2% alcohol; generally, they are 2.5% or 2.6%.

Breweries do not have to display the % alcohol on the cans. Proposed federal legislation is attempting to require breweries to display the % alcohol. The breweries are opposed.

---

volume. Fortified wines include sherry, port, and madeira. Fortified wines such as Cisco and Thunderbird are popular with young drinkers because they have a "kick."

3. *Beer and ale*: made by controlled fermentation of cereal grains and malt. Hops are added to give these drinks a distinctive flavor. Lager beer contains 3% to 4% alcohol; malt liquor, 4% to 5%; and high-powered beer such as ale, porter, and stout, 6% to 7% alcohol.

Figure 12.5 shows the per-capita consumption of alcohol by types between 1977 and 1989. Figure 12.6 gives the percentage alcohol content in selected beverages.

Wine often accompanies meals and is used to flavor certain foods. Alcoholic beverages are consumed during social gatherings to relax, to feel more convivial, and to escape from pressures. Wine is part of sacred rites in some religious ceremonies. Alcoholic beverages are used socially to celebrate occasions such as weddings, births, graduations, anniversaries, family reunions, and sporting events. Alcohol slows or depresses the central nervous

KEY TERMS

Nicotine patch a pad worn on the arm that delivers a steady amount of nicotine through the skin as an aid to quitting

Ethyl alcohol a colorless liquid and central nervous system depressant made by the process of fermentation and found in alcoholic beverages

Proof amount of alcohol in a beverage, expressed as twice the percent of alcohol

---

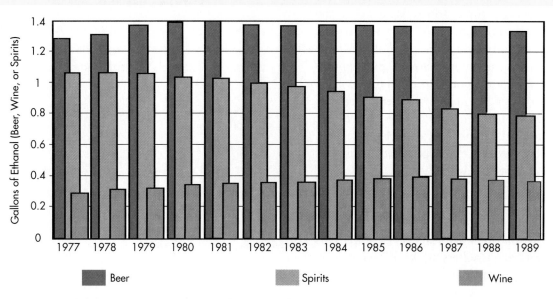

Apparent Per Capita Alcohol Consumption: National, State, and Regional Trends, 1977–1989, by G. D. Williams, F. S. Stinson, S. D. Brooks, D. Clem, and J. Noble (NIAAA Surveillance Report No. 20, DHHS Publ. No. (ADM)281-00001) (Washington, DC: Government Printing Office, 1991).

Figure 12.5 Per-capita alcohol consumption by type of beverage, 1977–1989

system and reduces inhibitions in some people, allowing them to be more expressive and explorative.

Prevalence

More than 60% of adults in the United States are regular drinkers. According to the National Institute on Alcohol Abuse and Alcoholism (NIAAA), 68.3% of Anglos, 64.5% of Hispanics, and 55.6% of African Americans used alcohol in 1990.

African Americans have higher rates of abstinence than Anglos, yet have higher rates of medical problems and death from alcoholism. A California study revealed that African Americans had higher rates of mortality from alcoholic cirrhosis than either Anglos or Asian Americans. The latter had the lowest rates of drinking, alcohol abuse, and death from alcohol-related causes.

The same California study reported that Hispanics had similar or lower mortality rates than

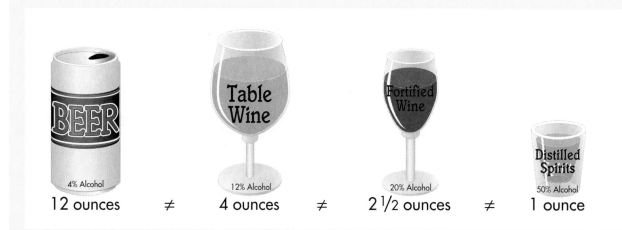

Figure 12.6 Percentage alcohol content in various beverages

Anglos. The mortality rate of Hispanics from alcohol-related motor vehicle crashes, however, was significantly higher than the rates for either Anglos or African Americans.

For American Indians alcohol abuse is a factor in five leading causes of death: motor vehicle crashes, alcoholism, cirrhosis, suicide, and homicide. The stereotype of the "drunken Indian" that has persisted since Colonial times is pervasive. Contrary to popular belief, the American Indian population is heterogeneous. For example, alcohol-related death rates varied in 1982 from 6 per 100,000 among the Cherokee Indians to 239 per 100,000 among the Cheyenne-Arapaho. Additionally 60% of the Navajos abstain completely, compared with 35% of the general population. Indian men are three times more likely than Indian women to be heavy drinkers. Still, one in every four deaths among Indian women is caused by alcoholic cirrhosis (liver disease), 37 times the rate among Anglo women. The main thing, however, is not to generalize statistics for American Indians as a category to any one of the more than 500 tribes in the United States.

Societal Effects of Drinking Alcohol

Abuse of alcohol continues to be a major societal problem. It can lead to problems in the family and contribute to irresponsible and dangerous sexual encounters (pregnancy, HIV/AIDS infection, and other STDs). Alcohol is a contributing factor in:

— motor vehicle crash injuries and deaths
— accidents
— violence — fighting, assaults, abuse, homicides
— absenteeism from work and school
— dissension and disharmony in the community and workplace
— decreased productivity
— job loss, discharge, and wage garnishment
— skyrocketing benefit costs (insurance).

Figure 12.7 shows the percentages of various societal problems that are alcohol-related. An estimated 25% of all people admitted to general hospitals have drinking problems. Moderate to heavy alcohol consumption is a major risk factor in injury and trauma, contributing to approximately 5% of all deaths. Ten percent of all deaths in the United States is linked to alcohol, including those caused by illness, accidents, and homicide.

Alcohol use is associated closely with violent crimes. When people are under the influence of alcohol, their reasoning and judgment are impaired, so they more often resort to aggressive behavior and violence. In about half of all homicides and serious assaults, and a high percentage of sex-related crimes, robberies, and domestic violence incidents, alcohol is found in the offender, the victim, or both.

Alcohol is used all too often to "anesthetize" the thinking processes — to try to block out pain, fears, unpleasant thoughts, and feelings of inadequacy, loneliness, and low self-esteem. In addition, people may use alcohol as a crutch to escape problems associated with the family, job, and social relationships.

Alcohol can have detrimental psychological consequences by altering feelings, perceptions, and moods. Many drinkers do not realize that alcohol is a depressant. Individuals with low self-esteem

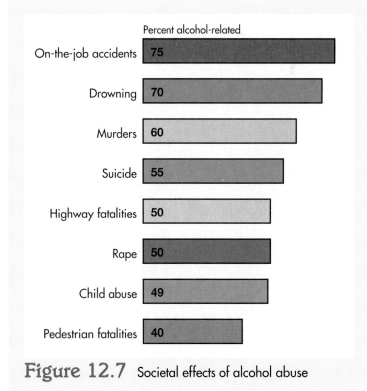

Figure 12.7 Societal effects of alcohol abuse

may turn unpleasant feelings and anger toward themselves. For example, alcohol often is a factor in suicide attempts.

In recent years, alcohol has been the drug of choice of high school and college students. Both groups are showing an increase in **binge drinking,** defined as drinking five or more consecutive drinks (men) or four consecutive drinks (women).

In a study published in the *Journal of the American Medical Association* in December 1994, 50%

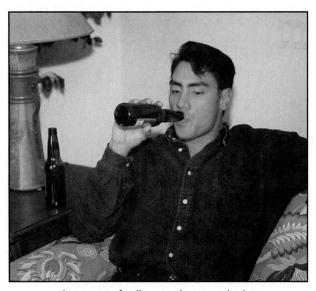

About 84% of college students are drinkers.

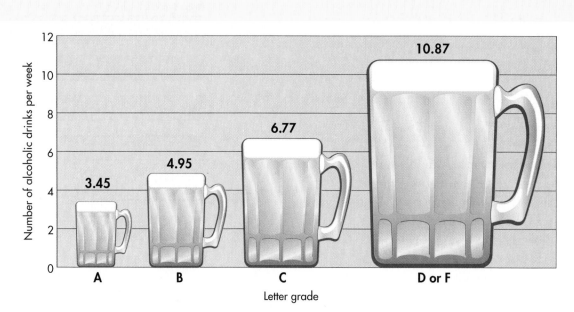

Table 12.2
Binge Drinking by College Students

	Men	Women
Drank on 10 or more occasions in the past 30 days	24%	13%
Usually binges when drinks	43	38
Drinks to get drunk	44	35
Was drunk three or more times in the past month	28	19

Source: Harvard School of Public Health.

of the men and 39% of the women said they had binged at least once in the last 2 weeks. Other statistics on college binge drinking are given in Table 12.2. Today's college student, on the average, spends more money on alcohol than on books. Drinking alcohol is a factor in about 28% of college dropouts. Gradepoint average is related to drinking, as shown in Figure 12.8. In one self-reporting survey, 36% of the students indicated driving while intoxicated. Of the current 12 million college students in the United States, 2% to 3% will die from alcohol-related causes.

Adapted from *Lifetime Physical Fitness & Wellness,* Werner W. K. Hoeger and Sharon A. Hoeger. (Englewood, CO: Morton Publishing, 1994).

Figure 12.8 Average number of drinks associated with college letter grades

Physical Effects of Drinking Alcohol

Once ethyl alcohol is swallowed, it has a direct effect on the mouth, esophagus, stomach, and small intestines. Alcohol is not a nutrient. It is not digested; however, it is partially broken down in the stomach.

The alcohol consumed is absorbed into the bloodstream quickly through the stomach wall and small intestine. Absorption is influenced by several factors such as the concentration of alcohol in the beverage, quantity consumed, rate of consumption, amount of food in the stomach, carbonation of the beverage or mixer, age, sex, and body weight (see Figure 12.9). The larger the body, the lower the concentration of alcohol in the blood will be. Individuals with more body weight have more body fluid, which disperses the alcohol consumed in a larger volume of blood. Therefore, they will not become intoxicated as rapidly as individuals who weigh less and consume the same amount of alcohol at the same rate.

Women and men respond differently to alcohol. Women have smaller quantities of the enzymes in the stomach tissue that aid in breaking down alcohol. This translates to women's absorbing 30% more alcohol into their bloodstream than men. This is the main reason for a higher incidence of liver damage among women drinkers than men drinkers. Alcohol also interferes with the absorption of some major nutrients and minerals, especially calcium, in the woman's body. As menopausal and older women start to lose calcium, this loss causes bones to become brittle and thin (osteoporosis). In addition, women taking oral contraceptives remain inebriated longer. Their bodies metabolize alcohol more slowly than women who are not on the pill.

KEY TERMS

Binge drinking consuming five or more drinks consecutively (men) and four consecutively (women)

# of Drinks	Body Weight							
	100–119	120–139	140–159	160–179	180–199	200–219	220–239	240 >
10	.38	.31	.27	.23	.21	.19	.17	.16
9	.34	.28	.24	.21	.19	.17	.15	.14
8	.30	.25	.21	.19	.17	.15	.14	.13
7	.26	.22	.19	.16	.15	.13	.12	.11
6	.23	.19	.16	.14	.13	.11	.10	.09
5	.19	.16	.13	.12	.11	.09	.09	.08
4	.15	.12	.11	.09	.08	.08	.07	.06
3	.11	.09	.08	.07	.06	.06	.05	.05
2	.08	.06	.05	.05	.04	.04	.03	.03
1	.04	.03	.03	.02	.02	.02	.02	.02

Blood Alcohol Concentration

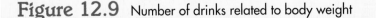 Reasonably safe   Unsafe   Illegal in all states

Figure 12.9 Number of drinks related to body weight

Mixing Alcohol and Medicines:

Sometimes alcohol increases the effects and the risks of a medicine to potentially dangerous levels. About 100 prescription medicines can produce unwanted effects when mixed with alcohol. A few examples are:

Analgesic pain medication

❋ salicylates (aspirin)

❋ ibuprofen (Advil, Motrin)

stomach and intestinal bleeding, bleeding ulcers

Antidiabetic agents

❋ chlorpropamide (Diabinese)

❋ tolbutamide (Orinase)

❋ insulin

altered control of blood sugar, most often hypoglycemia

Barbiturates

❋ secobarbitol (Seconal)

❋ phenobarbital (Barbita)

❋ pentobarbital (Nembutal)

greater sedative effect, drowsiness, confusion

Benzodiazepines

❋ alprazolam (Xanax)

❋ diazepam (Valium)

❋ triazolam (Halcion)

greater sedative effect, impaired motor coordination (such as driving ability)

Monamine oxidase (MAO) inhibitors

❋ isocarboxazid (Marplan)

❋ phenelzine (Nardil)

❋ tranylcypromine (Parnate)

certain alcoholic beverages contain tyramine, which can cause severe high blood pressure; may be fatal

Furthermore, alcohol can interact harmfully with some common nonprescription medicines such as aspirin and allergy medicines.

Adapted from National Council on Patient Information and Education, 666 Eleventh St. N.W., Suite 810, Washington, DC 20001.

In males, metabolism of alcohol by the liver produces a chemical substance that speeds destruction of testosterone. Sex problems such as impotence and testicle atrophy are common among heavy drinkers.

In addition, absorption may be influenced by body chemistry, emotions, and individual tolerance. When the liver becomes more efficient in metabolizing alcohol, because of repeated consumption, the body becomes more tolerant. As more alcohol is consumed and metabolized, more alcohol is needed to get the desired effect ("buzz") one got initially. The rate at which alcohol enters the bloodstream is the key factor in **blood alcohol concentration (BAC)**, or **blood alcohol level (BAL)**, which is the percentage or ratio of alcohol present in the blood as it relates to the total volume of blood.

Once absorption occurs and alcohol enters the bloodstream, it is distributed uniformly throughout the body, extending to all body fluids and tissues. The brain has a large blood supply; therefore, it absorbs alcohol quickly. If a woman is pregnant and is drinking alcohol, it is distributed within the fetal circulation.

Ninety-five percent of alcohol in the blood has to be metabolized. It must be converted to carbon dioxide and water so it can be removed from the body. Recent research indicates that as much as 30% of alcohol consumed by nonalcoholic males may be metabolized in the stomach. The liver is capable of metabolizing approximately .25–.3 ounces of liquor per hour. The additional 5% of alcohol, which is not metabolized and therefore is unchanged, is excreted via urination, perspiration, and respiration.

In all states a person is considered legally intoxicated if the BAC measures between 0.08% and 0.10%. BAC is measured scientifically with a **breathalyzer** or by testing blood or urine samples. When the BAC reaches 0.02%, an individual may feel mild relaxing effects from alcohol. Typically, more definite impairment begins when the BAC ranges between 0.03% and just under 0.10%. These effects include impairment of mental function including judgment. In addition, voluntary muscle control decreases,

Males' Use of Alcohol Hurts Sperm

New animal research shows that males who drink before conception may have adverse effects on the fetus, as much as alcohol consumption by pregnant women can. A single large dose of alcohol given to male rats before mating had the effect of reducing the number of pregnancies by 50%, said neuro-pharmacologist Theodore H. Cicero of Washington University School of Medicine in St. Louis. Unlike the fetal alcohol syndrome, in which the fetus is bathed in alcohol consumed by the mother, the male rat experiments suggest that alcohol affects sperm adversely, resulting in abnormalities.

Pups whose sires had been given alcohol also were smaller than normal and had a higher death rate, Cicero reported in the Journal of Life Sciences.

causing some difficulty when performing fine-motor skills.

As the BAC increases, alcohol causes the central nervous system to alter behavioral and physical body function. The changes can include diminished psychomotor performance and severe depression of areas responsible for motor control in the brain. The results are disorientation, slurred speech, visual and hearing difficulty, confusion, poor judgment, and euphoria.

When alcohol is consumed more rapidly than the liver can metabolize it, the BAC rises. The alcohol impairs brain functions, causing **intoxication,** which is a temporary state of mental confusion. Physical and behavioral dysfunctioning also results from intoxication. Other complications can include depressed reflexes, anesthesia, unconsciousness, and coma. BAC 0.50% to 0.60% may lead to

KEY TERMS

Blood alcohol concentration (BAC) or blood alcohol level (BAL) ratio of alcohol measured in the blood to total blood volume

Breathalyzer device used to measure blood alcohol

Intoxication temporary state of mental confusion

Alcohol poisoning death attributed to BAC at 0.50% and above

❋ Table 12.3
Effects of Alcohol Related to Blood Alcohol Content

Blood Alcohol Concentration % (BAC)	Effects
0.01	Mild, if any. Slight changes in feeling, mood elevation.
0.03	Feelings of relaxation and exhilaration; slight impairment of mental function.
0.08	Diminished inhibitions, difficulty performing motor skills, impaired judgment, impaired visual and hearing acuity; meets DUI (driving under the influence) criteria in several states
0.10	Typically, little or no judgment and poor condition. Legal evidence of DUI in all states
0.12	Difficulty performing gross motor skills, impaired vision, definite impairment of mental function
0.15	Major impairment of physical and mental functions, erratic and irresponsible behavior, distorted judgment, feeling of euphoria, difficulty responding to stimuli
0.20	Confusion, decreased inhibitions, inability to move without assistance, inability to maintain upright position; may fall asleep
0.30	Severe mental confusion, difficulty in comprehension and perception, difficulty responding to stimuli, extreme distortion of sensibility; produces sleep in most people
0.40	Nearly complete anesthesia, severely depressed reflexes, possible unconsciousness or coma
0.50	Unconsciousness or deep coma; possibly death
0.60	Total depression of nerves that control heart and breathing centers; death

death by **alcohol poisoning**. Table 12.3 summarizes the effects of alcohol related to the BAC.

Drinking and Driving

Alcohol was involved in one-half of all fatal traffic crashes in 1990. Alcohol-related motor vehicle accidents also can result in serious personal injury, property damage, and economic cost. Drinking drivers are lethal weapons on the road. They have visual impairment, poor judgment, impaired coordination, and unrealistic sensations of speed and perceptions. As the BAC rises, the danger and risk of being involved in an alcohol-related motor-vehicle accident increase.

To curtail this carnage on our roads, some states have taken various precautionary measures including identifying repeat offenders, confiscating drivers' licenses and license plates, immobilizing vehicles, strongly publicizing the dangers of drinking and driving, utilizing prevention methods, and incarcerating the offenders. In addition, many states are passing harsher laws and incorporating larger fines when individuals drive under the influence of alcohol. Several states have passed laws lowering the legal BAC from .10% to .08%.

The Hangover

For some people a **hangover** follows excessive drinking. It clearly signals to the drinker the unpleasant side effects associated with overindulging. Symptoms vary from one person to another. They include a throbbing headache, slurred speech, gastritis, nausea, vomiting, poor circulation, dizziness, thirst, irritability, fatigue, and mental depression. Alcohol acts as a **diuretic**, speeding the elimination of fluid from the body. This causes the drinker to be thirsty and dehydrated after drinking excessively. When alcohol is present in the bloodstream, recovering from a hangover takes time. Showering, taking aspirin, and drinking coffee or more alcoholic beverages will not help speed recovery. Drinking

📞 Call for information ⎯⎯⎯⎯⎯⎯

> Mothers Against Drunk Driving (MADD)
> 800-438-6233
> (24-hour hotline for victims only)

Tips for action

* Legal drinking age in all states is 21 years. If you are not 21, refrain from the use of alcoholic beverages.

* A "40-ounce" (Beer) is not one drink; it is equal to 3–12 ounce cans of beer plus 4 extra ounces. Know the concentration of alcohol by volume and the amount of any alcoholic beverage you are consuming. When using distilled spirit, use a shot (1.25-ounce) glass as the standard.

* Do not drink and drive. For most people two drinks in one hour can raise blood alcohol level to .10% which is the tolerance level for driving under the influence in most states.

* Choose a designated driver (who will not drink) *before* drinking begins.

* If you are hosting a party offer alternative beverages for those who will not be drinking alcohol.

* Be aware that your drinking partners tolerance level may be higher than yours. Do not drink in competition.

* Do not ever participate in drinking contests. Blood alcohol can rise to lethal levels (.40%+) and produce alcohol poisoning and possible death.

* Accept the definition of heavy drinking as five or more drinks once or twice each weekend. If your drinking pattern is suspect, you may have a drinking problem.

* Recognize the warning signs of alcohol abuse given in this chapter.

How Much is Too Much

Moderate drinking for some individuals may not be moderate for others. There is no set amount. Some characteristics of moderate drinkers are:

❋ Moderate drinkers are aware that alcoholic beverages have a time and a place.

❋ Moderate drinkers have control over the amount of alcoholic beverage they consume and the rate at which they consume it.

❋ Moderate drinkers do not gulp drinks and do not consume several drinks in a short time.

❋ Moderate drinkers drink slowly.

❋ Moderate drinkers do not drink because they *need* to.

❋ Moderate drinkers understand the importance of eating nutritious foods and not replacing food with alcohol.

plenty of water, however, can restore needed body fluids more quickly and prevent further dehydration.

Passing out after excessive consumption can be extremely dangerous. If a person vomits while unconscious, the airway can be blocked, causing death. Alcohol intoxication can cause shock and death. Obstruction of the air passage and alcohol intoxication are medical emergencies and should be treated as such.

Chronic Effects of Alcoholism

Recent reports indicate that *moderate* intake of alcohol may be beneficial to health. Research reported in the September, 1994, *Journal of the American Medical Association* suggests that alcohol thins the blood and moderate drinking may help prevent blood clots from forming. One member of the American Medical Association opined via radio that 31,000 more people would die yearly in the USA of cardiovascular disease if Americans would become teetotalers. Many studies have found that people who drink moderately reduce their risk of dying from heart disease by

about 40%. At the same time, the lower risk was offset by the greater risk of dying from cancer (see Table 12.4).

Alcoholism has been called the "most untreatable disease in America." Alcoholism is apparent when consumption of alcoholic beverages is no longer merely social or controllable. Its use exceeds social norms and results in inappropriate drinking patterns. The user becomes physically dependent on alcohol. As drinking opportunities are presented, drinking episodes occur more frequently and periods of intoxication lengthen. Excessive drinking may cause the drinker not to be able to recall what happened the day before or recall events in which the drinker was physically present. This is called a **blackout**, or temporary amnesia.

The person rationalizes drinking behavior, physical problems, destruction of peer and family relationships, and encounters with law enforcement personnel. Drinkers sometimes attempt to modify excessive drinking behavior by switching brands and limiting their drinking to certain times of day.

❋ Table 12.4
Drinking and Death Rates

Amount drunk	Overall death rate	Heart Disease death rate	Cancer death rate
1 drink/week	16% lower	11% lower	21% lower
2–4 drinks/week	22% lower	20% lower	5% lower
5–6 drinks/week	21% lower	46% lower	7% higher
1 drink/day	1% higher	4% lower	12% higher
2 or more/day	63% higher	62% higher	123% higher

Source: Harvard Medical School, 1994.

KEY TERMS

Hangover aftereffects of drinking excessively including headache, nausea, vomiting, dizziness

Diuretic any drug that speeds up elimination of salts and water from kidneys and other body organs

Alcoholism the chronic, progressive condition of dependence on alcohol characterized by consumption above social and controllable limits

Blackout inability to remember recent events

Signs of Alcoholism

The following are signals that drinking has become excessive and that the person may be an alcoholic.

❋ *Secret drinking.* Alcoholics sneak drinks so other people will not know how much they are drinking.

❋ *Guilt feelings about drinking.* Alcoholics realize they have lost control over drinking and start to rationalize drinking behavior, feel remorseful, and avoid any discussion about alcohol.

❋ *Gulping the first few drinks.* Alcoholics want a quick "buzz," so they gulp down the first drinks rapidly. They want the soonest possible effects.

❋ *Periods of total abstinence.* Occasionally alcoholics go "on the wagon." They do not drink for some time. This reassures them that they can "take it or leave it." Most will resume drinking though.

❋ *Hiding bottles.* Alcoholics want to be certain they will not run out of alcohol.

❋ *Neglecting proper nutrition.* Alcoholics do not eat properly. They have little interest in food because alcohol comprises a substantial portion of their dietary intake.

❋ *Effects on family and friends.* In some cases the family and friends become embarrassed because of the alcoholic's behavior. Family members may change their socialization patterns.

❋ *Decrease in sexual drive.* Alcohol is a depressant drug, so it represses sexual drive and sexual activity along with other functions.

Long Term Effects of Excessive Alcohol Use

As alcohol consumption becomes more excessive, the individual develops a drug dependency, losing control over drinking. Chronic alcohol consumption lowers resistance to disease, damages the liver, the cardiovascular system, the central nervous system, and causes severe nutritional deficiencies that lead to further problems. Prolonged heavy drinking is also linked to increased risks of cancer of the bladder, mouth, stomach, and esophagus. Figure 12.10 illustrates parts of the body affected by long-term alcohol use. Figure 12.11 relates physical and psychological effects to the length of time a person has engaged in excessive drinking. Some of the more common alcohol-related disorders are listed below.

1. **Malnutrition** occurs when prolonged consumption of alcohol depresses the appetite and attacks the mucosa in the stomach. Heavy drinkers often do not obtain the needed calories. Without needed nutrients the alcohol depresses protein synthesis, interferes with the transfer of glucose into energy, increases mineral loss, and increases fatty acids.

2. **Alcoholic pellagra** is caused by a deficiency of protein and niacin. Symptoms of alcoholic pellagra are gastrointestinal disorders, mental and nervous disturbances, inflammation of the skin (dermatitis), and diarrhea.

3. Alcohol affects the heart and blood vessels by increasing the heart rate and constricting the arterial blood flow to the heart. Prolonged,

HEALTHY PEOPLE 2000 | OBJECTIVES FOR ALCOHOL USE

❋ Reduce deaths caused by alcohol-related motor vehicle crashes.

❋ Reduce the proportion of young people who have used alcohol, in the past month.

❋ Reduce the proportion of high school seniors and college students engaging in heavy drinking of alcoholic beverages.

❋ Reduce alcohol consumption by people aged 14 and older.

❋ Extend to 50 states legal blood alcohol concentration tolerance levels of .04 percent for motor vehicle drivers age 21 and older and .00 percent for those younger than age 21.

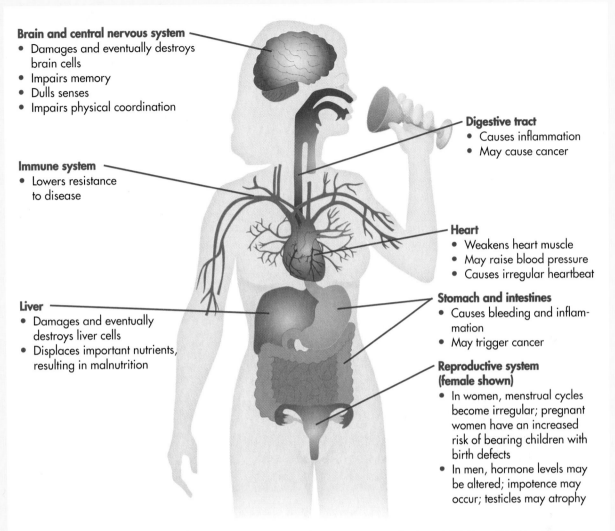

Brain and central nervous system
- Damages and eventually destroys brain cells
- Impairs memory
- Dulls senses
- Impairs physical coordination

Immune system
- Lowers resistance to disease

Liver
- Damages and eventually destroys liver cells
- Displaces important nutrients, resulting in malnutrition

Digestive tract
- Causes inflammation
- May cause cancer

Heart
- Weakens heart muscle
- May raise blood pressure
- Causes irregular heartbeat

Stomach and intestines
- Causes bleeding and inflammation
- May trigger cancer

Reproductive system (female shown)
- In women, menstrual cycles become irregular; pregnant women have an increased risk of bearing children with birth defects
- In men, hormone levels may be altered; impotence may occur; testicles may atrophy

Source: *Wellness: Guidelines for a Healthy Lifestyle*, by Brent Q. Hafen and Werner W. K. Hoeger (Englewood, CO: Morton Publishing, 1994), p. 288.

Figure 12.10 Long-term effects of chronic alcohol use

excessive drinking can weaken the heart and contribute to **cardiomyopathy**, a disease of the heart muscle. In addition, excessive drinking can cause abnormal heart rhythms and heart failure. Alcoholics also tend to have higher blood pressure, which can lead to stroke.

4. Alcohol causes blood vessels in the kidneys to dilate. This in turn produces an increase in urine output. An acute effect is dehydration. Prolonged and excessive use of alcohol can cause irreversible damage to the kidneys.

5. Cigarette smoking and alcohol drinking enhance the development of cancers of the oral cavity, larynx, esophagus, and pancreas.

Tobacco contains known carcinogens. Whether carcinogens are found in alcohol is not conclusive.

6. Liver disorders and diseases are common among heavy drinkers. When the effects of alcohol become toxic, this causes **hepatotoxic**

KEY TERMS

Malnutrition effects on body due to prolonged deficiency of necessary nutrients

Alcoholic pellagra condition caused by deficiency of protein and niacin due to prolonged alcohol consumption

Cardiomyopathy a disease of the heart muscle

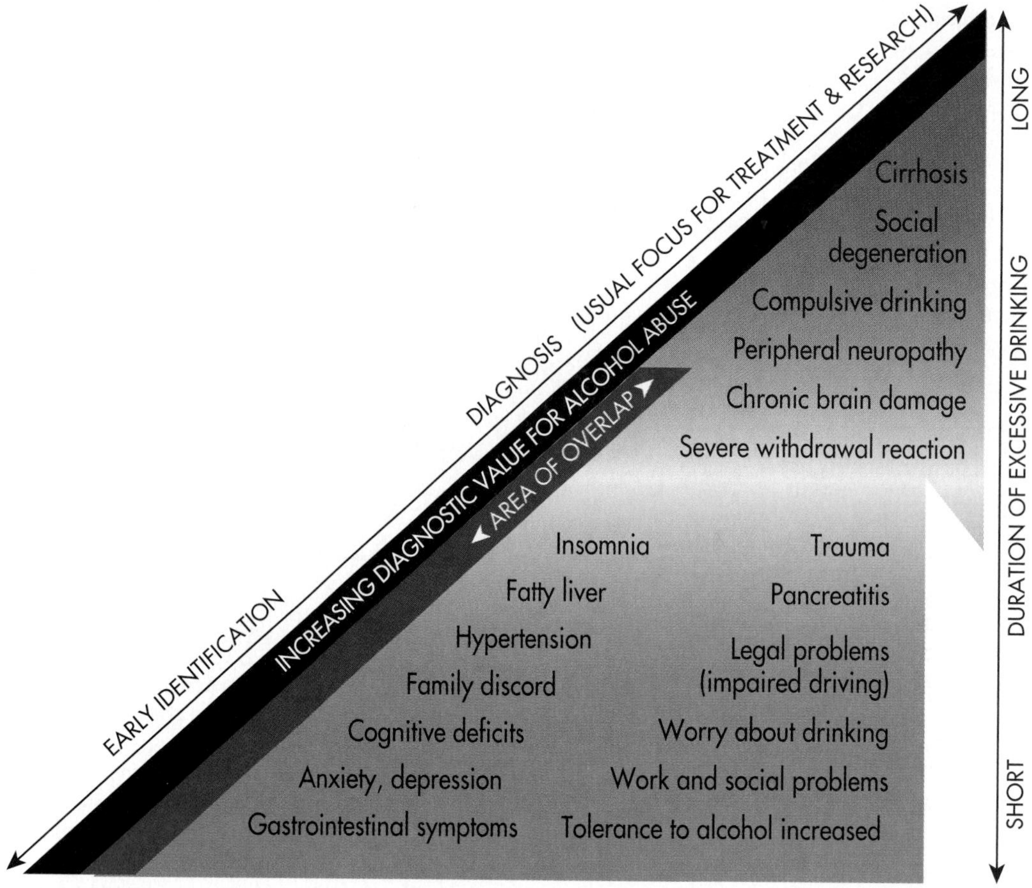
DIAGNOSIS (USUAL FOCUS FOR TREATMENT & RESEARCH)
EARLY IDENTIFICATION
INCREASING DIAGNOSTIC VALUE FOR ALCOHOL ABUSE
AREA OF OVERLAP
Cirrhosis
Social degeneration
Compulsive drinking
Peripheral neuropathy
Chronic brain damage
Severe withdrawal reaction
Insomnia
Trauma
Fatty liver
Pancreatitis
Hypertension
Legal problems (impaired driving)
Family discord
Cognitive deficits
Worry about drinking
Anxiety, depression
Work and social problems
Gastrointestinal symptoms
Tolerance to alcohol increased
LONG
DURATION OF EXCESSIVE DRINKING
SHORT

Source: "Early Intervention for Alcohol and Drug Problems: Core Issues for Medical Education," *Australian Drug and Alcohol Review* 5 (1986), 69–74.

Figure 12.11 Disorders as related to duration of excessive drinking

trauma, commonly termed "fatty liver" (90%-100% of heavy drinkers show evidence of fatty liver). If the person stops drinking, this condition can be reversed. **Alcoholic hepatitis**, a chronic inflammation of the liver tissue, develops in 10% to 35% of heavy drinkers. Alcoholic hepatitis is often fatal. When it is not, it can develop into **alcoholic cirrhosis**. Cirrhosis, which occurs in 10% to 20% of heavy drinkers, is characterized by scarring, shriveling, and hardening of the liver tissue. The scar tissue replaces functioning liver cells and blocks the flow of blood to cells that are still alive. This impairs liver functioning and the metabolism of alcohol. Fatty liver is reversible if the person stops drinking, and the progression of cirrhosis can be halted.

7. Chronic alcohol consumption affects the central nervous system mainly because prolonged drinking depresses the appetite. When drinkers do not take in needed nutrients, they are predisposed to several neurological conditions.

   a. **Wernicke's disease** is caused by a thiamine deficiency. Symptoms include rapid, involuntary oscillation of the eyeballs and double vision, severe decrease in mental functioning, and lack of muscular coordination.

   b. **Polyneuritis** is another condition caused by thiamine deficiency. It is characterized by inflammation of several peripheral and central nerves, which causes the drinker to become weak and have tingling sensations.

c. **Korsakoff's syndrome** is caused by a deficiency of B-complex vitamins, specifically B_{12} and thiamine. Symptoms of this type of psychosis include severe amnesia and, more specifically, loss of contact with reality and personality alterations. The person is apathetic and has difficulty walking.

d. **Alcoholic hallucinosis** is a mental disorder commonly found in chronic alcoholics. Symptoms of this condition include seeing images ("pink elephants," snakes, spiders), mood disturbances, and alcohol-related depression.

8. Chronic alcohol use alters the hormones that regulate the pituitary, hypothalamus, and the gonads (ovaries and testes). This can cause men to have lower levels of testosterone, shrinking testicles, loss of facial hair, low sex drive, impotence, and infertility. Women may encounter menstrual disturbances, atrophying ovaries, and infertility.

9. A small amount of ethyl alcohol stimulates stomach activity. Alcohol can irritate the mouth, throat, esophagus, stomach, small intestines, and pancreas. Two common gastrointestinal disorders found in alcoholics are **gastritis**, chronic inflammation of the stomach lining, and **gastric ulcers**, chronic inflammation of the lower end of the esophagus and stomach.

10. **Fetal alcohol syndrome (FAS)** is a group of physical and behavioral defects believed to be caused by maternal use of alcohol during fetal development. When mothers drink, babies drink. Alcohol crosses the placenta and becomes part of fetal circulation. Each year many infants born to drinking and alcoholic mothers have distinct aberrant patterns of growth and development including:

— growth deficiency before and after birth
— lower than average intelligence or mental retardation
— hyperactivity
— sleep disorders
— extreme nervousness
— poor attention span
— abnormalities of the head and face such as a small head, small, slanted eyes, flat or sunken nasal bridge, short, "pudgy" nose

— defects in the heart and other major organs
— malformed arms, legs, and genitals

Overall rates for FAS in the United States are one to three per 1,000. The prevalence of FAS in Southwestern Plains Indians was found to be 10.7 in one study reported by the National Institute on Alcohol Abuse and Alcoholism (NIAAA). The incidence of FAS in African Americans is about seven times higher than in Anglos, even though more African American women are nondrinkers.

11. **Fetal alcohol effect (FAE)** is another result of the mother's alcohol consumption during pregnancy. Aberrant patterns of development are not as distinct in infants diagnosed with FAE as in FAS. FAE symptoms, however, include some physical and behavioral dysfunctioning, such as lower birthweight, jittery and irritable newborns, and permanent abnormal emotional and mental functioning.

12. Alcoholics are 21 times more likely than nonalcoholics to receive a diagnosis of antisocial personality disorder. The rates are four and six times higher for schizophrenia and mania, respectively. Between 10% and 30% of alcoholics have panic disorders. In addition,

KEY TERMS

Hepatotoxic trauma disease of the liver caused by alcoholism; commonly called "fatty liver"

Alcoholic hepatitis chronic inflammation of the liver tissue

Alcoholic cirrhosis scarring, shriveling, and hardening of liver tissue

Wernicke's disease caused by thiamine deficiency; due to excessive alcohol consumption

Polyneuritis inflammation of several peripheral and central nerves caused by thiamin deficiency due to alcoholism

Korsakoff's syndrome psychosis caused by deficiency of B vitamins due to alcoholism

Alcoholic hallucinosis mental disorder characterized by mental disorientation and mood disturbance

Gastritis chronic inflammation of stomach lining

Gastric ulcers chronic inflammation of lower end of esophagus and stomach

Fetal alcohol syndrome (FAS) group of physical and behavioral defects in a newborn caused by the mother's alcohol use during pregnancy

Fetal alcohol effect (FAE) aberrant behavior pattern in newborns resulting from mother's alcohol consumption during pregnancy

alcoholism often is associated with bulimia, depression, and overuse of other drugs including sedatives, hallucinogens, stimulants, and marijuana.

Genetic Influences

Certain ethnic minorities may have genetic traits that either predispose them to or protect them from becoming alcoholic. The differences may relate to variants of the genes for enzymes involved in alcohol metabolism by the liver. One enzyme found in Japanese people, for example, has been associated with faster elimination of alcohol from the body, as compared to Anglos. Table 12.5 points out some of the specific risk factors by ethnic group. Acculturation also plays a large role in drinking patterns among various ethnic groups. For example, studies of Asian Americans suggest that, as they become assimilated into the American culture, their drinking rates increase and eventually conform to those of the U. S. population as a whole.

Treatment of Alcoholism

An estimated 18 million American adults currently have problems as a result of alcohol overconsumption. The success of any treatment approach depends upon the alcohol-dependent person. The alcoholic must desire and be willing to stop drinking. He or she must take the first step. Treatment may consist of:

✳ *Detoxification.* In most cases the first step in treatment and rehabilitation of alcoholism is detoxification, a process of removing toxic substances from the body. During this period certain drugs are given to prevent the patient from having convulsions. In addition, vitamins are administered to increase the appetite, and the person is given a highly nutritious diet so the body organs will receive proper nutrients and start to heal from damage that may have occurred during the drinking period.

✳ *Drug therapy.* Several drugs have been used in treating alcoholism. Once the patient has been detoxed, tranquilizers are given for several weeks to decrease symptoms associated with agitation, anxiety, and tremors. In **aversion therapy** the prescription drug disulfiram (Antabuse) is administered. This drug blocks the metabolism of acetaldehyde. If the patient takes Antabuse and drinks alcohol, the combination causes extremely unpleasant reactions such as breathing difficulty, intense headache, nausea, vomiting, and pounding heart.

In early 1995 the Food and Drug Administration approved the first new drug in 47 years to treat alcoholism. The drug, maltrexone, works by blocking the craving for alcohol and also the pleasure derived from drinking alcohol. In clinical trials maltrexone combined with behavior modification enabled as many as three-fourths of alcoholics to avoid a relapse.

✳ *Psychotherapy.* Psychotherapy is as individualized as the personality. It can be effective for some alcoholics by helping the person discover or uncover an underlying conflict that is

✳ Table 12.5
Alcohol-Related Health Risks in Minority Groups

Ethnic Group	Risk Factors from Alcohol Abuse
African Americans	High risk for cirrhosis of the liver, heart diseases, nutritional deficiencies, neurological disorders, and cancer of the tongue, mouth, esophagus, and larynx; extremely high accident and homicide rates
Hispanics	High risk for liver disorders and diseases, neurological disorders caused by nutritional deficiency, cancer of the tongue, mouth, esophagus, and larynx
American Indians	Very high mortality rates; cirrhosis of the liver, suicide, homicide, cancers, and emotional and neurological disorders
Asian Americans	Low rates and risks of drinking-related health problems. Recent research does indicate that about half carry a gene that affects metabolism in the liver, causing a build-up of a toxic metabolite, manifested by the "flushing" response of the face, sweating, and nausea.

contributing to or has precipitated the drinking behavior. Most psychotherapists include the family in therapy, as successful treatment may well depend upon the understanding and support the alcoholic receives from family members. The alcoholic and the family should understand fully that alcoholism is an illness, a disease, and the alcoholic must accept the fact that he or she needs help.

✳ *Nutrient Supplements.* Some supplements that may be helpful in the treatment of alcoholism are:

vitamin A	vitamin B$_1$	vitamin B$_2$
vitamin B$_6$	vitamin B$_{12}$	choline
folic acid	niacin	pangamic
pantothenic acid	vitamin C	acid
vitamin E	vitamin K	vitamin D
iron	magnesium	chromium
zinc	unsaturated	manganese
glutamine	fatty acids	

Organizations Dealing with Alcoholism

Alcoholics Anonymous (AA) is a well organized, long-established, supportive fellowship of alcohol-dependent people. Their sole purpose is to get sober and remain sober. Members decide to turn over their lives and will to a power greater than their own. They have to desire to stop drinking, admit they are unable to stop drinking and need help, and be honest with themselves. AA has at least 19,000 affiliated groups and more than 350,000 members across the United States.

Al-Anon and **Alateen** are organizations that help families cope with alcohol-dependent family members. Al-Anon is for mates and other relatives. The family members are encouraged and supported by other families. They learn that they are not alone. Alateen is a supportive organization of teenagers of alcoholic parents.

☎ Call for information _____

Alcoholic Anonymous
(212) 870-3400

Al-Anon Family Group Headquarters
800-344-2666

Additional organizations that are helpful and supportive include the Salvation Army, the National Institute of Alcohol Abuse and Alcoholism (NIAAA), and the National Council on Alcoholism (NCA). Work-based programs are available to give assistance in your area.

An AA Poem

We drank for happiness
and became unhappy.
We drank for joy and
became miserable.
We drank for sociability
and became argumentative.
We drank for friendship
and made enemies.
We drank for sleep and
awakened without rest.
We drank for strength and
felt weak.
We drank "medicinally"
and acquired health problems.
We drank for relaxation and
got the shakes.
We drank for bravery
and became afraid.
We drank to make conversation
easier and slurred our speech.
We drank to feel heavenly
and ended up feeling like hell.
We drank to forget and were
forever haunted.
We drank for freedom
and became slaves.
We drank to erase problems
and saw them multiply.
We drank to cope with life
and invited death.

–Author Unknown

KEY TERMS

Detoxification process of removing toxic substances, such as alcohol, from the body

Aversion therapy treatment in which a person is given the drug antabuse which blocks metabolism of acetaldehyde

Alcoholics Anonymous (AA) supportive fellowship of alcohol-dependent people

Al-Anon, Alateen two organizations that help families cope with alcohol-dependent family members

Summary

1 Tobacco use has been declining since 1942, with the exception that teens are smoking just as much or more.

2 Tobacco contains some 4,000 gases and tars. Nicotine is the addictive ingredient.

3 Tobacco is a major contributor to lung and other cancers, emphysema, chronic bronchitis, and many other diseases.

4 Secondhand smoke can produce harmful effects to the lungs of those who live with smokers and those who are around smokers a good share of the time.

5 Quitting smoking can be done cold turkey or gradually, utilizing medical and social supports.

6 Alcoholic beverages are of three basic types — distilled liquor, wine, and beer and ale — involving different processes and containing varying amounts (proof) of ethanol or grain alcohol.

7 More than half of all Americans are regular drinkers. Moderate drinking may be beneficial to health.

8 Overconsumption of alcohol has led to societal problems in relationships, accident rates, increased violence, decreased productivity, and other problems.

9 Of all deaths in the United States, 10% are linked to alcohol, including deaths caused by illness, accidents, and homicide.

10 Binge drinking among college students has assumed epidemic proportions.

11 Absorption of alcohol in the bloodstream depends on variables such as the blood alcohol concentration, quantity consumed, rate of consumption, amount of food in stomach, age, sex, and body weight.

12 Because the liver is involved in metabolizing alcohol, it often is the first organ damaged by chronic alcohol drinking. Other potential problems among many are: malnutrition, pellagra, kidney damage, some cancers, Wernicke's disease, Korsakoff's syndrome, hormonal deficiencies, gastrointestinal disorders, and fetal alcohol syndrome, as well as psychiatric and psychological problems.

13 A genetic factor may be involved in how the body metabolizes alcohol, causing disproportionate effects in some minority groups.

Select Bibliography

"Alcohol and Minorities." *Alcohol Alert*, 23 (January 1994). (a National Institutes of Health publication)

Cole, Richard. "Study: Black Smokers' Cancer Risk Higher." *Journal of the American Medical Association*, 266:11, (September 1991).

Cohen, S. "Alcohol and the Indian." *Drug Abuse and Alcoholism Newsletter*, 11:4 (May 1992).

Difranza, J. R. and Richards, J. Jr. "RJR Nabisco's Cartoon Camel Promotes Camel Cigarettes to Children." *Journal of the American Medical Association*, 266 (1991), 3149–3153.

Dixon, Barbara. *Good Health for African Americans*. New York: Crown, 1994.

Dunne, Lavon, J. *Nutrition Almanac*, 3d edition. New York: McGraw-Hill, 1990.

Johnson, R. C., and C. T. Nagoshi, "Asians, Asian-Americans and Alcohol." *Journal of Psychoactive Drugs*, 22:1 (1990), 45, 52.

Steenland, K. "Passive Smoking and the Risk of Heart Disease." *Journal of the American Medical Association*, 267 (1992), 94–99.

U. S. Department of Health and Human Services. *Eighth Special Report to the U. S. Congress on Alcohol and Health*. Washington, DC: Government Printing Office.

Why Do You Smoke?

NAME _____ DATE _____

COURSE _____ SECTION _____

	Always	Fre-quently	Occa-sionally	Seldom	Never
A. I smoke cigarettes in order to keep myself from slowing down.	5	4	3	2	1
B. Handling a cigarette is part of the enjoyment of smoking it.	5	4	3	2	1
C. Smoking cigarettes is pleasant and relaxing.	5	4	3	2	1
D. I light up a cigarette when I feel angry about something.	5	4	3	2	1
E. When I have run out of cigarettes I find it almost unbearable until I can get them.	5	4	3	2	1
F. I smoke cigarettes automatically without even being aware of it.	5	4	3	2	1
G. I smoke cigarettes to stimulate me, to perk myself up.	5	4	3	2	1
H. Part of the enjoyment of smoking a cigarette comes from the steps I take to light up.	5	4	3	2	1
I. I find cigarettes pleasurable.	5	4	3	2	1
J. When I feel uncomfortable or upset about something, I light up a cigarette.	5	4	3	2	1
K. I am very much aware of the fact when I am not smoking a cigarette.	5	4	3	2	1
L. I light up a cigarette without realizing I still have one burning in the ashtray.	5	4	3	2	1
M. I smoke cigarettes to give me a "lift."	5	4	3	2	1
N. When I smoke a cigarette, part of the enjoyment is watching the smoke as I exhale it.	5	4	3	2	1
O. I want a cigarette most when I am comfortable and relaxed.	5	4	3	2	1
P. When I feel "blue" or want to take my mind off cares and worries, I smoke cigarettes.	5	4	3	2	1
Q. I get a real gnawing hunger for a cigarette when I haven't smoked for a while.	5	4	3	2	1
R. I've found a cigarette in my mouth and didn't remember putting it there.	5	4	3	2	1

Scoring Your Test:

Enter the numbers you have circled on the test questions in the spaces provided below, putting the number you have circled to question A on line A, to question B on line B, etc. Add the three scores on each line to get a total for each factor. For example, the sum of your scores over lines A, G, and M gives you your score on "Stimulation," lines B, H, and N give the score on "Handling," etc. Scores can vary from 3 to 15. Any score 11 and above is high; any score 7 and below is low.

A _____ + G _____ + M _____ = _____ Stimulation

B _____ + H _____ + N _____ = _____ Handling

C _____ + I _____ + O _____ = _____ Pleasure Relaxation

D _____ + J _____ + P _____ = _____ Crutch: Tension Reduction

E _____ + K _____ + Q _____ = _____ Craving: Psychological Addiction

F _____ + L _____ + R _____ = _____ Habit

A score of 11 or above on any factor indicates that smoking is an important source of satisfaction for you. The higher you score (15 is the highest), the more important a given factor is in your smoking.

From *A Self-Test for Smokers.* U.S. Department of Health and Human Services, 1983.

Why You Smoke	What to Do Instead
Stimulation You smoke to keep from slowing down, for a lift, to pep you up.	Find something else to pep you up — a hobby, brisk walks, simple exercises.
Handling You like the ritual of smoking, to have something in your hands and mouth.	Pick something else to handle: coins, pen or pencil, "worry beads"; try doodling, or chew on paper straws or minted toothpicks.
Relaxation You enjoy smoking; it's a reward, a time you feel good about yourself.	Consider the harm cigarettes cause you and the reward of quitting. Substitute social or physical activity; prove self-control and feel good about yourself.
Crutch You smoke to deal with problems and negative feelings.	Prove to yourself smoking doesn't solve problems. Reduce tension other ways: Take deep breaths, call a friend, talk over feelings. Work on keeping your "cool."
Craving You feel "hooked" and begin to think of the next cigarette before you put out present one. You're aware of the need to smoke.	Recognize that quitting will be difficult and prepare to "see it through." Plan to try to stop "cold turkey," abstaining completely. The day before quitting, smoke to the point of distaste.
Habit You smoke automatically, often without realizing what you're doing.	Become aware of every cigarette you smoke and ask yourself why you're smoking and if you really want it. Wrap up your cigarettes or put them in a place difficult to get.

Audit

NAME _____ DATE _____

COURSE _____ SECTION _____

AUDIT is a brief structured interview, developed by the World Health Organization, which can be incorporated into a medical history. It contains questions about recent alcohol consumption, dependence symptoms, and alcohol-related problems.

BEGIN the AUDIT by saying: "Now I am going to ask you some questions about your use of alcoholic beverages *during the past year*." Explain what is meant by alcoholic beverages (i. e., beer, wine, liquor [vodka, brandy, etc.]).

Record the score for each question in the box on the right side of the question [   ].

1. How often do you have a drink containing alcohol?
   - ❏ Never (0) [   ]
   - ❏ Monthly or less (1)
   - ❏ 2 to 4 times a month (2)
   - ❏ 2 to 3 times a week (3)
   - ❏ 4 or more times a week (4)

2. How many drinks containing alcohol do you have on a typical day when you are drinking?
   - ❏ None (0) [   ]
   - ❏ 1 or 2 (1)
   - ❏ 3 or 4 (2)
   - ❏ 5 or 6 (3)
   - ❏ 7 or 9 (4)
   - ❏ 10 or more (5)

3. How often do you have six or more drinks on one occasion?
   - ❏ Never (0) [   ]
   - ❏ Less than monthly (1)
   - ❏ Monthly (2)
   - ❏ Weekly (3)
   - ❏ Daily or almost daily (4)

4. How often during the last year have you found that you were unable to stop drinking once you had started?
   - ❏ Never (0) [   ]
   - ❏ Less than monthly (1)
   - ❏ Monthly (2)
   - ❏ Weekly (3)
   - ❏ Daily or almost daily (4)

5. How often during the last year have you failed to do what was normally expected from you because of drinking?
   - ❏ Never (0) [   ]
   - ❏ Less than monthly (1)
   - ❏ Monthly (2)
   - ❏ Weekly (3)
   - ❏ Daily or almost daily (4)

6. How often during the last year have you needed a first drink in the morning to get yourself going after a heavy drinking session?
   - ❏ Never (0) [   ]
   - ❏ Less than monthly (1)
   - ❏ Monthly (2)
   - ❏ Weekly (3)
   - ❏ Daily or almost daily (4)

Reprinted with permission World Health Organization.

7. How often during the last year have you had a feeling of guilt or remorse after drinking?

    ❑ Never   (0)   [ ]
    ❑ Less than monthly   (1)
    ❑ Monthly   (2)
    ❑ Weekly   (3)
    ❑ Daily or almost daily   (4)

8. How often during the last year have you been unable to remember what happened the night before because you had been drinking?

    ❑ Never   (0)   [ ]
    ❑ Less than monthly   (1)
    ❑ Monthly   (2)
    ❑ Weekly   (3)
    ❑ Daily or almost daily   (4)

9. Have you or someone else been injured as the result of your drinking?

    ❑ Never   (0)   [ ]
    ❑ Less than monthly   (1)
    ❑ Monthly   (2)
    ❑ Weekly   (3)
    ❑ Daily or almost daily   (4)

Record the total of the specific items   [   ]

A score of 8 or greater may indicate the need for a more in-depth assessment.

Psychoactive Drugs

13

OBJECTIVES

* Describe what psychoactive drugs are and what effects they have in the brain.
* Describe the depressants and their effects.
* Describe the narcotics and their effects.
* Identify the stimulants and their effects
* Describe the forms and effects of marijuana.
* Identify the properties of inhalants.
* Identify some hallucinogenic drugs.
* Explain "designer drugs."
* Outline various treatment options.

*D*rugs can be your best friend or your worst enemy. They play a major role in the treatment of medical and psychological conditions. Prescription and over-the-counter (OTC) medications are capable of curing diseases, easing pain, calming fears, alleviating anxiety and frustration, relieving sleeplessness, and treating many health problems. Improved drug technology and the availability of prescribed and OTC medications have dramatically improved the health status of millions. In addition, as medications improve health, they aid in extending life

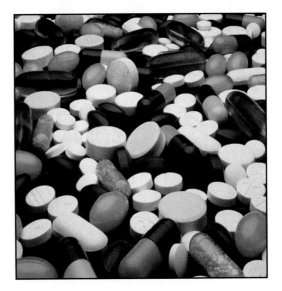

expectancy. Even when carefully monitored, however, drugs can cause adverse reactions, **iatrogenic** (medically induced) **illnesses**, and death. One must be aware constantly of the potential for **physical dependence** as well as **psychological dependence** with the use of any medication or psychoactive drug.

Drug abuse and **drug misuse** cause deleterious effects on the health and well-being of millions of people daily. Despite a decline in overall drug use, Americans continue to light-up, shoot-up, snort, guzzle-down, and spit in the wind. Figure 13.1 shows the percentages of various groups using illicit drugs within the month surveyed. The damaging effects that can be caused by misuse and abuse of drugs, whether prescribed, OTC, or illicit (illegal), include:

— drug dependency
— physical and mental dysfunctioning
— disruption of family units
— criminal and destructive behavior
— premature and accidental death
— disruption of career goals and aspirations
— incarceration.

Tragically, drug use among teenagers in the United States is rising after a period of decline beginning in the late 1970s. The 20th annual survey by the University of Michigan Institute for Social Research in 1994 showed that nearly half of all high school seniors had experimented with psychoactive drugs — marijuana, hallucinogens, inhalants, stimulants, barbiturates, steroids, and cocaine and crack — with the sharpest increase for marijuana. The trend over the past 12 years for grades 8 through 12 is shown clearly in Figure 13.2. The trend was observed in all regions of the country and ethnic groups including Anglo Americans, Hispanics, and African Americans, in males and females, and in all social classes. Table 13.1 shows the percent of students using illicit drugs by ethnicity in one study. Alcohol and tobacco (Chapter 12) are included. Although caution always should be exercised in generalizing statistics from a small study to a larger group, if this study is representative at all, the drug problem is real and it cuts across all ethnic groups.

One theory is that teenagers are growing less afraid of the effects of drugs as the culture glamorizes drug use. Rap and grunge groups talk openly about their own drug use. Another theory, proposed by national talk radio host and physician Dean Edell, is that we are not being honest with our youth. We do not admit what they already know — that drugs *do* make them feel better. What teens are not considering, however, are the devastating effects that drugs can have on them and the difficulty in overcoming the addiction. For example, the Substance Abuse and Mental Health Services Administration reported that about two-thirds of emergency room patients test positive for some intoxicant, an 8% increase over 1992.

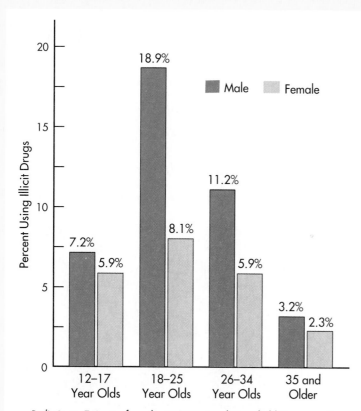

Preliminary Estimates from the 1993 National Household Survey on Drug Abuse (Washington, DC: U.S. Department of Health and Human Services, Public Health Service , 1994), p. 10.

Figure 13.1 Illicit drug use during past month, 1993

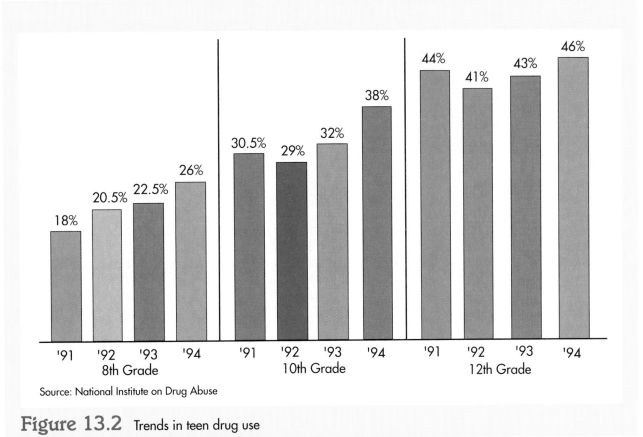

Figure 13.2 Trends in teen drug use

Source: National Institute on Drug Abuse

KEY TERMS

Iatrogenic illnesses medically induced sickness caused by adverse reactions to drugs

Physical dependence a biochemical need to repeat administration of a substance

Psychological dependence a state in which individuals crave drugs to satisfy some personality or emotional need

Drug abuse the use of chemical substance that results in physical, mental, emotional, or social impairment

Drug misuse the occasionally inappropriate or unintentional use of a medication

HEALTHY PEOPLE 2000

OBJECTIVES FOR DRUG USE

❋ Reduce drug-related deaths.

❋ Reduce drug abuse-related hospital emergency room visits.

❋ Reduce the proportion of young people who have used marijuana and cocaine in the past month.

❋ Increase the proportion of high school seniors who perceive social disapproval associated with occasional use of marijuana and experimentation with cocaine.

❋ Increase the proportion of high school seniors who associate risk of physical or psychological harm with regular use of marijuana and experimentation with cocaine.

Table 13.1
Percent of Students Using Various Drugs, by Ethnicity, Grades 7–12

Substance	American Indian (n=216)	African American (n=2084)	Chicano Mexican American (n=43)	Puerto Rican Latin American (n=58)	Asian Oriental American (n=215)	White Caucasian (n=4162)
Alcohol	58.4	44.8	64.1	56.9	39.2	68.9
Cigarettes	48.5	20.6	60.0	43.4	29.7	48.9
Marijuana	34.0	22.7	48.7	20.8	14.9	27.9
Snuff	15.2	3.4	27.5	11.3	7.4	15.1
Chewing Tobacco	23.6	3.8	35.0	13.2	9.9	16.6
Inhalants	13.2	2.1	32.5	15.1	8.9	8.6
Amphetamines	8.9	1.6	30.0	11.3	5.5	6.2
Clove Cigarettes	9.8	1.9	32.5	13.2	7.4	9.6
Stimulants	13.8	2.2	35.0	13.2	9.0	12.0
Nitrite	5.9	1.1	20.5	9.4	5.4	2.9
Cocaine	10.8	3.1	35.0	11.3	7.0	6.3
Tranquilizers	10.8	1.5	25.0	11.3	5.4	5.3
Hallucinogens	11.8	1.3	35.0	9.4	7.0	9.1
Methadone	8.8	1.2	23.1	7.5	4.5	3.4
Opiates	6.4	0.9	20.0	9.3	5.5	3.1
Barbiturates	9.3	1.4	20.0	7.5	5.5	3.9
PCP	8.3	1.2	35.0	7.5	6.0	4.1
Ecstacy	7.4	1.0	22.5	9.4	5.0	3.6
Steroids	8.3	2.4	17.5	9.6	6.0	4.1
Needle Use	5.9	1.4	23.1	5.7	6.5	3.1
Mean	16.0	6.0	32.1	14.8	9.8	13.1

Source: *Cultural Competence for Evaluators*, by the Office for Substance Abuse Prevention (Washington, DC: Public Health Service, 1992).

In addition to the largely physical effects discussed in this chapter, a strong relationship exists between drug abuse and sociological factors including delinquency and violence.

HOW DRUGS AFFECT THE BRAIN

The brain sends and receives messages via a network of nerve cells, or **neurons**, depicted in Figure 13.3. To receive information, each neuron has branches, called **dendrites**, and on these branches are **receptors** that receive the messages. The cell body on each neuron decides if the information is important and, if so, sends it to another neuron. To send information, each neuron has a long cable called an **axon**, which acts like a telephone wire, receiving the message from the cell body and sending it to the receptors on the dendrites of another neuron. In this way, messages are passed from neuron to neuron throughout the nervous system.

Between each neuron and the next one is a gap called a **synapse**, which requires special chemicals to get a message across the gaps. These chemicals called **neurotransmitters**, take the message from the axon of one nerve cell and send it to the receptors of another nerve cell. A neurotransmitter is like a key, and a receptor is like a lock. When the key fits, the nerve cell is turned on and sends the message. If it does not fit, the nerve cell cannot send or receive a message. The entire nervous system depends on these neurotransmitters and receptors.

Psychoactive drugs disrupt the way messages are sent to and from the brain. Some drugs slow down or completely shut down message transmission. Other drugs speed the number of messages so much that the brain cannot make sense of them. Sometimes this is a good thing. For example,

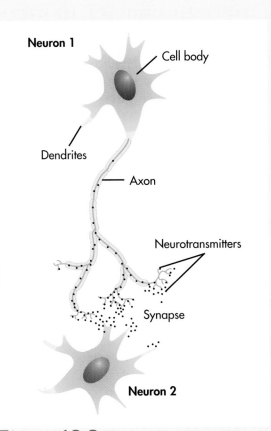

Figure 13.3 Physiological effects of psychoactive drugs on the brain

are the narcotics (opium, morphine, heroin); the depressants (barbiturates, quaaludes, tranquilizers); the stimulants (cocaine/crack, amphetamines, caffeine); the hallucinogens (LSD, PCP); cannabis (marijuana and hashish); inhalants; and over-the-counter (OTC) medications. Tobacco and alcohol, the topics of Chapter 12, are also psychoactive substances.

ROUTES OF ADMINISTRATION

Routes of administration are ways or methods in which drugs are introduced into the bloodstream and central nervous system (CNS). Common routes of administration are:

1. *Inhalation*: introduction of a vapor or gas into the respiratory tract via the nose and mouth or a powder through the nose. Sniffing vapors from drugs is one example of inhalation.

2. *Injection*: introduction of drugs into the body subcutaneously (injecting drugs just below the surface of the skin), intramuscularly (injecting drugs into large muscles), or intravenously (injecting directly into the vein). Injecting drugs directly into the vein is the most rapid route for introducing drugs into the bloodstream.

3. *Oral ingestion*: introduction of the drug into the body through the mouth or oral cavity. These

certain drugs can stop pain by blocking the pain messages going from the painful area into the brain. Sometimes, though, changing the brain through psychoactive drugs can be harmful. By unlocking the pleasure center, the drugs may start the person on the road to **addiction**, a state of biochemical and psychological dependence produced by habitual drug taking. If the person is physically addicted to a drug and discontinues it, various **withdrawal** symptoms occur, such as: flulike symptoms, diarrhea, abdominal pain, delirium tremens (DTs), hallucinations, paranoia, and sometimes death, depending on the actual substance.

WHAT ARE PSYCHOACTIVE SUBSTANCES?

A **psychoactive substance** is any agent that has the ability to alter mood, perception, or behavior. The psychoactive substances discussed in this chapter

---

KEY TERMS

Neuron a nerve cell

Dendrite branch of a neuron that conveys impulses to the cell body

Receptor component of the neuron that combines with the neurotransmitter to receive messages from another neuron

Axon a long cable connected to the neuron, receiving information from the cell body, relaying it to another neuron

Synapse a gap between each neuron that requires a special chemical to send messages across

Neurotransmitters chemicals that send messages across a synapse from the axon of a nerve cell to another nerve cell

Addiction a state of biochemical and/or psychological dependence produced by habitual drug-taking

Withdrawal physical and psychological symptoms that occur when an individual who is addicted to a drug discontinues its use

Psychoactive substance any agent that has the ability to alter mood, perception, or behavior

---

routes may include between the cheek and gum (buccal surface) and under the tongue (sublingual). By these routes a drug such as LSD is introduced rapidly into the bloodstream via the capillaries.

4. *Rectal or vaginal route:* introduction of drugs into the body via the vascularized openings, utilizing suppositories, enemas, and similar forms.

NARCOTICS

According to *The Bantam Medical Dictionary*, a **narcotic** is a drug that induces stupor and insensibility. The term is used particularly for morphine and other opium derivatives. In legal terms a narcotic is any addictive drug subject to illegal use. **Opiates** are obtained from the juice of the opium poppy, *Papaver somniferum*. **Opioids** are synthetic narcotics. Narcotic drugs induce sleep, relieve acute pain, and treat coughs, diarrhea, and various other illnesses. They are divided into four categories:

1. Natural opiates, including opium, morphine, and codeine.

2. Semisynthetic opiates, including heroin, Dilaudid, and Percodan.

3. Synthetic narcotics, including Demerol, methadone, and Darvon

4. **Endorphins** and **enkephalins**, naturally occurring narcotics in the body produced by the immune system.

Opium

Opium, the "mother drug," is the base compound for all of the natural narcotics. It is a resin derived from the unripe seed pods of the poppy plant. Ancient Egyptian physicians used opium nearly 6,500 years ago to kill pain. When the opiates were found to relieve anxiety, create **euphoria**, and provide an escape from reality, people began to use opium recreationally.

Opium usually is smoked, though sometimes it is eaten. However it enters the body, it has the potential to produce stupor, sleep, coma, and death. With repeated use the person may develop a strong **tolerance** and physical dependency. The first law banning opium use was passed in 1875 in San Francisco, where smoking opiates was prohibited in opium houses or dens. Opium has been taken off the market in the United States.

Morphine

The reason for the scant use of opium in the United States today relates largely to its successor, morphine. Around 1800, **morphine** was extracted from

To Legalize or Not to Legalize?

The debate concerning legalization of drugs is heating up. Should we or shouldn't we legalize currently illegal substances of abuse? Here's what proponents of legalization say.

❋ People have always used and always will use mood-altering drugs. They have the right to do this as long as it does not harm others.

❋ Funds currently used for enforcement of drug laws could be diverted to prevention, education, and treatment.

❋ Current policy has little impact on criminal activities and very little influence on the millions who use illicit drugs.

❋ The failure of Prohibition can serve as a model; it didn't work with alcohol and it won't work with other drugs.

❋ Workable models exist in other countries that permit drug use.

The counterarguments go as follows.

❋ Enforcement has not been pursued forcefully enough, so we cannot dismiss it as a failure.

❋ Allowing drug use sends the wrong message. Therefore, it would rise dramatically if sanctions were lifted.

❋ Prohibition actually may have reduced alcohol-related problems, and many illicit drugs have far greater potential for addiction problems than alcohol.

❋ Use of drugs in the privacy of one's own home still implies health and social costs to society, just as the problems related to alcoholism do.

The moral stigma attached to drug use is still strong. And even without that factor, the absence of hard evidence makes the predictions of both sides of the debate only speculation.

Source: *The Facts About Drug Use* by Barry Stimmel and the Editors of Consumer Reports Books (Washington, DC: Public Health Service, 1993), pp. 312–313.

opium and became known as a "wonder drug" because it brought quick relief from pain. It is 10 times stronger than opium and therefore exerts rapid depressing effects on the brain receptors that control analgesic (pain killing) action. In addition, it causes euphoria and sedation. When some 250,000 injured Civil War soldiers became addicted, it came to be known as the "soldier's disease." Because it was such a useful drug, however, it continued to be prescribed for everything from headaches to skull fractures. Patent medicines containing morphine were readily available, and cough medicine containing morphine was even given to infants. Its most effective uses are to anesthetize patients during heart surgery, to control pain associated with postoperative surgery and cancer, and to suppress cells that cause viral infections and cancer.

Illicit morphine is produced mostly in powder form and also as tablets, cubes, and capsules. It may cause light sensitivity, nausea, vomiting, and decreased respiration, to the point where death may occur. When morphine is injected using non-sterile techniques pathogens introduced into the bloodstream can cause HIV infection, abscesses, cellulitis, liver disease and other problems.

Heroin

In 1898 chemists produced a new, "safe" drug from morphine and introduced it as a drug that could cure opium and morphine addiction. Later it came to be known as **heroin**, also called "junk," "smack," and "horse." During the early 1900s the use of heroin spread rapidly. Because it is 35 times stronger than morphine, and an even more potent painkiller, it made people feel even more euphoric.

Unfortunately, heroin is more addictive than morphine. Laws were passed in the early 1900s prohibiting the use of heroin. The Harrison Act of 1914 introduced the term *narcotics* to describe all habit-forming, nonprescription drugs used for pleasure. The law did little to abate heroin use because of its extremely addictive properties. During the 1960s heroin use was widespread among American soldiers stationed in Vietnam. Heroin continues to be the most frequently

"China White" is a sinister new kind of heroin that is up to 90% pure and extremely dangerous.

abused narcotic. Ironically, it is no longer used medicinally in the United States.

In its purest form heroin is a white powder with an extremely bitter taste. When sold illegally, it is almost always diluted or "cut" with other substances, such as sugar or starch. Heroin usually is liquefied and injected intramuscularly ("muscling"), just under the skin ("skin popping"), or intravenously ("mainlining"). It also is "snorted" (sniffed) or smoked — methods that are becoming increasingly popular because they do not require a needle for injection. Like other narcotic drugs, heroin affects the nerve cells of the brain and spine, dulling pain and clouding the senses. Heroin in the body produces immediate euphoria (a "rush"), constricted pupils, lowered sex drive, less tension, and loss of appetite. The euphoria from heroin may last 3 to 8 hours. After it wears off, the user must continue taking the drug to prevent withdrawal symptoms.

Users tend to become addicted within 2 weeks of consistent use. Many develop a tolerance to the drug over time, with stronger and more frequent cravings. Withdrawal symptoms occur 8 to 24 hours after the last "fix" (dose). Sometimes serious, these may include watery eyes, runny nose, nausea and vomiting, diarrhea, chills, excruciating cramps in the abdomen and legs, and tremors. Symptoms associated with heroin withdrawal get progressively worse for approximately 3 to 4 days. The person becomes more irritable and experiences episodes of severe sneezing and coryza (inflammation

KEY TERMS

Narcotic a drug that induces stupor and insensibility; in legal terms, any addictive drug subject to illegal use

Opiates drug obtained from the juice of the opium poppy

Opioids synthetic narcotics

Endorphins and enkephalins naturally occurring narcotics in the body produced by the immune system

Opium base compound for all natural narcotics

Euphoria a heightened sense of well-being associated with drug use

Tolerance condition in which an individual must increase drug dosage to experience the same effects over time

Morphine main alkaloid found in opium; used medically to kill pain and sedate

Heroin narcotic drug derived from morphine that is 35 times stronger than morphine

of nasal passage coupled with profuse nasal discharge).

Pregnant women who have drugged their embryo or fetus with heroin will likely cause the infant to suffer withdrawal symptoms shortly after birth, called the **neonatal abstinence syndrome (NAS)**. Newborns with NAS are highly sensitive to noise, are irritable, have poor coordination, sneeze and yawn excessively, and have uncoordinated sucking and swallowing reflexes. Research using ultrasound measurements raises questions about the rate of brain growth in fetuses exposed to narcotics. The head circumference tends to be slightly smaller than usual. Even though the head size catches up to that of nonexposed babies within 6 months or so, possible long-term effects of prenatal harm to the brain remain a concern.

HIV/AIDS is the deadly "injectable STD" that is ravaging the African-American community.

AIDS is now the fourth leading cause of death in women of childbearing age in the United States, most of which is attributable to the woman's use of contaminated needles in conjunction with her drug use or having sex with an HIV-infected injecting drug user.

HIV infection and AIDS are especially prevalent among African American injectable drug users. African Americans are twice as likely as Anglo-Americans to have used drugs intravenously. While representing about 12% of the U. S. population, African Americans account for 27% of all people with AIDS, and of those cases, 44% reported injecting an illicit substance prior to the AIDS diagnosis, according to the Centers for Disease Control and Prevention (CDC). In addition, African Americans accounted for 31% of heroin and morphine deaths in 1989.

The CDC reported that more than 30,000 Hispanics had developed AIDS as of July, 1991, and almost half of these cases involved injectable drug use. Of the Hispanics using drugs intravenously, 74% never used bleach or alcohol to clean their needles before injecting.

Other Narcotics

Codeine is a natural alkaloid derivative of opium, though it is produced more often from morphine. Medically, it is used as a cough suppressant or mild painkiller in combination with other drugs such as acetamenophin and cough medicines. Although codeine is less effective than morphine, it is a widely abused prescription drug with the potential for physical dependence.

Dilaudid is derived from morphine. Though short-acting, it is two to eight times more potent than morphine. Dilaudid is used legitimately as a cough suppressant and as an analgesic for treating severe pain. When the drug is used nonmedically, it is taken in tablet form or injected. Dilaudid has high potential for physical dependence.

Percodan is an extremely potent semisynthetic narcotic used medically as an antidirrheal, antitussive (cough-suppressing), and analgesic medication. Its potential for analgesic, sedative, and respiratory depressant effects is more than a thousand times greater than that of morphine. Percodan has high potential for physical dependence.

Demerol is a short-acting synthetic drug that usually is injected. It is used as an analgesic or a painkiller. It, too, has high potential for physical dependence.

DEPRESSANTS

Depressants, informally called "downers," are drugs that inhibit neural activity and slow physical and mental functions. They do this by decreasing awareness and incoming stimuli to the brain cells and spinal cord. Depressants cause drowsiness, relax muscles, and if taken in excessive quantities, can even cause death.

Sedative — Hypnotics

Barbiturates

In the early 1900s, two German chemists derived a substance from barbituric acid that had a calming and relaxing effect and even could put a person to sleep. Since then, scientists have developed more than 2,500 **barbiturates**, 15 or so of which are still in use to treat conditions such as anxiety, insomnia, epilepsy, and peptic ulcers.

Many uses, however, are illicit. Most popular during the 1960s, barbiturates were distributed through the black market and were widely abused. The short-acting pentobarbital (Nembutal), secobarbital (Seconal), and amobarbital (Amytal) were the drugs of choice.

Today, barbiturates are prescribed most often as sleeping pills, although this sleep is not ideal as it has less rapid eye movement (REM) than normal sleep and the person dreams less. Doctors also prescribe barbiturates to relieve anxiety, tension, and irritability.

Abusers quickly develop a tolerance to the drug and typically take 20 times the amount recommended by the medical profession. Heroin addicts often resort to barbiturates if they cannot obtain the narcotic. Overdose is a real danger. Effects include cold, clammy skin, a weak, rapid pulse, and difficulty breathing. The usual treatment is to pump the stomach and administer CPR if necessary. Otherwise the person may lapse into a coma and die.

Barbiturates become even more dangerous when they are combined with other depressants such as alcohol. This speeds the absorption of barbiturates into the bloodstream and adds to the drug's physically depressing effects on the body.

Withdrawal symptoms are similar to those from alcohol: anxiety and agitation, loss of appetite, nausea and vomiting, sweating, rapid heartbeat, tremors, and cramping. These symptoms peak during the second or third day or longer after discontinued use. The person may go into convulsions and even become delirious. Some people have hallucinations. The withdrawal symptoms that follow excessive, prolonged, heavy barbiturate use may be more serious than those of any other drug. Withdrawal symptoms caused by using barbiturates are difficult to treat and create true medical emergencies.

Chloral Hydrate

Chloral hydrate is a drug rapidly metabolized to trichloroethanal, the active hypnotic agent. This nonbarbiturate sedative-hypnotic is a liquid marketed as soft capsules and as a syrup. It takes effect approximately a half hour after ingestion. Given in equal doses, chloral hydrate does not depress the central nervous system as much as barbiturates. Its potential for abuse and physical dependence is moderate. Chloral hydrate will irritate the stomach and cause serious gastric disturbances. This drug is not widely used. Brand names are Somnos and Noctec.

Methaqualone

Another form of depressant is methaqualone, a nonbarbiturate sedative-hypnotic. It is also a painkiller. **Quaalude** is the most familiar trade name. This drug often has been used interchangeably with barbiturates, as it has similar effects and was believed to be nonaddictive — a supposition that has proved to be false. Quaaludes have high potential for both physical and psychological dependence. High doses may cause headaches, abdominal cramping, major motor convulsions, insomnia, and possible coma and death. Although they are no longer marketed in the United States, large amounts of illicit Quaaludes are imported for black market sale.

Tranquilizers

In the 1940s the American Medical Association began to search for a substitute for barbiturates ("thrill pills"), and the pharmaceutical companies developed a new class of drugs known as benzodiazepines or **tranquilizers**. These "antianxiety drugs" depress the central nervous system but have milder effects than the other classes. The most popular tranquilizers are Valium and Librium. Used medically as anticonvulsants and muscle relaxants, they reduce tension, irritability, and stress and sometimes are prescribed to manage panic disorders.

Although benzodiazepines are milder than the other forms, they may have serious side effects and toxic reactions including confusion, muscular

---

KEY TERMS

Neonatal abstinence syndrome (NAS) set of withdrawal symptoms occurring shortly after birth in newborns that have been exposed to heroin in utero

Codeine a natural derivative of opium used as a cough suppressant or mild painkiller

Dilaudid derived from morphine, legitimately used as a cough suppressant and as an analgesic for treating severe pain

Percodan a cough-suppressing and analgesic medication

Demerol short-acting synthetic narcotic used as an analgesic or a painkiller; usually injected

Depressants a drug that inhibits neural activity and slows physical and mental functions; "downers"

Barbiturates substances that have calming and depressant effects

Quaalude a depressant often used interchangeably with barbiturates; high potential for physical and psychological dependence

Tranquilizers psychoactive drugs that depress the central nervous system but have milder effects than the other depressants

---

incoordination, nausea, lethargy, skin rashes, and constipation. They may alter the sex drive, cause menstrual irregularities, and produce blood cell abnormalities. Benzodiazepines have the potential to cause physical and psychological dependence.

A person quickly develops a tolerance to benzodiazepines. Used in conjunction with alcohol, barbiturates, opiates, or other depressant drugs, the outcome can be life-threatening. Drug overdose is common.

The typical abuser is Anglo-American, female, and 20-40 years old. Taking three or four tablets of Valium a day for about 6 weeks is enough to cause addiction. Addicts frequently take the tablets with alcohol or marijuana to ensure a high. Withdrawal symptoms last about 7 to 10 days. The withdrawal is like that from the barbiturates.

STIMULANTS

Cocaine

Cocaine, the most powerful of the natural stimulants, is found in the leaves of several species of *Erythroxylum coca* or coca plant native to the Andes Mountains of South America. When the Spanish conquistadores entered that area in the early 16th century, they found the indigenous people chewing the leaves. They had discovered the pleasure (and possibly the addiction) that cocaine brings.

After cocaine enters the body, the user feels the first effects in a matter of seconds or minutes, depending upon the route of administration — an intense "flash" or "rush." The heart beats faster, and the blood pressure rises. The drug makes users feel more energetic and alert. The key to cocaine's addiction is **dopamine**, a neurotransmitter that controls pleasure sensations. Cocaine causes the release of more dopamine but also blocks reuptake from the brain. As a result, neurons make less and less of it and gradually the user tries larger and more frequent doses of cocaine to recapture the feeling of pleasure.

With cocaine use the sense of euphoria lasts only a few minutes, after which the user "crashes." To relieve the resulting depression (dysphoria), the person takes another dose of the drug. The cycle continues.

The active ingredient cocaine was first isolated in the mid-19th century. Famed psychoanalyst Sigmund Freud partook of cocaine and advocated its use to treat a variety of ills including asthma, digestive upset, and morphine addiction. He suggested that it might be used as an **aphrodisiac**. Freud participated in the events leading to the discovery of the one valid medical use of cocaine: as a local anesthetic. It is still used as a local anesthetic in throat, nose, eye, and ear surgery. Novocaine and Xylocaine are cocaine synthetics.

Another user was William Halstead, often called the Father of American Surgery. One of the four founders of the Johns Hopkins Medical School, his experiments with cocaine led to an intense addiction that threatened his career. Scientists at that time used themselves as guinea pigs, so he injected himself often and as a result developed a dependence on the drug. He finally was able to overcome his dependence and resume his illustrious work. History shows, however, that he turned to

Facts About Cocaine

❋ Damage and deaths from crack use are most often caused by brain hemorrhage or lung failure brought on by cocaine-induced blockage of the heart and blood vessels.

❋ Men have a higher rate of cocaine use than women.

❋ African American women are more likely than women in any other racial/ethnic group to have used crack cocaine.

❋ African Americans and Hispanics have higher rates of cocaine use than Anglo-Americans.

❋ Almost 57% of the cocaine emergency room cases involved African American patients; of the emergency room deaths, 41% were African Americans.

❋ Cocaine use is more prevalent in the West than in other regions of the United States.

❋ The cocaine-using population is aging. In 1979, 12% of patients with cocaine episodes were age 35 or older. By 1985 the proportion was 19%, and by 1992 it was 34%.

❋ Rates of cocaine use are highest between ages 18 and 34.

❋ Cocaine use is correlated with educational status; those who have not completed high school have the highest rates, and college attendees the lowest.

Sources: *National Household Survey on Drug Abuse*, National Institute on Drug Abuse, Public Health Service, 1991, 1993; preliminary estimates, July 1994.

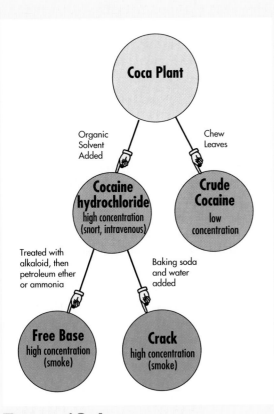

Figure 13.4 Forms of cocaine

Chart labels:
- Coca Plant
- Organic Solvent Added
- Chew Leaves
- **Cocaine hydrochloride** high concentration (snort, intravenous)
- **Crude Cocaine** low concentration
- Treated with alkaloid, then petroleum ether or ammonia
- Baking soda and water added
- **Free Base** high concentration (smoke)
- **Crack** high concentration (smoke)

Act in 1914. This law made cocaine available only by medical prescription, although that did not put an end to its illicit use.

To make cocaine, the leaves of the coca plant are stripped and mixed with an organic solvent, which forms a coca paste. The paste is synthesized into cocaine hydrochloride (see Figure 13.4), the white crystalline powder known by users as white lady, blow, snow, and nose candy, among other names.

Cocaine often is sniffed ("snorted" or "tooted"). It also can be injected intravenously alone or mixed with heroin, the latter of which is called "speedballing." Cocaine that is smoked has been converted into freebase by treating the cocaine powder with an alkaloid and then with petroleum ether or ammonia. The more popular cocaine freebase method is to mix cocaine hydrochloride with baking soda and water. A base forms and is dried into small pieces called "rocks" or **crack**. When a piece of rock cocaine is heated in a glass pipe, cocaine vapors are produced and inhaled. "Space-basing" refers to smoking crack mixed with phencyclidine (PCP or angel dust, discussed later).

Chronic use of cocaine has a number of adverse effects on the body.

✳ It can constrict the blood vessels and cause angina, irregular heart rhythm (ventricular fibrillation), and heart attacks.

✳ It causes the heart to beat too fast (tachycardia), which can cause it to stop functioning.

✳ It can raise blood pressure, and some suggest it may cause arterial constriction in the brain, leading to a stroke.

✳ With repeated use over time it can cause long-term psychological effects such as restlessness, excitability, anxiety, insomnia, irritability, mood swings, paranoia, and depression.

morphine to subdue the cocaine addiction and remained addicted the rest of his life.

The fictional Sherlock Holmes's use of cocaine suggests that it was well known during the time Sir Arthur Conan Doyle penned his classic mysteries. Some speculate that Robert Louis Stevenson may have written *Dr. Jekyll and Mr. Hyde* while under the influence of cocaine because he was so prodigious despite suffering from tuberculosis. He was taking morphine for that condition, so cocaine could have been prescribed routinely as well. In the late 19th century and the early 20th century, Cole Porter referred to cocaine in his popular tune "I Get a Kick Out of You."

During that period ground coca leaves were sold as "tonics." Coca-Cola took half of its name from the cocaine in it. When the dangers of the drug became obvious, cocaine was removed from the beverage just before the Pure Food and Drug Act was passed in 1907. The federal government erroneously classified cocaine as a narcotic and outlawed its use with passage of the Harrison Narcotic

---

KEY TERMS

Cocaine most powerful of the natural stimulants; includes several forms

Dopamine brain chemical that controls pleasure sensations; the key to cocaine's addiction

Aphrodisiac a substance that stimulates sexual desire

Crack small pieces or "rocks" formed from a dried mix of cocaine hydrochloride, baking soda, and water

Call for information

Cocaine Anonymous (CA)
Hotline: 1-800-COCAINE

Alcohol, Drug & Pregnancy Help Line
Monday-Friday 9-5 Central
800-638-2229

❋ The mucous membrane in the nasal passages dries and deteriorates. Cilia (the hairlike projections that protect the nasal lining) are destroyed, producing nasal discomfort, hemorrhaging, and perforation of the nasal septum (the cartilage that separates the nostrils).

❋ Chronic, long-term cocaine use can result in the inability of men to retain an erection for orgasm and ejaculation and the inability of females to reach orgasm.

❋ Crack users may have severe chest congestion and a chronic cough in which they expel a black phlegm.

Crack can cause serious problems with pregnant females. Cocaine-addicted women are four times as likely as drug-free women to experience premature separation of the placenta from the uterus, which causes hemorrhaging and threatens the lives of both mother and fetus. Cocaine also can precipitate miscarriage or premature delivery by promoting uterine contractions. Maternal cocaine use endangers the fetus by constricting arteries leading to the uterus, which in turn diminishes the blood supply and, hence, oxygen to the fetus. Embryos and fetuses robbed of oxygen and nutrients are called **crack babies** after they are born. Crack babies exhibit various characteristics including prematurity, irritability, neurological disorders, and strokes. They bond poorly, have difficulty sucking, and experience short, irregular periods of restless sleep.

Cocaine and crack use are allied closely with drug-related crimes including homicides and shootouts among gang members and organized crime groups, as crack makes the user more aggressive, dangerous, and paranoid. Unfortunately, children often are enlisted to work in the crack distribution network. They are being lured into gangs and into the streets as "lookouts" (to alert crack dealers when police are nearby), to "run" (transport drugs between dealers), and to "deal" (actually sell crack).

According to the National Institute on Drug Abuse (NIDA), the number of illegal users of cocaine today is about 1.6 million, down from a peak of 5.3 million in 1985. Statistics are misleading without differentiating occasional versus steady users, and this may indicate the extent of problems arising from addiction. Figure 13.5 shows the trends in cocaine use in recent years. Although occasional users clearly are becoming fewer, the prevalence of chronic users remains about the same.

Amphetamines

Amphetamines are groups of synthetic amines that stimulate the body's own epinephrine (adrenaline

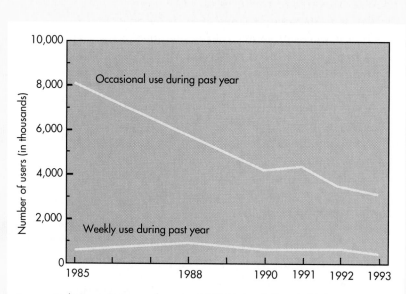

Source: *Preliminary Estimates from the 1993 National Household Survey on Drug Abuse* (Washington, DC: U.S. Department of Health and Human Services, Public Health Service, 1994), p. 11.

Figure 13.5 Trends in cocaine use, 1985–1993

hormone) and norepinephrine (neurotransmitter hormone). They affect the portion of the brain that controls breathing, heart rhythm, blood pressure, and metabolic rate. They act directly on the central nervous system by inducing feelings of well-being, exhilaration, wakefulness, confidence, excitement, and talkativeness.

Amphetamines have a number of medicinal uses. The first, still used, was to treat narcolepsy (a sleep disorder). Later, amphetamines became a component of nasal inhalants, as well as an agent to counteract fatigue and enhance alertness. Because they were found to curb the appetite, they were marketed with weight-loss programs. They still are used for short-term treatment and management of obesity and weight control. Amphetamines are administered to individuals who have attention deficit disorder (ADD), a condition characterized by extreme motor restlessness, poor attention span, and impulsivity. Appropriate doses also can enhance physical performance.

Amphetamine use became widespread during the 1920s, eroding the popularity of cocaine. Amphetamines produced a similar high and their effects lasted longer. More important, they were cheap and easy to obtain. Legal amphetamine use peaked about the end of World War II, when billions of pills prepared for army use became surplus and were made available to Japan. Within 10 years, Japan, a country with no history of drug abuse, had an epidemic of amphetamine dependency.

As with the other wonder drugs, the downside to amphetamines became apparent. Drivers who took amphetamines ("pep pills") to stay awake ended up having more accidents when the pills' effects wore off suddenly. Students who took the pills to stay up all night cramming for exams displayed bizarre behavior. Executives who used the pills to stay alert discovered that their judgment and decision-making ability were impaired. The same problems are present with amphetamines today, particularly when they are not controlled. Additional effects of amphetamines include elevated body temperature, dry mouth, irritability, slurred speech, repetitive movements, nausea, vomiting, blurred vision, aggressive behavior, and insomnia. Most users take amphetamines in capsules, also called uppers, bennies, dexies, jolly beans, and copilots.

The average American drinks about 34 gallons of soda and 28 gallons of coffee each year.

Probably the most dangerous form of **methamphetamine** is "ice," which is smoked in a glass pipe or injected. It looks like a lumpy crystal of ice (hence the nickname "crystal"). It first brings on intense euphoria, which may be followed by nausea and vomiting. Over time it is associated with aggressive behavior, paranoia and psychosis, weight loss, kidney and lung failure, and possible death. Many first-time users become addicted instantly. The high can last as long as 24 hours in a regular user and as long as 7 days in a novice user. When deprived of the drug, regular users feel strong cravings for it. Withdrawal symptoms cover a wide range and can include depression, cramps, sleepiness, apathy, irritability, mental confusion, and hallucinations.

Mothers who ingest ice during pregnancy can damage their unborn babies irreparably. These infants, called "ice babies," have tremors and may cry up to 24 hours nonstop. They tend to avoid any type of closeness, bonding, or contact with other people.

Caffeine

Caffeine, one of the world's most widely used drugs, has been ingested by humans for centuries. It is an alkaloid substance found in beverages such as coffee, tea, cola, and other soft drinks, as well as chocolate, and in prescription and over-the-counter medications. The average American drinks about 34 gallons of soda and 28 gallons of coffee each year.

Among the 63 natural sources from which caffeine is extracted are seeds of *Coffea arabica* (coffee), roasted leaves of the *Camellia sinensis*, which is an evergreen shrub (tea), the West African kola or guru nut, and the Brazilian soapberry plant. Table 13.2 shows the amount of caffeine in various substances.

KEY TERMS

Crack babies newborns who were exposed to cocaine and deprived of oxygen because of maternal cocaine use during pregnancy

Amphetamines group of synthetic amines affecting portions of the brain that control breathing, heart rhythm, blood pressure, and metabolic rate

Methamphetamines powerful stimulants that induce intense euphoria

Caffeine a legal drug with stimulant properties

Table 13.2
Caffeine Content of Selected Items

Product	Amount	Average Caffeine (mg)
Coffee		
Drip	6 oz	137
Brewed	6 oz	117
Instant	6 oz	60–117
Decaffeinated	6 oz	3
Cola	12 oz	30–45
Chocolate		
Cake	1 slice	25
Baking chocolate	1 oz	25
Milk chocolate	1 oz	6
Chocolate milk	8 oz	5
Hot cocoa	6 oz	5
Tea		
5-minute steep	6 oz	50
Decaffeinated	6 oz	1
Instant	6 oz	33
Medications		
Pain relief	Standard dose	41
Diuretics	Standard dose	167
Alertness	Standard dose	150
Diet	Standard dose	168
Cold/Allergy	Standard dose	27

Caffeine levels peak in the body within an hour after consumption, and more than half of the caffeine is metabolized (broken down, becoming inactive) in 3 to 7 hours. A stimulant, caffeine produces a feeling of well-being and alertness. It is a diuretic, so too much of it will deplete the body's water content. The effects of caffeine are hard to study because the response varies from person to person. Some people are caffeine-sensitive and should not consume it at all. Generally, however, the effects of lower doses may include:

* increased muscle capacity
* stimulation of learning
* heightened intellectual processes
* improvement in certain motor skills
* faster heartbeat
* relaxed bronchial muscles
* increased output of urine
* increased metabolic rate (BMR)

* increased blood levels of glucose and lipids (fats)
* stimulation of the respiratory center

Higher doses of caffeine have the following potential effects:

* constricted blood vessels in the brain (usually associated with hypertensive headaches)
* irregular heartbeat
* extreme nervousness
* flushed appearance
* muscle twitching/tremor
* irritability
* tinnitus (ringing in the ears)
* insomnia

Rarely does anyone die of a caffeine overdose. To overdose, a person would have to drink more than 80 cups of coffee in a short time.

No consensus has been reached as to whether caffeine is addictive. Although it has been consumed throughout history, evidence has not proven any dangers in moderate consumption for most people. Nevertheless, the scientific community often has investigated linkages between caffeine and

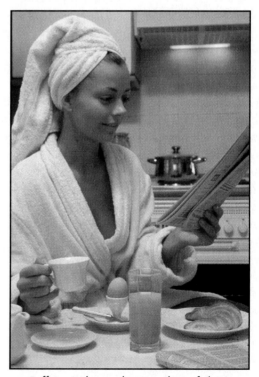

Caffeine is the number-one drug of choice for many Americans.

heart disease, cancer of the pancreas, and, in women, problems associated with reproduction, aggravated PMS, fibrocystic breast disease, and calcium depletion and bone loss. In 1985 the National Institute of Mental Health (NIMH) reported that caffeine can cause panic attacks in some people. These attacks are characterized by irrational feelings of anxiety, accompanied by heart palpitations, shortness of breath, sweating, and mental confusion.

Conflicting studies about the risks of consuming caffeine during pregnancy have been published. Researchers discourage consumption of more than 300 milligrams (2–3) cups of coffee) per day, and even lower levels may not be safe. The potential risk to the fetus posed by caffeine is small but real. To be safe, pregnant women should avoid caffeine altogether or keep their intake to a minimum.

CANNABIS

Marijuana is a preparation of chopped leaves, flowering tops, stems, and seeds of the hemp plant *Cannabis sativa*. To prepare for smoking, all of the plant is dried, and rolled into paper, called a joint or a reefer. Other common names for marijuana are pot, grass, bo, bud, Mary Jane, and gold. Marijuana also is eaten in foods such as brownies, cakes, and cookies. Other popular uses include stuffing it in cigar leaves ("blunt") and adding cocaine ("primo").

Marijuana contains more than 400 chemicals, the primary psychoactive ingredient being THC (Delta-9-tetrahydrocannabinol). The highest concentration of THC is found in the plant resin. Potency of marijuana ranges from less than 1% in the weakest form to as much as 15% in some forms of hashish, a concentrated form of THC is extracted from the flowers of the plant. Hashish oil contains even more highly refined THC. A drop or two of the oil smoked on a tobacco cigarette has a more potent effect than smoking a whole marijuana joint.

Nearly 5,000 years ago doctors in ancient China recommended marijuana as a remedy for gout, rheumatism, malaria, constipation, loss of appetite, melancholy, and as an aid in childbirth. Every civilization has used cannabis medically as well as recreationally. Currently limited medicinal

Home Alone

Middle school students left home alone 2 or more days a week are more likely to use drugs, particularly marijuana, earlier in life and more often than supervised kids — and not to perform as well academically. Latchkey kids are four times more likely to have gotten drunk in the past month than supervised peers and more likely to use cigarettes, inhalants, and marijuana. Overall, the rate of experimentation was twice as high as the rate for supervised kids. The rate for marijuana use only was six times greater.

Source: From a study by researchers at the University of Illinois, based on a survey of 636 male and female students, grades five through seven, in cities and rural areas in Illinois.

uses include treatment for glaucoma by relieving pressure in the eyes, and for relief from nausea in people undergoing chemotherapy.

Marijuana is the most widely used illegal drug in the United States. By 1970 an estimated 50 million people used marijuana. Its use subsequently declined to an estimated 9 million, or 4.3% of the U.S. population age 14 and older. The most significant trend is a resurgence of use by high school students. According to the National Institute on Drug Abuse, the number of eighth-graders who have sampled marijuana has doubled since 1991.

Marijuana affects users in different ways. Some become ebullient, gaining an exaggerated sense of well-being and a feeling of self-confidence. Others become reflective and quiet. Marijuana usually enhances social interaction and bestows what many users refer to as "mellowing out" — a dreamy sense or state. The user may have more intense and vivid sensory perceptions of sight, taste, hearing, and smell. The sense of time is distorted. Thoughts may become fragmented, and moods vary from calm to argumentative and violent.

The most immediate physical change is reddening of the eyes. The long-term effects are more sobering. These include loss of motor coordination, difficulty concentrating, and trouble learning new facts and remembering old ones. Memory lapses are common. The possibility of measurable brain damage is being researched. People often describe regular users as "slow" and "dull." Among the most severe physical problems is permanent damage to the reproductive organs, including sterility in males. Also, heavy marijuana use by pregnant women is associated with low birthweight and

Driving and Drugs

Reckless drivers who don't seem drunk may well be high on cocaine or marijuana, according to roadside tests that indicate drugs may rival alcohol as a hazard on the highways. Police in Memphis, Tennessee, gave urine tests to reckless drivers who appeared not to be drunk. They found that more than half were on cocaine or pot.

On-the-spot testing for drugs other than alcohol is rare, because it requires taking a urine specimen. Memphis police put together a "drug van," a former ambulance fitted out with toilet, interview area, and videotape equipment. They gave drug tests on the spot to any reckless drivers who were not obviously drunk. Police took urine samples from 150 drivers; 89 of them, or 59%, tested positive for cocaine or marijuana use.

The tests, widely available from several manufacturers, can give results in 10 minutes. Individuals who use large amounts of cocaine or marijuana regularly may flunk the tests even though they have been off drugs for days. The effects of cocaine can last that long. Those withdrawing from the drug may drive worse than people who are still high.

Drugged driving is hard to detect, because it has no clear pattern. For instance, drivers on cocaine may act sleepy and slow, happy and talkative, or combative and paranoid. When asked to take the standard curbside sobriety test, which involves measuring coordination and attention, cocaine drivers actually can perform better than sober ones.

"We saw people who did great on the sobriety test," said Daniel Brookoff, Methodist Hospital, Memphis. "The problem was, they were driving 90 miles an hour on the wrong side of the road with their lights off." They show poor judgment, he said. Typically they are wildly over-confident of their abilities, taking turns too fast or weaving through traffic. Police inspector Charles Cook calls this "diagonal driving." "They are just as involved in changing lanes as they are in going forward."

He said drivers on marijuana can be inattentive and have poor reflexes. In this way they are similar to drunks, although their impairment is usually less extreme.

While the study was going on, Memphis police made 111 arrests for driving under the influence of drugs. During the same period in 1992, they made only six arrests, five of them after serious accidents.

From "Study: Drug Highway Hazard," by Daniel Q. Haney, *Denver Post*, August 25, 1994.

possible abnormalities in children born to them. In short, evidence continues to accumulate that long-term marijuana use has a harmful effect on the heart, lungs, brain, and reproductive system.

Because marijuana causes a temporary rise in pulse rate, heartbeat, and blood pressure, its use may be more dangerous for African Americans because they have higher rates of hypertension than other ethnic groups. Marijuana increases the appetite (the "munchies"), which is a pitfall for overweight people who are trying to manage their weight. Finally, the combined effects of marijuana and alcohol are greater than when either substance is used alone.

Effects of marijuana are not limited to the person using it. Intoxication by marijuana alone is responsible for 16% of auto accident fatalities. The drug is involved in 20% of all traffic accidents. In one study, marijuana was detected in the blood of 37% of young adults killed in auto accidents.

HALLUCINOGENS OR PSYCHEDELICS

Hallucinogens are a group of mind-altering drugs that affect the brain and nervous system, bringing about changes in thought, self-awareness, emotion, and sensation. The synonymous term **psychedelic** was coined by scientist Humphrey Osmond in 1956. It means "revealing to the mind." These drugs create a distorted perception of reality, irrational thinking patterns, and modified states of consciousness. The most pronounced effect may be sensory: Sounds become louder, colors brighter, smells stronger.

True to their name, these drugs produce hallucinations. This happens because hallucinogenic drugs cause the blood vessels in the brain to constrict, limiting the amount of blood that reaches the brain and thus depriving it of its normal amount of oxygen. Some hallucinations are pleasant. Others are "bad trips" or "bummers." Occasionally a user gets a panic reaction. Impurities in street drugs may alter or exacerbate the effects.

Because of the nature of hallucinations, users have been known to jump out of windows and walk in front of cars. Another common reaction is the **flashback**, recurrence of the "trip," which can happen unexpectedly during drug-free periods. Long-term reactions from using hallucinogens include recurrent anxiety, depression, and mental disturbance or psychosis.

Natural sources of hallucinogens include morning glories, jimsonweed, nutmeg, mace, and the fly agaric mushroom. The use of hallucinogens has been traced back at least 3,500 years. They often played a part in early religious ceremonies. In modern times **mescaline**, or **peyote**, derived from the peyote cactus, is still part of religious ceremonies of American Indians of the southwestern United States. Mescaline users experience vivid color imagery, distortions in the perception of time, and enhanced senses.

LSD

During the 1960s and 1970s the traditional uses of hallucinogens changed dramatically. LSD and PCP became major drugs of abuse. In 1938 the Swiss scientist Albert Hofmann, while searching for a headache remedy, created the compound that came to be known as **LSD**, lysergic acid diethylamide-24. Although it did not cure headaches, he was interested in its potential research associated with mental illness. Over the next 20 years other scientists discovered that LSD could cause severe psychoses (rarely), possibly damage the chromosomes, and produce abnormalities in developing embryos and fetuses. In 1960, Harvard psychologist Timothy Leary began to publicize the attractiveness of LSD for recreational use, and its use skyrocketed.

LSD is a colorless, odorless, tasteless liquid. It can be made from lysergic acid, found in the ergot fungus *Claviceps puppures*, which grows on rye and other grains, or it can be made synthetically. For many years a drop of LSD was placed on a sugar cube and ingested in that form. Today it appears more often as a tablet or soaked into heavy blotter paper, from which it is licked off or placed under the tongue for absorption. LSD takes effect in 40 minutes to an hour or more. The effects continue 12 hours or more.

Physical reactions include dilation of the pupils, sometimes trembling and shaking, a rise in blood pressure, and dry mouth. Some people may experience nausea, an aching body, tingling, and sweating. Research with

Designer Drugs

A relatively recent classification of psychoactive substances is called **designer drugs**. These are **structural analogs**, or drugs that mimic the psychoactive reactions of controlled drugs. They are produced in clandestine laboratories and sold on the black market. Use of designer drugs is increasing.

The best known designer drug is **China white**. Initially promoted as a safe alternative to heroin, it turned out to be a thousand times more potent. Many cases of fatal overdoses have been reported.

Another category is MDA, which combines methamphetamine and mescaline analogs. On the street it is known as the "love drug," because it makes people more sociable. It, too, can be fatal.

Ecstasy, or MDMA, is chemically similar to both methamphetamine and mescaline. It has hallucinogenic effects. It may be a mood elevator, or it may cause panic, anxiety, paranoia, rapid heart rate, involuntary twitching, and shaking. An overdose is life-threatening.

In the 1980s states began to regulate the manufacture of drug analogs. Still, the underground manufacture continues, and new designer drugs emerge. Needless to say, they pose grave dangers to users.

animals indicates that LSD may cause genetic damage, manifested in children born to users.

Bad "trips" and other unpleasant side effects led to the declining popularity of LSD. Some substituted mescaline, which is not as powerful as LSD but has similar effects. Largely, however, PCP took the place of LSD.

KEY TERMS

Hallucinogens a group of mind-altering drugs that affect the brain and nervous system

Psychedelic literally, "revealing to the mind"

Flashback recurrence of a drug "trip"

Mescaline hallucinogen derived from peyote cactus

Peyote a type of cactus that yields mescaline

LSD lysergic acid diethylamide-24, a psychedelic drug that produces distorted reality

Designer drugs manufactured drugs that mimic the effects of other drugs

Structural analog a designer drug that mimics the effects of another drug

China white a designer drug with more potent effects than heroin

PCP

PCP, or phencyclidine hydrochloride— also known as angel dust, peace pills, tranq, hay, hog, killer weed, and rocket fuel — is an anesthetic that blocks nerve receptors from pain and temperature without producing numbness. It was first synthesized in 1959 and used as an intravenous surgical anesthetic. Its harmful side effects of confusion, delirium, intense anxiety, and depression quickly became apparent. For these reasons it was discontinued for use with humans in 1967, although it came to be used as a relaxant and an anesthetic in veterinary medicine.

PCP became a popular drug in the mid-1960s because of its low cost and ready availability, though at least one physician called PCP the most dangerous drug to hit the streets. Taken in small doses, it induces feelings of euphoria. Moderate doses cause blurred vision, slurred speech, sleepiness, heavy sweating, and rapid breathing. Higher doses cause intoxication accompanied by mental confusion, hallucinations, and trouble speaking. Still higher dosages can produce symptoms of serious mental illness. A massive overdose will result in coma and death. Most PCP deaths stem from mental confusion. Abusers have drowned in shallow pools because they did not think to stand up, or died in fires because they could not feel the flames or could not figure out how to escape.

One of the most serious consequences is the loss of inhibitions and ensuing threat of harm to others. PCP can cause extreme, unpredictable rages. Many particularly gruesome murders have been committed by people under the influence of PCP.

Psychedelic Mushrooms

Psilocybin is the primary psychoactive agent in the mushroom *teonanacatl*, the "magic mushroom," of which several species grow in damp meadows and pastures in the United States. Sold illegally, it is called "shrooms." It is taken orally.

INHALANTS

Inhalants are chemicals containing volatile solvents that produce mind-altering vapors. To gain the most effect, inhalants are placed in plastic or paper bags, or soaked into rolls of toilet tissue, absorbent cotton balls, or pieces of fabric or paper, and sniffed. For many years the most popular inhalant was the glue used in making model airplanes. Today, inhalants used more often are gasoline, paint thinner, transmission fluid, lighter fluid, liquid shoe polish, and fingernail polish remover. Almost any substance that is volatile (evaporates quickly) and can be inhaled will produce some effect. Inhalants tend to be used most often by children, some as young as 7 or 8, and young teens because they are easy to obtain and most are legal substances.

The chemical fumes from inhalants act as depressants on the central nervous system. The inhaler gets an almost immediate high. Low doses produce giddiness, excitement, and silliness. Higher doses render the user less inhibited and out of control.

Many of the effects are similar to those of alcohol. Users may have slurred speech, lose coordination, and have blurred vision. The user's judgment may become impaired, which may lead to intense physical fights and other risky or dangerous acts. Unlike alcohol, however, these effects last only about half an hour.

Effects of inhaling over time include gastroenteritis, depressed muscle tone, lead poisoning, damage to the liver and kidneys, nervous system dysfunction, and bone marrow disorders. Chronic use of solvents such as gasoline can lead to leukemia. Inhaling chemicals also decreases the appetite, which often is related directly to nutritional deficiencies.

About half of chronic sniffers suffer brain damage, which may be irreversible depending on which substance is sniffed. A few gases, such as methylene chloride (found in spray paint, for example), are extremely dangerous, and sudden deaths have followed first-time use. The oxygen level of the blood drops suddenly, producing an irregular heartbeat and heart failure. Inhaling a solvent in a plastic bag has caused some deaths by suffocation.

Inhalants are not believed to produce physical dependence. Their use, however, is associated with negative effects such as school failure. Users also tend to drink alcohol as they get older, followed by the abuse of sedatives and other illegal drugs.

Table 13.3 summarizes the drugs and their routes of administration.

KEY TERMS

PCP an anesthetic that blocks nerve receptors from pain and temperature without producing numbness; angel dust

Psilocybin primary psychoactive agent in psychedelic mushrooms

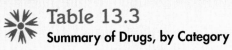

Table 13.3
Summary of Drugs, by Category

Drug	Other Names	Appearance	Route of administration
Narcotics			
Opium	Paregoric, Dover's powder, Parepectolin	Dark brown chunks, powder	Smoked, eaten, injected
Morphine	Pectoral syrup	White crystals, hypodermic tablets, injectable solutions	Taken orally, injected, smoked
Heroin	Smack, horse, stuff, junk, black tar, big H, downtown	White to dark-brown powder or tarlike substance	Injected, smoked, inhaled
Codeine	Empirin compound with codeine, Tylenol with codeine, Codeine in cough medicine	Dark liquid varying in thickness, capsules, tablets	Taken orally, injected
Depressants			
Barbiturates	Downers, barbs, blue devils, red devils, yellow jacket, yellows, Nembutal, Tuinals, Seconal, Amytal	Red, yellow, blue, or red and blue capsules	Taken orally
Chloral hydrate		Soft capsules; syrup	Taken orally
Methaqualone	Quaaludes, ludes, sopors	Tablets	Taken orally
Tranquilizers	Valium, Librium, Miltown, Serax, Equanil, and Tranxene	Tablets or capsules	Taken orally
Cocaine			
Cocaine	Coke, snow, nose candy, flake, blow, big C, snowbirds white lady, ready rock.	White crystalline powder	Inhaled, injected
Crack cocaine	Crack, rock, freebase	White to tan pellets or crystalline rocks that look like soap	Smoked
Stimulants			
Amphetamines	Speed, uppers, black beauties, pep pills, copilots, hearts, benzedrine, dexedrine, footballs	Capsules, pills, tablets	Taken orally, injected, inhaled
Methamphetamines	Crank, crystal meth, crystal methedrine, speed	White powder, pills, rock that resembles a block of paraffin	Taken orally, injected inhaled.
Caffeine	ingredient in coffee, soda, chocolate, and other food items		Taken orally
Cannabis			
Marijuana	"chronic," reefer, grass, weed, bo, primo, joint, bud	Like dried parsley, with stems and/or seeds; rolled into cigarettes	Smoked or eaten
Tetrahydro-cannabinol	THC	Liquid; tablets	Taken orally

(Continued)

Table 13.3
Summary of Drugs, by Category *(Continued)*

Drug	Other Names	Appearance	Route of Administration
Cannabis (cont.)			
Hashish	Hash	Brown or black cakes or balls	Smoked or eaten
Hashish oil	Hash oil	Concentrated syrup liquid varying in color from clear to black	Smoked — mixed with tobacco
Hallucinogens			
Phencyclidine	PCP, hog, angel dust loveboat, lovely, killer weed rocket fuel, peace pill	Liquid, white crystalline powder, pills, capsules	Taken orally, injected, smoked (sprayed on joints or cigarettes
Lysergic acid diethylamide	LSD, acid, white lightning, blue heaven, sugar cubes	Colored tablets, blotter paper, clear liquid, thin squares of gelatin	Taken orally, licked off paper, gelatin and liquid can be put in the eyes
Mescaline and peyote	Mesc, buttons, and cactus	hard, brown discs, tablets, capsules	Discs — chewed, swallowed, or smoked Tablets and capsules — taken orally
Psilocybin	Magic mushrooms 'shrooms	Fresh or dried mushrooms	Chewed or swallowed
Designer Drugs			
Analog of fentanyl (Narcotic)	Synthetic heroin, China white	White powder	Inhaled, injected
Analog of meperidine (Narcotic)	MPTP (new heroin), MPPP, synthetic heroin	White powder	Inhaled, injected
Analog of amphetamines or methamphetamines (hallucinogens)	MDMA (ecstasy, XTC, Adam, essence), MDM, STP, PMA, 2, 5-DMA, TMA, DOM, DOB, EVE	White powder, tablets or capsules	Taken orally, injected, or inhaled
Analog of phencyclidine (PCP)	PCPy, PCE	White powder	Taken orally, injected, or smoked
Inhalants			
Nitrous oxide	Laughing gas, whippets	Small 8-gram metal cylinder sold with a balloon or pipe, propellant for whipped cream in aerosal spray can	Vapors inhaled
Amyl nitrite	Poppers, snappers	Clear yellowish liquid in ampules	Vapors inhaled
Butyl nitrite	Rush, bolt, bullet, locker room, climax	In small bottles	Vapors inhaled
Chlorohydrocarbons	Aerosol sprays, cleaning fluids	Aerosol paint cans	Vapors inhaled
Hydrocarbons	Solvents	Cans of aerosol propellants, gasoline, glue, paint thinner	Vapors inhaled

OVER-THE-COUNTER (OTC) DRUGS

Thousands of drugs can be purchased without a prescription. These over-the-counter, or OTC drugs are self-prescribed, self-administered, and usually used without a physician's knowledge or supervision. Nonprescription products are capable of alleviating various symptoms, disorders, and diseases and also capable of producing ill effects, dependency, and in some cases, addiction.

Two serious potential hazards are improper self-diagnosis and overmedication. Also, drugs can interact unfavorably with other medications taken, with substances in the diet, and with one's own body chemistry. When self-prescribing, a person always should follow the directions printed on the product, inquire about the product from the pharmacist, or read the *Physician's Desk Reference* (PDR) *for Nonprescription Drugs* to be completely informed about the medication.

Consumers are bombarded with more than 300,000 advertised OTC products. The **Food and Drug Administration (FDA)** is the federal regulatory agency charged with establishing criteria for all drugs and reviewing active ingredients in all 26 classes of OTC drugs listed below.

1. Analgesics
2. Antacids
3. Antidiarrheal products
4. Antiemetics
5. Allergy treatment products
6. Antimicrobial products
7. Antiperspirants
8. Antirheumatic products
9. Antitussives
10. Bronchodilators and antiasthmatic products
11. Cold remedies
12. Contraceptive products
13. Dandruff products
14. Dentifrices and dental products
15. Emetics
16. Hematinics
17. Hemorrhoidal products
18. Laxatives
19. Miscellaneous internal products
20. Miscellaneous dermatologic products for external use

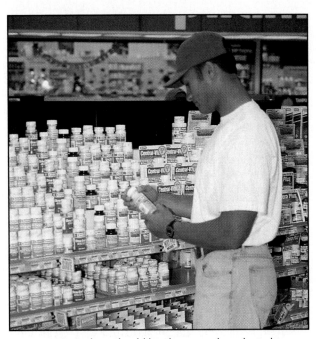

OTC products should be chosen and used wisely

21. Ophthalmic products
22. Oral hygiene aids
23. Sedatives and sleep aids
24. Stimulants
25. Sunburn prevention and treatment products
26. Vitamin-mineral products

The FDA initiated certain rules for regulating safety, effectiveness, and honesty in labeling OTC products. The FDA uses the following descriptives:

1. GRAS: generally recognized as safe
2. GRAE: generally recognized as effective
3. GRAHL: generally recognized as honestly labeled

Functions of the FDA are discussed further in Chapter 15.

TREATING DRUG ADDICTION

Drug addiction surfaced as a social problem in the United States after the Civil War, when wounded

KEY TERMS

Food and Drug Administration (FDA) the regulatory agency charged with establishing criteria for all drugs and reviewing active ingredients in all OTC drugs

veterans came home hooked on the morphine they had received to relieve pain. With the invention of the hypodermic needle came the legal — and illegal — intravenous use of drugs. American homemakers became addicted to various prescription drugs. By the beginning of the 20th century, the public was raising questions about the misuse of drugs.

In the 1930s the federal government opened the first two drug treatment hospitals, in Lexington, Kentucky, and in Fort Worth, Texas. In the 1950s Riverside Hospital in New York City opened the first drug treatment facility designed especially for juvenile addicts. Synanon was founded on the West Coast in 1958. Programs and facilities began to multiply in the 1970s, in response to the increasing abuse of drugs by middle-class youth, a rise in the crime rate resulting from drug use, and the return of many addicted soldiers from Vietnam.

In approaching the practicalities of treatment, drugs differ in how widespread their use is and how addictive the various drugs are. Figures 13.6 and 13.7 clearly illustrate these characteristics. Alcohol and tobacco, discussed in the previous chapter, remain in Figure 13.6, for comparative purposes. Table 13.4 summarizes the effects of various drugs on the body.

The treatment programs available in the United States today are outlined briefly below. No one best method exists. Some work better with some forms of addiction, and the goal is to find the treatment plan that works best for each individual. Regardless of the type of addiction, the key to success is personal motivation, backed by an ongoing support system.

Traditional Treatment

Most drug experts view chemical dependence as a medical condition, just as diabetes or heart disease. Therefore, in some forms of addiction, medication

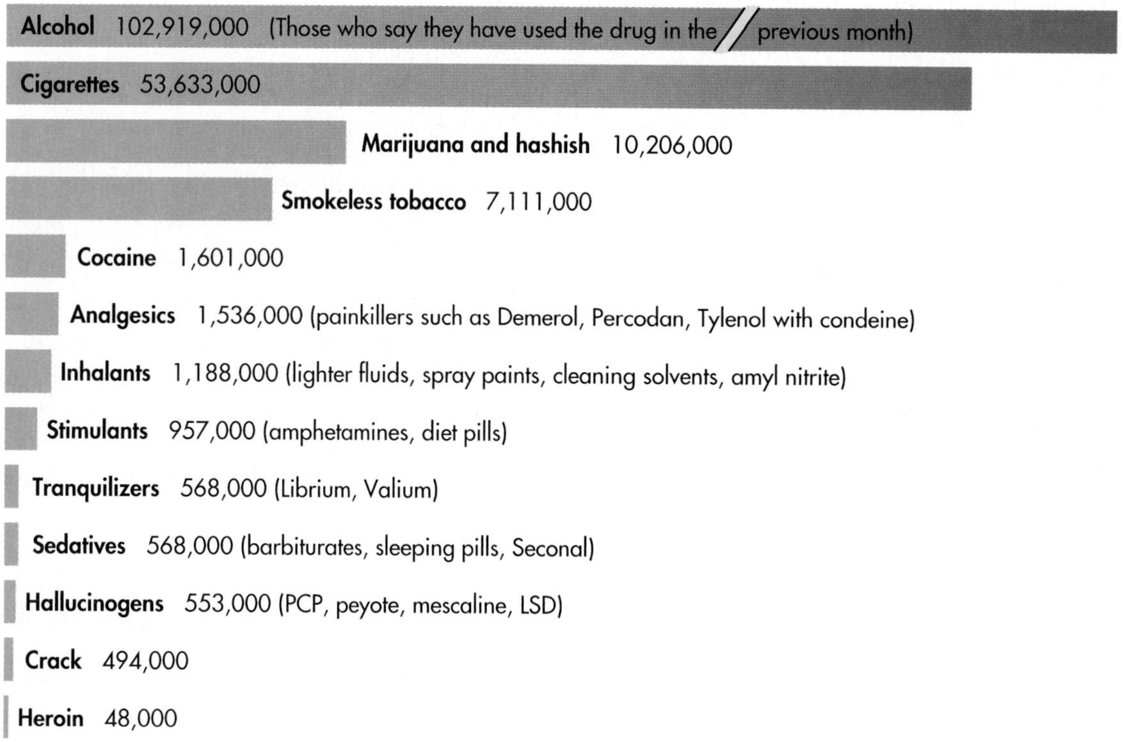

Alcohol 102,919,000 (Those who say they have used the drug in the // previous month)

Cigarettes 53,633,000

Marijuana and hashish 10,206,000

Smokeless tobacco 7,111,000

Cocaine 1,601,000

Analgesics 1,536,000 (painkillers such as Demerol, Percodan, Tylenol with condeine)

Inhalants 1,188,000 (lighter fluids, spray paints, cleaning solvents, amyl nitrite)

Stimulants 957,000 (amphetamines, diet pills)

Tranquilizers 568,000 (Librium, Valium)

Sedatives 568,000 (barbiturates, sleeping pills, Seconal)

Hallucinogens 553,000 (PCP, peyote, mescaline, LSD)

Crack 494,000

Heroin 48,000

Note: Estimates are for Americans over age 12 who say they have used drugs for nonmedical reasons (prescription drugs are not included).

Source: National Institute on Drug Abuse, *Washington Post Health*, March 26, 1991.

Figure 13.6 Relative use of drugs in the United States

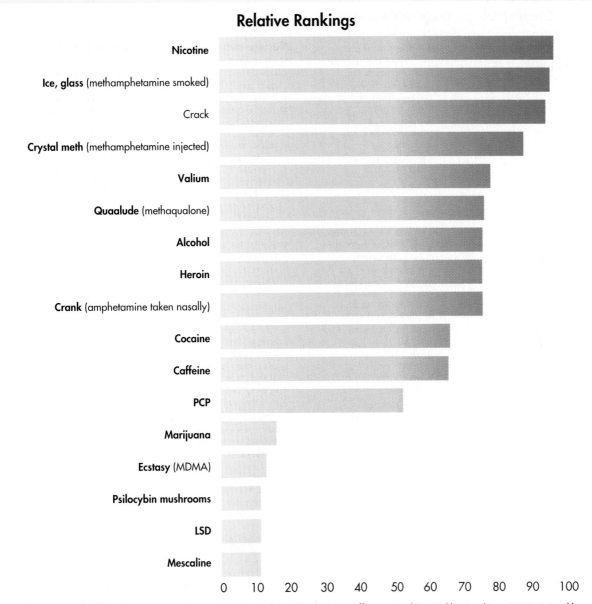

Relative Rankings

Nicotine
Ice, glass (methamphetamine smoked)
Crack
Crystal meth (methamphetamine injected)
Valium
Quaalude (methaqualone)
Alcohol
Heroin
Crank (amphetamine taken nasally)
Cocaine
Caffeine
PCP
Marijuana
Ecstasy (MDMA)
Psilocybin mushrooms
LSD
Mescaline

0 10 20 30 40 50 60 70 80 90 100

Source: Researched by John Hastings, "Easy to Get Hooked On, Hard to Get Off," reprinted in *Health*, Nov./Dec. 1990. © Health. Reprinted by permission.

Figure 13.7 Addictive properties of various drugs

is appropriate in the treatment plan. The best known of these prescribed medications is **methadone**, a synthetic narcotic used in the treatment of heroin addiction. Among its advantages are that it can be taken orally (rather than having to be injected), its effects last 24 hours (compared to 5 hours or so for heroin), the person taking methadone is functional and has no withdrawal symptoms, and methadone is inexpensive. Experts claim that clients on methadone commit fewer crimes than they did previously when they were injecting heroin and that they are better able to hold jobs.

KEY TERMS

Methadone a synthetic narcotic used as a heroin substitute

Table 13.4

Effects of Selected Drugs on the Body

	Narcotic	Cocaine and Crack	Amphetamines
Type of Drug	✳ poppy derivatives (opium, codeine, morphine, heroin) and synthetics (Demerol, Methadone, Dilaudid, Percodan) ✳ smoked, eaten, or injected ✳ ancient painkillers used medicinally ✳ deaden pain; produce euphoria and drowsiness	✳ derived from South American coca bush (still chewed in Andes to offset fatigue) ✳ *cocaine hydrochloride* is white powder ("coke," "C," "flake," "snow") ✳ crack is mixture of cocaine and baking soda ✳ used until 1920 in many medicines ✳ stimulant action — like amphetamine, but now legally classed as a narcotic	✳ synthetically produced: *amphetamine* (speed), *dextroamphetamine* (Dexedrine), *methylamphetamine* or "Ice," *methylphenidate* (Ritalin), etc. ✳ used as pills, inhaled, or injected (speed) ✳ CNS stimulants that resemble action of adrenaline (natural body hormone)
Short-Term Effects (after a single dose)	✳ briefly stimulate, then depress higher brain centers ✳ give quick pleasure surge (for few minutes), then stupor (which mutes hunger, pain, sex drive) ✳ taken by mouth, effects slower, no initial pleasure surge ✳ pupils tiny, body warm, limbs heavy ✳ mouth dry, skin itchy ✳ users may "nod" off, alternately awake or asleep, oblivious to surroundings	✳ short-acting, powerful CNS stimulant; also a local anesthetic ✳ effects vary depending on whether drug is "snorted" (inhaled), injected, put in mouth, rectum, or vagina, or smoked (as crack) ✳ transient euphoria and increased energy ✳ loss of appetite ✳ rise in heart rate and breathing ✳ dilated pupils ✳ agitated, restless talkative ✳ brief rise in sex drive	✳ nervous system briefly stimulated ✳ reduces appetite ✳ increases energy, offsets fatigue ✳ talkative, restless, more alert ✳ faster breathing ✳ rise in heart rate and blood pressure (with risk of burst blood vessels and heart failure) ✳ temperature raised, mouth dry, skin sweaty ✳ pupils dilated ✳ alleviates stuffy nose (original medicinal use)
With Larger Doses and Longer Use	✳ extremities heavy ✳ permanent drowsiness ✳ pupils become pinpoints ✳ skin cold, moist, bluish ✳ progressively slower breathing ✳ depressed breathing ✳ dangers increase with alcohol intake	✳ permanently stuffy nose (if snorted) and risk of perforated nasal septum ✳ brief euphoric effect followed by "crash" — depression ✳ anesthetic effect can depress brain function ✳ bizarre, erratic, perhaps violent actions ✳ paranoid "psychosis" (disappears if drug is discontinued) ✳ sensation of "crawling under the skin" ✳ convulsions, disturbed heart action, even death	✳ bizarre behavior, talkative, restless, tremors, excitability ✳ sense of power, superiority, aggression ✳ illusions and hallucinations ✳ some users become paranoid, suspicious, panicky, violent ✳ elevated blood pressure ✳ insomnia
Long-Term Effects	✳ constipation ✳ moodiness ✳ risk of endocarditis (heart infection) and other infections (AIDS) from needle-sharing ✳ hormone upsets (menstrual irregularities) ✳ liver damage ✳ damaged offspring ✳ strong dependence	✳ weight loss, malnutrition ✳ destroyed nose tissues (if sniffed) ✳ restlessness, mood swings, insomnia, *extreme* excitability, suspiciousness/paranoia, delusions ("psychosis") ✳ depression ✳ impotence ✳ risk of heart attacks ✳ strong *psychological* dependence	✳ malnutrition, emaciation (owing to appetite loss) ✳ anxiety states ✳ "amphetamine-psychosis" (with schizophrenia-like hallucinations) ✳ kidney damage ✳ susceptibility to infection ✳ sleep disorders ✳ *psychological* dependence
Withdrawal Symptoms	✳ striking withdrawal effects (4-5 hours after last dose), sweating, anxiety, diarrhea, "gooseflesh," shivering, tremors	✳ little or no withdrawal sickness; sleepiness ✳ extreme exhaustion ✳ possibly "cocaine blues" (depression)	✳ long sleep, chills ✳ ravenous hunger ✳ depression

LSD Hallucinogens	Cannabis	Inhalants	Caffeine
❋ derived from mushrooms *(psilocybin)* or cactus *(mescaline)* or synthetically — e.g., *lysergic acid* (LSD) or "acid" and *phencyclidine* (PCP) ❋ structures resemble *catecholamines* —normal brain neurotransmitters ❋ hallucinogens can distort reality and produce severe delusions	❋ derived from *cannabis sativa;* preparations vary in potency; hash most potent, marijuana least ❋ smoked in joints or chewed (sometimes with food) ❋ medicinally used for epilepsy, glaucoma, against nausea	❋ volatile organic hydrocarbons from petroleum and natural gas (e.g., gasoline, toluene, hexane, chloroform, carbon tetrachloride, nail polish remover or acetone, lighter fluid, paint thinners, cleaning fluid, airplane cement, plastic glue) ❋ hallucinogenic effects	❋ derived from tea, coffee beans, kola nuts, chocolate ❋ used in many medicines (e.g., with painkillers, cold/cough, pain remedies, antihistamines) ❋ average cup of coffee contains 60-75 mg caffeine, colas about 35 mg (per 250 ml) ❋ CNS stimulant
❋ unpredictable effects — at first like amphetamine ❋ excitation, arousal ❋ temperature raised ❋ altered sense of smell, shape, size, color, distance ❋ exhilaration, "mind-expansion" or anxiety — depending on user ❋ rapid pulse, dilated pupils, blank stare ❋ exaggerated power sense with possibly violent behavior ❋ later – dramatic perceptual distortions ❋ occasionally convulsions	❋ produces dreamlike euphoria, laughter, relaxation ❋ alters sense of space, time ❋ increases heart rate ❋ reddens eyes ❋ dreamy, "stoned" look ❋ at later stages, users are quiet, reflective, sleepy ❋ combined with alcohol, increased effects, distorted behavior ❋ impairs short-term memory, thinking, and ability to drive car or perform complex tasks	❋ exhilaration, light-headedness, excitability, disorientation ❋ confusion, slurred speech, dizziness ❋ distorted perception ❋ visual and auditory hallucinations ❋ impaired muscular control ❋ possible nausea, increased saliva, sneezing ❋ dampened reflexes ❋ recklessness, feelings of power, invincibility	❋ stimulates brain, speeds nerve-cell transmission ❋ elevates mood and alertness ❋ stimulates mental activity ❋ speeds up breathing, metabolism ❋ enhances mental performance ❋ postpones fatigue ❋ shortens sleep ❋ more urine output ❋ rise in blood fats ❋ increases stomach acidity ❋ decreases appetite
❋ anxiety, panic attacks, paranoid delusions, occasionally psychosis (like schizophrenia) ❋ injury or accidents because of drug-induced delusions or distance misjudgment ❋ increased risk of fetal abnormalities ❋ tolerance develops rapidly but also disappears fast with renewed drug sensitivity ❋ with PCP, high fever, muscle spasm, erratic behavior, psychosis lasting weeks or more	❋ slowed digestive (gastrointestinal) activity ❋ time misjudgment ❋ sharpened or distorted sense of color, sound ❋ thinking slow and confused ❋ apathy, loss of motivation/drive ❋ large doses can produce severe confusion, panic attacks ❋ hallucinations (even psychosis)	❋ drowsiness and possible unconsciousness ❋ severe disorientation ❋ risks increase with fume concentration ❋ irregular heartbeat, heart action disturbed ❋ large doses may cause heart failure (especially with spot removers or airplane cement)	❋ nervousness, hand tremors ❋ delayed sleep onset, reduces depth of sleep; insomnia ❋ abnormally rapid heartbeat ❋ jitteriness ❋ mild delirium possible ❋ convulsions (rare) ❋ suspected cancer-causing agent
❋ long-term medical effects not known ❋ may include muscle tenseness, "flashbacks" — brief, sponta-neous recurrence of prior LSD (hallucinogenic) experiences ❋ prolonged, profound depression ❋ panic attacks ❋ no *physical* dependence	❋ loss of drive, reduced energy ❋ regular heavy use increases risk of — bronchitis, lung cancer —reduced sex hormones —impaired learning —memory loss —possible decrease in immunity ❋ *psychological* dependence	❋ pallor, thirst, nose, eye, mouth sores ❋ irritability, hostility, forgetfulness ❋ may damage liver, kidney, and brain ❋ nosebleeds, impaired blood cell formation ❋ depression, weight loss ❋ other drugs compound damage ❋ dependence possible	❋ raised blood cholesterol level ❋ risk of stomach ulcers ❋ suspected cancer-inducing agent ❋ *possible* damage to unborn baby ❋ regular coffee use (more than 5 cups daily) can lead to dependence
❋ few withdrawal effects, possible flashbacks, anxiety	❋ withdrawal symptoms mild — somnia, anxiety, irritability	❋ restlessness, anxiety, irritability, headaches ❋ stomach upsets ❋ delirium (rare)	❋ severe headache ❋ irritability ❋ tiredness

Adapted by permission from *Health News*, a publication of the University of Toronto Faculty of Medicine. Subscriptions and back issues can be obtained by writing 109 Vanderhoof Ave., Suite 205, Toronto, Ontario M4G 2H7 or by calling 416-978-5411.

On the minus side, methadone is an addictive substance itself. It can produce some unpleasant side effects such as weight gain, constipation, nausea, and insomnia. Because it does not cure addiction, addicts often relapse once treatment ends. Finally, if the people taking methadone consume alcohol at the same time, as is often the case, the combination is deadly. In most cases the first step in traditional treatment and rehabilitation of psychoactive drug abuse is **detoxification**, which means ridding the body of toxic substances or the effects of the toxins. It has three basic steps:

1. Get the person completely off drugs as quickly as possible.
2. Relieve both the physical and psychological distress of the withdrawal process.
3. Achieve and maintain abstinence — a drug-free life.

Detoxification usually requires "cold turkey" withdrawal rather than gradually tapering off. Tranquilizers and other drugs usually are prescribed to reduce anxiety and tension. Most people in these "detox" programs are treated on an outpatient basis, and the treatment usually lasts about 3 weeks. Long-term results are not encouraging. One study found that the average addict is back on drugs in about 8 days after treatment. Detoxification works best if it is part of a treatment program that includes counseling and psychotherapy.

Nondrug Therapies

Counseling and psychotherapy are part of most drug abuse treatment programs. These programs usually are based on behavior modification principles. The costlier programs are residential, and others are administered on an outpatient basis. Of the approximately 10,000 drug and alcohol rehabilitation centers in the United States, the average stay is 28 days. The programs are tailored to deal with emotional problems that triggered the drug abuse in the first place. Again, the results are mixed and not entirely promising.

Therapeutic Communities

Independent **therapeutic communities** such as Phoenix House and Gateway have shown some success in turning around the lives of addicts. Staffed largely by former addicts and graduates of the program, they stress a self-help approach. Encounter group sessions and confrontational therapy techniques based on peer pressure are part of the program. Treatment can last from 3 months to 2 years. The average duration of treatment is less than 6 months, but those who have gone through treatment continue to be considered members of the therapeutic community.

Self-Help Groups

Many addicts participate in **self-help groups** with others who have similar experiences and thus can offer personal support. Examples are Narcotics Anonymous (NA), Pills Anonymous (PA), and Cocaine Anonymous (CA). These groups are based on the twelve-step program developed by the founders of Alcoholics Anonymous (AA), one of which is the recognition of a higher power. If that premise makes a potential member uncomfortable, an alternative group that excludes the spiritual element is Rational Recovery (RR). Another alternative is Secular Organizations for Sobriety (SOS). Although this group advocates total abstinence, it, unlike the others, does not adhere to the disease theory. Rather, the theme is independence, building on one's inner strengths.

Participation in these self-help groups is voluntary. Members are there because they want to be — which points toward greater success. At the meetings, people talk about their past experiences with drugs, and their fears and hopes. Listening to

☎ Call for information

National Association of Alcoholism and Drug Abuse Counselors
703-920-4644

National Clearinghouse for Alcohol & Drug Information
800-729-6686

National Council on Alcoholism and Drug Dependence
800-622-2255

Rational Recovery
916-621-4374

Substance Abuse Prevention
301-443-0365

World Service Office of Narcotics Anonymous
818-780-3951

others and exchanging accounts seems to help relieve the compulsions. Because the commonality is drug abuse, these groups tend to be multiracial.

Private Medical Professionals

Physicians (including psychiatrists) who specialize in addiction and withdrawal treatment are certified by the American Society of Addiction Medicine (ASAM) or the American Academy of Psychiatrists in Alcoholism and Addiction (AAPAA). In conjunction with their therapy, they highly recommend self-help support programs.

Some psychologists treat drug addiction. They emphasize the psychological aspects of anger, depression, anxiety, and other feelings that underlie the addiction. They, too, should be trained in this area of specialty. In choosing the professional to see, the person should always look for someone who puts the addiction issue first.

KEY TERMS

Detoxification ridding the body of poisons or the effects of poisons

Therapeutic communities self-help group homes programmed to assist addicts in remaining drug-free

Self-help groups addicts participating with others who have similar experiences and can offer personal support

Summary

1 Psychoactive drugs affect the brain by disrupting the messages sent by the neurotransmitters.

2 The routes of drug administration are: inhalation, injection, oral, and the rectal or vaginal route.

3 The narcotic drugs are natural derivatives of opium — morphine and codeine — as well as semisynthetic opiates such as heroin and synthetic narcotics such as Demerol and methadone.

4 The depressant classification of drugs includes sedative-hypnotics (barbiturates, chloral hydrate, and methaqualone) and tranquilizers.

5 The stimulants encompass cocaine/crack, amphetamines, and caffeine.

6 Hallucinogens are mind-altering drugs such as mescaline, LSD, PCP, and psychedelic mushrooms.

7 The designation of cannabis covers marijuana, THC, and hashish.

8 Inhalants are volatile solvents that produce mind-altering effects.

9 Over-the-counter drugs fall into 26 different drug categories and have the potential for misuse and abuse.

10 Drug addictions are treated through medication and by nondrug therapies such as therapeutic communities, self-help groups, and private physicians.

Select Bibliography

Bell, Peter. *Chemical Dependency and the African-American*. Center City, MN: Hazelden, 1990.

Editors of Market House Books Ltd. *The Bantam Medical Dictionary* (rev. ed.). New York: Bantam, 1990.

Flynn, John C. *Cocaine*. Secaucus, NJ: Carol Publishing Group, 1993.

Kantrowitz, Barbara. "The Crack Children." *Newsweek*, February 12, 1990.

Kemper, Donald W., Jim Giuffré, and Gene Drabinski. *Pathways: A Success Guide for a Healthy Life*. Boise, ID: Healthwise Inc., 1985.

Lerner, Michael A. "The Fire of 'Ice'." *Newsweek*, November 27, 1989.

Phibbs, C. S., D. A. Bateman, and R. M. Schwartz, "The Neonatal Costs of Maternal Cocaine Use," *Journal of the American Medical Association*, 266:11 (September 1991).

"The Safe Use of Medications," *Mayo Clinic Health Letter*, 7:2 (February, 1989).

Schlaadt, Richard, and Peter T. Shannon. *Drug Use, Misuse and Abuse*. Englewood Cliffs, NJ: Prentice Hall, 1994.

Schwebel, R. *Saying No Is Not Enough: Raising Children Who Make Wise Decisions About Drugs and Alcohol*. New York: Newmarket Press, 1989.

Stimmel, Barry, and Editors of Consumer Reports Books. *The Facts About Drug Use*. New York: Haworth Press, 1993.

U. S. Department of Health and Human Services. *Cultural Competence for Evaluators*. Washington, DC: Office for Substance Abuse Prevention, 1992.

Drugs: Can You Tell The Difference?

NAME _____ DATE _____

COURSE _____ SECTION _____

Differentiate the psychoactive substances listed below in terms of category, source, and route of administration.

Substance	Category	Source	Route of Administration
barbiturates			
benzodiazepines			
caffeine			
"crack"/cocaine			
heroin			
marijuana			
mescaline			
methamphetamine/"ice"			
morphine			
psilocybin			

Are You An Addict?

NAME _____ DATE _____

COURSE _____ SECTION _____

The following questions were written by recovering addicts in Narcotics Anonymous.

	Yes	No
1. Do you ever use alone?	☐	☐
2. Have you ever substituted one drug for another, thinking that one particular drug was the problem?	☐	☐
3. Have you ever manipulated or lied to a doctor to obtain prescription drugs?	☐	☐
4. Have you ever stolen drugs or stolen to obtain drugs?	☐	☐
5. Do you regularly use a drug when you wake up or when you go to bed?	☐	☐
6. Have you ever taken one drug to overcome the effects of another?	☐	☐
7. Do you avoid people or places that do not approve of you using drugs?	☐	☐
8. Have you ever used a drug without knowing what it was or what it would do to you?	☐	☐
9. Has your job or school performance ever suffered from the effects of your drug use?	☐	☐
10. Have you ever been arrested as a result of using drugs?	☐	☐
11. Have you ever lied about what or how much you use?	☐	☐
12. Do you put the purchase of drugs ahead of your financial responsibilities?	☐	☐
13. Have you ever tried to stop or control your using?	☐	☐
14. Have you ever been in a jail, hospital, or drug rehabilitation center because of your using?	☐	☐
15. Does using interfere with your sleeping or eating?	☐	☐
16. Does the thought of running out of drugs terrify you?	☐	☐
17. Do you feel it is impossible for you to live without drugs?	☐	☐
18. Do you ever question your own sanity?	☐	☐
19. Is your drug use making life at home unhappy?	☐	☐
20. Have you ever thought you couldn't fit in or have a good time without using drugs?	☐	☐
21. Have you ever felt defensive, guilty, or ashamed about your using?	☐	☐
22. Do you think a lot about drugs?	☐	☐
23. Have you had irrational or indefinable fears?	☐	☐
24. Has using affected your sexual relationships?	☐	☐
25. Have you ever taken drugs you didn't prefer?	☐	☐
26. Have you ever used drugs because of emotional pain or stress?	☐	☐
27. Have you ever overdosed on any drugs?	☐	☐
28. Do you continue to use despite negative consequences?	☐	☐
29. Do you think you might have a drug problem?	☐	☐

Are you an addict? This is a question only you can answer. Members of Narcotics Anonymous found that they all answered different numbers of these questions "yes." The actual number of *yes* responses isn't as important as how you feel inside and how addiction has affected your life. If you are an addict, you must first admit that you have a problem with drugs before any progress can be made toward recovery.

Reprinted from *Am I an Addict?*, revised copyright © 1986, World Service Office, Inc. Reprinted by permission of World Service Office, Inc. All rights reserved.

Aging, Death, and Dying

14

OBJECTIVES

* Describe the profile of America's aging population.
* List three different ways of determining age.
* Discuss the impacts of aging on the body.
* Identify diseases that are common in the elderly population.
* List factors that can enhance health during advanced years.
* Discuss the need for proper medical care and appropriate use of medications by the elderly.
* Discuss safety issues involving the elderly.
* Discuss the issues involved in care-giving.
* Identify the stages of dying.
* Give pros and cons associated with euthanasia.
* Contrast a living will and a holographic will.
* Discuss factors involved in planning a funeral or memorial service.
* Identify the stages of grief.

Nothing in life is constant. All of nature changes, and so do we as human beings. We are born and, if we are blessed, we will live through childhood, adolescence, and adulthood. Some people live healthy lives relatively unmarred by health problems to the age of 100 or even older. Other people, troubled by health problems, live a much briefer time.

Aging is perhaps the least understood of all human processes. It differs from one person to another. Although most people start to

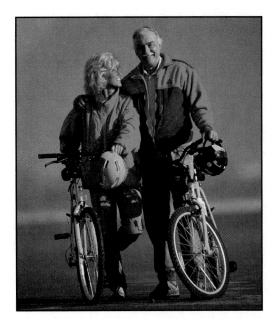

show signs of aging in their 40s, 50s, or 60s, some begin aging in their teens or 20s. A much smaller number stay hale and hearty into their 70s and 80s. The aging process can vary even within a single person. Some organs remain healthy and robust at the same time other organs deteriorate.

In this chapter we present the myriad of issues involved in aging — the way the body changes, factors that enhance health, the specialized medical care, and the importance of planning for the later years. It also explores the many issues that surround dying and death.

Tips for action

Dare To Be 100
by Walter M. Bortz

1. **Aim for 100.** Set your mind to living out your entire 100+ lifespan. Don't stop at 75. Dare to be 100.

2. **Use it or lose it.** Keep active physically and mentally.

3. **Keep a positive attitude.** Fill your life with hope, caring, and creativity.

4. **Know your family medical history.** Accept the good you've inherited, and commit to changing the not-so-good. Get regular check-ups and enlist your doctor's help in your prevention program.

5. **Let nature provide.** The fewer processed foods in your diet, the better. Especially watch for foods processed with salt and sugar.

6. **Trim the fat** — especially saturated fat. It's a burden that weighs you down physically and emotionally.

7. **Get your vitamins from foods** whenever possible. Don't rely on pills.

8. **Don't let 200 be your unlucky number.** Have your cholesterol checked then use diet to keep it in check.

9. **Lighten up.** Keep your sense of humor, and don't let temporary problems get you down. Laughter has healing properties.

10. **Slow down aging** by sticking to a strength and flexibility program.

11. **Keep your brain sharp** by using it. Read. Visit a planetarium. Take a class. You're never too old to learn.

12. **Don't be put out to pasture.** You, not your age, decide when to retire. Keep your job skills up-to-date. When you do retire, keep active. Return to *LIFE*!

13. **Stay fit.** Take advantage of every opportunity to use your body and mind.

14. **Get the sleep your body needs.**

15. **Walk every chance you get.** Take the stairs. Park farther away. Take a brisk walk through the mall the next time you shop.

16. **Take care of your heart** with regular cardiovascular exercise, reduced salt intake, and a low-cholesterol diet.

17. **Choose a doctor** who shares your philosophy of prevention and health promotion. But remember, the best healer is you.

18. **Don't end sexual activity** until you want to. Staying in shape can help keep you looking and feeling sexy. See your doctor when you have problems.

19. **Don't smoke.** It not only shortens your life, but it also ages your skin.

20. **It's your choice.** You have the tools to lengthen and improve your life. Use them!

Adapted with permission from A.H. Belo Corporation for *Cooking Light*, October 1993, pp. 33–40. Reprinted by permission of the author.

AN AMERICAN PROFILE

Americans are living longer than ever, despite the epidemics of heart disease and cancer and the outbreak of AIDS. **Life expectancy** is the average length of time that members of a population can expect to live. Statisticians determine life expectancy by averaging the ages of death of all the people in a group for a certain period. **Lifespan**, on the other hand, refers to the *potential* maximum number of years a person could probably live if everything goes well. Thanks to advanced technology, the potential lifespan now is approximately 110 years.

At the beginning of this century, the average life expectancy for an American was 47 years. Today, it is approximately 76 years. The result is what some social scientists have called "the graying of America." Figure 14.1 shows the increasing proportion of people over age 65. Projections for the year 2030 are that one in five people in the United States will be over age of 65.

Statistically, life expectancy differs along cultural and racial lines. According to the Centers for Disease Control and Prevention, the highest life expectancy is for Anglo women, at 79.6 years. Life expectancy for African American women is 73.8 years. Anglo men in America can expect to live 72.9 years, and African American men 64.6 years. Figure 14.2 shows life expectancy trends in the United States by sex.

During the first half of the 21st century the elderly population will have much ethnic diversity. According to the National Council on the Aging, the minority elderly population was about 4.5 million at the beginning of this decade. That number is expected to reach 23 million by the year 2050 — including 10 million African Americans and 8 million Hispanics.

How does the United States compare with the rest of the countries of the world? Life expectancy in the United States is twentieth in the world. Sweden has the highest percentage of people over the age of 65. Norway, Belgium, Italy, and the United Kingdom round out the top five.

An increase in average life expectancy is good news in many ways. It means we have reduced infant mortality rates, improved medical care, made progress in controlling pathogens that cause infectious diseases, improved nutrition, and made excellent strides in sanitation and disease prevention. The graying of America has a challenging aspect, too. More and more elderly people will rely on government programs for food, housing, and medical care. Longevity can bring with it poverty, illness, inadequate health and medical care, and loneliness.

The need to plan for old age is perhaps most pressing for women. Statistically, women can expect to outlive men. According to the Administration on Aging, by the year 2000 there will be five women for every two men over age 75. Longevity puts women at social and financial disadvantages.

For example, many pensions are cut off when the person who paid into the fund dies. Traditionally, that was the man. More women, however, have private pensions because many of them are working full time throughout their lives but are paid less than men. Therefore, the older woman

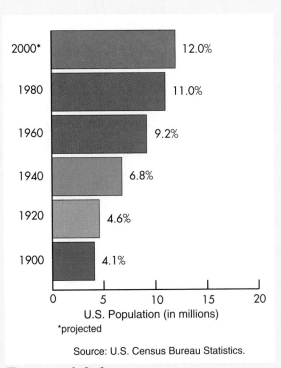

2000*   12.0%
1980   11.0%
1960   9.2%
1940   6.8%
1920   4.6%
1900   4.1%

0   5   10   15   20
U.S. Population (in millions)
*projected

Source: U.S. Census Bureau Statistics.

Figure 14.1 Percentage of persons living to be over age 65 years, 1900–2000

KEY TERMS

Life expectancy average length of time members of a population can expect to live

Lifespan potential maximum number of years members of a population could live

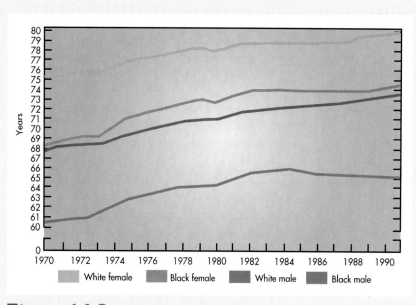

Figure 14.2 Life expectancy by sex

Legend: White female | Black female | White male | Black male

a person may have a relatively young psychological age, determined by sense of self-sufficiency and ability to meet life's challenges.

PHYSICAL AGING

With each passing year the body shows signs of aging, the decline traditionally associated with getting older. Elderly people have decreased homeostasis, the body's ability to restore itself to its normal state once it has been disturbed. When elderly people are injured or become ill, they take longer to recover. **Comorbidity**, having two chronic health problems at the same time, is more common among elderly people.

Physical decline is subtle and gradual for some people and rapid for others. Regardless of how quickly it occurs, certain changes eventually affect various body organs and systems.

who survives her husband often comes face-to-face with poverty. According to the Older Women's League, almost half of American women today over age 65 have less than $10,000 a year to live on.

DETERMINING AGE

How do you determine your age? That may seem like a simple, almost foolish, question, but it is not. **Gerontologists**, (professionals who study the aging process) have identified different ways of determining "age." Only one involves the simple calculation of birth date. The others rely on more complex factors:

❋ *Biological age:* a measure of the relative condition of the body. A 76-year-old man who has participated in cardiovascular conditioning for 3 decades may have a biological age of 40 years. A 32 year-old woman crippled with arthritis may have a biological age of 60 years.

❋ *Functional age:* a measure of how a person compares with contemporaries — in seeing, hearing, walking, endurance, and reflexes.

❋ *Psychological age:* a measure of how well a person adapts to changing circumstances. Even if impaired by physical illness or advanced years,

The Skin

The skin's aging process involves a slow decline in structure and function. Major changes that accompany physical aging include the following:

1. Elasticity decreases, and the underlying support structure gradually changes, resulting in wrinkles and sagging.

2. Skin cells reproduce more slowly and have a shorter life, so injuries take longer to heal.

3. Skin color becomes less even.

4. The skin becomes less effective as a barrier. Its ability to protect against sunlight, substances that cause allergic reaction, detergents, and other harmful elements is reduced.

5. The number of sweat glands decreases, as does the activity of oil glands. As a result, the skin gets dry and itchy.

Exposure to the sun is a major cause of premature aging of the skin. Sun-related damage can

Tips for action

Balding: Not Just For Men

Men might *expect* to go bald, as they get older. About half of all men experience some balding as they age. Surprisingly, so do half of all women. A woman's baldness usually is more evenly distributed and less extensive. To save as much hair as you can:

❋ Eat a well-balanced diet. Crash dieting causes hair loss.

❋ Wear hats or tight wigs only occasionally.

❋ When your hair is wet, comb it. Don't brush it.

❋ As often as possible, let your hair dry naturally. Curling irons, blow dryers, and hot curlers all damage hair.

❋ Avoid styles that pull your hair, such as cornrows and braids.

❋ Protect your hair from sunlight and harsh chemicals such as the chlorine in swimming pools.

❋ Use a mild shampoo and a gentle conditioner after every shampoo.

cause wrinkles, sagging skin, discoloration, and brown "age spots." Researchers have shown that sun exposure and damage to the skin early in life have the greatest impact on skin later in life.

Overexposure to the sun causes not only premature aging but skin cancer as well (see Chapter 7). The chance of developing skin cancer increases with advancing age, especially in people who live in sunny regions and those who have jobs requiring them to work outside. When detected early and treated promptly, most cases of skin cancer can be cured.

The Head

The head actually changes size with age. The skull grows thicker and the head increases in size by an average of one inch per decade, even though brain mass decreases slightly. All facial features get bigger especially the nose, which gets wider and longer.

Hearing and Eyesight

Hearing, especially the ability to hear high-pitched tones, diminishes with age. Most hearing loss involves the inability to distinguish sounds in extreme ranges, not the ability to distinguish conversational tones.

Beginning in the 30s, the eyes undergo gradual and progressive changes that often result in difficulty reading small or fine print, limited visibility in areas that are not lighted well, problems with depth perception, colorblindness, and farsightedness. These progressive changes involve hardening of the lens, yellowing of the lens, loss of transparency in the lens, and shrinking of the pupil.

Elderly people are also more prone to **glaucoma**, a disorder marked by increased pressure within the eye, and **cataracts**, in which the lens becomes opaque (cloudy), causing partial or total blindness.

Taste

Structural changes in the tongue affect the ability to taste as one ages. By age 70, the tongue has only about one-third the functioning taste buds as it did at the age of 25. Elderly people gradually lose the

KEY TERMS

Gerontologist professional who studies the aging process

Comorbidity having two chronic health problems simultaneously

Glaucoma a disorder marked by excessive pressure within the eye

Cataracts an eye disease in which the lens becomes opaque (cloudy), causing partial or total blindness

ability to distinguish between sweet, sour, and salty tastes. As a result, they may use too much salt and sugar to enhance the flavor of their food. A diminished sense of smell and decreased production of saliva also affect the sense of taste.

Bones and Joints

The composition of bones changes continually throughout life as minerals are added and depleted. Sometime during the 40s, mineral loss starts to exceed mineral gain. As a consequence, the bones become porous and brittle. Although mineral loss occurs in both sexes, older women are at highest risk for osteoporosis, severe calcium loss in the bones. The loss of bone density and calcium increases the risk for bone injuries in the elderly population, including fractures and breaks. Osteoporosis will be discussed in greater detail later in the chapter.

Sickness comes suddenly, but goes slowly
—saying from West Indies

The Heart

As a person ages, the heart pumps less blood because the heart muscle (myocardium) begins to deteriorate and weaken. Atherosclerosis, a narrowing of the arteries caused by a buildup of fatty deposits on artery walls, further restricts blood circulation. Arteries blocked by atherosclerosis are a common cause of heart attack and strokes in elderly people. A common complicating factor is high blood pressure. When blood pressure is elevated, the heart is forced to work harder to pump blood more forcefully against resistant arteries. The extra load causes a heart already weakened by age to simply wear out. These cardiovascular problems are covered in depth in Chapter 8.

The Lungs

The elasticity of the lungs decreases with age. The breathing rate slows, and the amount of air circulating in and out of the lungs decreases. As a result, the blood flowing through the pulmonary vessels is not as richly oxygenated, and cells throughout the body are gradually deprived of oxygen.

The Kidneys and Bladder

Kidney cells die as a person ages. Therefore, the kidneys filter waste products from the blood more slowly. By age 70, the kidneys work half as fast as they did four decades earlier. Aging can present a "domino effect" for the kidneys as well. As other organs and systems deteriorate, the kidneys have to work harder to keep wastes removed from the bloodstream. The resulting overexertion of aging kidneys can lead to kidney failure.

Bladder capacity also decreases with age. The average bladder holds 2 cups of urine at age 30. By age 70, bladder capacity averages only half that amount, one cup of urine.

Sexual Functioning

Sexual enjoyment can last throughout old age if a couple acknowledges changes in sexual functioning and can adjust to those physical changes. The rate and degree of physical change varies from one person to another, but women can generally anticipate these changes:

1. The tissues of the vulva and vagina become thinner, making intercourse more painful.
2. The walls of the vagina lose their elasticity, which also makes intercourse more painful.
3. The amount of vaginal secretions diminishes, making it difficult to lubricate sufficiently for penile penetration.
4. The strength of vaginal orgasmic contractions is reduced.
5. The external genitals gradually get smaller.
6. The breasts lose firmness and fatty tissue.

In men the following changes occur:

1. More time is required to achieve an erection.
2. An erection is more difficult to maintain.
3. The angle of the erection decreases.
4. Ejaculation is less forceful and contains less ejaculate fluid. Sperm production decreases. The orgasm is briefer than previously.
5. More time is required between orgasms.

Certain medications — such as tranquilizers, antidepressants, and some medications for high blood pressure — interfere with sexual function. A physician may be able to prescribe a drug that has fewer side effects. One drug that affects sexual performance often is alcohol, which is known to delay orgasm.

Tips for action

When You Can't Take Estrogen

If you and your doctor have decided against estrogen replacement therapy:

✳ When a hot flash strikes, drink a glass of cold juice or icy water.

✳ Try meditation, biofeedback, deep breathing, or yoga to beat hot flashes.

✳ Dress in clothing made of natural fibers — cotton, linen, or wool.

✳ Sleep in a cool room and use cotton sheets.

✳ Open the windows and lower the thermostat.

✳ Exercise! Women who exercise have half as many hot flashes as those who don't.

✳ Steer clear of alcohol, caffeine, and spicy foods.

✳ Eat tofu, tempeh, and other soybean products. They contain plant estrogen.

✳ If intercourse is painful, use estrogen creams or vaginal lubricants that do not contain petroleum jelly.

✳ Get plenty of calcium (ask your doctor about supplements).

Prostate surgery in men and hysterectomies in women affect the sexual performance of some. Diabetes, stroke, arthritis, heart disease, and some other chronic debilitating diseases can also interfere with sexual activity among the elderly. Even the most serious diseases rarely warrant discontinuing sexual activity completely, however. For example, the joint pain of rheumatoid arthritis responds to medication and surgery. Exercising, resting, taking warm baths, changing position, and changing the timing of sexual activity (avoiding the time of day when discomfort is worst) can help restore sexual enjoyment.

Menopause

Menopause, often called the "change of life," is a natural part of the female life cycle. The ovaries stop producing eggs, and levels of female hormones—estrogen and progesterone—decrease. The "normal" range for onset of menopause varies widely — between ages 42 and 56. If the ovaries are surgically removed, menopause occurs at that time, regardless of the woman's age.

The lack of estrogen during menopause causes an increase in cholesterol levels, which places a woman more at risk for heart disease. In addition, most women have some symptoms, which may include:

— changes in the menstrual cycle, such as lighter bleeding or irregularity in the time menstruation occurs each month; gradually periods stop completely.
— hot flashes or flushes (short episodes of heat that spread over the upper body, sometimes accompanied by sweating).
— vaginal dryness, itching, or burning.
— incontinence.
— increase in facial and body hair.
— headaches.
— fatigue.
— sleep disturbances.
— mild depression, irritability, anxiety, or mood swings.
— mild memory loss and inability to concentrate.

For most women the symptoms associated with menopause are mild and require no medical

KEY TERMS

Menopause stage in the life cycle when the ovaries stop functioning and hormone levels decrease

treatment. For those who have more severe problems, treatments are available that can relieve discomfort. A physician may suggest hormone replacement therapy (HRT) to relieve the symptoms of menopause. HRT, discussed in more detail later in the chapter, also slows the age-related bone loss that can lead to osteoporosis and protects against heart disease. Because HRT carries risks as well as benefits, the pros and cons of HRT should be weighed carefully.

COMMON DISEASES IN ELDERLY PEOPLE

Several conditions that are of particular concern to the aging are osteoporosis, Alzheimer's disease, urinary incontinence, influenza and pneumonia, and depression.

Osteoporosis

Osteoporosis is a condition in which decreasing bone mass results in thinner, more porous bones that fracture easily (see Figure 14.3). Some degree of bone loss is normal in both men and women of advancing age, but the sharp decrease in estrogen following menopause accelerates the rate of bone loss in women. Osteoporosis is the major cause of bone fractures in women over age 50. Experts estimate that half of all women over age 65 have osteoporosis. Of the approximately 25 million Americans who have osteoporosis; four of five are women.

A major risk factor for osteoporosis is early menopause (either naturally or from a hysterectomy). Additional factors include a small, thin frame, delicate bone structure, physical inactivity, low calcium intake, cigarette smoking, excessive use of alcohol, and a family history of osteoporosis. Anglo Americans are at highest risk. Women who have never had a baby are at increased risk. Certain drugs, such as cortisone, heparin, and several anticonvulsants, also weaken the bones and can aggravate osteoporosis.

Overweight women are *less* likely to develop osteoporosis because estrogen is stored in body fat. Even after

Milk: It Really *Does* Do a Body Good!

Calcium alone won't prevent or cure osteoporosis but it is important in keeping bones healthy and strong.

✳ **Men and nonmenopausal women** need 1,000 mg a day, the equivalent of three 8-ounce glasses of skim milk.

✳ **Menopausal women who are taking estrogen** need the same amount as nonmenopausal women.

✳ **Menopausal women who are not taking estrogen** need 1,500 mg a day, the equivalent of five 8-ounce glasses of skim milk.

the ovaries stop producing estrogen, it is produced in the body's fat layer.

Osteoporosis is sometimes called a "silent disease" because it has no symptoms during its early stages. For that reason, the condition usually is not recognized until it reaches an advanced stage. At that point fractures start occurring— most often in the spine, wrists, and hips. In its later stages, osteoporosis causes debilitating pain, permanent disfigurement, and lasting disability.

Ordinary x-rays do not show bone loss until about 30% of the bone density has been lost but

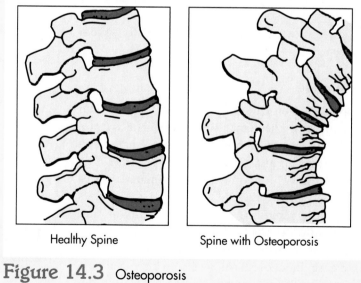

Healthy Spine   Spine with Osteoporosis

Figure 14.3 Osteoporosis

Tips for action

To prevent osteoporosis:

✳ Get regular weight-bearing exercise throughout your life: walking, jogging, running, cross-country skiing, racquetball, tennis, stair climbing, dancing, and light weight training. A recent study done at Tufts University in Boston shows that weight training using five machines, done twice a week, is more effective in preventing osteoporosis than estrogen replacement therapy.

✳ Eat plenty of calcium-rich foods throughout your life, including low-fat milk, low-fat cheese, and yogurt.

✳ Stop smoking, and reduce alcohol and caffeine consumption.

✳ Get vitamin D every day — from 15 minutes of sunshine or from fortified milk.

three medical tests are available for diagnosing osteoporosis:

✳ Single- and dual-photon absorptiometry

✳ Dual-energy x-ray absorptiometry

✳ Computerized tomography (CT scan)

The type of test chosen depends on the area of the body to be examined, the available equipment, and the patient's ability to pay (insurance coverage). Blood and urine tests usually are done first to rule out other diseases that can weaken the bones.

Many doctors believe that routine testing to predict the chance of developing osteoporosis-related bone fractures is not warranted. A person at high risk for osteoporosis, however, may want to ask about bone density measurement.

Estrogen replacement therapy can protect post-menopausal women from osteoporosis. Because estrogen slows bone loss and improves the body's

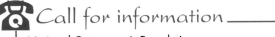

Call for information

National Osteoporosis Foundation
202-223-2226

ability to absorb and retain calcium, it often is prescribed for women who are at risk for developing osteoporosis. The drug calcitonin also is used by both men and women to slow bone breakdown and reduce the pain associated with osteoporosis. Other treatments include a calcium-rich diet (see Table 14.1) and a program of weight-bearing exercise.

Alzheimer's Disease

Alzheimer's disease is an incurable mental impairment associated with elderly people, though it has been diagnosed in individuals as young as the late 40s. The disease gradually destroys the brain cells that allow people to concentrate, reason, and perform ordinary tasks, such as driving a car. Alzheimer's is irreversible and cuts remaining life expectancy in half.

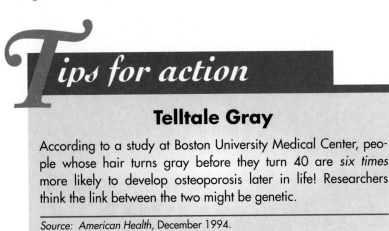

Tips for action

Telltale Gray

According to a study at Boston University Medical Center, people whose hair turns gray before they turn 40 are *six times* more likely to develop osteoporosis later in life! Researchers think the link between the two might be genetic.

Source: American Health, December 1994.

KEY TERMS

Osteoporosis a condition in which the bones lose calcium and become brittle

Alzheimer's Disease a progressive, incurable disease in which nerve cells in the brain die

Table 14.1

Table 14.1
Sources of Calcium

Food	Amount	Calcium (milligrams)	Calories
Dairy Products			
Milk			
Whole, 3.5%	1 cup	288	159
Nonfat (skim)	1 cup	296	88
Cheese			
Cheddar	1-inch cube	129	68
Cottage	4 oz.	107	180
Swiss	1-inch cube	139	56
American	1-inch cube	122	65
Custard, baked	1 cup	297	305
Ice cream	1 cup	194	257
Ice milk			
Hardened	1 cup	204	199
Soft serve	1 cup	273	266
Pudding			
Chocolate	1 cup	250	385
Vanilla	1 cup	298	283
Yogurt			
from whole milk	1 cup	272	152
from partially skimmed milk	1 cup	294	123
Meat, Poultry, and Seafood			
Clams	3 oz.	53	65
Salmon, pink canned	3 oz.	167	120
Sardines, canned in oil, drained	3 oz.	372	174
Tuna, canned in water	3 oz.	17	135
Vegetables			
Beans			
Lima	1 cup	80	189
Red kidney	1 cup	74	218
Snap (green or yellow)	1 cup	72	31
Broccoli, cooked	1 stalk	158	47
Collards, cooked	1 cup	289	51
Mustard greens	1 cup	193	32
Spinach	1 cup	200	41
Turnip greens, cooked	1 cup	252	28
Fruit and Fruit Products			
Oranges, fresh	1 medium	54	71
Grain Products			
Bread	1 slice	23	74
Pancakes, plain or buttermilk	1 cake	58	61
Nuts and Beans			
Tofu, soybean curd	3 oz.	110	61

Alzheimer's affects more women than men, probably because women live longer. An estimated 4 million older Americans have the disease. Alzheimer's strikes an estimated one in twenty people between ages 65 and 75. By the age of 80, the rate is up to one in five. Researchers believe that the number of Alzheimer's victims will rise to 14 million by the middle of the 21st century, especially because technological advances are enabling people to live longer.

The risk for developing Alzheimer's disease is greater if one or both parents develop the disease. Also, individuals with Down syndrome are four times more likely than the general population to develop Alzheimer's disease.

Experts say that Alzheimer's disease is now the third costliest health problem affecting Americans, exceeded only by heart disease and cancer. Medical bills, nursing homes, home health care, and lost productivity from Alzheimer's cost an average of $47,000 a year for each Alzheimer's patient, for a total of almost $90 billion.

The areas of the brain that seem particularly affected by Alzheimer's disease are:

1. The *cerebral cortex*, or outer layer, which is responsible for cognitive functions such as language.

2. The *hippocampus*, located deep in the brain, believed to play an important role in memory.

The death of neurons in these areas of the brain has a severe impact on memory, thinking ability, and behavior. The three general "stages" of the disease are:

Stage 1   Forgetfulness and disorientation become noticeable. Victims also may be depressed, lack interest in their surroundings, and show poor judgment. During the first stage of Alzheimer's disease, victims become

☎ Call for information

Alzheimer Association
800-272-3900

Tips for action

Active Mind = A Healthy Mind

Recent studies — one involving a group of nuns in their 90s and older — have found that a lifetime of "mind exercises" can help delay the dementias so common in old age. To start protecting your mind:

* Strive for a broad range of experiences.

* Be willing to try new things.

* Stay flexible — mentally and physically.

* Get to know a wide variety of people.

* Surround yourself with people who are smarter than you are.

* Seek out challenging activities.

The TV magazine 20/20 aired a segment featuring people who were not only living but were living well after age 100. The interviewees had three commonalities:

1. They were *engaged* in living. They all had interests and meaningful activities.
2. They were *physically active*. One taught a dance class. Another raced automobiles.
3. They had the ability to face and bounce back from losses. One interviewee had just lost her 70-year-old daughter but insisted that the interview go on as scheduled. In it, she related fond memories of her daughter.

---

progressively unable to take care of routine tasks such as grocery shopping and doing the laundry.

Stage 2 Existing symptoms worsen, and victims become restless and agitated. They often perform repetitive actions. Eyesight, hearing, taste, smell, and touch gradually diminish.

Stage 3 The victims become completely dependent on caregivers. During this final stage they gradually lose all control of physical functions and become completely disoriented.

No definitive diagnosis for the condition is possible. When every other condition is ruled out, the physician makes a "diagnosis of exclusion." Unfortunately, the only certain diagnosis for Alzheimer's is during autopsy. Doctors examine the brain of a dead person for **plaques** (dense deposits of a certain protein) and **tangles** (bunches of twisted nerve cell fibers in the neurons). Scientists do not yet know whether the plaques and tangles are a *cause* or a *result* of the Alzheimer's disease.

At present, no test is available to diagnose Alzheimer's disease in living patients. A *probable* diagnosis of Alzheimer's is made, based on:

— medical history.
— physical examination.
— tests of mental ability.

When a person has symptoms of mental impairment, thorough medical, psychiatric, and neurological evaluations should be done. This is especially important because many *reversible* conditions mimic Alzheimer's disease. Symptoms resembling those of Alzheimer's disease can be caused by poor nutrition, stroke, adverse drug reactions, high fever, viral infection, minor head injuries, anxiety, boredom, loneliness, and depression. Physicians consider previous illnesses and use of medications,

KEY TERMS

Plaques dense deposits of protein found in the brain of Alzheimer's patients during autopsy

Tangles bunches of twisted nerve cell fibers found in the neurons of Alzheimer's patients during autopsy

neurological tests that detect anatomical changes in the brain, and psychological tests that measure memory.

Scientists doing Alzheimer's disease research have identified mutations in several genes in Alzheimer's patients. They also have identified several enzymes and unique changes in the way the body processes proteins. Armed with this and continuing research, they are working toward developing a way to diagnose Alzheimer's disease in the living.

Presently, no established treatment has been developed for Alzheimer's patients. The National Institutes on Health, the National Institute on Aging, and other governmental and private foundations have funded research into several possible treatments. So far, the most promising are several drugs, vitamin E, and a group of plant extracts being tested in India.

Urinary Incontinence

Urinary incontinence, the loss of voluntary bladder control, affects more women than men. An estimated 40% of all women over age 60 have problems ranging from slight loss of urine to severe and frequent wetting.

Most commonly, incontinence in elderly people is caused by weakened pelvic muscles. This is a common aftereffect of pregnancy and childbirth, which is why the condition is more common among women. A common cause in men is obstruction or inflammation that can accompany prostatitis.

Urinary incontinence is not an inevitable consequence of aging. Instead, it is caused by specific changes in body function. Most often it stems from disease or is a side effect of certain kinds of medication.

The two general kinds of incontinence are:

1. *Urge incontinence.* The person has a sudden, strong urge to urinate and is unable to hold the urine long enough to reach a toilet.

2. *Stress incontinence.* Urine leakage occurs during physical exertion or when the person strains, laughs, coughs, or sneezes. Stress incontinence is the type caused by weakened pelvic muscles.

In most cases urinary incontinence responds to treatment. Among the wide variety of available treatments are:

— surgery to correct structural problems (such as abnormalities in the position of the bladder) and severely weakened muscles; most cases of stress incontinence can be corrected surgically.

— a set of specific exercises to strengthen pelvic muscles.

— medication to control urination or improve the bladder's capacity to hold urine.

— bladder training, which involves urinating at specific time intervals. A type of behavior modification, it often is combined successfully with other techniques such as restricting liquids after a certain time of day.

Influenza and Pneumonia

Although influenza (the "flu") and pneumonia strike people of every age, they are most serious in older people. According to the Centers for Disease Control and Prevention, of the approximately 60,000 adults who die every year from influenza and pneumonia, 95% are over age 65. Combined, influenza and pneumococcal pneumonia are the sixth leading cause of death in the United States. The influenza virus attacks the respiratory tract and can lead to bronchitis or pneumonia. Pneumococcal pneumonia affects an estimated half-million Americans a year. Caused by a strep bacteria, it results in severe inflammation and infection in the lungs. Influenza initially exhibits the same symptoms as a cold, with a stuffy or runny nose and a cough. The flu is more severe, however, and lasts longer.

The drugs *amantadine* and *rimantadine* can reduce flu symptoms in nine of ten people if it is taken within 48 hours of the first symptoms. Pneumococcal pneumonia is treated with aggressive doses of antibiotics to kill the strep bacteria.

Vaccinations are available against both influenza and pneumococcal pneumonia, and are recommended for people in high-risk groups, including all those over age 65. People over age 60 who get a flu shot are only half as likely to develop the flu as those who do not get vaccinated.

Because the viruses that cause the flu mutate constantly, becoming resistant to existing vaccines, a person should get a flu shot every year. Most doctors recommend getting the vaccine in late October or November. Flu vaccines may become slightly less effective in preventing the flu entirely as people age, but they still protect a high percentage of the elderly population from infection. Of those who do get infected, the flu vaccine makes symptoms less severe.

The pneumonia vaccine is required only once. Booster shots are given annually to those at highest risk for developing the disease (including those with chronic respiratory disease). Although the vaccination does not prevent pneumonia in all people who receive it, those who are vaccinated and still develop pneumonia usually have milder symptoms and quicker recoveries.

Influenza and pneumonia vaccinations *do not*:
— cause the illness or symptoms of the illness.
— make any existing illnesses worse.
— interfere with other medications.
— cause side effects other than temporary soreness or redness at the injection site.

Depression

Although depression strikes people of all ages, it is more common in elderly people. They are particularly vulnerable to life events that lead to depression, such as loss of a spouse, deterioration of health, financial pressures, the transitions involved in retirement, and the challenge of living alone. Depression also a common side effect of drugs older people take for conditions such as arthritis, hypertension, and heart disease. An estimated 15% of all older Americans have symptoms of serious depression, and more than two-thirds of them are not diagnosed or treated properly. Depression is a concern in older people, too, because it often is dismissed as a "natural part of aging" or misdiagnosed. For example, forgetfulness and confusion are

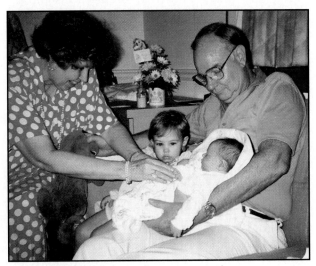

Grandchildren can be a great antidepressant.

symptoms of depression, and these also are symptoms of Alzheimer's disease. The symptoms presented in Chapter 2 apply to the elderly population.

As many as 80% of people with depression can be treated successfully outside of a hospital with either therapy alone or a combination of therapy and medication. Short-term psychotherapy ("talk therapy") has proven successful in a number of cases, reducing the cost and the involvement of treatment for depression.

HEALTH PROMOTION AND AGING

Developing good health habits should start early in life, but it is never too late. Adopting healthy habits, even later in life, offers many health benefits. Among them are improved general physical condition, enhanced mental well-being, and slowed physical decline.

Adopting a healthy lifestyle is especially important for elderly people who live in rural or isolated areas. They more often have to face inadequate medical facilities, fewer economic resources, transportation problems, and a scarcity of health services.

Eating for Health and Fitness

Almost everyone can get all the needed nutrients by eating a variety of nutritious foods every day. For older people, the experts recommend the amounts presented Table 14.2.

Little research has been done to define how aging changes the body's use of various nutrients. Some studies show that aging may affect the need for certain vitamins and minerals. For example, the body's ability to absorb calcium and vitamin D decreases with age. Although Daily Values have been published for infants, children, and adults, guidelines for the specific nutritional needs of older people are scarce.

Preliminary results of a study recently conducted at Boston's Tufts University did show that the current recommendations for protein actually may be *less* than what elderly people need. Older

KEY TERMS

Urinary incontinence loss of bladder control

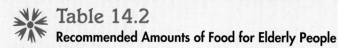

Table 14.2
Recommended Amounts of Food for Elderly People

Recommendations	Examples
At least two servings of dairy product	Low-fat or skim milk, reduced-fat cheese, low-fat cottage cheese, low-fat or non-fat yogurt
Two servings of protein	Poultry, tuna, salmon, mackerel, lean meat, dried beans or peas, nuts
Four to five servings of fruits and vegetables	Apples, bananas, pears, plums, strawberries, oranges, grapefruit, broccoli, cauliflower, carrots, squash, beans, corn, tomatoes, spinach; include at least one citrus fruit or juice and at least one dark green leafy vegetable
Four servings of bread and cereal products	Whole-grain bread, whole-grain pasta, rice, oatmeal

of diseases common in the elderly population, including diabetes, hypertension, coronary artery disease, and arthritis.

The body's need for protein, carbohydrates, vitamins, and minerals stays the same as we age, but the need for *calories* decreases significantly. Therefore, elderly people have to make a special effort to eat foods that provide a good ratio of nutrients to calories. Fruits, vegetables, and natural grains are among the best. They should try to avoid "empty calories," foods laden with calories but minimal nutrients. The most notorious culprits are processed foods high in fat, sodium, and refined sugar.

people may need more protein because of weakened muscles and reduced ability to respond to physical stress.

Maintaining a Healthy Weight

Maintaining a healthy weight, important at all ages, becomes more difficult for elderly people, who tend to be less active and expend fewer calories. The USDA Human Nutrition Research Center on Aging suggests that maintaining a healthy weight may be especially difficult for elderly men. When they gain weight, they retain the extra pounds, and when their weight drops below normal, they often are unable to regain it. Either way, the failure to adjust can increase the risk of serious illness. Poor weight control can worsen the effects

Exercise

Good health depends on staying physically active in later years. Although older people may have to gradually modify the type and duration of exercise sessions, even those who have never exercised can improve their health by exercising regularly.

Exercise also can prolong life. According to studies conducted at Stanford, middle-aged people who took up exercise for the first time gained an average of a year and a half of life.

People who exercise regularly, even into their 90s, report more energy, endurance, and flexibility. They move more easily, sleep better, and are less anxious. Exercise even may help delay the physical effects of aging, which, according to some researchers, is not as much a function of passing

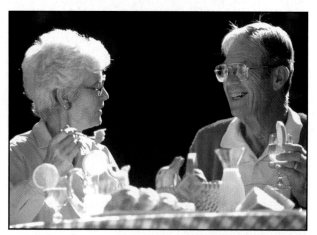

Good nutrition promotes health as people age.

Heart-Healthy Vitamins

According to a recent study by the National Institute on Aging, older adults who take vitamins C and E are less likely to die of a heart attack.

Most of the benefit apparently comes from vitamin E, which cut the chances of dying from a heart attack by more than 60 percent over a period of 12 years.

Check with your doctor before using any nutritional supplement: vitamin E can accumulate in body fat if the dose isn't right. And, since it thins the blood, you shouldn't take it if you are prone to excess bleeding.

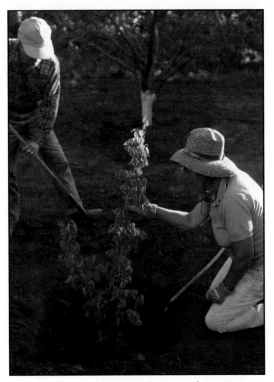

Gardening is one good means of exercise for elderly people.

years as it is of disuse. Author Walter Bortz coined the term "disuse syndrome" to describe the ways in which a lack of physical activity leads to premature aging. Some of the common signs of "aging" — stooped posture, shriveled muscles, memory loss — actually are effects of inactivity, not a function of advancing years.

Current evidence from research shows that exercise strengthens the heart and lungs, lowers blood pressure, reduces the risk of diabetes, lowers the level of certain fats in the bloodstream, improves mobility of the joints, and strengthens the bones, thus reducing the risk of osteoporosis. Recent studies show that moderate exercise such as walking or gardening helps elderly people avoid stomach and intestinal bleeding. Exercise improves overall health and boosts resistance to disease.

Smoking

Cigarette smoking—dubbed by a former U.S. Surgeon General C. Edward Koop the number-one preventable cause of death in the United States — is a risk to good health for people of any age. A person who smokes one pack of cigarettes a day deducts twelve years from his or her life.

Smoking is even more serious among older people. As people age, the blood flow to the lungs and oxygen exchange diminish. Cigarette smoking makes that already compromised situation even worse. In addition, smoking is the major cause of chronic obstructive pulmonary diseases, which are much more common among the elderly.

Alcohol in Moderation

As with smoking, alcohol can be detrimental to health for people of all ages. As we age, physical changes in the body affect the way alcohol is metabolized and eliminated. The body retains less body fluid, so alcohol is not readily diluted. With less body fluid, the concentration of alcohol in the blood (BAC) increases much more rapidly. The brain is affected more profoundly by lower levels of alcohol in the blood. Also, older people have a lower ratio of lean muscle mass, and, thus, less mass in which the alcohol can be distributed (alcohol is not distributed in body fat). The liver, too, works more slowly to metabolize the alcohol, delaying the removal of alcohol from the body.

How Do Medications and Alcohol Mix

The following reactions can occur when alcohol is mixed with:

❋ **Aspirin**: an increase in stomach irritation and bleeding.

❋ **Pain relievers**: mental confusion, excessive drowsiness, impaired coordination, loss of consciousness, and impaired breathing

❋ **High blood pressure medication**: dizziness, fainting, lightheadedness, loss of consciousness

❋ **Diabetes medication**: weakness, headache, nausea, vomiting, rapid heartbeat, difficulty breathing

Mixed with sleeping pills, tranquilizers, antidepressants, some cough and cold products, and monoamine oxidase inhibitors, alcohol can be fatal.

Source: *Medication Education for Seniors and The Consumer's Guide to Drug Interactions* (New York Collier Books/Macmillan, 1993).

Alcohol consumption worsens many of the chronic disease conditions common among elderly people. Alcohol interferes with and diminishes the functioning of the most common medications taken by people over age 65. When alcohol is mixed with some medications, such as barbiturates, tranquilizers, certain cough and cold products, the result can be fatal.

The same drink that had few effects at 50 may have considerably more harmful effects at 75. Depending on existing health problems, regular medications, and physical condition, some elderly people may need to stop drinking. Others need to limit their intake of alcohol.

MEDICAL CARE FOR THE ELDERLY

Regular medical examinations are more important during later years than at almost any other time of life. Physical changes that take place during aging can result in chronic illnesses that demand frequent ongoing attention. Diseases that are common in the elderly population — glaucoma, diabetes, hypertension, and cancer — have few symptoms in their early stages and may go unnoticed by elderly individuals and their caregivers. Regular medical check-ups, including eye examinations, allow early diagnosis and aggressive care, which can slow the deterioration these conditions cause.

Prior to age 65, healthy adults should have a complete physical exam every 3 years. The U. S. Preventive Services Task Force recommends an annual physical after age 65. Those at high risk for specific diseases, such as heart disease, cancer, or diabetes, may need a more frequent check-up as advised by a physician.

In deciding which screening tests to recommend, experts take three factors into consideration: cost of the test, potential risks posed by the test, and whether knowing test results will enable doctors to start treatment that will prolong life. Using those criteria, medical experts have identified several screening tests that should be done throughout adult life and more frequently in elderly people. After age 50, *healthy* adults should have the following medical tests done annually:

> The man who views the world at 50 the same as he did at 20 has wasted 30 years of his life.
>
> — Muhammad Ali

* Rectal exam
* Test for *occult* (hidden) blood in the stool
* *Proctosigmoidoscopy* (an internal examination of the colon to detect abnormalities or cancerous growths)
* Blood pressure measurement

Healthy women over age 50 should have an annual mammogram, Pap smear, and breast exam. Every woman should perform a breast self-exam every month. Healthy men should have a prostate exam and a testicular exam and also do a testicular self-exam every month. All adults should be tested for glaucoma annually from the age of 25.

MEDICATIONS AND THE ELDERLY

Elderly people take more medications than any other segment of the population. Of over-the-counter medications, aspirin and laxatives are the ones purchased most often. Because the elderly population has the highest rate of chronic or long-term illnesses (such as arthritis, diabetes, hypertension, and heart disease), they also tend to take many different drugs at the same time. Prolonged use of multiple drugs, increases the risk of dangerous drug interactions. Damage to major organs, drug overdose, drug dependency, and death may result.

Because of the normal changes that occur with aging, drugs act differently in the body in later years than they do earlier in life. Those changes can affect the length of time a drug remains in the body and the amount of drug absorbed by body tissues. To reduce the risks of adverse drug reactions, the elderly should follow the same guidelines as people of any age:

* Take the exact dosage the physician prescribes.
* Ask the doctor or pharmacist any questions *before* beginning to take the medication.
* Never take medication prescribed for someone else.
* Tell the doctor about all other medications being taken, including over-the-counter medications.

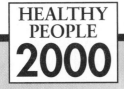

HEALTHY PEOPLE 2000
OBJECTIVES FOR AGING

✳ Reduce the proportion of all people age 65 and older who have difficulty in performing two or more personal care activities.

✳ Report any problems with specific medications to the doctor who prescribed them. A doctor can often substitute another medication that will be just as effective.

✳ Immediately report any unusual reactions to the prescribing doctor.

Estrogen

A drug that deserves special mention is estrogen. It often is used in **estrogen replacement therapy (ERT)** for menopausal women (or those who have had their ovaries removed surgically). The recommendation for estrogen replacement therapy is based on two distinct advantages of estrogen: It seems to reduce the risk for osteoporosis and for heart attack.

The bone loss of osteoporosis accelerates rapidly after menopause because of the lack of estrogen, which maintains bone mass and helps protect the calcium reserves in the bones. Lack of estrogen is the major cause of osteoporosis after menopause. ERT has proven to be one of the most effective ways of preventing the fractures associated with osteoporosis in women. According to the Arthritis Foundation, long-term estrogen use can reduce the risk of fracture by as much as 50%.

Researchers also have found that estrogen offers women protection against heart disease. According to the American Heart Association, the risk of heart disease in women begins to rise steadily after menopause. The risk for heart disease increases much more sharply if menopause is caused by hysterectomy rather than by natural cessation of estrogen production.

Recent studies sponsored in part by the American Heart Association show that post-menopausal women who take estrogen have 50% less risk of stroke and coronary heart disease. Although researchers are not sure why estrogen affects heart disease risk, they do know that estrogen seems to increase levels of high density lipoprotein ("good") cholesterol and reduce levels of low density lipoprotein ("bad") cholesterol implicated in heart disease. A second female hormone — progesterone (and its synthetic form, progestin) — also may help provide protection against heart disease.

Even with all of its benefits, estrogen replacement therapy is not for all women. Those with a personal or family history of breast or uterine cancer probably should not take estrogen. The decision to start estrogen replacement therapy should be based on a woman's medical history and risk factors. Those who may benefit the most are women at high risk for heart disease because of family history, blood cholesterol levels, or other factors.

CAREGIVING ISSUES

The medical technology that is enabling more and more people to reach old age is bringing with it a crisis in the caregiving arena. With the lifespan extending well into the 80s and 90s, people in their 60s and older are finding themselves caring for a parent, an aging spouse, or a friend. **Caregivers** may be defined as people who help others who are unable to fulfill the tasks of daily living such as eating, bathing, dressing, or using the bathroom.

Caregiving has become a critical issue. The number of people over age 85 — those in greatest need of daily help — is increasing rapidly and is expected to more than double in the next 15 years.

KEY TERMS

Estrogen replacement therapy hormone treatment after menopause or after the ovaries have been removed

Caregiver a person who renders services to another person who is unable to take care of the activities of daily living

This rapid growth, combined with a declining birth rate and an increasing number of women in the workforce, has resulted in more diverse groups taking on the responsibility for caregiving. As the population continues to age, more men and women, especially those who themselves are aging, will face the responsibility of caring for older relatives and friends.

SAFETY IN OLD AGE

Accidents are more frequent, and accidental injuries generally more serious, later in life. The most common causes of fatal injuries in older people are falls and automobile accidents. Elderly people are more prone to accidents because:

* Poor eyesight and hearing decrease awareness of hazards.

* Arthritis, neurological disease, and impaired coordination or balance cause elderly people to be unsteady.

* Changes in bones, muscles, and joints affect the ability to move quickly and easily.

* Diseases and medication, along with the natural aging process, can cause dizziness.

* Illness or use of some medications can cause drowsiness.

* Reflexes and reaction time are slowed.

Many of the accidents involving elderly people can be prevented by staying in good physical and mental health and by improving safety habits.

Every year in the United States, falls cause serious fractures in more than 200,000 older people; of those, 20% die within the first year following the injury. People with osteoporosis have an increased risk for fracture when they fall. Potential consequences include long-term pain and confinement and possible institutionalization.

☎ Call for information

National Safety Council
800-621-7619

National Institute on Aging
800-222-2225

The age-related change most likely to cause automobile accidents among the elderly population is probably the change in eyesight. As the eyes age:

* Distance vision is less acute, so curves in the road and traffic intersections are difficult to anticipate.

* Gauges on the dashboard are difficult to read.

* Night vision becomes reduced dramatically, and the eyes become much more sensitive to the glare from oncoming headlights (resistance to glare deteriorates by about 50% every 12 years after age 17).

* Peripheral (side) vision narrows, requiring the driver to turn to the side more often.

* Switching focus from objects in the distance to those that are close, (from the roadway to the speedometer, for example) takes longer.

* Distinguishing traffic signs on a crowded street gets more difficult.

Partly because of chronic illness and deteriorating health, automobile accidents not only are more frequent but also are more serious for older drivers. Data on car injuries released by General Motors shows that if a car driven by a 20-year-old is involved in an accident with a car driven by a person over 65, the elderly person is five times more likely to be killed in the accident.

PLANNING FOR OLD AGE

The changes that occur as part of aging are not limited to physical and mental changes; most elderly people also have to adjust to changes in finances and possible changes in housing.

Facing Financial Challenges

Many older people are able to enjoy their retirement years with enough money to meet their basic needs and enjoy some leisure activities. Others face poverty for the first time in their lives. Retirement savings often must be used for expensive medical treatment not covered by insurance or Medicare. Many older people simply outlive their assets.

Even when benefits are available to elderly people who qualify for them, many do not take advantage of them. Some are too proud to accept assistance. Many more either do not know about the benefits or do not know how to get them. Others, especially those for whom English is a second language, may not understand the complicated paperwork required. As a result, only about half of those who are eligible for Supplemental Security Income (SSI) actually receive the benefits allowed them.

Getting educated about benefits, and how to apply for them, is only part of what has to be done. Planning should start early, in the 20s and 30s, so adequate amounts of money can be put into interest-earning accounts for retirement income. Younger people would be wise to take advantage of tax-deferred savings plans such as the 401(k)

When I Am an Old Woman
by Jenny Joseph

When I am an Old Woman . . .
I shall wear purple
With a red hat which doesn't go, and doesn't suit me.
And I shall spend my pension on brandy and summer gloves
And satin sandals, and say we've no money for butter
I shall sit down on the pavement when I'm tired
And gobble up samples in shops and press alarm bells
And run my stick along the public railings
And make up for the sobriety of my youth.
I shall go out in my slippers in the rain
And pick the flowers in other people's gardens
And learn to spit.
You can wear terrible shirts and grow more fat
And eat three pounds of sausages at a go
Or only bread and pickles for week.
And hoard pens and pencils and beermats and things in boxes.
But now we must have clothes that keep us dry
And pay our rent and not swear in the street
And set a good example for the children.
We must have friends to dinner and read the papers.
But maybe I ought to practice a little now?
So people who know me are not too shocked and surprised
When suddenly I am old and start to wear purple.

plan and other tax shelter annuities to prepare for the financial challenges of retirement.

Elderly people often have to reconsider where they are living because of:

— costly maintenance and utility bills.
— the desire to live closer to children and other family members.
— the desire to live in a smaller home.
— the need to move from a home that has stairways and other structural barriers.
— the desire to move from an unsafe neighborhood.
— the need for regular nursing attention.

Before making any move, issues of cost, independence, availability of medical care, and other aspects of personal concern have to be considered. Many types of housing offer support services such as nursing homes and continuing care communities. Other people arrange "in-home" services that may include nursing care, home-delivered meals, transportation services, or escorts.

Options for the elderly encompass a broad range of possibilities, including:

✳ Staying in their own home and renting out part of it to a caregiver or helper.

✳ Moving to a smaller home.

✳ Moving in with family members.

✳ Moving to a group home where older people share a single residence.

✳ Moving to an apartment building where elderly residents share communal dining facilities and on-call nursing assistance.

✳ Moving to a community designed especially for older people.

DEFINITIONS OF DEATH

When the body can no longer adapt to the changes involved in disease or aging, it stops functioning and death occurs. Traditionally, death was identified when a person stopped breathing and the heart stopped beating. Because of the ethics and issues surrounding organ transplants and other medical procedures, however, the medical and legal professions have had to devise more precise definitions of death.

Three general definitions of death are used to determine when death occurs: brain death, clinical death, and cellular death.

Brain death

Brain death occurs when the brain stops functioning completely. To measure whether the brain has stopped functioning, medical scientists use the following criteria:

❋ whether the person has any reflexive movement

❋ whether the person reacts to stimuli (such as being pinched)

❋ whether the person is breathing spontaneously (without the aid of a respirator) or shows any kind of spontaneous muscle movement

❋ whether there is any activity on an electroencephalogram, which measures and records brain waves; a flat line indicates brain death.

According to standards established by the Harvard Medical School, two sets of readings must be taken 24 hours apart to establish brain death.

A person can be brain dead while oxygenated blood is being circulated through the body with life-support equipment. In this way, vital organs can be kept alive for transplant after a person has been declared brain dead.

Clinical death. When a person stops breathing and the heart stops beating, **clinical death** has occurred. This determination is adequate in cases where medical procedures are not at issue.

Cellular death. The gradual breakdown of the body that occurs after the heart stops beating signals **cellular death**. Deprived of oxygen, body cells and tissues gradually stop functioning. All metabolic processes cease. Eventually the muscles stiffen (**rigor mortis**), and blood pools in whatever body parts are resting against a surface.

DYING

After interviewing hundreds of people who were dying, Dr. Elisabeth Kubler-Ross wrote her landmark work, *On Death and Dying*. In it she identified the five stages people go through when they learn they are dying. Not everyone who is dying experiences all five stages. Among those who do,

not everyone experiences them in the same order. Some even go through two stages at the same time or bounce back and forth among the stages, repeating one or more. The stages are: denial, anger, bargaining, depression, and acceptance.

1. *Denial.* The first stage is marked by a sense of shock and disbelief that death may be imminent. Denial may last a few seconds or a few years. It is actually a defense mechanism that at first refuses to acknowledge a stressful situation, and later allows a temporary way of confronting the stress.

2. *Anger.* "Why me?" a dying person shouts. Denial has passed, and the situation is now real. Few people want to surrender to death. For them, anger is a natural and expected reaction to losing all they have known. Many lash out in anger at family members, friends, caregivers, physicians, the environment, or God.

3. *Bargaining.* When the anger finally subsides, many people gather up whatever hope remains and try to strike a bargain with God. "If you get rid of the cancer, I'll devote my life to the homeless," promises one. "If you'll just let me live long enough to see Michael graduate from college, I'll never take another drink," says another. Others launch a desperate search for a miracle, and end up being victimized instead by peddlers of medical fraud.

4. *Depression.* At this stage the person begins to lose hope. Maybe God isn't going to accept the bargain. Maybe papaya leaves and crushed juniper berries are *not* going to cure the cancer after all. A very real personal grieving begins. The person may refuse to eat, talk, or have visitors. Many cry much of the time. Of all the stages of dying, this can be the most difficult.

5. *Acceptance.* At last the person accepts what is about to happen. "I'm ready to die," the person sighs. Hope returns, but this time it is hope for the end of a struggle, hope for an existence beyond this one. During the final stage, the person actually welcomes death.

Choosing When to Die

Euthanasia is a means of allowing death to occur by taking no extraordinary measures to prolong

Probably the most famous euthanasia case was that of Karen Ann Quinlan, who was admitted to an intensive care unit in 1975 at the 22. She was in a coma when admitted. Placed on a respirator, she remained in a vegetative state. Her parents, convinced that she would never recover or come out of the coma, asked her physicians to turn off the respirator. They refused. A legal battle ensued. The New Jersey Supreme Court finally ruled that the respirator keeping Karen Ann Quinlan alive could be turned off.

life or by providing the means to end life. The two different types of euthanasia are:

1. **Active euthanasia** or **direct euthanasia.** Also known as "assisted suicide," it involves taking steps to speed death. Most often it involves the use of strong chemical compounds that depress the central nervous system and induce death. Active euthanasia is illegal in the United States and most other countries, so it usually is done under secretive conditions. One public exception is Dr. Jack Kevorkian, dubbed "the suicide doctor," who has been arrested and jailed briefly on several occasions for assisting terminally ill people to end their own lives.

2. **Passive euthanasia** or **indirect euthanasia.** Medical treatment or life-sustaining procedures (such as intravenous feeding or oxygen therapy) are withheld, or the decision is made not to initiate medical treatment (such as heart surgery) needed to save a patient's life. In most states mentally competent adults have the legal right to refuse medical treatment. The most impassioned controversies occur when patients are not responsive and family members or physicians have to make that decision on their behalf.

Euthanasia is shrouded in controversy. Proponents believe that terminally ill people who have no hope of recovery — and who are suffering degrading and demoralizing illness — should be allowed to "die with dignity." Opponents believe that all life has meaning, and that no one — including the patient — has the right to determine when that life has lost value. Beyond the proponents and the opponents are the legal experts, who struggle to determine who exercises the ultimate decision to end a life.

The Living Will

Because of the controversies surrounding euthanasia and the right to die, most states have enacted legislation that allows people to draft a **living will**, a document that expresses what they want done if they become terminally ill or critically injured and unable to speak for themselves. Because people have the right to make decisions concerning their own medical treatment, a living will can take the moral, legal, and ethical pressure off survivors if a decision about treatment has to be made.

In essence, the living will directs that life-sustaining procedures be withheld or withdrawn if the patient is in a terminal condition. Although the laws vary slightly from one state to another, the will must generally be:

— drafted by a mentally competent adult.

— drafted in the person's handwriting.

— signed by the person making it; if the person is physically unable to sign but is mentally competent, it may be signed by someone else in the person's presence.

— dated.

— witnessed by two adults. Neither can be the person who signed the will; neither can stand to benefit financially from the person's death. (For example, a witness could not be named as a beneficiary on the person's life insurance policy.)

— delivered by the person or at the person's direction to his or her physician.

— in accordance with the form prescribed by state law.

Once drafted, a living will stands forever. Unless the person who drafts it decides to revoke it. In

KEY TERMS

Brain death complete loss of brain function

Clinical death cessation of heartbeat and breathing

Cellular death cessation of all metabolic processes

Rigor mortis stiffening of the muscles after death

Euthanasia allowing terminally ill patients to die either by active or direct means and withholding life-saving treatment (passive or indirect)

Living will legal written document stating what kind of treatment should or should not be given in the event of a terminal illness or critical condition

Sample Living Will Declaration

Declaration made this _____ day of _____

(month and year)

I, _____, being of sound mind willfully and voluntarily

(Print full name)

make known my desires that my dying shall not be artificially prolonged under the circumstances set forth below, do hereby declare:

If at any time I should have an incurable injury, disease, or illness certified to be terminal condition by two physicians who have personally examined me, one of whom shall be my attending physician, and the physicians have determined that my death will occur whether or not life-sustaining procedures are utilized and where the application of life-sustaining procedures would serve only to artificially prolong the dying process, I direct that such procedures be withheld or withdrawn, and that I be permitted to die naturally with only the administration of medication or the performance of any medical procedure deemed necessary to provide me with comfort care.

In the absence of my ability to give directions regarding the use of such life-sustaining procedures, it is my intention that this declaration shall be honored by my family and the physician(s) as the final expression of my legal right to refuse medical or surgical treatment and accept the consequences from such refusal.

I understand the full import of this declaration and I am emotionally and mentally competent to make this decision.

Signed _____

City, County and State of Residence _____

Date _____

The declarant has been personally known to me and I believe him or her to be of sound mind. I did not sign the declarant's signature above for or at the direction of the declarant. I am not related to the declarant by blood marriage, entitled to any portion of the estate of the declarant according to the laws of intestate succession or under any will of declarant or codicil thereto, or directly financially responsible for declarant's medical care.

Witness _____

Witness _____

Date _____

Figure 14.4 A sample of a living will

that case, the person can destroy the will, issue a written revocation, or verbally revoke it in the presence of an adult witness. That witness must sign and date a notification of the revocation, then deliver it to the person's physician. Figure 14.4 provides an example of a living will.

Some states also allow a person to give **power of attorney** to a trusted family member or friend. This proxy is entitled legally to speak on your behalf, make medical decisions for you, and see that your wishes are carried out.

The Holographic Will

A **holographic will** is a legal, completely hand-written document (in most states), in which the writer gives directives concerning his or her decisions and wishes in the event of the writer's death. The document usually contains.

— a person named as executor;
— a list of personal items or property and a list stating to whom the items and property are to be given;
— a selectee or guardian should the writer have young children;
— memorial, funeral, or burial arrangements;
— the location of the holographic will.

When a person does not have a will and dies, he or she dies *intestate*. When no will exists, the state in which the dead person resides makes decisions concerning the welfare of the children and the dead person's property.

CHOOSING HOSPICE CARE

In addition to choosing *when* to die, people may be able to choose *where* to die. Advances in technology have enabled most dying patients to choose to die either in the hospital or at home. Much of that choice is made possible by **hospice care**, a concept that originated in England.

Whether the patient is at home, in a hospital, or at a hospice center, hospice care provides comforting, kind, caring, humane services to people who are dying and to their families and caregivers. The hospice team focuses on the physical, social, emotional, and spiritual needs of the terminally ill person. The patient is made as comfortable as possible and is given personalized attention.

Though hospice care can be offered in an institutionalized setting, most hospice patients are cared for in their own homes.

The hospice team also supports the family of the dying person by helping family members accept and prepare for the death. Family members are taught how to care for the dying person physically and emotionally; hospice team members visit on a regular basis to provide extra nursing care, emotional support, or other help.

Organ Donations

Approved in 1968 and legal in all fifty states, the **Uniform Anatomical Gift Act** provides for donation of the body or specific parts of the body when the donor dies. Most commonly, the donor carries a **uniform donor card**, which specifies the donor's wishes and is signed and witnessed. The card is considered a legal document in all fifty states. Uniform donor cards are available from the National Kidney Foundation, and in some states they are available where driver's licenses are issued.

Although some people are disturbed by the thought of "harvesting" organs, the procedures used to remove organs are similar to those used in standard autopsies. Depending on the organs being donated, the process may not vary significantly from what has to be done to prepare the body for burial.

The uniform donor card allows donors to specify whether they want any needed organs or parts donated, whether the body can be used for anatomical study, or whether specific organs or parts can be used. Many organs and parts can be transplanted successfully. Those used most often are the heart, lungs, liver, kidneys, bones, skin (used for grafting), and corneas.

KEY TERMS

Power of attorney appointment of a friend or relative to make legal decisions for another

Holographic will a legal handwritten document in which the writer leaves instructions to be carried out upon his or her death.

Hospice care services for terminally ill patients and their families focusing on their comfort and social, emotional, and spiritual needs

Uniform Anatomical Gift Act provision that provides for the donation of the body or organs upon death

Uniform donor card card that specifies the wishes of a person to donate organs after death

---

PLANNING A FUNERAL

Funeral services are a rite of passage for people who have died. These services recognize the value of the dead person, comfort survivors, and play an important role in the grieving process by helping survivors break all physical and social contact with the person who died.

Specific kinds of services vary and are dictated by cultural beliefs. Some are somber occasions in which the dead person is paid tribute and eulogized. Others are joyous occasions (called "wakes") in which survivors celebrate the person's life. In some cases, terminally ill people plan their own funerals, choosing the type of ceremony and those who will participate. Costs of funerals vary substantially and can include the casket, services of funeral home staff, use of facilities and equipment, the cemetery plot or crypt, the vault or liner, grave site care, services of the clergy, and flowers. Costs also vary depending on how the body is disposed of — whether it is embalmed or cremated.

Embalming involves draining blood and body fluids, then injecting the body with formaldehyde and alcohol. The embalming procedure preserves the body for an indefinite time after burial, allowing funeral participants to view the corpse. In some states embalming is not required by law but in most cases a body must be buried within a strict time period if it is not embalmed or cremated.

Cremation is a technique whereby the body is incinerated in a specialized furnace where the intense heat reduces the body to ashes. When a body is cremated, the survivors generally honor the deceased person with a memorial service instead of a funeral. In some cases, the ashes are kept in an urn or other container instead of being buried in a cemetery. Some cemeteries have special vaults where the container of ashes can be stored.

THE STAGES OF GRIEVING

Grief is a way of responding to something that has been lost. Significant losses include the loss of a job, a relationship, status, sense of security, or loved one. Regardless of what has been lost, the stages of grief are the same. No two people react to grief in the same way, however. For some, grief becomes painful or debilitating. Others manage to cope reasonably well. The way in which a person handles grief tends to be a reflection of how the person copes with stress in general.

Even though every reaction is individual, the general stages of grief are the same from one person to another. They are:

1. *Shock and disbelief.* The initial reaction to news of a loss is shock and disbelief: "No way!" "I don't believe it!" Lasting from several minutes to several days, this stage is characterized by

Tips for action

Coping with Bereavement

To stay healthy while you grieve:

❋ Keep things in your life as *status quo* as possible. The death of a loved one is a major source of stress so do what you can to cut down on other stressors (a new job, moving to a new house, going on vacation).

❋ If you can, postpone making decisions that can wait until later.

❋ Keep in touch with other people; social support is especially important now.

❋ Avoid the temptation to use alcohol or drugs.

❋ Get plenty of rest. Take naps if you need to, and try to maintain your normal sleeping pattern at night.

❋ Eat a balanced diet.

❋ Drink plenty of fluids, but steer away from alcohol, caffeine, and drugs.

❋ Exercise regularly.

numbness and denial. The feeling of shock is actually a defense mechanism that allows the body time to gear up for coping with the stress of the loss.

2. *Awareness.* As the person becomes aware of the loss, he or she may cry, scream, become silent, want to be alone, or lash out in anger at others.

3. *Restitution.* During this third stage, the mourner relies on spiritual or religious beliefs, cultural tradition, or various other rituals that help him or her come to terms with the loss. Funerals, wakes, and memorial services help the mourner face the loss and accept its reality. The restitution stage also begins the long process of being able to utilize coping techniques. The survivor may begin to talk about the dead person and recall the person's personality, attributes, and mannerisms. By remembering things as simple as a gesture or a smile, the mourner begins to categorize the memories that eventually lead to healing.

4. *Idealization.* The mourner thinks constantly of the dead person's good qualities, and may even try to emulate certain beliefs, behaviors, and attributes of the dead person. In this stage, which usually lasts several months to several years, the mourner gradually directs his or her feelings toward other survivors.

5. *Resolution.* At last the healing process is finished. The survivor reestablishes former contacts, readjusts to ordinary activities, establishes relationships other than those shared with the dead person, and accepts the environment without the dead person. The mourner still remembers the dead person's attributes and accomplishments but finally can also remember the deceased's failures and disappointments.

Even though grief is normal and natural and necessary, it can cause illness because it involves intense emotions and is so inseparably connected to loss. A special kind of grief is **bereavement,** the process of "disbonding" from someone who played an important role in one's life and who is now gone. The intense grief involved in bereavement has been shown to pose significant health risks, ranging from immune system disorders to suicides, sudden deaths, and increased death rates from all causes.

KEY TERMS

Funeral rite of passage for those who have died

Embalming procedure in which blood and body fluids are drained and formaldehyde and alcohol are injected

Cremation incineration of a body in specialized furnace

Grief emotional reaction to a significant loss

Bereavement intense grief associated with the process of "disbonding" from a significant person who has died

Summary

1 Lifespan and life expectancy are lengthening, giving rise to new issues surrounding the growing population of the elderly.

2 Age may be thought of in three ways: biological, functional, and psychological.

3 Physical aging takes its toll on the skin, the brain, hearing and eyesight, bones and joints, the heart, the lungs, the kidneys and bladder, and sexual functioning.

4 Conditions of particular concern in the elderly population include osteoporosis, Alzheimer's disease, urinary incontinence, influenza and pneumonia, and depression.

5 To counteract the ill effects of aging, people should eat for health and fitness, maintain a healthy weight, get enough exercise, and not engage in smoking or overindulge in alcohol drinking.

6 Elderly people are more prone to accidents (in the home and on the road) because of poor eyesight, diminished hearing acuity, decreased coordination and balance, slower reactions, and the physical limitations posed by any disease.

7 Death has been classified by the medical and legal communities in three ways: brain death, clinical death, and cellular death.

8 Upon learning of pending death, the five stages a person goes through are: denial, anger, bargaining, depression, and acceptance.

9 Euthanasia has two forms: active or direct and passive or indirect.

10 The living will allows a person to state the conditions for continuing his or her life. The holographic will is a legally binding, handwritten will giving various instructions to be followed upon the writer's death.

11 Funeral options range widely in cost and require decisions regarding embalming, cremation or burial.

12 The stages of grieving are: shock and disbelief, awareness, restitution, idealization, and resolution.

Select Bibliography

Bortz, Walter. "We Live Too Short and Die Too Long." *Cooking Light*, October 1993.

Duffy, Mary E. "Determinants of Health-Promoting Lifestyles in Older Persons." *Image: Journal of Nursing Scholarship*, 25:1 (Spring 1993), 23-28.

Dyer, Kristi. "Reshaping Our Views on Death and Dying." *Journal of American Medical Association*, March 4, 1992.

Ezell, Gene, et al. *Dying and Death: From a Health and Sociological Perspective*. Scottsdale, AZ: Gorsuch Scarisbrick, 1987.

Johnson, Kirk A. "The Color of Health Care." *Heart and Soul*, Spring, 1994.

Kubler-Ross, Elisabeth. *On Death and Dying* (New York: Macmillan, 1969).

Levy, Doug. "Pumping Iron Helps Bones of Older Women." *USA Today*, December 28, 1994, p. D1.

Morganthau, Tom. "The Clinton Solution." *Newsweek*, September 20, 1993.

National Council on the Aging. *Perspective on Aging*, July-September 1994, p. 23.

Speake, Dianne L., Marie E. Cowart, and Rebecca Stephens. "Healthy Lifestyle Practices of Rural and Urban Elderly." *Health Values*, 15:1 (January/February 1991), pp. 45-57.

Staudacher, Carol. *Beyond Grief: A Guide for Recovering from the Death of a Loved One*. Oakland, CA: New Harbinger Publications, 1991.

"Time For an Update?" *Looking Forward*, 4:3 (Fall 1994), p. 7.

Walsh, Froma, and Monica McGoldrich. *Living Beyond Loss: Death in the Family*. New York: Norton, 1991.

York, Jeffrey. "FDA Ensures Equivalence of Drugs." *FDA Consumer*, September, 1992.

Osteoporosis
Can It Happen To You?

NAME _____ DATE _____

COURSE _____ SECTION _____

Complete the following questionnaire to determine your risk for developing osteoporosis.

QUESTION	YES	NO
1. Do you have a small, thin frame, or are you Caucasian or Asian?	☐	☐
2. Do you have a family history of osteoporosis?	☐	☐
3. Are you a postmenopausal woman?	☐	☐
4. Have you had early or surgically induced menopause?	☐	☐
5. Have you been taking excessive thyroid medication or high doses of cortisone-like drugs for asthma, arthritis, or cancer?	☐	☐
6. Is you diet low in dairy products and other sources of calcium?	☐	☐
7. Are you physically inactive?	☐	☐
8. Do you smoke cigarettes or drink alcohol in excess?	☐	☐

The more times you answer "yes," the greater your risk for developing osteoporosis. See your physician, and contact the National Osteoporosis Foundation for more information.

Source: National Osteoporosis Foundation.

How Well Will I Age?

NAME _____ DATE _____

COURSE _____ SECTION _____

The following are factors that will affect you life as you get older .Check each box that applies to you.

❑ I eat nutritional foods.

❑ My weight is within the recommended range.

❑ I exercise regularly and according to sound principles.

❑ I do not smoke cigarettes or misuse drugs.

❑ I get regular physical check-ups and conduct self-exams.

❑ I get enough sleep.

❑ I stimulate my mind and stay mentally active.

❑ I have a good sense of self-worth and self-esteem.

❑ I have learned ways to deal with stress effectively.

❑ I maintain friendships and nurture interpersonal relationships.

❑ I help others and participate in volunteer activities.

❑ I buckle my seatbelt, have an operational smoke detector in my home, and adhere to safety regulations and standards.

❑ I respect the environment and do what I can to preserve it by recycling and not being wasteful.

❑ I am planning financially for my retirement.

❑ I have a legal will covering disposition of my desires upon my death.

The more boxes you checked, the better off you will be as you get older. Reread the items you did not check, and make a commitment to work on them.

Consumerism and Environmental Health

15

*Y*our health is your responsibility, and taking responsibility for your health starts with wise self-care. This requires you to know when it is no longer smart to self-diagnose and self-treat. You need to familiarize yourself with the type of health care provider you need and how to find a good one. In addition, you need to know how to use medicines correctly, whether your doctor prescribes them or you buy them over-the-counter; what your options are for paying for health care; and how to avoid fraud.

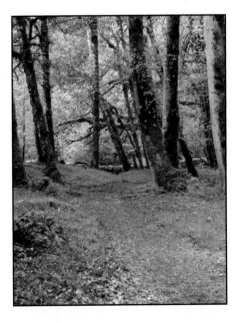

When you take responsibility for yourself, you also take responsibility for the conditions in which you live and that involves the planet we all share. It means first being aware of what causes pollution and then doing your part to reduce pollution and the other things that are posing a threat to the earth.

A number of government agencies can help in your quest to be responsible for yourself and your environment; this chapter lists some of them. You also can take many steps individually.

BEING A SMART HEALTH CONSUMER

Your level of wellness is dynamic. Throughout your life many factors — some controllable, some not — influence your state of wellness. It depends in part on:

— inherited conditions and your health at birth.
— your environment.
— your access to regular professional health care.
— your behavior and lifestyle.

You can do many things to influence your health, even to compensate for the factors you cannot control, such as heredity.

Among the many resources for information about your health are:

— your health-care professional (if your doctor does not volunteer the information, ask him or her).
— the library.
— information in newspapers, magazines, news programs, and health programs on radio or television.
— government agencies, such as the National Institutes of Health, the Centers for Disease Control and Prevention, the Environmental Protection Agency, and the Food and Drug Administration.
— voluntary health agencies, such as the American Heart Association and the American Cancer Society.
— labels on food and medications (by federal law, these labels, which provide certain health-related information, must be truthful and accurate).

— consumer action groups, which provide information on health-care fraud often will send up-to-date information as requested.

Self-Care

The growing trend toward **self-care** has stemmed from several factors.

❋ People want to be in control of their health, and more Americans than ever are learning the basics.

❋ The cost of health care has skyrocketed over the last decade, making self-care a necessity for many.

❋ *Prevention* has become a household term, and disease prevention entails many steps people can take on their own.

That does not mean you should stop going to the doctor. What it *does* mean is that you may be able to do some of the things you previously relied on health-care professionals to do. It also means being wise enough to know the difference. *Responsible* self-care involves:

— knowing whether you are sick enough to need a physician.
— checking your own vital signs (such as your pulse and your temperature).
— using home health tests that determine pregnancy and those that detect hidden blood in the stool.
— managing certain kinds of illnesses and injuries, such as common colds, indigestion, and minor abrasions.
— administering your own therapy, such as allergy shots, insulin for diabetes, and asthma treatments.
— preventing illness and injury.
— performing regular self-exams (such as monthly breast self-exam or testicle self-exam).
— promoting your own health and wellness — starting an exercise program, losing weight, or reducing stress.

Part of responsible self-care is knowing when self-care is no longer safe or smart. Knowing when you need to consult a health care provider is not always easy. Generally, you should seek medical help for any unusual symptoms that keep coming back, any serious injury or accident, unexplained

Using Home Health Tests

A number of health test kits on the market can be administered in the privacy of your own home. Used properly, most are accurate a high percentage of the time. To get the best results:

✳ Ask your pharmacist or physician about the test before you buy it; these pros are qualified to give advice and answer questions.

✳ Check the expiration date on the test before you buy it; expired test kits may not yield accurate results.

✳ Check the label before you leave the store; some test kits should be protected from heat, cold, or light.

✳ Read the instructions all the way through first, then follow directions carefully. If you're unsure about anything, talk to your pharmacist or doctor before using the test.

✳ If the test has to be timed, use a watch with a second hand.

✳ Write down your test results in case you need to compare against a second test later.

Note: As useful as home health tests can be, *they are not a substitute for professional testing or medical care.*

changes in weight, or any unexplained bleeding. You also should consult a health professional if you develop any sudden, severe, or persistent symptoms, including:

✳ Chest pain.

✳ Shortness of breath.

✳ Bluish skin, lips, or fingernails.

✳ Yellowing of skin or whites of the eyes.

✳ High fever (102°F in adults, 103°F in children).

✳ Any significant and persistent change in bowel or bladder habits.

✳ Diarrhea or vomiting that lasts more than 2 days or that comes back.

✳ A sore that does not heal.

✳ A lump, thickness, or swelling that gets bigger.

✳ Numbness, paralysis, or slurred speech.

✳ Allergic reactions to medication or an insect sting (severe swelling, dizziness, difficulty breathing, widespread hives, swelling of the throat or tongue).

✳ Injury to the head followed by loss of consciousness, vomiting, or blurred vision.

Over-the-Counter Medication

A number of medications once available only by prescription have been approved for use without a prescription. Examples are a medication to treat vaginal yeast infection and one for lice infestation. More than half a million products are available without a prescription, including cold remedies, laxatives, sleeping pills, antacids, pain medication, vitamin supplements, and athlete's foot lotion. That does not mean, however, that they are safe or effective in all situations.

All over-the-counter (OTC) medications are regulated by the Food and Drug Administration. For consumer protection the FDA requires that all OTC medications be packaged with a tamper-proof seal and that the package include information about:

— active ingredients
— strength
— amount of medication in the container
— appropriate dose
— indications for use
— side effects
— warnings
— expiration date

Further discussions of OTC medications is found in Chapter 13.

Access to Health Care

Health care in the United States is not available equally to all residents. One serious barrier is income. Many of the nation's poor cannot afford to go to the doctor, are too far from a health clinic, live in isolated areas, or cannot qualify for Medicaid or other subsidized programs. For some, the only health-care that is available is the hospital emergency room, using this facility for nonemergency health care. This adds to the problem of health care delivery from an already overburdened hospital staff. Figure 15.1 shows the percentage of various groups lacking a source of primary health care in 1992.

KEY TERMS

Self-care taking responsibility for one's own basic health care

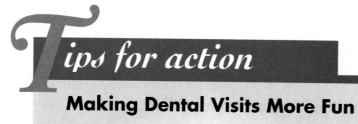

Making Dental Visits More Fun

American Health magazine offers the following tips.

❋ Use lip balm to keep your lips moist.

❋ Wear sunglasses to reduce glare from the dentist's lamp.

❋ Bring a portable stereo with headphones to distract you. Slow, rhythmic music is most relaxing.

of dentistry to earn a D.D.S. (Doctor of Dental Surgery) or a D.M.D. (Doctor of Medical Dentistry) degree. The dentist then must pass a state or regional licensing examination.

Some dentists choose to specialize, much like physicians do. Dental specialization requires additional coursework and clinical practice in the area of specialty. The specialties include:

❋ *Endodontics:* treating the interior of the tooth, including the pulp and root ("root canals")

❋ *Orthodontics:* straightening irregularities of the teeth (installing braces)

❋ *Periodontics:* treating diseases of the gum and bone, such as gingivitis and dental pyorrhea

❋ *Oral surgery:* operating to correct problems of the mouth, face, and jaw (such as removing impacted wisdom teeth)

The **dental hygienist** is a person who takes x-rays of the teeth, cleans and polishes the teeth, and teaches patients how to take care of their mouth and teeth.

Selecting a dentist requires just as much attention as selecting a physician, including recommendations from friends and family. The county dental society is another source for recommendations. If a dental school is established in your area, it can provide referrals. Again, the prospective patient should seek information concerning the office location, office hours, after-hours emergency care, billing procedures, and payment options. The dentist should examine your mouth thoroughly, explain all treatment options, and answer questions carefully in understandable terms. The dentist's office should be clean, and

Fluoride Alert

If children drink only bottled water, they may not be getting enough *fluoride*, the mineral that strengthens tooth enamel and prevents tooth decay. Researchers at the University of Texas in Houston found that only six brands of bottled water provide the recommended level of fluoride. Reverse osmosis home water filters can take most of the fluoride out of your drinking water.

Source: *American Health*, December 1994.

Tips for action

Boosting Oral Health

To maintain healthy teeth and gums:

❋ Brush and floss the right way every day — after every meal, if possible.

❋ Eat more whole-grain products, fresh fruits and vegetables, low-fat dairy products, lean meats, and dried peas and beans. Cut down on sugars, sweetened drinks, sweet snacks, and foods that stick to your teeth.

❋ Watch for signs of trouble — chronic bad breath, a persistent bad taste in the mouth, aching teeth, loose teeth, or gums that are red, swollen, or bleeding.

❋ Get regular dental check-ups and attend to necessary dental work.

anyone who touches the inside of the mouth — the dentist, any assistants, and the dental hygienist — should wear a mask and latex gloves to prevent the transmission of pathogens.

Podiatrists

Podiatrists diagnose and treat conditions of the feet, including corns, bunions, calluses, and malformations. Podiatrists complete an undergraduate degree, then a 4-year academic and clinical program at an accredited school of podiatry. They earn either a D.P.M. (Doctor of Podiatric Medicine) or D.P. (Doctor of Podiatry) degree. Podiatrists can take x-rays, prescribe medication, prescribe therapies and therapeutic devices (such as corrective shoes), and perform surgery on the foot.

Optometrists

Optometrists complete an accredited academic and clinical program and receive an O.D. (Doctor of Optometry) degree. Then they must be licensed to practice. These practitioners examine the eyes, diagnose defects in eyesight, and prescribe eyeglasses or contact lenses to correct vision. They are *not* trained physicians, like ophthalmologists, who can prescribe medication, treat diseases of the eye, and perform surgery.

Psychologists

Clinical **psychologists** complete both an undergraduate and a graduate program leading to the Ph.D. (doctorate in psychology). In most states psychologists also must be certified or licensed before they can practice. In many states they must meet further requirements. Many also earn credentials from professional societies and organizations. Psychologists specialize in treating a variety of emotional and behavioral disorders *without* medication. They work with patients in individual or group settings and many practice family or marriage counseling. Unlike psychiatrists, who hold the M.D. degree, psychologists are not allowed to prescribe or dispense medication.

Chiropractors

Chiropractors employ a variety of techniques to manipulate the spine and relieve pain. As a science, **chiropractic medicine** is founded on the belief that vital life forces flow from the spine to all parts of the body and misalignment of the spine interrupts these life

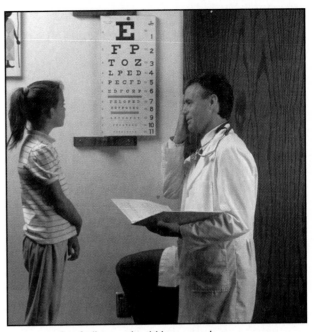

People of all ages should have regular eye exams.

forces. Chiropractic methods often are successful in treating certain disorders, such as pain in the neck or lower back.

Chiropractors complete an intensive 6-year academic program — emphasizing anatomy, physiology, biochemistry, and nutrition — combined with hands-on experience. They earn a D.C. (Doctor of Chiropractic) degree. They are licensed and regulated by the states in which they practice. They are not allowed to prescribe or dispense medication or perform surgery. Chiropractors should adhere to standard chiropractic regimens, though specific techniques may differ.

Nurses

Nursing is concerned with providing information and services that restore, maintain, or promote

KEY TERMS

Dental hygienist health-care specialist who takes x-rays, cleans and polishes the teeth and teaches proper dental care

Podiatrist Specialist who diagnoses and treats problems of the feet

Optometrist licensed practitioner who examines the eyes, diagnoses problems, and prescribes eyeglasses or contact lenses

Psychologist specialist in treating emotional and behavioral disorders without medication

Chiropractor health-care practitioner who manipulates the spine to relieve pain

Chiropractic medicine science founded on the belief that life forces flow from the spine to the rest of the body

What to Expect During an Examination

What should you expect from your next check-up? Your doctor should:

- ☐ Quiz you about major illnesses you've had, complaints you have now, drugs you're taking, any risky behaviors you engage in, allergies you have.
- ☐ Check your skin for moistness, elasticity, and sores.
- ☐ Check your pulse and blood pressure.
- ☐ Check your eyes, ears, mouth, and nose with a flashlight, looking for signs of infection or disease.
- ☐ Check your neck for lumps in the thyroid gland or swollen lymph nodes.
- ☐ Listen to your heart and lungs with a stethoscope.
- ☐ Probe your abdomen for tenderness, rigidity, or hernia.
- ☐ Use a gloved finger to feel inside your rectum (a check for rectal cancer and an enlarged prostate gland).
- ☐ Check your joints for reflexes, swelling, or deformity.

If you're a woman, you can also expect a breast exam (the doctor will check for abnormal lumps) and a pelvic exam (the doctor will check the vagina and cervix for signs of disease).

---

wellness and prevent illness. Nursing services are generally provided in a hospital, clinic, school, work site, or private physician's office. As with other disciplines, nursing has specialty areas that require additional classroom and clinical preparation.

The **registered nurse**, or R.N., completes an academic and clinical program at a college or school of nursing. The nurse then must pass a state licensing examination. In most areas the entry-level requirement for nursing is a college degree (B.S.N.) or associate degree in nursing.

Registered nurses who specialize in a clinical area and who diagnose and treat patients independent of a physician are called **nurse practitioners**. Examples are the family planning nurse practitioner and the certified nurse midwife. Nurse practitioners are required to complete advanced academic and clinical training. Many have master's or doctoral degrees in nursing. While they work under a physician's supervision, they perform many basic diagnostic and treatment procedures and prescribe medications, freeing physicians to handle more complex cases.

The **licensed practical nurse** (LPN) and **licensed vocational nurse** (LVN) have fewer educational requirements and a much shorter training period than the registered nurse — usually 12 to 18 months in a hospital-based program. Each must pass a state board examination

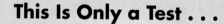

Tips for action

This Is Only a Test . . .

Before you agree to any medical test, find out:

- ❋ *Exactly* why the test is necessary.
- ❋ What the doctor expects to learn from the test.
- ❋ Whether the doctor could learn the same thing some other way.
- ❋ How long the test will take.
- ❋ What the test is going to feel like. (How much pain is involved? Will you be restricted afterward? How long before you can get back to your normal activities?)
- ❋ What risks are involved.
- ❋ How reliable the test is.

before being able to work as a nurse. Their scope of practice is limited, and they must be supervised by a registered nurse or a physician.

Allied Health-Care Professionals

Some of the allied health-care professionals and paraprofessionals who help patients maintain and restore health are:

❋ nursing aides and physician assistants

❋ medical technologists

❋ emergency medical technicians

❋ x-ray technicians

❋ occupational therapists

❋ physical therapists

❋ operating room technicians

❋ phlebotomists

❋ respiratory and inhalation therapists

Although not all of these areas of specialization require a college degree, all do require from 1 to 5 years of specialized post-high school training. Many programs provide hospital-based training that leads to a college degree or associate degree. Most allied health-care professionals must pass state or national licensing examinations before they are allowed to work in their field.

HOW TO CHOOSE HEALTH-CARE FACILITIES

People who live in rural areas may have access to only a single health-care facility. Those who live in urban areas may be able to choose from a private physician's office, a clinic, a nonprofit hospital, a for-profit hospital, a teaching hospital, a college health center, an outpatient surgery center, and a freestanding emergency center. Home health care may be available in some situations. The choice of a facility should be based on availability, convenience, the specific medical needs, ability to pay, and whether your physician has staff privileges at the facility.

Important distinctions between health-care facilities are given in Table 15.2.

Prescription Jargon

Here's a quick translation of the abbreviations on your prescription:

R$_x$	take
c̄	with
a.c.	before meals
p.c.	after meals
cap.	capsule
tab.	tablet
gtt.	drop
h.s.	at bedtime
q.4.h.	every four hours
in.d.	daily
b.i.s.	twice a day
t.i.d.	three times a day
q.i.d.	four times a day
p.r.n.	as the circumstances may require

Prescription Medication

Prescription medications are drugs legally available only with the permission of a physician or other health practitioner who is authorized to make a diagnosis and prescribe a medication for treatment. Prescription medications regulated by both the Food and Drug Administration and the Drug Enforcement Agency are those that have psychoactive properties and the potential to be abused. All prescription drugs bear the following warning on the label: *Caution: Federal law prohibits dispensing without prescription.* That does not apply only to practitioners. Strictly speaking, it is against the law for anyone to share prescription medication with

---

KEY TERMS

Registered nurse health care practitioner who provides information and services that promote or restore health and wellness

Nurse practitioner registered nurse who diagnoses and treats patients independent of a physician

Licensed practical nurse (LPN) and Licensed vocational nurse (LVN) nurses with shortened training period and limited responsibility

Prescription medications drugs that are legal only when authorized by a physician or qualified health care practitioner

---

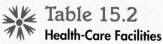

Table 15.2
Health-Care Facilities

Facility	Description
Clinics	A group of practitioners work together in a single facility; they may cover only one specialty (such as internal medicine) or many specialties. Some include dental offices, x-ray facilities, and a pharmacy.
Nonprofit Hospitals	Generally administered by religious or other humanitarian groups, these hospitals provide care for patients regardless of whether the patient can pay for services.
For-Profit Hospitals	These hospitals are owned by a group of people or shareholders. They provide far less care for patients who are unable to pay. They generally stabilize such patients, then transfer them to nonprofit facilities.
Teaching Hospitals	Affiliated with schools of medicine, these facilities provide a setting where students can study and practice alongside their professors. "Experimental" treatments and medications often are more available at teaching hospitals, used as part of studies and research programs. Teaching hospitals generally treat patients regardless of their ability to pay.
College Health Centers	These facilities are affiliated with colleges and universities. Some provide services only to students; others extend services to staff, faculty, students, and family members. They range in size from small dispensaries to large multispecialty clinics. Patients generally receive treatment at a discount or for a co-pay.
Outpatient Surgery Centers	These facilities handle minor, low-risk surgical procedures that do not require the patient to stay overnight, such as vasectomies, breast biopsies, cataract removal, tonsillectomies, cosmetic surgery, hernia repair, D&Cs, and therapeutic abortions. Approximately 40% of all surgical procedures can be handled in these facilities. Those requiring prolonged anesthesia, complex skills, or extensive post-surgery care must be handled in a traditional hospital.
Freestanding Emergency Centers	These are "emergency rooms" that usually are not part of a hospital but tend to be affiliated with one. Patients can get urgent care quickly and at less cost than traditional emergency room, where they must become part of the hospital system.
Home Health Care	In some situations, physicians and other practitioners can arrange for patients to be cared for at home. Procedures such as dialysis and chemotherapy can be administered at home at a much lower cost than in the hospital. Approximately 80% of all insurance companies now pay for health aides, nurses, and other practitioners who give care in the home.

someone else. The only person who is legally permitted to take a prescription drug is the one for whom it was prescribed (Caution: Federal law prohibits transfer of this drug to any person other than the patient for whom prescribed).

For a consumer to get a prescription medication legally, the practitioner writes an order that the patient takes to a pharmacist to be filled. The order is commonly called the **prescription**. Prescriptions are written in a type of "shorthand" of the profession that pharmacists are trained to translate.

To get the intended benefits from prescription medications, these must be taken exactly according to the directions on the prescription label. The doctor should explain how to take the medication. Upon obtaining the medication from the pharmacist, the patient should ask for any additional information that is important to know. Some medications, for example, must be taken with food or milk, others on an empty stomach. The most important advice is: *Finish taking your prescription.* Many antibiotics, for example, help a person feel better within a few days, but they must be continued for a full 10 days to completely kill the pathogen that caused the illness. Otherwise the infection may recur.

Tips for action

A Spoonful of Sugar . . .

. . . helps the medicine go down. Try these suggestions:

❋ **To take tablets or capsules:**

Stand or sit up straight. Sip some water to moisten your mouth and throat first, then swallow the tablet with a mouthful of water. Follow up with a glass of water. If the tablet feels "stuck," eat a piece of bread or a banana, then drink more water. Capsules float, so tilt your head slightly forward for easier swallowing.

❋ **To use nose drops:**

Tilt your head back. Breathing through your mouth, put the drops in your nostrils. Gently breathe in through your nose. Keep your head tilted back a few minutes.

❋ **To use eye drops or ointment:**

Tilt your head back. Pull your lower eyelid down and look toward the ceiling. Put the drops or ointment in the "pouch" formed by your lower lid, then close your eye gently. Wipe away any excess with a tissue.

❋ **To use ear drops:**

Tilt your head so the ear points up; grasp your ear lobe and pull it down and back to straighten the ear canal. Put in the drops. Keep your head tilted a few minutes, then place a loose cotton plug at the opening of your ear to keep the drops from running out.

Note: Wash your hands thoroughly before and after using any nose, eye, or ear drops, and never let the dropper touch your body.

To keep medications potent, they should be stored away from direct sunlight, hot temperatures, and humidity. The prescription should be kept in its original container so the directions for use will be handy and others (family members, roommates) will not take the medication by mistake.

Avoiding Problems With Prescription Drugs

When the doctor prescribes a drug, patients should mention any other medications they are taking. Serious problems can arise when some medications are taken at the same time. The same concept applies to food and drink. Serious (even life-threatening) interactions can take place if a person drinks or eats certain foods when taking certain medications. The doctor and the pharmacist can provide the needed information.

In general, problems with prescription drugs can be avoided by:

❋ Taking any current medications along to a doctor's appointment; these drugs may have affected your current symptoms and may make a difference in what your doctor prescribes.

❋ Taking only the prescribed amount of medication at the prescribed times. If you have problems remembering when you take the medication, write it down.

❋ Checking with the doctor or pharmacist before opening capsules or crushing tablets. Some medications are not supposed to dissolve in the mouth.

❋ Asking about possible food interactions. If you are supposed to take the medicine on an empty stomach, take it at least an hour before you eat or 2 hours *after* you eat.

❋ Never drinking alcohol or hot beverages when you take medication.

KEY TERMS

Prescription written order authorizing a pharmacist to dispense medication

✳ Watching for signs of an allergic reaction. Although reactions are not common, they can be serious. Call your doctor if you develop nausea, vomiting, weakness, a widespread rash or hives, or pale (ashy) skin after taking medication.

Brand-Name Versus Generic Medication

A **generic drug** is a medication that is chemically equivalent to the brand-name drug for which it is a substitute. It is also **bioequivalent**, which means the body absorbs and uses it at the same rate and to the same extent as the brand-name drug. Generic drugs also must deliver the same amount of active ingredients into the patient's bloodstream in the same amount of time, and they must be approved by the FDA.

Certain generic medications may not work as well as the brand name originals.

Generic drugs in general are less expensive, mostly because manufacturers of generic drugs do not have to repeat the extensive clinical trials that were used in developing the brand-name drug. Though the active ingredients are the same, the fillers and binders used in generic drugs usually differ from those in brand-name drugs — which can affect how quickly they are absorbed or can make them less potent. Some people are allergic to the binders and fillers used in the generic substitute.

When a drug is first placed on the market, it is patented for 17 years. That means no one can manufacture another drug with the same chemical formulation during the first 17 years. Only when the patent has expired can other pharmaceutical companies manufacture generic versions of brand-name drugs. For that reason, some drugs currently on the market do not have generic versions.

Certain generic medications may not work as well as the brand-name originals. Doctors generally advise patients to stick with brand names for drugs to control epilepsy, other seizure conditions, heart problems, and psychiatric conditions.

CONSUMER FINANCING: WHO PAYS FOR HEALTH CARE?

More than 80 million Americans have chronic health problems that should be monitored and treated regularly by a physician. All Americans have the potential of needing professional medical care at some time in their lives. Some people can afford to pay cash for the medical or dental services they need, but they are certainly the exception. Most people in this country need help covering the skyrocketing cost of medical care. Some qualify for Medicaid, Medicare, or other government programs. Others have private health insurance and pay **premiums** (regular payments) to an insurance company, which then covers a percentage of the cost for surgery, hospitalization, or other medical care that may be needed.

Enrollment in a health insurance plan does not guarantee quality health care. For one thing, the insurance plan restricts the kind of care the insured person can receive. Clients must have prior authorization for many procedures, and almost all insurance plans have limits on what they will pay. In addition, few insurance plans will pay for preventive services, and almost none pay for what they consider "experimental" procedures (such as bone marrow transplants). Health insurance *does* help cover the cost of medical care if all the necessary requirements are met.

Health Insurance

Health insurance policies are either **individual policies** (on your own) or **group policies** (combining the buying power of others, such as those at a place of employment). Health insurance does not automatically pay all the costs for a person's health care. All plans have certain restrictions. Depending on the health insurance, some or all of the following may apply:

✳ *Waiting period:* the amount of time that must pass after purchasing the policy before the insurance company will pay. For example, the waiting period may be 3 months; the newly insured would have to pay the full cost of any health care during that time.

✳ *Exclusion for preexisting conditions:* the circumstances under which the insurance company will pay the cost of medical conditions the insured person had at the time the policy was bought. Some companies specify a waiting time; for example, they will begin to pay for

Making Health Insurance Work for You

To get the most out of your monthly premium to your health insurance company:

❋ Obtain necessary approvals ahead of time. If you don't, you'll end up paying the whole amount.

❋ Follow the rules. If a particular claim form is provided, use it. If you are required to go to certain doctors, choose them.

❋ Keep the company informed about changes in your life, such as marriage, divorce, or addition of a child. A waiting period may be involved.

❋ Plan ahead. Don't cancel one insurance policy before you've satisfied the waiting period for another one.

❋ Keep good records. If your insurance company refuses to pay a claim that it should, you have the right to dispute it and will need the documentation.

❋ Pay all your premiums on time. You can't afford to be canceled.

❋ Be absolutely truthful. If you lie or withhold important health information, your company can refuse to pay your claim or cancel your policy.

---

preexisting conditions after 6 months. Others never will pay for preexisting conditions.

❋ *Deductible:* the part of the bill that has to be paid before the insurance starts to pay. For example, the insured might have to pay for the first $200 in medical care for each family member each year before the insurance will pay anything.

❋ *Co-payment:* a set dollar amount the insured is required to pay for each doctor's visit. For example, the insured may have to pay $10 or $20 for each visit to the doctor, and the insurance pays the rest of the bill.

❋ *Co-insurance:* shared cost of medical care between the insured and the insurance company on a set percentage determined by the insurance company. For example, the insured may be required to pay 20% of all medical costs, regardless of how high they are, and the insurance company will pay the other 80%.

❋ *Fixed indemnity:* a limit the insurance company will pay for certain procedures. For example, the company may have a limit of $1,200 for prenatal care; if the

cost of prenatal care is $1,500, the insured will have to pay the additional $300.

❋ *Exclusions:* the procedures for which the insurance will not pay. For example, the insurance company may not pay for infertility testing and treatment.

❋ *Major medical coverage:* an amount the insurance will pay if the insured has a catastrophic condition and has exceeded the regular benefits.

❋ *Lifetime limit:* the total amount the insurance company will pay. For example, the policy may have a lifetime limit of $300,000; once the company has paid $300,000 of the medical costs, it will pay no more.

KEY TERMS

Generic drug chemically equivalent medication substituted for a brand-name drug

Bioequivalent generic drug that the body can absorb and use at the same rate and level as a brand-name drug

Premiums payments to an insurance company for a percentage coverage of future medical expenses

Individual policy health insurance purchased by a person

Group policy health insurance purchased by a group of individuals, usually through a place of employment, and at a reduced rate

The three general types of health insurance plans are: private fee-for-service plans; private prepaid group plans; and public/governmental plans.

Private Fee-For-Service Plans

With this kind of plan, the insured pays a premium to the insurance company. The insurance company then pays its part of the insured's medical bills directly to the people or facilities that provide them. The practitioner or the facility sets the fees. The insured is free to use any practitioner or facility that accepts that insurance.

A variety of the fee-for-service plan is the **PPO**, or **preferred provider organization**. Simply, the insurance company contracts with various physicians and hospitals; those physicians and hospitals in turn agree to charge a set fee for the services provided. The patient must receive any health care from a doctor or hospital that has contracted with the insurance company or the insurance company will not pay for the health care.

Private Prepaid Group Plans

In group plans the insured pays a monthly fee to a group practice, such as an **HMO (health maintenance organization)**. Once the insured has paid that monthly fee, he or she can use the services of practitioners in the HMO as many times as needed. The insured is not charged a fee for each service but is limited, of course, to the physicians who participate in the HMO. HMOs traditionally have been able to provide medical care at reduced cost because they emphasize preventive behaviors and they try various treatments before hospitalizing patients.

The trend is toward "open" HMOs, which allow their members to seek medical care from physicians outside the HMO. Patients who choose another doctor usually pay between 20% and 30% of the bill to that physician, and the insurance policy pays the remainder.

Public/Governmental Plans

One example of a public insurance plan is **Medicare**, established in 1965 by President Lyndon Johnson to help people over the age of 65 to pay their hospital bills. Part A of Medicare, which covers hospital room

and board, is paid by Social Security taxes and is available to anyone over 65 who qualifies. Part B, which covers fees to doctors and other medical services during hospitalization, is optional; the consumer must pay the premium for Part B.

In an attempt to contain costs of Medicare, the federal government in 1983 instituted a system of paying the hospital bill called **diagnosis-related groups** (DRGs). When a Medicare patient is admitted to the hospital, the price of the care is determined already by the DRG under which the patient is admitted. If the actual cost for the patient is less than the preset DRG, the hospital makes money. If the hospital stay is longer than expected or the bill exceeds the set amount, the hospital loses money. The federal government has developed almost 500 DRGs.

A second public health plan is **Medicaid**. This plan provides limited coverage for people who cannot afford to pay for medical services — the medically indigent. It is financed through funds from the federal government combined with contributions from each state. Eligibility for Medicaid is based on income. Figure 15.2 shows the percentage of health insurance coverage for people age 64 and younger by type of coverage.

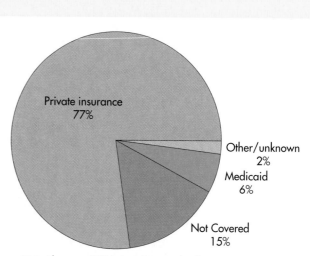

Note: These are 1986 data. Percent distribution is approximate because of overlap among categories.

Source: *Healthy People 2000: Summary Report*, based on *Health, United States, 1989* and *Prevention Profile* (U.S. Department of Health and Human Services, Public Health Service).

Figure 15.2 Health insurance coverage, age 64 and younger, by type of coverage

MEDICAL QUACKERY AND HEALTH CARE FRAUD

Caveat Emptor (Let the Buyer Beware)

Millions of dollars are lost each year to medical and health fraud — much of it to **quackery**, unproven practices that claim to cure diseases. In some cases people are desperate and searching for a miracle when traditional medicine has failed them. In other cases patients (often elderly or less educated people) are taken advantage of intentionally by unscrupulous practitioners known as **quacks**. Regardless of the reason, the patients lose money. They also lose time — time that could mean the difference between successfully managing the health problem and death.

Those engaging in health care fraud promote devices, treatments, medication, and services that are worthless. Some are licensed practitioners, but most have little or no training in the medical field. Quacks have the ability to convince consumers that they are concerned about a patient's health status, and that the product or service they offer will effect a cure.

According to the FDA, which is charged with protecting consumers against health fraud, the ten most common health frauds in the United States are:

1. Arthritis products
2. Cancer clinics
3. AIDS cures
4. Weight-loss schemes
5. Sexual aids
6. Baldness remedies
7. Nutritional cures
8. Chelation therapy
9. Muscle stimulators
10. Candidiasis hypersensitivity

Contrary to popular belief, almost anyone can be the victim of a quack. Regardless of income, level of education, and experience, a person can be taken in. The best defense is sound knowledge about the products and services you are seeking — and the ability to spot the common signs of medical quackery. In general, a medical quack may:

* promise a quick cure or guarantee

* diagnose a health problem by mail
* change office locations or mailing addresses often
* try to sell you one product to cure a wide variety of conditions
* say a product will cure a condition for which no known cure exists (such as AIDS or certain kinds of cancer)
* claim to be persecuted or harassed by the government or the medical community
* say you must pay in advance
* use testimonials from previous "patients" or "clients" (a legitimate medical practitioner knows that what patients say is confidential)
* try to frighten you about legitimate products or services
* use titles such as "professor" or "specialist" that could be confused with legitimate credentials.

Nutritional Fraud

Americans are bombarded with so much conflicting information about nutrition that knowing what to believe is difficult. The best sources of accurate, current information are:

* registered dietitians
* college faculty members who teach food science or nutrition
* licensed dietitians in colleges, businesses, hospitals, and nursing homes
* cooperative extension agents in county extension offices

KEY TERMS

Preferred provider organization (PPO) insurance plan in which the insured must obtain medical treatment from health-care workers with whom the insurance company has contracted services

Health maintenance organization (HMO) name denoting a group practice with emphasis on preventive medicine

Medicare public insurance plan for people over age 65

Diagnosis-related groups (DRG) a system of predetermined payment made by Medicare based on the patient's diagnosis

Medicaid public insurance plan for people who cannot afford medical care

Quackery/quack use of unproven methods of curing diseases/ unqualified practitioners who take advantage of patients for their money

---

Protect Yourself from Quacks

To avoid being a victim of medical fraud:

✱ Don't abandon medical treatment even if you think it's not working. If you want to try something else, do it *in addition* to what your doctor has prescribed.

✱ Don't agree to pay in advance for *anything*. Quacks want you to pay up front because they know your insurance policy will not pay — and neither will you when you catch on.

✱ Don't agree to unorthodox tests to diagnose disease.

✱ Ignore testimonials. Ask for published reports in legitimate journals that confirm the claim.

✱ If you have questions about a new treatment, ask your doctor or write to a professional organization such as the American Cancer Society.

In general, people should avoid anyone who is prescribing or selling vitamins out of an office or door-to-door; suggesting hair analysis as a basis for determining nutritional needs; using a computer-scored nutrition deficiency test as a basis for prescribing vitamins; or offering nutritional tests and products through the mail. Health food stores often offer unsound nutritional advice, and some chiropractors, doctors, and dentists venture outside their practice, using unproven diagnostic tools and treatments.

AGENCIES THAT PROTECT CONSUMERS

Various official agencies and organizations have been created to protect consumers against health and medical fraud. Their scope varies. Governmental agencies are charged with enforcing regulations, making inspections, and suspending the services of violators. Voluntary and nongovernmental organizations monitor, advise, and provide consumer information and education.

Governmental or Official Agencies

The agencies discussed next have the primary responsibility for consumer protection.

Food and Drug Administration (FDA)

Part of the U. S. Public Health Service, the FDA ensures the safety of foods and food products and the safety and effectiveness of drugs, cosmetics, and medical devices and equipment. The FDA has jurisdiction over all products sold in interstate commerce. It has the authority to:

✱ approve new drugs

✱ inspect plants where products are made

✱ set safety standards for diagnostic equipment

✱ set regulations for the proper labeling of foods, drugs, and cosmetics

✱ issue warnings to the public when a product is found to be unsafe

✱ request manufacturers to recall products

✱ take legal action against those in violation of the law

Environmental Protection Agency (EPA)

The U.S. **Environmental Protection Agency** has broad-based regulatory and enforcement powers over environmental matters. Its jurisdiction covers indoor and outdoor air pollution, pollution of water supplies, chemical waste, pesticides, radiation, electromagnetic fields, nuclear waste, radon gas, and noise pollution.

Federal Trade Commission (FTC)

The **FTC** is an independent federal agency organized to protect consumers through the Bureaus of Consumer Protection, Competition, and Economics.

One of the most vital functions of the Bureau of Consumer Protection is to control advertising. If the FTC decides that a company's advertising methods are deceptive or false, the FTC has the authority to investigate, then seek a court order to stop the advertising if the company will not do it voluntarily.

U.S. Postal Service

The Postal Service is responsible for protecting consumers from mail fraud and deception. It has the authority to file complaints and seek legal remedies to prevent unscrupulous vendors from using the U.S. mail to advertise or ship worthless products and services.

Nongovernmental/Voluntary Agencies

The **Better Business Bureau (BBB)** is a not-for-profit organization composed of member businesses that operate to ensure fair and reputable business practices in a locality. It has offices in the major cities and is listed in the White Pages of the telephone directory. One of its functions is to share with its members and consumers information about companies and their business practices.

Because the BBB is a voluntary agency, it has no legal powers. It is a clearinghouse for information and a place where consumers may register complaints. The BBB does not endorse or recommend products or services. If consumers have concerns or doubts about a business, a promoter, or a business practice, however, they can call the BBB for information before making a decision to purchase. In addition, the BBB offers a wide variety of pamphlets for consumer education and mediation services.

PROTECTING OUR ENVIRONMENTAL HEALTH

Our environmental resources are abundant, but they are limited. They must be protected and preserved today so they will not be depleted for future generations. Various threats to life on earth are

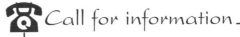

Call for information

Environmental Protection Agency
202-260-2090

Council on Environmental Quality
202-395-5750

explored in the following pages. The common thread running through all these threats is pollution — the pollutants we release into the environment as a result of the cars we drive, the products we manufacture and use, and the wastes we generate.

Air Pollution

Exhaust from gasoline engines, black clouds belched out of industrial smokestacks, and chemicals released during manufacturing processes hang in the air over the earth, clogging it with **particulates** (tiny solid or liquid particles) that can contribute to respiratory disease, heart disease, cancer, and life-threatening changes in the immune system. Elderly people, people with chronic health problems, cigarette smokers, and people with existing respiratory diseases are at even greater risk.

The problem worsens when Mother Nature deals a blow known as **thermal inversion**. In thermal inversion a layer of warm air covers a layer of colder air, trapping pollutants and smog so they cannot rise from lower levels. Dangerous pollutants in the air remain close to the earth's surface, where they increase health risks.

KEY TERMS

Environmental Protection Agency (EPA) federal office with regulatory and enforcement powers over environmental matters

Federal Trade Commission (FTC) U.S. Agency organized to protect consumers

Better Business Bureau (BBB) not-for-profit organization composed of member businesses that promote fair and reputable business practices in a locality

Particulates tiny solid or liquid particles in the air that can cause serious health problems

Thermal inversion atmospheric condition that occurs when a layer of warm air covers a layer of cold air and holds particulates at lower levels

Another serious problem is **acid rain**, rain that falls through air polluted by sulfur dioxide and nitrogen dioxide. It is gradually acidifying the water in lakes and streams, making them unable to support life. Pollutants — most significantly nitric acid and sulfuric acid that result from burning fossil fuels and smelting nickel and copper ore — rise into the atmosphere and can be carried far from their source. Eventually they fall to earth in rain, sleet, and snow, or hang in the air in the form of mist or fog. This polluted precipitation is destroying some forests, acidifying lakes and streams, and corroding manmade structures such as buildings and monuments.

The form of air pollution most familiar to Americans is probably **smog**, a brownish or grayish fog produced by chemical pollutants in the air. Smog develops when pollutants in the air react with sunlight, resulting in a dense, foggy cloud. Smog has been known to irritate the eyes and lungs and impair immunity. It can be hazardous to people with chronic respiratory diseases (such as emphysema, bronchitis, and lung cancer).

Smog comes in two different "colors":

1. Gray smog (called **sulfur-dioxide smog**) results from burning oil that has high sulfur content. It is most common in the eastern United States and Europe.

2. Brown smog (called **photochemical smog**) results when the nitric oxide in automobile exhaust reacts with oxygen in the air. The end

What's Polluting Our Air?

The top sources of air pollution are:

❋ **Carbon monoxide and hydrocarbons** from internal combustion engines.

❋ **Sulfur dioxide** from coal-powered smelters, refineries, industrial plants, and electrical generating stations.

❋ **Ozone** produced from the reaction of nitrogen dioxide and hydrogen chloride.

❋ **Nitrogen dioxide** from motor vehicle exhaust and coal-powered electrical boilers.

❋ **Lead** from motor vehicle exhaust and lead smelter emissions.

❋ **Smog** from a combination of smoke and fog.

product is nitrogen dioxide, which becomes a brownish haze when exposed to sunlight. Exposure to sunlight also results in the formation of other pollutants, most notably ozone. (Among its other effects, ozone reduces plant yields in tomato, bean, soybean, snap bean, peanut, and corn crops; causes premature leaf dropping and lower growth rates in forests; and causes cracking of rubber products, weakening of textiles, changes in dyes, and premature cracking of paint.) Photochemical smog is most common in densely populated traffic centers of the world.

Tips for action

Mixing Exercise and Air Pollution (of course not)

When the air is polluted, think twice about exercising outside. Deep breathing and increased blood circulation involved in exercise circulate pollutants more quickly through the body. Instead:

❋ Keep workouts brief.

❋ Avoid heavy exertion.

❋ Stay off heavily congested streets, especially between noon and 4 p.m.

❋ Exercise early in the morning or late at night, when most traffic has cleared.

If you have asthma, chronic bronchitis, other chronic lung disease, or heart disease, limit your workouts to indoors.

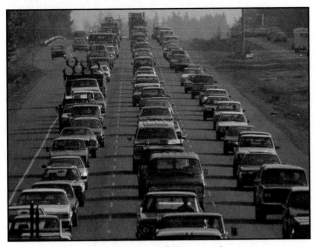

The number-one air pollutant in urban areas is automobile exhaust.

To Prevent Carbon Monoxide Poisoning

❋ Have your furnace checked by a professional before you turn it on for the season.

❋ Have all natural gas appliances and wood-burning stoves professionally installed and maintained.

❋ Never use an oven to heat your home, cabin, or recreational vehicle.

❋ Never burn charcoal inside — not even in a small hibachi grill.

❋ Make sure you have proper fresh-air ventilation when using a wood-burning stove, fireplace, space heater, or gasoline-powered engine.

Indoor Air Pollution

Pollution that occurs indoors can impair health seriously. The tendency for people to conserve energy by insulating their homes well has increased the risk for indoor air pollution. The problem is worse during cold weather, when people take extra precautions to seal and insulate their homes. Indoor pollution is suspected as a cause in the increase in asthma cases in recent years.

Carbon monoxide poisoning A colorless, taste-less, odorless, poisonous gas, **carbon monoxide** results from the incomplete combustion of fuel in furnaces, water heaters, space heaters, and engines. When inhaled, it reduces the oxygen level of the blood. If breathed in high enough concentrations, it is fatal. In its early stages carbon monoxide poisoning causes symptoms much like those of the flu: dizziness, weakness, fatigue, nausea, and vomiting. Carbon monoxide poisoning should be suspected if all members of a family are stricken.

Asbestos A mineral that once was widely used as an insulating material and fire retardant in build-ings, **asbestos** now has been banned in new construction. In addition, materials containing asbestos have been removed from schools and other public buildings. Researchers finally discov-ered that microscopic asbestos particles and fibers were being released into the air, where unsuspect-ing victims inhaled them. The result sometimes was lung cancer and **asbestosis**, a progressive and fatal lung disease. Because this disease did not appear

for 20 to 30 years, countless people were exposed to the hazard in the meantime.

Asbestos was used most commonly in attics and crawl spaces, around furnaces, and to insulate pipes. People should never touch asbestos. If its presence in a house is suspected, it should be profes-sionally inspected. A professional can recommend whether to seal the asbestos or to have it removed.

Lead Lead — once used in gasoline, paint, and food containers — has been shown to cause major health problems, especially in children. An esti-mated 98% of the lead in the atmosphere comes from burning leaded gasoline. Other common sources of lead are:

❋ Paint (an estimated 57 million houses and apartment buildings still have lead paint)

KEY TERMS

Acid rain rain that falls through air polluted by sulfur diox-ide and nitrogen dioxide and carries it into groundwater

Smog brown or gray fog caused by chemical pollutants

Sulfur-dioxide smog gray smog caused by burning oil with a high sulfur content

Photochemical smog brown smog caused when auto-mobile exhaust containing nitric oxide reacts with oxygen and forms nitrogen dioxide

Carbon monoxide colorless, tasteless, odorless, poison-ous gas

Asbestos a mineral formerly used in construction as an insulator; now known to be toxic

Asbestosis progressive and fatal lung disease caused by inhaling microscopic asbestos particles

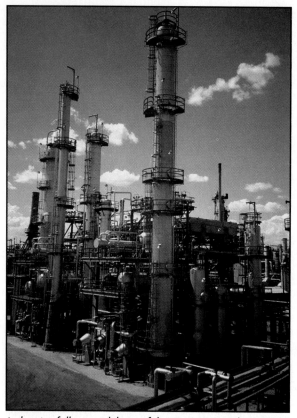

Industries follow guidelines of the Environmental Protection Agency (EPA) to prevent air and water pollution.

of blood for adults, and 10 micrograms per deciliter for children. The average American probably has 5 to 6 micrograms per deciliter in the blood.

For some reason, lead poisoning affects African Americans disproportionately. African American male children have the highest lead exposure and blood lead levels of any measured group in the United States.

Mercury Prior to 1990, when it was banned, mercury was added to latex paints to prevent the growth of mold and mildew. Researchers now have documented cases of **mercury poisoning** among those who use latex paint containing mercury. Health effects include peeling skin, aching limbs, hand tremors, profuse sweating, and racing pulse. Although some concern has been expressed over amalgam dental fillings, which contain mercury, long-term studies have not confirmed that these fillings pose a health threat.

Formaldehyde **Formaldehyde** is an invisible gas used in home insulation, building materials (including plywood and particle board), carpet backing, and some furniture. The vapors and emissions from these materials have been shown to cause eye and lung irritation, headache, dizziness, and nausea. In tests on animals, formaldehyde has caused cancer.

※ Pipes (water that flows through lead pipes or pipes soldered with lead becomes contaminated with lead)

※ Glazes on some ceramic cookware and dishes

※ Imported metal cans (lead is used in the solder)

Once lead enters the body, it is absorbed by the bones. In high enough concentrations, it causes **lead poisoning**. The results are damage to the liver, kidneys, and major systems — including the nervous, cardiovascular, gastrointestinal, reproductive, and immune systems. In children, lead can retard intellectual development, resulting in impaired math and language skills, motor skills, and the ability to concentrate.

Lead is a natural metal, and it lasts forever in the environment. For most, lead in the body has come from past exposure to products such as leaded gasoline or leaded paint dust. Lead toxicity is associated with levels as low as 30 micrograms per deciliter

Does Pollution Cause Breast Cancer?

Only 1 in 20 American women contracted breast cancer 50 years ago. Today the number has jumped to 1 in 8. Pollution may be partially at fault.

All the established risk factors for breast cancer have one thing in common: total lifetime exposure to estrogen. The following chemical pollutants act like estrogens in the body:

※ Plastics

※ Fuels

※ Pharmaceuticals

※ Chlorine-based chemicals such as DDT and PCBs

※ Chlorofluorocarbons

These pollutants accumulate in body fat for years, mimicking the activity of estrogen in the body, including the ability to cause breast cancer. Although all women run some risk because of widespread pollution in the United States, those who work in the chemical industry or live near hazardous waste sites have the highest risk.

The vapors are worse when materials containing formaldehyde are exposed to heat and humidity.

Federal regulations have not yet been passed against materials containing formaldehyde. Many manufacturers, however, have stopped using it voluntarily in light of known health risks. State and county health departments offer formaldehyde testing to people who are concerned about exposure in their homes.

Cigarette smoke The dangers of secondhand smoke are becoming well-publicized, and much legislation against public smoking is being enacted. Chapter 12 includes a discussion of passive smoking and its effects on health. Following a report on environmental tobacco smoke by the U.S. Surgeon General, most states have passed laws and ordinances that severely restrict or ban smoking in public buildings.

Radon Radon, a naturally occurring radioactive gas, comes from the natural breakdown of uranium. High concentrations of radon are found in soil and rock containing uranium, granite, shale, phosphate, and pitchblende. It also is found in soils contaminated with certain kinds of industrial wastes, such as byproducts from uranium or phosphate mining. In recent years well-insulated houses have tested positive for radon, most often in basements.

Radon is attracted to dust particles, which may lodge in the lungs. Late in 1994 researchers backed off somewhat on earlier warnings regarding radon, saying the levels of radon in most homes do not warrant fear of illness. Exposure to very high levels of radon, however, have been known to cause cancer. Those who are concerned about the level of radon in their home should contact the state or local health department to measure the radon levels and receive information on how to bring down high levels.

Water Pollution

Nearly three-fourths of the earth's surface is covered by some kind of water: seas and oceans, lakes, rivers, and streams. Reservoirs of groundwater even exist beneath what we consider to be dry land. More than 2,000 contaminants have been found in America's waters, and almost 100 of them are known to cause cancer. Pollution in these waters affects all of us, and poses a significant threat to the nation's water supply.

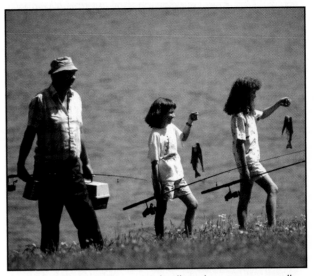

Anything put in the air or soil will work its way eventually into the water and back into the human body.

The most common sources of water pollution in the United States are:

❋ Human and animal wastes, largely a result of poorly designed or structurally inadequate sewage treatment plants or improperly installed septic systems.

❋ Improperly located landfills, which allow biological waste, industrial waste, household garbage, and other contaminants to leak into the water supply

❋ Corroded underground storage tanks for gasoline and petroleum products, many of them located near gas stations

❋ Oil, resulting both from tanker accidents and from the seepage of crude oil into the soil, then the groundwater

❋ Excessive **fluoride** or **chlorine**, added to the water to prevent tooth decay and to kill microorganisms in the water

KEY TERMS

Lead poisoning damage to liver, kidneys, and other body systems caused by absorption of lead into the body

Mercury poisoning deleterious effects on the body caused by overexposure to mercury

Formaldehyde an invisible gas used in home construction materials whose vapors may cause eye and lung irritations

Radon naturally occurring radioactive gas

Fluoride chemical compound added to drinking water to prevent tooth decay

Chlorine chemical used to purify water

* The decay of vegetation and dead fish that fill ponds, lakes, and streams

* Mercury, lead, hydrocarbons, pesticides, arsenic, industrial byproducts, and other toxic chemicals

* Natural sediments, such as sand and clay.

Simply stated, anything that enters the air or soil can work its way eventually into the water and should be considered as a source of pollution. Any pollutant can contaminate the water we drink — and can cause illnesses that range in seriousness from indigestion to cancer.

Since 1977, federal law has required that suppliers of drinking water periodically sample and test the water supplied to household taps. Federal law also requires that the supplier correct any problems and that customers be notified. If a violation poses an acute risk to human health, notification must take place within 72 hours. Notification is made by:

— a letter from your water supplier

— a letter from your local health department

— a notice in the newspaper, or

— an announcement on radio or television

Along with notification of the problem is notification of what the supplier is doing to correct the problem, and what the people notified can do to protect themselves. Finally, a person never should drink water directly from a lake, pond, river, or stream, no matter how clean it looks, without disinfecting it first.

Noise Pollution

If noise is loud enough or persistent enough, it is classified as pollution. Loud, prolonged noise can hurt a person. Taken to extremes, it can result in permanent hearing loss. Sounds so loud they hurt include a jet taking off from the runway and a jackhammer slamming through thick slabs of asphalt. Noises in the harmful range include loud arguing, a crying baby, the whir of a food blender, and the hum of a vacuum cleaner.

Sound is measured in *decibels*. Every ten-point increase in decibels represents a tenfold jump in intensity of the sound. Thus, traffic speeding along

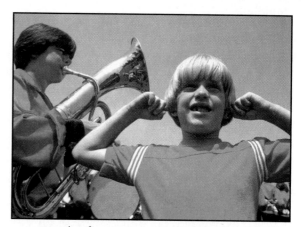

Even brief exposure to extremely loud sounds can cause hearing loss.

ips for action

How to Purify Water

These methods won't get rid of many pollutants, but they *will* kill bacteria, viruses, and parasites:

* **Household bleach:** use four drops per quart of water; wait 30 minutes before drinking

* **2% tincture of iodine:** use ten drops per quart of water; wait 20 minutes before drinking

* **Iodine tablets:** use two tablets per quart of water; wait 20 minutes after the tablets dissolve before drinking

* **Chlorine tablets:** use five tablets per quart of water; wait 30 minutes after the tablets dissolve before drinking

Saturated iodine is not recommended for disinfecting drinking water.

Tips for action

How to Save Your Hearing

To save yourself from noise pollution, avoid *repeated* or *prolonged* exposure to:

* freeway traffic and other heavy traffic
* car and truck horns
* construction equipment
* motorcycles
* emergency vehicle sirens
* lawnmowers and weed-eaters
* chainsaws
* farm equipment
* rock concerts and loud stereo music
* factory noise
* air traffic
* large crowds
* cheering at sporting events

Cutting Down on Noise Pollution

Whenever you can, avoid *making* noise: Turn down the volume on the stereo, tune up your lawnmower, stop shouting. To protect yourself from noise made by others:

* Wear foam, wax, or soft plastic ear plugs in noisy places or when working with lawn care equipment, power tools, and other machinery.

* Close the windows of your house or car to block out as much noise as possible.

* Cut down on the use of noisy appliances such as blenders, food processors, electric grain grinders, and electric juicers.

* Place rubber mats under the noisy appliances you do use, including the washing machine.

* Insulate your home from noise by installing drapes and carpets.

* Avoid drinking alcohol or taking aspirin if you're exposed to high noise levels. Both increase the risk of damage to the ears.

a highway (at 70 decibels) is 500 times more intense than someone whispering (at 20 decibels). Researchers have concluded that repeated exposure to noise measuring 80 decibels or above causes temporary hearing loss. If prolonged, the hearing loss is permanent. Even brief exposure to extremely loud sounds (such as an explosion) can cause immediate, permanent hearing loss.

As many as 20 million Americans are exposed chronically to health-harming levels of noise. More than half of those people have partial hearing loss already. By the time they are 65, one-third of all Americans have hearing loss bad enough to interfere with communication. This is not strictly a function of age. In societies with less noise pollution, the incidence of hearing loss also is significantly lower in elderly people.

Hearing impairment caused by noise pollution can occur at any age, even during early infancy. It can range from a mild form such as **tinnitus** (ringing in the ears) to permanent damage. Temporary hearing impairment usually disappears a few hours after the noise stops, but gradual damage to the delicate structures of the inner ear can result in permanent hearing loss eventually. Noise pollution also can increase levels of stress, raise blood pressure, produce anxiety, cause insomnia, and damage the nervous system.

Chemicals and Pesticides

Pesticides — chemicals used to kill the insects, rodents, and plants that destroy crops — have become a significant source of pollution, partly because of overuse and partly because small amounts of pesticides are absorbed into the food we eat. Some pesticides known to be

KEY TERMS

Tinnitus ringing in the ears

Pesticides chemicals used to kill insects, rodents, and weeds

harmful to people, such as DDT, have been banned from the market. Other pesticides are regulated fairly strictly by the Environmental Protection Agency. Pesticides work their way through the entire food chain by contaminating the soil, the groundwater, and eventually the food we eat.

Although the long-term effects of many pesticides are unknown, pesticides are known to accumulate in the human body. The effects in children are much more pronounced than adults. Some pesticides have been shown to cause birth defects and cancer. The chemicals in pesticides also may be related to nervous system disorders, liver damage, and kidney disease.

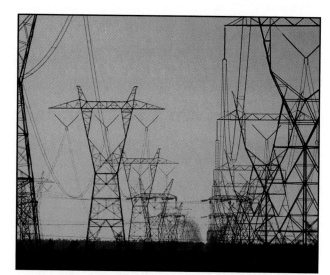

Overhead power lines generate electromagnetic fields that may pose health risks.

Radiation and Electromagnetic Fields

Radiation is not confined to nuclear power plants or atomic bombs. People are exposed to radiation every day. It is in video display terminals, microwave ovens, x-rays, and even in the ultraviolet rays of the sun. Food is bombarded with radiation to kill bacteria, prolong shelf life, destroy insects, inhibit sprouting, and delay ripening. Although the potential for a nuclear accident always exists, daily exposure to low levels of radiation from a variety of sources is a greater concern.

Another problem is radioactive waste. Most of the waste generated by nuclear plants, commercial industry, and military operations is still being stored "temporarily" in vats or barrels (many of them under water) at sites all over the country. A permanent solution to the problem has not been found; yet more radioactive waste is generated every year. Some of the waste that is stored will not be considered "safe" for tens of thousands of years.

We are not sure about some of the health effects of common sources of radiation. For example, the jury is still out on video display terminals; studies have shown that more harmful rays are emitted from the sides and back than from the front. You might suffer more harm from the computer *next* to you than from the one in *front* of you! Microwave ovens are relatively safe. The biggest potential danger comes from the chemicals in the plastic wrap used to cover food in the microwave. The damage from x-rays can be considerable.

Moderate radiation exposure can damage the eyes and skin, affect egg and sperm production, and cause birth defects. Regular or prolonged exposure can cause cancer. Exposure to high levels of radiation can cause **radiation sickness**, characterized by nausea, vomiting, diarrhea, hemorrhage, and hair loss. In large enough doses, radiation can kill a person.

Of special concern are **electromagnetic fields (EMFs)**, invisible fields (spaces that contain energy) caused by electrically charged conductors. Electromagnetic fields are generated by a variety of common household products including light fixtures, electrical wiring, telephone lines, computers, household appliances, refrigerators, radio and television signals, microwave ovens, hair dryers, electric blankets, waterbed heaters, and overhead power lines.

Scientists think the fields that are emitted interfere with the electromagnetic fields created by the body's own cells. Early studies showed a statistical link between high-voltage power lines and cancer — especially in electrical workers and in children who live under overhead lines. More studies are needed. The Science Advisory Board of the Environmental Protection Agency says that current evidence is insufficient to prove that electromagnetic fields cause cancer.

Other possible health consequences of electromagnetic fields include infertility, spontaneous abortion, developmental problems, growth retardation, and mood disorders. The association between spontaneous abortion and slow fetal growth and use of electric blankets is so strong that federal officials urge pregnant women to use electric blankets with "prudence."

Waste Disposal

Possibly the greatest impact from pollution comes not from automobile exhaust or pesticides but, rather, from the wastes and garbage people generate daily. As the population increases, so does the amount of waste. In the United States alone, each person produces approximately a ton of garbage every year — more than 4 pounds every day. Almost half of this waste is paper; a fourth is plastic, glass, and metal; and a fifth originates in yards. All of it has to go somewhere.

Solid Wastes

Solid wastes cover the spectrum of the American lifestyle: disposable diapers, newspapers, and the mulch that grinds out of our garbage disposals. Traditionally, people have coped with solid wastes in four ways:

1. *Putting it in a sanitary landfill.* A **sanitary landfill** is a huge open pit where trash is compacted and buried. Landfills are supposed to be dug away from streams, ponds, and sources of groundwater to lessen the likelihood that water sources will be polluted by the garbage. Unfortunately, contaminants often *do* filter into the soil and surrounding groundwater, creating a pollution source. Trash dumped in sanitary landfills is compacted. Each day a fresh layer of dirt is spread over any new trash. When the landfill is full, it is covered with a heavy layer of dirt, and trees and grass often are planted over it. About 80% of the trash we generate is buried in sanitary landfills.

2. *Burning it.* Various **incinerators** are used to burn solid waste. These include furnaces, cement kilns, and commercial incinerators designed for that purpose. Poorly designed incinerators contribute to air pollution by releasing particulates into the air. Approximately 10% of trash is incinerated.

3. *Dumping it in open pits.* In some areas solid waste is compacted, then dumped into open pits. The garbage in open pits rarely decomposes properly, smells putrid, and can be scattered by birds, animals, and the wind. Many urban areas have outlawed dumping garbage into open pits.

4. *Dumping it into the ocean.* Shoreline communities sometimes compact solid wastes, then ship

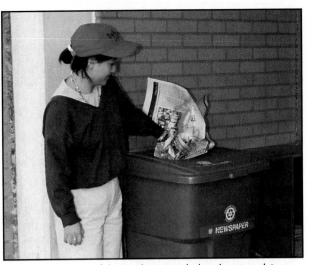

Only about 10% of the trash is recycled in the United States.

it by barge to dump sites. Offshore sites have the potential for polluting the oceans, and their capacity is limited.

Because our resources for disposal are being depleted, we are beginning to transport trash to sites in rural and unpopulated areas of the country and to developing countries. Only about 10% of the trash we generate is **recycled** — collected, reprocessed, and marketed — though officials estimate that eight to nine times that much actually could be recycled. More and more communities are starting programs to recycle newspaper, other paper products, aluminum, glass, and plastics. Others are encouraging homeowners to **compost**, or mix leftover food and vegetable peels with lawn clippings and leaves. When bacteria eat the organic material, the result is a rich soil that is useful in gardening.

KEY TERMS

Radiation energy from waves and particles such as ultraviolet rays and x-rays

Radiation sickness illness caused by overexposure to radioactive substances; characterized by nausea, hemorrhage, hair loss, and possibly death

Electromagnetic fields (EMFs) invisible spaces of energy caused by electrically charged conductors

Sanitary landfill large, open pit where trash is buried

Incinerator container used to burn solid waste

Recycling collecting, reprocessing, and reusing trash

Compost rich soil resulting from the decomposition of leftover food mixed with lawn clippings and leaves

Tips for action

Preserving the Environment

To conserve and preserve:

✳ Don't pour household chemicals or pesticides down the drain. Take them to a collection site.

✳ Use low-phosphate detergents.

✳ Leave lawn clippings on the lawn; compost yard trimmings.

✳ Never use your toilet as a trash can. The septic system is designed to handle liquid and solid human waste, not materials meant for the trash can.

✳ Install water-saving faucets and shower heads.

✳ Use a bucket — not a running garden hose — when washing your car at home.

✳ Carpool or use public transportation if you can.

✳ Never pour used oil and antifreeze down the drain or into drainage ditches. Take them to a service station.

✳ Get involved in neighborhood and community clean-up projects.

✳ Recycle!

Hazardous Wastes

Some of the waste products generated by industry, laboratories, and medical facilities are classified as **hazardous wastes**, waste products contaminated with toxic substances or pathogens that can cause cancer or other diseases. By law, hazardous wastes cannot be dumped in a sanitary landfill.

Before federal laws were enacted to regulate the disposal of hazardous wastes, these toxic materials were dumped in canals, open pits, and other areas that now are called **hazardous waste sites**. The worst of these sites have been scheduled for clean-up by the federal government under the Superfund law. The government has identified 1,219 sites as hazardous and an additional 32,000 as potentially hazardous.

As many as 40 million Americans live within 4 miles of the nation's worst hazardous waste sites. As a result they have birth defects, nervous system disorders, cancer, cardiovascular problems, respiratory irritation, and skin irritation. Poor people and minorities are affected more profoundly by the placement of landfills and the disposal of toxic waste in proximity to where they live. A 1987 study published by the United Church of Christ's Commission for Racial Justice found that three in five African Americans and Hispanics live in communities with uncontrolled toxic waste sites, including abandoned production operations and unregulated dumps.

Liquid Waste

Liquid wastes — generally, what is flushed down the toilet — are handled in most cities and municipalities by sewage treatment plants. At these treatment facilities, sewage is processed, removing bacterial contaminants and **polychlorinated biphenyls** (PCBs), chemicals that cause cancer and damage the central nervous system. Once treated, the water is returned to the river or lake from whence it came. In areas that do not treat liquid wastes responsibly, these present a huge pollution problem for water and soil alike.

FOOD SAFETY

We all want our food to be safe as well as nutritious, but a number of safety hazards have been identified by **food toxicologists** (specialists who

Is Peeling the Best Defense?

If you're worried about chemical and pesticide residues on produce, you might be tempted to peel fresh fruits and vegetables before you eat. Random annual testing by the Food and Drug Administration, however, shows that 99% of the produce we eat either has no residue at all or amounts well below safe limits.

Besides, you need the fiber and nutrients found in the skin of potatoes, apples, pears, plums, and other fresh produce.

The FDA advises that you simply scrub fruit and vegetable skins with a stiff-bristle brush under running tap water, a technique that will get rid of any residue that might be present.

---

detect toxins in food). The foods we buy are often adulterated with:

— pesticides, used to kill the pests that destroy crops

— antibiotics, used to prevent infections in animals intended for slaughter

— hormones, used to increase milk production in cows

— radiation, used to prolong the shelf life of canned food, inhibit the sprouting of vegetables, and delay the ripening of some fruits

Food Additives

Every time you sit down to a delicious meal, you may be getting more than you bargained for. In a single year the average person eats 160 pounds of food additives and 140 pounds of sweeteners.

Additives (sometimes called **preservatives**) are chemical substances added to food to lengthen storage life, prevent the growth of microorganisms, prevent nutrients from breaking down, alter taste, enhance color, and make foods more appealing to consumers. Processed foods purchased at the grocery store may contain:

❊ Sodium and calcium propionate, sodium benzoate, sodium nitrate, potassium sorbet, and sulfur dioxide, to prevent the growth of bacteria, yeast, and mold in baked goods

❊ Sulfites, to prevent browning

❊ Nitrites and nitrates, to prevent botulism and improve the color and flavor of meats

❊ Antioxidants (such as BHA, BHT, citric acid, and vitamin E), to prevent fats and oils from turning rancid and fruits and vegetables from turning brown

❊ Emulsifiers (such as lecithin, diglycerides, monoglycerides, and polysorbates), to keep oil and water suspended in foods such as mayonnaise, ice cream, and salad dressings

❊ Monosodium glutamate (MSG) and disodium guanylate (GMP), to improve the natural flavors of food

❊ Acetone peroxide (a bleaching agent) and azodicarbonamide (a maturing agent), to bleach flour white and improve its baking qualities

❊ Agar, gelatin, pectin, carrageenan, locust bean gum, sodium alginate, and carboxymethylcellulose, to thicken foods and improve their texture

❊ Wax coatings (made of fats, mineral oil, vegetable oil, shellac, beeswax, paraffin, or synthetic resin), to preserve the moisture in fresh fruits and vegetables

KEY TERMS

Hazardous waste trash contaminated with toxic substances

Hazardous waste site any area where toxic waste was dumped before laws existed to regulate proper disposal of toxic substances

Polychlorinated biphenyls (PCBs) industrial chemicals found in sewage that cause cancer and central nervous system damage

Food toxicologist specialist who detects dangerous substances in foods

Additives (preservatives) chemical substances added to foods to make them safer and more appealing to consumers

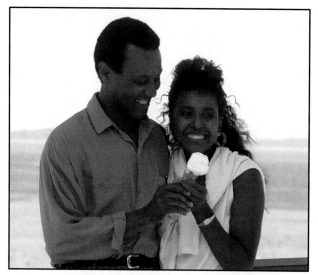

In one year the average person eats 160 pounds of food additives and 140 pounds of sweeteners.

and vegetables, including those in salad bars, because of fatal allergic reactions in sensitive individuals. The FDA also requires labeling foods containing sulfites. Nitrites and nitrates, which can be converted into a cancer-causing agent called nitrosamine in the digestive tract or during the cooking process, have been reduced by law in products including bacon, luncheon meats, and sausage.

The federal government also discourages the use of **fungicides** (agents that kill fungi) in wax coatings used on fruits and vegetables. According to the National Academy of Sciences, 90% of all fungicides can cause cancer.

Although many food additives are safe, some are under scrutiny by the Food and Drug Administration because of their potential health risks. The FDA has banned the use of sulfites on fresh fruits

KEY TERMS

Fungicides agents that kill fungi

HEALTHY PEOPLE 2000 OBJECTIVES FOR ENVIRONMENTAL HEALTH

❋ Eliminate blood lead levels above 25 μg/dL in children under age 5.

❋ Increase protection from air pollutants so at least 85% of people live in counties that meet EPA standards.

❋ Reduce human exposure to air pollutants.

❋ Increase the proportion of people who receive a supply of drinking water that meets the safe drinking water standards established by the Environmental Protection Agency.

❋ Establish programs for recyclable materials and household hazardous waste.

❋ Increase the proportion of pharmacies and other dispensers of prescription medications that use linked systems to provide alerts to potential adverse drug reactions among medications dispensed by different sources to individual patients.

❋ Increase the proportion of primary care providers who routinely review with their patients age 65 and older all prescribed and over-the-counter medicines taken by their patients each time a new medication is prescribed.

Summary

1 One's state of wellness is controlled by inheritance, environment, access to regular health care, and lifestyle.

2 Traditional or orthodox medicine is based on scientifically validated procedures developed over time.

3 Health-care facilities may be clinics, nonprofit hospitals, for-profit hospitals, teaching hospitals, and college health centers, outpatient surgery centers, freestanding emergency centers, and home health care.

4 Health insurance may be private fee-for-service, preferred provider, private prepaid group plans, or public/governmental plans.

5 People should guard against quackery, particularly promised cures for progressive diseases such as arthritis, cancer, and AIDS.

6 Governmental agencies that protect consumers are the Food and Drug Administration, Environmental Protection Agency, Federal Trade Commission, and U.S. Postal Service. The Better Business Bureau is a consumer protection organization without legal powers of enforcement.

7 Air pollution and smog cause respiratory irritation and damage, in addition to other ill health effects.

8 Indoor air pollution can be caused by carbon monoxide, asbestos, lead, mercury, formaldehyde, and radon.

9 The most common sources of water pollution are human and animal wastes, improperly located landfills, corroded storage tanks, oil, excessive fluoride or chlorine added to the water, decaying vegetation and dead fish, natural sediments, and toxic chemicals.

10 Continuing elevated noise pollution levels can cause permanent hearing loss.

11 Food additives, some of which may be harmful, are regulated by the Food and Drug Administration.

Select Bibliography

Bredin, Alice. "On Ill Health and Air Pollution." *New York Times Good Health Magazine*, October 7, 1990.

Breslin, Karen. "In Our Own Backyards: The Continuing Threat of Hazardous Waste." *Environmental Health Perspectives*, 101 (November 1993), p. 6.

Cunningham, W., and B. Saigo. *Environmental Science: A Global Concern*, 2d edition. Dubuque, IA: Wm. C. Brown, 1992.

Greeley, Alexandra. "Getting the Lead Out . . . Of Just About Everything," *FDA Consumer*, July-August 1991.

Johnson, Kirk A. "The Color of Health Care." *Heart and Soul Magazine*, Spring 1994.

Martin, D. L., and G. Gershuny, editors. *The Rodale Book of Composting: Easy Methods for Every Gardener*. Emmaus, PA: Rodale Press, 1992.

Miller, G. T. *Living in the Environment*, 7th edition. Belmont, CA: Wadsworth, 1992.

Mushak, Betty. "Environmental Equity: A New Coalition for Justice." *Environmental Health Perspectives*, 101 (November 1993), p. 6.

Roter,. D. L., and J. A. Hall. *Doctors Talking with Patients/Patients Talking with Doctors*. Westport, CT: Auburn House, 1992.

Are You a Savvy Health Consumer?

NAME _____ DATE _____

COURSE _____ SECTION _____

Answer each of the questions below. For each Yes, give yourself 1 point. For each No, give yourself 2 points. If a question does not apply to your situation, leave it blank and score 0 points.

1. Do you know which signs and symptoms indicate that you are sick enough to see a physician? ❑ Yes ❑ No

2. Do you know how to check your own vital signs, such as temperature and pulse? ❑ Yes ❑ No

3. When appropriate, do you purchase and use home health tests? ❑ Yes ❑ No

4. Do you know how to manage most minor illnesses and injuries, such as a common cold, temporary indigestion, or a minor abrasion? ❑ Yes ❑ No

5. If appropriate, do you administer your own therapy, such as allergy shots? ❑ Yes ❑ No

6. Do you regularly perform monthly self-exams, such as breast self-exams or testicular self-exams? ❑ Yes ❑ No

7. Do you participate in a regular exercise program? ❑ Yes ❑ No

8. Is your weight within 10% of the range considered ideal for your age, gender, and height? ❑ Yes ❑ No

9. If you need to lose or gain weight, are you actively involved in an appropriate nutrition and exercise program? ❑ Yes ❑ No

10. Before you take any over-the-counter medications, do you read the label and carefully check instructions for use? ❑ Yes ❑ No

11. Before you take any prescription medication, do you check the label carefully for the physician's instructions? ❑ Yes ❑ No

12. Do you follow instructions on medications strictly, taking only the recommended dose and using the medication only as long as recommended? ❑ Yes ❑ No

13. Do you check for expiration dates on over-the-counter and prescription medication and do you discard medications when they expire? ❑ Yes ❑ No

14. If your symptoms persist or get worse while you are taking medication, do you check with your physician? ❑ Yes ❑ No

15. Do you have a primary-care physician? ❑ Yes ❑ No

16. Have you checked your physician's credentials, such as years of training, years of practice, and licensing compliance? ❑ Yes ❑ No

17. Before visiting your physician do you write a list of your symptoms or your questions ahead of time? ❑ Yes ❑ No

18. If your physician recommends medical tests, do you question the need for tests and explore alternatives with your physician? ❑ Yes ❑ No

19. Do you have regular physical and dental check-ups? ❑ Yes ❑ No

20. Do you have some type of health insurance, either private, group, or government-funded? ❑ Yes ❑ No

21. If you have health insurance, do you get necessary approvals before visiting the doctor and follow up with proper claim forms? ❑ Yes ❑ No

22. If a practitioner offers you an unorthodox diagnosis or treatment, do you insist on seeing published reports in legitimate sources first? ❑ Yes ❑ No

23. If you live in an area of heavy traffic, do you try to avoid outdoor exercise and exposure between the hours of noon and 4 p.m.? ❑ Yes ❑ No

24. If you live near a smelter, refinery, industrial plant, or coal-powered furnace, do you take measures to protect yourself from possible air pollution? ❑ Yes ❑ No

25. Do you resist smoking yourself, and do you avoid exposure to the cigarette smoke of others? ❑ Yes ❑ No

26. Has your home been checked for asbestos — and, if appropriate, has the asbestos been removed or sealed? ❑ Yes ❑ No

27. If you have natural gas appliances, were they installed professionally and are they checked before seasonal use? ❑ Yes ❑ No

28. If your home was built prior to 1950, has it been checked for lead in the paint and pipes? ❑ Yes ❑ No

29. Has your home been checked for radon gas? ❑ Yes ❑ No

30. Do you take regular measures to protect yourself from loud noise, including turning down the volume on your stereo? ❑ Yes ❑ No

Add up your scores. If you scored:

20–30 Congratulations! You're a savvy health consumer. Continue to do what you can to protect yourself against threats from the environment and to practice good preventive health practices.

32–46 Some of the areas in your life could use improvement! Go back over the assessment and review the questions to which you answered No. Those questions will give you a blueprint for improving your consumer health.

48–60 You're not doing everything you can to protect your health and wellness. Review the suggestions in this chapter, then work to design a plan that will help you be a better health consumer.

Glossary

Ablative techniques any of several techniques of destroying malfunctioning heart tissue

Acid rain rain that falls through air polluted by sulfur dioxide and nitrogen dioxide and carries it into groundwater

Acquired immune deficiency syndrome (AIDS) an incurable, sexually transmitted viral disease

Acquired immunity protection from re-acquiring an infectious disease because the first occurrence triggered antibodies against it

Acute HIV infection having symptoms similar to flu or mono, which disappear within days or a few weeks

Addiction a state of biochemical and/or psychological dependence produced by habitual drug-taking

Additives (preservatives) chemical substances added to foods to make them safer and more appealing to consumers

Adrenocorticotropic hormone (ACTH) hormone released by the pituitary gland that stimulates the adrenal glands to release other hormones in the initial stage of stress

Aerobic exercises any activity that requires oxygen to produce energy

AIDS dementia deteriorated mental and motor capacity

Alcoholic hepatitis chronic inflammation of the liver tissue

Al-Anon, Alateen two organizations that help families cope with alcohol-dependent family members

Alcoholic pellagra condition caused by deficiency of protein and niacin due to prolonged alcohol consumption

Alcohol poisoning death attributed to BAC at 0.50% and above

Alcoholic cirrhosis scarring, shriveling, and hardening of liver tissue

Alcoholics Anonymous (AA) supportive fellowship of alcohol-dependent people

Alcoholism the chronic, progressive condition of dependence on alcohol characterized by consumption above social and controllable limits

Alcoholic hallucinosis mental disorder characterized by mental disorientation and mood disturbance

Alzheimer's disease a progressive, incurable disease in which nerve cells in the brain die

Amino acids chemical compounds that contain carbon, oxygen, hydrogen, and nitrogen

Amniotic sac (amnion) tough, transparent membrane that surrounds the fetus like a balloon

Amphetamines group of synthetic amines affecting portions of the brain that control breathing, heart rhythm, blood pressure, and metabolic rate

Anabolic steroids synthetic derivatives of the male hormone testosterone

Anaerobic exercise high-intensity activity that does not require oxygen to produce the desired energy

Anemia condition characterized by an insufficient quantity or quality of red blood cells

Aneurysm sac formed by distention or dilation of an artery wall

Anger temporary, negative emotion that combines physiological and emotional arousal

Angina pectoris chest pain that occurs when the heart doesn't get enough blood

Anorexia nervosa an eating disorder in which a person does not eat enough food to maintain normal body weight

Antigen a substance that triggers the immune response

Antibody a protein substance that interacts with an antigen and forms the basis of immunity

Antihypertensives medications used to lower blood pressure

Antioxidants disease-fighters that protect the body from the harmful effects of free radicals

Anxiety disorders psychological conditions characterized by exaggerated fear

Aorta artery through which oxygen-rich blood is transported from the heart to arteries that nourish the body systems

Apgar score an evaluation of baby's health at birth based on heart rate, respiration, color, reflexes, and muscle tone; maximum score is 10

Aphrodisiac a substance that stimulates sexual desire

Aplastic crisis interruption in the body's production of red blood cells; may occur in babies with sickle cell disease

Arrhythmia irregular heartbeat

Arthritis general classification of numerous diseases that cause swelling and pain in the joints, muscles, and bones

Artificial insemination medical procedure in which sperm are placed into uterus via a catheter

Asthma respiratory disease characterized by attacks of wheezing and difficulty breathing caused by narrowing of the bronchi

Asymptomatic without signs of illness

Asbestos a mineral formerly used in construction as an insulator; now known to be toxic

Asbestosis progressive and fatal lung disease caused by inhaling microscopic asbestos particles

Arteries blood vessels leaving the heart full of oxygen

Arterioles smaller blood vessels

Atherosclerosis condition that results when the blood vessel walls become coated with plaque, obstructing blood flow

Atria the two upper chambers of the heart that receive the blood

Atrophy to decrease in strength or size of tissue from disuse

Aura warning signals that may precede migraine headaches

Autoimmunity a disorder of the immune system in which the immune system attacks the body's own cells and tissues

Autoinnoculation spreading a virus to other parts of one's own body

Alveoli air sacs in the lungs where the exchange of gases takes place

Aversion therapy treatment in which a person is given the drug antabuse which blocks metabolism of acetaldehyde

Axon a long cable connected to the neuron, receiving information from the cell body, relaying it to another neuron

AZT a drug used to treat AIDS

B-cells a type of lymphocyte that produces antibodies capable of deactivating invading pathogens

Balloon angioplasty use of a catheter and balloon-tipped tube to expand artery and allow more blood to flow through it

Bacteria a type of disease-causing microorganism

Bacterial endocarditis infectious disease involving the heart valves or tissues

Barbiturates substances that have calming and depressant effects

Basal body temperature (BBT) method of NFP that incorporates a woman's temperature fluctuations to indicate when coitus is safe or unsafe

Basal cell carcinoma common type of skin cancer that usually does not metastasize

Basal metabolic rate (BMR) amount of energy (calories) a person uses when totally inactive

Behavioral psychology theory that all behavior is learned

Benign tumor that remains self-contained; noncancerous

Benign prostatic enlargement (BPH) enlargement of prostate gland, not related to cancer

Bereavement intense grief associated with the process of "disbonding" from a significant person who has died

Beta blockers medications prescribed to control high blood pressure and heart conditions

Beta-carotene plant source of vitamin A; helps guard against free radicals

Better Business Bureau not-for-profit organization composed of member businesses that promote fair and reputable business practices in a locality

Binge drinking consuming five or more drinks consecutively (men) and four consecutively (women)

Binge eating an eating disorder characterized by consuming a lot of food in a short time

Binging Consuming a large amount of food in a short time; gorging

Bioelectrical impedance method of determining body composition by analyzing electrical conduction through the body

Bioequivalent generic drug that the body can absorb and use at the same rate and level as a brand-name drug

Biofeedback training method of measuring physiological functions that usually are not noticeable

Biopsy microscopic examination of a small piece of tissue that has been removed with a special needle

Bisexuality/ambisexuality physical attraction to both the same sex and the opposite sex

Blackout inability to remember recent events

Blood alcohol concentration (BAC) or **blood alcohol level (BAL)** ratio of alcohol measured in the blood to total blood volume

Blood lipids/lipoproteins fatty substances carried through the blood

Body composition proportionate amounts of fat tissue and nonfat tissue in the body

Body mass index (BMI) Body weight in kilograms divided by the square of height in meters or BMI = kg/m2

Bradycardia heart rate less than 60 beats per minute

Brain death complete loss of brain function

Braxton-Hicks contractions normal uterine contractions that occur periodically throughout pregnancy

Breathalyzer device used to measure blood alcohol concentration

Breech presentation positioning of fetus so buttocks are seen first at birth

Bronchi two main passageways that connect to each lung from the trachea

Bronchitis inflammation of the bronchial tubes in the lungs

Bulimia nervosa an eating disorder in which a person consumes a lot of food in a short time, followed by self-induced vomiting or taking laxatives or diuretics

Burnout physical and mental exhaustion caused by chronic stress

Bursae fluid-filled sacs found among muscles, bones, ligaments, and tendons

Caffeine a legal drug with stimulant properties

Calendar method form of NFP that requires refraining from coitus during ovulation

Calcium an essential mineral

Caliper instrument used to measure the thickness of fat under the skin

Calorie a term meaning the same as kilocalorie

Cancer group of diseases characterized by uncontrolled growth and spread of abnormal cells that kill normal cells

Candida a common STD caused by a fungus; also known as candidiasis, moniliasis, and yeast infection

Capillaries extremely small blood vessels with thin walls that allow nutrients and oxygen to pass through

Carbohydrates compounds composed of carbon, hydrogen, and oxygen used by the body to create 90% of its energy

Carbon monoxide colorless, tasteless, odorless, poisonous gas

Carcinogen cancer-causing agent or substance

Carcinoma *in situ* an early cancer that does not extend beyond the surface

Cardiologist physician trained in the diagnosis and treatment of heart conditions

Cardiomyopathy a disease of the heart muscle

Cardiorespiratory endurance the ability of the heart, lungs, and blood vessels to deliver blood and nutrients to the cells efficiently during aerobic activity

Cardiopulmonary resuscitation (CPR) manual method of reversing sudden cardiac death

Carotid endarterectomy removal of fatty deposits from one of the two main arteries in the neck that supply blood to the brain

Carotid pulse pulse taken by locating the carotid artery in the neck

Cartilage elastic tissue at ends of bones that acts as a shock absorber and buffer between bones

Caudal anesthesia similar to an epidural, but injected at tip of the spine

Cataracts an eye disease in which the lens becomes opaque (cloudy), causing partial or total blindness

Caregiver a person who renders services to another person who is unable to take care of the activities of daily living

Cellular death cessation of all metabolic processes

Cellulite fat cells

Central nervous system the brain and spinal cord

Cerebral embolism moving blood clot that partially blocks a blood vessel in the brain

Cerebral hemorrhage bleeding from a ruptured blood vessel in the brain

Cerebral thrombus blood clot that gets caught on plaque in a blood vessel in the brain causing complete blockage of the blood vessel

Certified nurse-midwife registered nurse who specializes in caring for women during pregnancy and delivery

Cervical cap small rubber cap that fits over the cervix and is used with a spermicide to prevent fertilization

Cervical mucous method NFP that requires judging the thickness of cervical mucus to determine ovulation

Cervicitis inflammation of the cervix

Cervix lower portion of uterus that connects with vagina

Cesarean section (C-Section) delivery of fetus through opening in abdomen and uterus created by a surgical incision

Chancre a painless ulcer that develops at the site where infection enters the body and is the primary symptom of syphilis

Chemotherapy drugs taken intravenously to kill cancer cells

Child sexual abuse violation of a child's genitalia or sexually motivated acts toward a child

China white a designer drug with more potent effects than heroin

Chiropractic medicine science founded on the belief that life forces flow from the spine to the rest of the body

Chiropractor health-care practitioner who manipulates the spine to relieve pain

Chlamydia a common STD caused by the bacteria *Chlamydia trachomatis*

Cholesterol yellow, waxy substance produced by the liver and found in animal products; used by the body for metabolism and production of certain hormones

Chlorine chemical used to purify water

Chronic fatigue syndrome (CFS) a viral illness that produces extreme fatigue and other symptoms similar to mononucleosis

Chronic obstructive pulmonary disease (COPD) lung diseases characterized by decreased breathing functions that include chronic bronchitis and emphysema

Cilia hairlike projections lining wall of fallopian tubes

Circumcision surgical removal of foreskin of penis

Client-centered therapy a focus on clients and their beliefs and needs as more important than the counselor's

Clinical death cessation of heartbeat and breathing

Clinical depression extreme emotional low characterized by feelings of hopelessness, thoughts of suicide, and other symptoms

Clinical psychologist mental health professional with a Ph.D. in psychology who treats psychological problems through psychotherapy

Clitoris sensitive female sex organ, which becomes erect when sexually excited

Clove cigarettes cigarettes containing about 40% cloves, with a numbing ingredient, eugenol

Cluster headaches headaches that occur in groups and cycles; characterized by intense pain

Cocaine most powerful of the natural stimulants; includes several forms

Codeine a natural derivative of opium used as a cough suppressant or mild pain killer

Cohabitation living together as spouses without being married

Coitus sexual intercourse

Coitus interruptus withdrawal of the penis before ejaculation

Colitis recurring inflammation of the large intestine

Collagen fibrous protein found in connective tissue

Colon large intestine where wastes are processed

Colostrum yellowish liquid secreted from the breasts; contains antibodies and protein

Colposcopy an internal medical examination performed to detect the presence of genital warts in women who are asymptomatic

Common cold inflammation of the upper respiratory tract caused by a virus

Comorbidity having two chronic health problems simultaneously

Complex carbohydrates (starches) important source of energy for the body found in fruits, vegetables, and legumes

Compost rich soil resulting from the decomposition of leftover food mixed with lawn clippings and leaves

Computerized axial tomography (CAT scan) use of radiation to view internal organs that do not show up on x-ray

Conception the start of pregnancy, when a sperm cell fertilizes an egg cell

Condom thin sheath placed over the penis that prevents semen from entering the vagina

Congenital heart defects heart malformations present in about 1% of live births

Congestive heart failure condition caused when blood flow *from* the heart slows and blood returning *to* the heart backs up in the veins, causing blood to collect in the tissues

Congenital anomalies defects that are present in a baby at birth

Congenital syphilis a condition in which a baby is born with syphilis transmitted by the mother

Contraceptive any device, drug, or practice that prevents ovulation, fertilization, or implantation

Cool-down the ending phase of a workout that helps the body begin to return to its resting state

Coronary angiography a diagnostic method in which a catheter with radioactive dye, visible on x-ray, shows precise areas of coronary artery blockage

Coronary artery bypass graft surgery a procedure in which blood supplying the heart muscle is rerouted around the blockage

Corpus luteum enlarged follicle from which ovulation originated; secretes progesterone

Cortisol hormone released by the adrenal glands in the first stage of stress

Cowper's glands two pea-sized organs that produce pre-ejaculatory fluid

Crack small pieces or "rocks" formed from a dried mix of cocaine hydrochloride, baking soda, and water

Crack babies newborns who were exposed to cocaine and deprived of oxygen because of maternal cocaine use during pregnancy

Cremation incineration of a body in specialized furnace

Cross-training combining more than one activity to attain cardiorespiratory fitness

Crowning the top of the fetus's head appearing at the vaginal opening

Crucifers plant family that includes cabbage, broccoli, kohlrabi and cauliflower

Cyanotic defects heart defects characterized by too little oxygen in the blood pumped to the body

Daily values government food labeling that includes the percentage of recommended daily amounts of nutrients

Date rape sex without the consent of both partners

Defibrillator a device that delivers electrical shocks to the heart in an attempt to restore normal rhythm

Dehydration abnormal depletion of body fluids

Demerol short-acting synthetic narcotic used as an analgesic or a painkiller; usually injected

Dental hygienist health-care specialist who takes x-rays, cleans and polishes the teeth and teaches proper dental care

Dentistry practice involving diagnosis and treatment of teeth, gums, and oral cavity

Depo-Provera® contraceptive that is injected and lasts 3 months

Depressants a drug that inhibits neural activity and slows physical and mental functions; "downers"

Dendrite branch of a neuron that conveys impulses to the cell body

Deoxyribonucleic acid (DNA) found in the nucleus of cells and contains the body's genetic code

Designer drugs manufactured drugs that mimic the effects of other drugs

Detoxification ridding the body of poisons or the effects of poisons

Developmental tasks work to be done at various stages in a person's life

Diabetic coma unconsciousness induced by ketoacidosis

Diabetes mellitus chronic condition characterized by excessive amounts of glucose in the blood

Diagnosis-related groups (DRG) a system of predetermined payment made by Medicare based on the patient's diagnosis

Diaphragm rubber cup that fits over the cervix and prevents semen from entering the uterus and fallopian tubes; available only by prescription

Diastole relaxation of the heart between beats

Diastolic blood pressure lower pressure during the heart's relaxation phase

Dietary fiber (roughage) non-nutrient complex carbohydrate needed to keep the digestive system in order

Dietary Guidelines for Americans eating recommendations established by Department of Agriculture and Department of Health and Human Services

Digestion process of breaking down food and drink into substances the body can absorb

Digestive tract 30-foot long channel where breakdown and assimilation of food and drink take place in the body

Digital cardiac angiography/digital subtraction angiography modified form of MRI to generate internal images by computer

Dilation (dilatation) opening of the cervix to 10 centimeters; occurs during first stage of labor

Dilation and curettage (D & C) surgical procedure that removes the embryo and placenta from the uterus by scraping

Dilation and evacuation (D & E) procedure in which the cervix is dilated and the fetus removed by suction

Dilaudid derived from morphine, legitimately used as a cough suppressant and as an analgesic for treating severe pain

Disease-prone personality personality that tends toward illness

Distress negative stress

Diuretic any drug that speeds up elimination of salts and water from kidneys and other body organs

Diverticulosis painful condition caused by weakened places in the intestine that bulge, fill with fecal matter and become irritated

Dopamine brain chemical that controls pleasure sensations; the key to cocaine's addiction

Drug abuse the use of chemical substance that results in physical, mental, emotional, or social impairment

Drug misuse the occasionally inappropriate or unintentional use of a medication

Duodenum the first 10 inches of the small intestine

Dynamic (ballistic) stretching technique using rapid, bouncy, or bobbing movements to stretch muscle fibers

Dyspareunia painful intercourse

Echocardiography technique that uses sound waves to show functioning of the heart chambers and valves

Eclampsia high blood pressure during pregnancy

Ectopic pregnancy implantation outside of the uterus

Effacement thinning of cervix during labor

Ego the part of the psyche that controls and regulates basic drives

Ejaculation sudden discharge of semen from the penis as part of the sexual response

Electrocardiogram (EKG or ECG) measurement of electrical events in the heart

Electromagnetic fields (EMFs) invisible sources of energy caused by electrically charged conductors

Electophysiologic testing method of mapping electrical signals in the heart

ELISA (EIA) a blood test that diagnoses HIV be exposing the presence of HIV antibodies

Embalming procedure in which blood and body fluids are drained and formaldehyde and alcohol are injected

Embryo product of conception, from 2 weeks through 7

Emphysema progressive lung disease that eventually destroys the alveoli and greatly reduces lung functioning

Endocrine system body system that manufactures and secretes hormones

Endometriosis a condition in which pieces of the endometrium migrate to fallopian tubes, ovaries, or abdominal cavity

Endometrium inner lining of the uterus

Endorphins natural painkillers released by the brain

Endorphins and enkephalins naturally occurring narcotics in the body produced by the immune system

Energy-balancing equation formula stating that when caloric input equals caloric output, an individual does not gain or lose weight

Energy value the result of multiplying the number of grams of each energy nutrient in a serving of food by the caloric values per gram of carbohydrate, protein, and fat

Environmental Protection Agency (EPA) federal office with regulatory and enforcement powers over environmental matters

Epidermis top layer of skin

Epididymis storage structure along the top of each testicle where sperm cells mature

Epidural anesthesia spinal anesthesia administered over a period of hours

Epilepsy a seizure disorder caused by abnormal electrical activity in the brain

Epinephrine hormone released by the adrenal glands during the first stage of stress that affects metabolism, the muscles, and circulation

Episiotomy procedure in which an incision is made from the bottom of the vaginal opening toward the anus to prevent tearing of vagina

Erection the engorged, rigid state of the penis during sexual arousal

Essential fat body fat needed for normal physiological functioning

Esophagus the tube that carries the food to the stomach

Estrogen hormone that controls female sexual development

Estrogen replacement therapy treatment for women after menopause or after the ovaries have been removed

Ethyl alcohol a colorless liquid and central nervous system depressant made by the process of fermentation and found in alcoholic beverages

Euphoria a heightened sense of well-being associated with drug use

Eustress positive stress

Euthanasia allowing terminally ill patients to die either by suicide (active or direct) or by refusing life-saving treatment (passive or indirect)

Explanatory style the way people perceive the events in their lives — optimistic or pessimistic

Extrovert outgoing personality

Fake fat a substance that mimics the taste of fat

Fallopian tubes tubular passages leading from upper portion of uterus to each of the two ovaries

Family practitioner physician who treats all family members

Fat cell hypertrophy and hyperplasia theory stating that the quantity of fat in the body is the result of the size and number of fat cells a person has

Federal Trade Commission (FTC) U. S. agency organized to protect consumers

Female condom sheath inserted into the vagina to prevent fertilization and sexually transmitted diseases

Fertilization union of egg and sperm cells; conception

Fetal alcohol effect (FAE) aberrant behavior pattern in newborn resulting from mother's alcohol consumption during pregnancy

Fetal alcohol syndrome (FAS) group of physical and behavioral defects in a newborn caused by the mother's alcohol use during pregnancy

Fibroid tumor a mass of muscle and connective tissue growing in the uterus

Fibromyalgia disease that causes unexplained muscular pain

Fight-or-flight collection of physiological changes evoked by stress

Fimbriae finger like projections

FITT formula frequency, intensity, time, and type of workout applied to each of the physical fitness components

Flashback recurrence of a drug "trip"

Flexibility the ability of a joint to move freely through its full range of motion

Fluoride chemical compound added to drinking water to prevent tooth decay

Folic acid a B vitamin important in preventing neural tube defects of the fetus

Follicle egg sac in ovary

Follicle-stimulating hormone (FSH) a hormone that stimulates ovulation

Fomite an object contaminated with a pathogen

Food and Drug Administration (FDA) the regulatory agency charged with establishing criteria for all drugs and reviewing active ingredients in all OTC drugs

Food Guide Pyramid grouping of foods into 6 categories indicating serving sizes for each

Food toxicologist specialist who detects dangerous substances in foods

Forcible rape forced sex; assault

Formaldehyde an invisible gas used in home construction materials whose vapors may cause eye and lung irritations

Fraternal twins two babies conceived about the same time as the result of fertilization of two egg cells

Free Radicals chemicals produced when the body burns fuel for energy

Frostbite a condition caused by overexposure to cold temperatures

Funeral rite of passage for those who have died

Fungicides agents that kill fungi

Gallbladder stores bile and releases it into the small intestine as needed

Gamete intrafallopian transfer (GIFT) eggs and sperm are collected and inserted into fallopian tube

Gametes sex cells

Gastric ulcers chronic inflammation of lower end of esophagus and stomach

Gastritis chronic inflammation of stomach lining

General adaptation syndrome body's attempt to react to and adapt to stressors

Generic drug chemically equivalent medication substituted for a brand-name drug

Genetic predisposition theory stating that inherited genes influence weight

Genital (venereal) warts an STD caused by a virus that produces lesions on the genitals

German measles (rubella) viral infection that can damage eyes, ears, brain, or heart of the fetus during the pregnancy if the mother contracts the disease

Gerontologist professional who studies the aging process

Gestation period from conception to birth

Gestational diabetes form of diabetes (a metabolic disorder) that occurs only during pregnancy

Glans sensitive tip of the penis

Glaucoma a disorder marked by excessive pressure within the eye

Glucose tolerance test blood test used to diagnose diabetes

GnRH analogs drug treatment for endometriosis

Gonads sex glands; the primary reproductive organs

Gonorrhea bacterial STD; also called "clap"

Grief way of reacting to a significant loss

Group or communal marriage a marriage of three or more individuals who share all family functions

Group policy health insurance purchased by a group of individuals, usually through a place of employment, and at a reduced rate

Hallucinogens a group of mind-altering drugs that affect the brain and nervous system

Hangover aftereffects of drinking excessively including headache, nausea, vomiting, dizziness

Hardiness personality traits characteristic of people who are resistant to stress

Hassles various minor annoyances that occur daily

Hay fever mild respiratory ailment caused by environmental agents that provoke the body to produce histamines

Hazardous waste trash contaminated with toxic substances

Hazardous waste site any area where toxic waste was dumped before laws existed to regulate proper disposal of toxic substances

HDL "Good cholesterol" molecule containing high concentration of protein

Health the condition of being sound in body, mind, and spirit, free from pain or disease

Health maintenance organization (HMO) name denoting a group practice with emphasis on preventive medicine

Health-related fitness has four components; body composition, cardiovascular endurance, muscular flexibility, muscular strength/endurance

Heart rate reserve (HRR) the difference between resting heart rate and maximal heart rate

Heart transplant replacement of a damaged heart with the heart removed from another person who has died

Height/weight table assessment tool used to determine recommended body weight

Hemoglobin a chemical in the blood that carries oxygen and is responsible for the blood's red color

Hemoglobin the protein that makes the blood red and transports oxygen from the lungs to the rest of the body

Hemoglobin electrophoresis screening test to identify sickle cell gene carriers

Hemoglobinopathy abnormal hemoglobin

Hepatitis an inflammation of the liver caused by a virus

Hepatitis A a mild form of hepatitis transmitted by food or water contaminated with feces

Hepatitis B a form of hepatitis caused by a virus that lives in the bloodstream, in semen, and in vaginal secretions; transmitted through sexual contact or contaminated hypodermic needles

Hepatitis C a form of hepatitis caused by a virus similar to hepatitis B; commonly found among IV drug users and those who have received improperly screened blood

Hepatotoxic trauma disease of the liver caused by alcoholism; commonly called "fatty liver"

Heroin narcotic drug derived from morphine that is 35 times stronger than morphine

Herpes an STD caused by the herpes simplex virus (HSV), which produces distinctive lesions

Heterosexuality physical attraction to the opposite sex

High density lipoprotein (HDL) fatty substance that picks up cholesterol in the bloodstream and returns it to the liver; "good" cholesterol

High-impact aerobics aerobic exercise that has a running or jumping component

HIV-positive determined to have HIV infection by testing

Holistic treatment of patients that takes into account social and mental factors as well as physical condition

Holmes-Rahe Scale assessment used to determine who is at risk for developing a stress-related illness

Holographic will a legal handwritten document in which the writer leaves instructions to be carried out upon his or her death.

Homeostasis the body's internal sense of balance

Homophobe exaggerated fear and hatred for homosexuals

Homosexuality physical attraction to the same sex

Hospice care services for terminally ill patients and their families focusing on their comfort and social, emotional, and spiritual needs

Hostility exasperation; characterized by lack of trust in others

Human chorionic gonadotrophin (HCG) a hormone produced by the placenta that signals the pituitary gland is not to release FSH and LH

Human immunodeficiency virus (HIV) a fragile virus spread through the exchange of blood and semen that circulates freely in the bloodstream and always precedes the onset of AIDS

Humanistic psychology theory that behavior is motivated by a desire for personal growth and achievement

Hydrogenated hydrogen added to fats to increase shelf life and make the product more spreadable; increases saturation of the fat

Hydrostatic weighing method of determining body composition by measuring the amount of water displaced when a person exhales and sits under water

Hymen membrane partially covering the vaginal opening at birth; may or may not be intact

Hyperglycemia high blood sugar caused by the body's inability to process glucose from the blood

Hypertension high blood pressure

Hyperthermia abnormally high body temperature

Hypertrophy an increase in size and strength of muscles that are used regularly and vigorously

Hypoglycemia low blood sugar

Hypokinetic underactive

Hypothermia a condition in which body temperature drops below 95° and loses its ability to produce heat because heat is lost faster than it can be produced

Hysterectomy surgical removal of uterus

Hysterotomy surgical procedure in which the fetus and placenta are surgically removed through an abdominal incision

Iatrogenic illnesses medically induced sickness caused by adverse reactions to drugs

Id the part of the psyche that seeks pleasure and satisfaction of basic drives

Identical twins two babies conceived about the same time as the result of a single fertilized egg that divides into two cells that develop separately

Immune-prone personality personality that enables a person to handle pressure without becoming ill

Immune response body's reaction to first exposure to a pathogen

Immunity resistance to disease; may be natural or acquired

Immunodeficiency failure of the immune system to react to pathogens

Immunotherapy desensitization to allergen through periodic injections of weakened allergens

Immunotherapy use of the body's own immune system to fight cancer

Implantation attachment of embryo to lining of the uterus

Implants pieces of endometrium that have migrated to other areas

Impotence inability to obtain or maintain an erection for coitus

In vitro fertilization procedure in which a woman's eggs are placed in a glass dish and incubated with donor sperm

Incinerator container used to burn solid waste

Incontinence inability to control urination voluntarily

Incubation period the time between infection and appearance of signs of illness

Individual policy health insurance purchased by a person

Individuation separating from family and developing a self-identity

Infarct area of the heart muscle deprived of oxygen

Infectious diseases conditions in which a pathogen can be spread from person to person

Inflammation body's reaction to pathogen or trauma, characterized by redness, pain, and swelling

Influenza (flu) a viral infection of the nose, throat, bronchial tubes, and lungs

Insoluble not dissolvable in water

Insomnia inability to fall asleep or stay asleep

Insulin hormone essential for processing glucose in the body

Insulin reaction low blood sugar caused by too much insulin

Intimacy a close association, contact, or familiarity with someone

Interferon a protein produced by the body to fight viruses, injected to stimulate the body's own immune system to fight cancer

Intoxication temporary state of mental confusion

Intrauterine device (IUD) contraceptive device placed in the uterus by a health care practitioner to prevent implantation

Introitus vaginal opening

Introvert reflective, inner-centered personality

Invasive tumor a tumor that continues to grow and encroach upon surrounding tissues and organs

Iron-deficiency anemia anemia caused by too little iron in the blood

Islets of Langerhans cells in the pancreas that produce insulin

Isokinetic exercises isotonic concentric activities utilizing constant resistance machines that regulate movement and resistance to overload muscles

Isometric (static) muscle contraction muscle remains the same length and no movement occurs while a force is exerted against an immovable object

Isotonic (dynamic) muscle contraction muscle changes in length, either shortening or lengthening

Karvonen formula a method for determining if exercise is demanding enough to condition the heart and lungs by ascertaining the optimal target zone

Karyotype photograph of a cell during cell division; shows chromosomes in order of size from largest to smallest; used to detect chromosomes defect

Kawasaki disease childhood disease most common to Asian children; affects the heart in about 20% of the cases

Keloid raised scar that results from overgrowth of fibrous tissue following a cut or burn to the skin

Ketoacidosis (ketosis) accumulation of acid substances (ketones) caused by the incomplete burning of fat for energy

Kilocalorie the amount of energy required to raise the temperature of 1 gram of water 1°C

Korsakoff's syndrome psychosis caused by deficiency of B vitamins due to alcoholism

Labia majora two outer folds of tissue covering vaginal opening

Labia minora two folds of skin within labia majora

Labor regular contraction of the uterus and dilation of the cervix to expel the fetus

Lactose intolerance adverse reaction to dairy products because of lack of digestive enzyme

Lactovegetarian one who eats dairy products and plants but not meat, poultry, fish, or eggs

Lactation milk secretion from the breast

Laminaria wand made from dried seaweed used to expand the cervical opening as part of an abortion procedure

Laparoscopy a procedure that uses an optical device to view the abdominal cavity

LDL "Bad cholesterol" molecule containing large amounts of cholesterol

LSD lysergic acid diethylamide-24, a psychedelic drug that produces distorted reality

Lead poisoning damage to liver, kidneys, and other body systems caused by absorption of lead into the body

Lean body mass nonfat body tissue made up of muscle, bone, and organs

Leukoplakia a condition in which tissue in the oral cavity turns white, thickens, and hardens; a common effect of smokeless tobacco

Libido sex drive

Licensed practical nurse (LPN) and Licensed vocational nurse (LVN) nurses with shortened training period and limited responsibility

Life expectancy average length of time members of a population can expect to live

Lifespan potential maximum number of years members of a population could live

Lipids blood fats

Lipoprotein form of cholesterol combined with protein when transported through the body

Liver digestive organ that produces bile, removes some waste from the body, produces and stores glucose

Living will legal written document stating what kind of treatment should or should not be given in the event of a terminal illness or critical condition

Local infection an infection that remains in the area of the body where the invasion of the pathogen occurred

Lochia discharge of blood and mucus that may last several weeks after childbirth

Locus of control extent to which a person believes he or she can control the external environment

Loneliness feeling of emptiness when a person's social network is significantly lacking in quality or quantity

Low birthweight weighing less than 5½ pounds at birth

Low density lipoprotein (LDL) type of fat produced by liver; "bad" cholesterol

Low-impact aerobics activities that place minimal stress on the joints and are recommended for people with low fitness levels

Lupus chronic disorder of immune system accompanied by inflammation of various parts of the body

Luteinizing hormone (LH) a hormone that stimulates ovulation

Lyme disease a bacterial infection transmitted by a tick bite

Lymph nodes larger glands of the lymph system found in the head, neck, armpits, small of the back, and groin

Lymphatic system specialized groups of vessels that network throughout the body and cleanse body tissues

Lymphocytes specialized white blood cells produced in the bone marrow that identify pathogens and help macrophages fight pathogens

Macrominerals the seven major minerals the body needs in relatively large quantities daily (100 mg or less)

Macrophages specialized cells (phagocytes) that destroy pathogens

Macrosomia literally, "large body," referring to a condition in which fetus converts extra glucose from mother to fat

Magnetic resonance imaging (MRI) a diagnostic procedure using magnetic fields and radio waves to produce computer images that may reveal abnormalities within the body

Magnetic resonance imagery (MRI) use of radio waves and magnetic fields that produce a computer image of the body to locate abnormalities

Malignancy a tumor that is concerous

Malignant melanoma a more serious type of skin cancer in the form of a pigmented mole or tumor

Mammography an x-ray used to detect breast cancer

Malnutrition effects on body due to prolonged deficiency of necessary nutrients

Mantra word or phrase repeated silently during meditation

Marriage a legally and socially sanctioned union between a man and a woman

Masturbation self-stimulation of genitals or other erogenous areas

Maximal heart rate (MHR) the fastest heart rate obtained during all-out exercise

Mechanical heart a manmade device that attempts to duplicate natural heart functions

Medicaid public insurance plan for people who cannot afford medical care

Medicare public insurance plan for people over age 65

Meditation relaxation exercise that enables a person to control all thought

Melanocytes pigment-producing cells of the skin

Menopause stage in the life cycle when the ovaries stop functioning hormone levels decrease

Menstruation the discharge of blood from the uterus through the vagina

Mercury poisoning deleterious effects on the body caused by overexposure to mercury

Mescaline hallucinogen derived from peyote cactus

Metabolic rate (MR) total amount of energy the body expends in a given amount of time

Metabolism process of converting nutrients into body tissue and functions

Metastasis new cancers formed when cells from a malignant tumor break off, travel to other parts of the body, and form new cancers

Metazoa multicellular animals, the largest pathogens, that live as parasites in and on humans and animals

Methadone a synthetic narcotic used as a heroin substitute

Methamphetamines powerful stimulants that induce intense euphoria

Microminerals trace minerals, those the body requires daily in minute quantities (10 mg or less)

Migraine headaches vascular form of headaches characterized by severe pain

Minerals inorganic substances that make up 4% of our body weight

Monogamy marriage of a man and a woman

Mononucleosis ("mono") a contagious viral illness that attacks the lymph nodes in the neck and throat

Monounsaturated fats fats with only one double bond of unsaturated carbons in carbon atom chain

Mons pubis mound of fatty tissue covering the pubic bone

Mood disorder psychological condition characterized by emotional highs or lows

Morphine main alkaloid found in opium; used medically to kill pain and sedate

Mucous membranes tissues that help protect the interior surfaces of the body from invasion by pathogens

Multiple birth birth of twins, triplets, or more babies

Muscular endurance the ability of muscles to exert force or sustain a muscle contraction repeatedly for an extended period

Muscular strength the ability or capacity of a muscle or muscle group to exert maximum force against resistance

Mutation change in genetic material; variation in genetic structure

Myocardial infarction heart attack; occurs when blood supply to heart muscle is cut off for a long time

Myocardium heart muscle

Myomectomy surgical removal of uterine fibroid tumor

Myotonia intense muscular contractions during orgasm

Narcotic a drug that induces stupor and insensibility; in legal terms, any addictive drug subject to illegal use

Natural family planning (NFP) any method of preventing pregnancy based on avoiding coitus during ovulation

Neonatal abstinence syndrome (NAS) set of withdrawal symptoms occuring shortly after birth in newborns that have been exposed to heroin in utero

Neurons the foundation for electrochemical communication system in the brain

Neurosis emotional disorder caused by unresolved conflicts and characterized by irrational behavior

Neurotransmitters chemicals that send messages across a synapse from the axon of a nerve cell to another nerve cell

Nicotine an addictive chemical component in tobacco

Nicotine patch a pad worn on the arm that delivers a steady amount of nicotine through the skin as an aid to quitting

Nitrosamines cancer-causing substance found in tobacco

Nonaerobic exercises activities that have frequent rest intervals between outlays of energy

Nongonococcal urethritis (NGU) infection in the urethra of men usually caused by the chlamydia bacteria

Norepinephrine hormone released by the adrenal glands during the first stage of stress that affects circulation.

Norplant® long-lasting hormonal contraceptive implanted under the skin by a health care practitioner to prevent ovulation

Nurse practitioner registered nurse who diagnoses and treats patients independent of a physician

Nutrients chemical substances or nourishing elements found in food

Nutrition the sum of all the interactions between an organism and the food it consumes

Nutrition facts term found on the new food labels

Obesity a condition in which a person has an excessive amount of body fat

Obsessive compulsive disorder an anxiety disorder in which a person has constant unpleasant and unacceptable thoughts and performs repetitive acts that are unnecessary

Obstetrician medical doctor who specializes in the care of women during pregnancy, delivery, and the period immediately following birth

Occupational Safety and Health Administration (OSHA) government agency that regulates health and safety in the workplace

Omega-3 oils oils found in fish

Oncogenes genes that prompt uncontrolled cell division

Oncologist physician who specializes in treating cancer

Open-ended marriage one in which one partner gives the other permission to have sexual relations outside the marriage

Ophthalmologist physician (M.D.) who specializes in diseases of the eyes

Opiates drug obtained from the juice of the opium poppy

Opioids synthetic narcotics

Opium base compound for all natural narcotics

Opportunistic infections illnesses that normally would not be serious but take hold in a person's body because of a weakened immune system caused by HIV

Optometrist licensed practitioner who examines the eyes, diagnoses problems, and prescribes eyeglasses or contact lenses

Oral contraceptives hormonal tablets taken by women to prevent ovulation

Orthodox medicine traditional form of medical practice using scientifically validated procedures

Osteoarthritis most common form of arthritis affecting primarily the hands and weight-bearing joints

Osteopathic physician doctor trained to treat patients as a whole person

Osteoporosis a condition in which the bones lose calcium

Ova female gametes

Ovaries almond-shaped female sex glands that produce eggs, or ova and the hormones estrogen and progesterone

Overload principle gradually subjecting the body to more stress than it is accustomed to

Overweight body weight that exceeds the normal or standard weight for an individual

Ovolactovegetarian one who eats eggs, dairy products and plants but not meat, poultry, or fish

Ovulation the release of a mature egg from the ovary in the middle of the menstrual cycle

Pacemaker device implanted near the heart to regulate heartbeat

Pancreas digestive organ that secretes insulin and other digestive juices

Panic disorder a condition in which a person is overwhelmed by feelings of anxiety and loss of control

Pap test diagnostic test for cancer of the cervix performed by taking a sample of cells from the cervix for examination under a microscope

Paracervical block a local anesthetic injected around opening of the uterus

Paraphilia atypical sexual behaviors using unusual objects, acts, or imagery to achieve gratification

Particulates tiny solid or liquid particles in the air that can cause serious health problems

Parturition live birth at end of pregnancy

Passive smoking inhaling of smoke in the environment by the nonsmoker; involuntary smoking

Patent ductus arteriosus heart defect caused by a duct remaining open between the pulmonary artery and the aorta allowing the blood to mix

Pathogens disease-causing organisms

PCP an anesthetic that blocks nerve receptors from pain and temperature without producing numbness; angel dust

Pediculosis infection with lice

Pelvic inflammatory disease (PID) inflammation of the uterus, fallopian tubes, and ovaries

Penis male organ of sexual activity

Peptic ulcers irritations in the lining of the stomach or small intestine caused by the corrosive effect of digestive juices

Percodan a cough-suppressing and analgesic medication

Perineum area between lower portion of external genitalia and anus

Pernicious anemia anemia caused by a vitamin B_{12} deficiency that occurs when the body is unable to absorb it

Personality the total of all individual characteristics that make each person unique

Pesticides chemicals used to kill insects, rodents, and weeds

Peyote a type of cactus that yields mescaline

Phagocytosis the destruction of pathogens by macrophages (phagocytes)

Photochemical smog brown smog caused when automobile exhaust containing nitric oxide reacts with oxygen and forms nitrogen dioxide

Physical abuse an act of physical harm intentionally inflicted on another

Physical dependence a biochemical need to repeat administration of a substance

Physical fitness the general capacity to adapt and respond favorably to physical effort

Pituitary gland a pea-sized body in the brain, which releases hormones including FSH and LH

Placenta organ through which fetus receives nourishment and empties waste via mother's circulatory system; the afterbirth

Plaque pasty material that adheres to the walls of the blood vessels

Plaques dense deposits of protein found in the brain of Alzheimer's patients during autopsy

Pleurae membranes that line the chest cavity

Pneumonia an inflammation of the bronchial tubes and air sacs of the lungs

Podiatrist Specialist who diagnoses and treats problems of the feet

Polychlorinated biphenyls (PCBs) industrial chemicals found in sewage that cause cancer and central nervous system damage

Polyandry a marriage in which one woman has more than one husband simultaneously

Polygamy a marriage of more than two people

Polygyny a marriage in which one man has more than one wife

Polyneuritis inflammation of several peripheral and central nerves caused by thiamin deficiency due to alcoholism

Polyps small growths on the wall of the colon or rectum

Polyunsaturated fats fats that contain two or more double bonds between unsaturated fats along the carbon atom chain

Postpartum the first 3 months after childbirth

Post-traumatic stress disorder condition in which a person mentally reexperiences a violent event

Power of attorney appointment of a friend or relative to make legal decisions for another

Preferred provider organization (PPO) insurance plan in which the insured must obtain medical treatment from healthcare workers with whom the insurance company has contracted services

Pregnancy condition of having a developing embryo or fetus in the uterus

Premature ejaculation emission of semen and loss of erection within 30 seconds to 2 minutes of beginning coitus

Premenstrual syndrome (PMS) a condition occurring about 10 days before menstruation, characterized by all or some of the following: nervousness, irritability, emotional disturbance, headache, or depression

Premiums payments to an insurance company for a percentage coverage of future medical expenses

Prepuce single fold of skin over clitoris (also over the glans of uncircumcised penis)

Prescription written order authorizing a pharmacist to dispense medication

Prescription medications drugs that are legal only when authorized by a physician or qualified health care practitioner

Primary prevention doctor seen initially for treatment and management of health conditions of individuals or the family

Primary-care physician doctor who oversees the treatment of patients

Prodomal period the time during which an infectious disease is most communicable; characterized by nonspecific symptoms

Progression principle placing additional stress on the body once it has adapted to its current stress factor

Progressive relaxation exercise to relieve stress; involves tensing and relaxing muscle groups

Progesterone hormone that prepares uterus for pregnancy

Proof amount of alcohol in a beverage expressed as twice the percent of alcohol

Prophylactic penicillin therapy use of penicillin to prevent infections from occurring in infants and young children with sickle cell anemia

Proprioceptive neuromuscular facilitation (PNF) technique based on the contraction and relaxation of muscles

Prostaglandins hormone that causes the uterus to contract; used to induce abortion

Prostate gland organ that produces the most seminal fluid

Protease inhibitors new class of potential anti-AIDS drugs that target a later point in the viral life cycle

Proteins chains of amino acids

Protozoa one-celled animals that can live as parasites in humans

Psilocybin primary psychoactive agent in psychedelic mushrooms

Psyche all conscious and unconscious mental functions

Psychedelic literally, "revealing to the mind"

Psychiatric registered nurse a registered nurse (R.N. or B.S.N.) who has additional training in mental health and cares for the needs of patients in a clinical setting

Psychiatric social worker mental health professional with a Master of Social Work degree who coordinates patient resources

Psychiatrist physician who specializes in the diagnosis and treatment of mental disorders

Psychoactive substance any agent that has the ability to alter mood, perception, or behavior

Psychoanalysis literally, "analyzing the psyche"

Psychological dependence a state in which individuals crave drugs to satisfy some personality or emotional need

Psychological/emotional abuse negative and hostile verbal or nonverbal treatment of another

Psychologist specialist in treating emotional and behavioral disorders without medication

Psychology the study of the human psyche

Psychoneuroimmunology science of how the brain affects the immune system

Psychosis mental disorder characterized by loss of contact with reality

Pubic lice small insects that infest the host's pubic hair

Pudendal block a local anesthetic that eliminates feeling from the lower vagina

Purging self-induced vomiting

Quaalude a depressant often used interchangeably with barbiturates; high potential for physical and psychological dependence

Quackery/quack use of unproven methods of curing diseases/ unqualified practitioners who take advantage of patients for their money

Radial pulse pulse taken by locating the radial artery in the wrist

Radiation energy from waves and particles such as ultraviolet rays and x-rays

Radiation sickness illness caused by overexposure to radioactive substances; characterized by nausea, hemorrhage, hair loss, and possibly death

Radiologist physician specializing in the use of radiation

Radionuclide imaging injecting substances called radionucleides into bloodstream so computer-generated pictures can locate them in the heart

Radon naturally occurring radioactive gas

Rate of perceived exertion (RPE) an alternative method of determining the intensity of exercise

RICES standard recommended treatment for acute injuries: rest, ice application, compression, elevation, support, and stabilization

Receptor component of the neuron that combines with the neurotransmitter to receive messages from another neuron

Recycling collecting, reprocessing, and reusing trash

Refractory period the time immediately following orgasm when a male cannot be sexually stimulated

Reframing changing the way a person looks at things

Registered nurse health care practitioner who provides information and services that promote or restore health and wellness

Relaxation response an inborn bodily reaction that counteracts the harmful effects of stress

Resusceptibility vulnerability to reinfection with a disease after having recovered from it

Retrogression principle leveling of performance for a period of time before performance improves again

Reye's syndrome a disease that affects children from 2 to 16, which can be fatal

Rh factor chemical in bloodstream of most people that can cause complications during pregnancy when a mother who is Rh⁻ (no Rh chemical) carries an Rh⁺ fetus

Rheumatic diseases disorders that involve inflammation and swelling of the joints and restrict range of motion

Rheumatic heart disease damage to the heart caused by earlier, untreated strep throat

Rheumatoid arthritis more severe form of arthritis that affects all joints of the body, causing inflammation

RhoGAM vaccine to counteract complications of Rh incompatibility

Ribonucleic acid (RNA) nucleic acid found in the nucleus of cells that controls protein synthesis

Rickettsiae a type of pathogen transmitted to humans through insect bites

Rigor mortis stiffening of the muscles after death

RU-486 drug that blocks absorption of progesterone and prevents the lining of the uterus from supporting an embryo

Sanitary landfill large, open pit where trash is buried

Satiety feeling of fullness

Saturated fats fats found in animal product; increase levels of blood fat cholesterol

Scabies condition caused by parasite that burrows under the skin and lays eggs

Schizophrenic disorders psychological conditions characterized by severe disturbances in perceptions, thoughts, moods, and behaviors

Scrotum loose pouch of skin containing the testes

Seasonal affective disorder (SAD) form of depression caused by lack of exposure to sunlight during the winter

Secondary prevention early detection and intervention to reduce the consequences of a health problem

Self-actualization fulfillment of one's potential

Self-care taking responsibility for one's own basic health care

Self-esteem a way of looking at oneself; may be high or low

Semen fluid containing sperm

Seminal vesicles Glands that produce a fluid suitable for sperm mobility

Seminiferous tubules hollow, cylindrical structures that make up most of the testes and produce sperm

Semivegetarian one who eats plant food, dairy products, eggs, small amounts of poultry and fish, but no beef or pork

Septal defects heart defects characterized by abnormal blood flow between the left and right heart chambers

Septum wall that bisects the heart lengthwise

Setpoint theory stating that individuals have a weight-regulating mechanism in the hypothalamus of the brain that controls how much we weigh

Sex the quality of being male or female

Sexual harassment unwanted sexual pressuring of someone in a vulnerable or dependent position by another in a position of power

Sexual orientation determined by whether a person is physically attracted to members of the same sex or the opposite sex

Sexuality the total biological, psychological, emotional, social, environmental, and cultural aspects of sexual behavior

Sexually transmitted diseases illnesses caused by pathogens that are transmitted during sexual acts

Shingles herpes blisters appearing on the trunk of the body caused by herpes zoster virus

Sickle cell disease an inherited form of anemia that produces sickle-shaped cells that clump together and clog tiny blood vessels

Simple carbohydrates sugars found naturally in foods; contribute no nutritional value

Skinfold measurement method of determining body composition by measuring the thickness of fat under the skin

Smog brown or gray fog caused by chemical pollutants

Smokeless tobacco chewing tobacco and snuff

Soluble dissolvable in water

Specificity of training aiming overload specifically at the desired outcome of the fitness component

Sperm male gametes

Spermatogenesis sperm cell production

Spermicide chemicals in the form of creams, foams, or jellies that kill live sperm

Sphygmomanometer instrument used to measure blood pressure

Spinal anesthesia solution containing local anesthetic

Spontaneous abortion (miscarriage) termination of pregnancy prior to 20th week; contents of uterus are expelled

Spot-reducing exercising to reduce fat in a specific location of the body; does not work

Squamous cell carcinoma common type of skin cancer that affects the squamous layer of the epidermis

Stalking intent to harass, annoy, or alarm another person by repeated communications or actions

Static (slow-sustained) stretching technique in which muscles are relaxed and lengthened gradually through a joint's complete range of motion

Stenoses heart defects characterized by obstructions to a valve, artery, or vein

Sterilization surgical procedure that leaves a person infertile

Stomach the organ containing acids and enzymes that break down food

Storage fat fat found beneath the skin and around major organs that acts as an insulator, as padding, and as a source of energy for metabolism

Strep throat an extremely contagious infection caused by a bacteria and treated with antibiotics

Stress demand that places physical and emotional strain on an individual

Stressors factors that cause stress

Stroke (cerebrovascular accident) (CVA) disruption of blood flow to the brain, causing destruction of brain cells

Structural analog a designer drug that mimics the effects of another drug

Sudden cardiac death (SCD) result of an electrical malfunction that throws the heart off rhythm and ends with the abrupt loss of heart function

Sudden infant death syndrome (SIDS) death of a baby by an undetermined cause, usually while sleeping at night

Sulfur-dioxide smog gray smog caused by burning oil with a high sulfur content

Sun protection factor (SPF) the rating by number given to a product that tells the consumer how effectively the product protects from the sun's ultraviolet rays

Superego internal voice or conscience; determines acceptable and unacceptable behavior

Surgery removal of tumor and surrounding tissue

Superego internal voice or conscience; determines acceptable and unacceptable behavior

Swinging agreement by both partners in a marriage to engage in sexual experimentation outside the marriage

Synapse a gap between each neuron that requires a special chemical to send messages across

Synovial membrane lining of joint that releases a lubricating fluid

Syphilis a sexually transmitted disease caused by a spirochete bacterium

Systemic infection an infection that spreads throughout the body

Systole contraction segment of heartbeat

Systolic blood pressure pressure during the heart's contraction

Tachycardia heart rate more than 100 beats per minute

Tangles bunches of twisted nerve cell fibers found in the neurons of Alzheimer's patients during autopsy

Tar yellowish-brown, sticky residue in tobacco that causes cancer

Taxol new drug used in chemotherapy, obtained from the bark and needles of the Pacific yew

Tay-Sachs disease An enzyme deficiency occurring almost exclusively among children of Eastern European Jewish ancestry

T-cells lymphocytes that activate additional B-cells, stop B-cell activity when the pathogen is destroyed, kill normal cells that have become cancerous, and attack pathogens

Telomerase enzyme that allows the cells to reproduce indefinitely, forming a tumor

Tension headaches headaches characterized by generalized pain all over the head

Tertiary prevention taking care of a sick person

Testes almond-shaped male sex glands that produce sperm and testosterone

Testosterone hormone that regulates male sexual development

Therapeutic communities self-help group homes programmed to assist addicts in remaining drug-free

Thermal inversion atmospheric condition that occurs when a layer of warm air covers a layer of cold air and holds particulates at lower levels

Tinnitus ringing in the ears

Tobacco a plant, *Nicotiana tobacum* or *Nicotiana rustica*, in which the leaves are dried and processed for smoking

Tolerance condition in which an individual must increase drug dosage to experience the same effects over time

Total body fat (% body fat) adipose tissue as a percent of total body tissue

Toxic core group of personality traits most detrimental to physical health: cynicism, frequent anger, aggression

Toxoplasmosis parasitic disease resulting from exposure to uncooked meat or cat litter; can produce blindness or mental retardation in fetus

Trachea windpipe; tube that connects the larynx to the lungs

Training intensity the intensity that gives the best cardiorespiratory development results

Tranquilizers psychoactive drugs that depress the central nervous system but have milder effects than the other depressants

Transfatty acids (TFAs) product of hydrogenation; may increase risk of heart disease and cancer

Transient hemispheral attack form of TIA in which difficulty thinking and communicating occur along with numbness in one arm, leg, or the face because of less blood flow to one side of the brain

Transient ischemic attack (TIA) brief occurrence of stroke symptoms

Transient monocular blindness form of TIA characterized by blurred vision in one eye

Trichomoniasis an STD caused by a protozoan; also known as trich or TV

Triglycerides fatty substances used for energy or stored by muscle or fat cells

Trimestera a three 3-month period of pregnancy

Tubal ligation female sterilization procedure in which the fallopian tubes are cut, sealed, or blocked

Tubal ovum transfer retrieval and placement of a woman's eggs into the end of fallopian tube

Tuberculin test a skin test that diagnoses TB

Tuberculosis (TB) a bacterial infection in the lungs characterized by coughing blood, pain in the chest, fever, and fatigue

Tumor an abnormal growth of tissue that grows independently of surrounding tissue and serves no useful function; neoplasm

Type I (insulin-dependent) diabetes form of diabetes in which the pancreas does not produce insulin

Type II (noninsulin-dependent) diabetes form of diabetes in which pancreas produces some insulin but the body is not able to use it well

Type A personality characterized by being impatient, aggressive, ambitious, hot-tempered, and hard-driving

Type B personality characterized by being calm, casual, and relaxed

Ultraviolet (UV) rays rays from the sun that contribute to the development of skin cancer when a person is exposed to them

Umbilical cord strand of tissue connecting the fetus to the placenta, through which fetus receives nourishment

Uniform Anatomical Gift Act provision that provides for the donation of the body or organs upon death

Uniform donor card card that specifies the wishes of a donor

Urethra long duct running through center of penis, which carries and releases the urine and also the semen

Urethritis inflammation of the urethra

Urinary incontinence loss of bladder control

U. S. Recommended Dietary Allowances FDA food labeling replaced in 1993 by DVs

Uterus (womb) pear-shaped, muscular organ where fetus develops

Vacuum curettage (aspiration) induced abortion procedure in which uterine contents are removed by suction

Vagina tubular passage leading to internal reproductive area that connects with the uterus

Vaginal sponge foam sponge containing a spermicide, inserted in the vagina to prevent fertilization

Vaginismus strong, involuntary contractions in the muscles of the lower part of the vagina

Vaginitis inflammation of the vagina

Valsalva effect an increase in pressure in the abdomen and chest that results from holding one's breath during exercise

Vas deferens tubes that carry the sperm from the epididymis up the ejaculatory duct

Vasectomy male sterilization procedure in which vas deferens is cut and tied

Vasocongestion increased supply of blood to genitals during sexual excitement

Vegan one who eats only plant foods

Vegetarian person who eats foods of plant origin and not meat

Veins blood vessels that return the blood with waste products and carbon dioxide to the heart

Ventricles the two lower chambers of the heart that pump the blood

Vena cava largest vein in the body; brings the blood back to the heart for more oxygen

Venules smaller veins

Vernix waxy coating on skin of a fetus and newborn

Viruses microorganisms without their own metabolism that reproduce within the living cells of the person they invade

Vitamins organic substances essential for normal growth

Vitiligo an autoimmune skin disorder characterized by gradual destruction of the pigment-producing cells

VLDL largest of the lipoproteins; allows cholesterol to circulate in blood stream

Waist-to-hip ratio waist circumference measurement divided by measurement of the widest circumference around the hips

Warm-up the beginning phase of each workout session that helps the body progress gradually from rest to exercise

Wellness adoption of healthy lifestyle habits that enhance well-being and reduce the risk of disease

Wernicke's disease caused by thiamine deficiency due to excessive alcohol consumption

Western Blot a blood test performed after ELISA to confirm the results of the ELISA tests

Withdrawal physical and psychological symptoms that occur when an individual who is addicted to a drug discontinues its use

Yoga exercise performed to calm and stimulate the mind

Zygote fertilized egg.

Index